Neuro-Ophthalmological Disorders

NEUROLOGICAL DISEASE AND THERAPY

Series Editor

WILLIAM C. KOLLER

Department of Neurology
University of Kansas Medical Center
Kansas City, Kansas

1. Handbook of Parkinson's Disease, *edited by William C. Koller*
2. Medical Therapy of Acute Stroke, *edited by Mark Fisher*
3. Familial Alzheimer's Disease: Molecular Genetics and Clinical Perspectives, *edited by Gary D. Miner, Ralph W. Richter, John P. Blass, Jimmie L. Valentine, and Linda A. Winters-Miner*
4. Alzheimer's Disease: Treatment and Long-Term Management, *edited by Jeffrey L. Cummings and Bruce L. Miller*
5. Therapy of Parkinson's Disease, *edited by William C. Koller and George Paulson*
6. Handbook of Sleep Disorders, *edited by Michael J. Thorpy*
7. Epilepsy and Sudden Death, *edited by Claire M. Lathers and Paul L. Schraeder*
8. Handbook of Multiple Sclerosis, *edited by Stuart D. Cook*
9. Memory Disorders: Research and Clinical Practice, *edited by Takehiko Yanagihara and Ronald C. Petersen*
10. The Medical Treatment of Epilepsy, *edited by Stanley R. Resor, Jr., and Henn Kutt*
11. Cognitive Disorders: Pathophysiology and Treatment, *edited by Leon J. Thal, Walter H. Moos, and Elkan R. Gamzu*
12. Handbook of Amyotrophic Lateral Sclerosis, *edited by Richard Alan Smith*
13. Handbook of Parkinson's Disease: Second Edition, Revised and Expanded, *edited by William C. Koller*
14. Handbook of Pediatric Epilepsy, *edited by Jerome V. Murphy and Fereydoun Dehkharghani*
15. Handbook of Tourette's Syndrome and Related Tic and Behavioral Disorders, *edited by Roger Kurlan*
16. Handbook of Cerebellar Diseases, *edited by Richard Lechtenberg*
17. Handbook of Cerebrovascular Diseases, *edited by Harold P. Adams, Jr.*
18. Parkinsonian Syndromes, *edited by Matthew B. Stern and William C. Koller*
19. Handbook of Head and Spine Trauma, *edited by Jonathan Greenberg*
20. Brain Tumors: A Comprehensive Text, *edited by Robert A. Morantz and John W. Walsh*

21. Monoamine Oxidase Inhibitors in Neurological Diseases, *edited by Abraham Lieberman, C. Warren Olanow, Moussa B. H. Youdim, and Keith Tipton*
22. Handbook of Dementing Illnesses, *edited by John C. Morris*
23. Handbook of Myasthenia Gravis and Myasthenic Syndromes, *edited by Robert P. Lisak*
24. Handbook of Neurorehabilitation, *edited by David C. Good and James R. Couch, Jr.*
25. Therapy with Botulinum Toxin, *edited by Joseph Jankovic and Mark Hallett*
26. Principles of Neurotoxicology, *edited by Louis W. Chang*
27. Handbook of Neurovirology, *edited by Robert R. McKendall and William G. Stroop*
28. Handbook of Neuro-Urology, *edited by David N. Rushton*
29. Handbook of Neuroepidemiology, *edited by Philip B. Gorelick and Milton Alter*
30. Handbook of Tremor Disorders, *edited by Leslie J. Findley and William C. Koller*
31. Neuro-Ophthalmological Disorders: Diagnostic Work-Up and Management, *edited by Ronald J. Tusa and Steven A. Newman*
32. Handbook of Olfaction and Gustation, *edited by Richard L. Doty*
33. Handbook of Neurological Speech and Language Disorders, *edited by Howard S. Kirshner*

Additional Volumes in Preparation

Therapy of Parkinson's Disease: Second Edition, Revised and Expanded, *edited by William C. Koller and George Paulson*

Evaluation and Management of Gait Disorders, *edited by Barney Spivack*

Handbook of Neurotoxicology, *edited by Louis W. Chang and Robert S. Dyer*

Handbook of Autonomic Nervous System Dysfunction, *edited by Amos D. Korczyn*

Neurological Complications of Cancer, *edited by Ronald G. Wiley*

Handbook of Dystonia, *edited by Joseph K. C. Tsui and Donald B. Calne*

Etiology of Parkinson's Disease, *edited by Jonas Ellenberg, William C. Koller, and J. William Langston*

Neuro-Ophthalmological Disorders

Diagnostic Work-Up and Management

edited by

Ronald J. Tusa
Department of Otolaryngology, Ophthalmology, and Neurology,
University of Miami School of Medicine
Miami, Florida

Steven A. Newman
Department of Ophthalmology and Neurological Surgery,
University of Virginia Health Sciences Center
Charlottesville, Virginia

Marcel Dekker, Inc. **New York • Basel • Hong Kong**

Library of Congress Cataloging-in-Publication Data

Neuro-ophthalmological disorders : diagnostic work-up and management / edited by Ronald J. Tusa, Steven A. Newman.
p. cm. — (Neurological disease and therapy ; 31)
Includes bibliographical references and index.
ISBN 0-8247-8839-7 (alk. paper)
1. Neuro-ophthalmology. 2. Neuro-ophthalmology—Diagnosis.
I. Tusa, Ronald J. II. Newman, Steven A.
III. Series: Neurological disease and therapy ; v. 31.
[DNLM: 1. Eye Diseases—diagnosis. 2. Eye Diseases—therapy.
3. Peripheral Nervous System Diseases—diagnosis. 4. Peripheral Nervous System Diseases—therapy. W1 NE33LD v. 31 1995 / WW 140 N4935 1995]
RE725.N456 1995
617.7'1—dc20
DNLM/DLC
for Library of Congress 94-27026
CIP

The publisher offers discounts on this book when ordered in bulk quantities. For more information, write to Special Sales/Professional Marketing at the address below.

This book is printed on acid-free paper.

Marcel Dekker, Inc.
270 Madison Avenue, New York, New York 10016

Current printing (last digit):
10 9 8 7 6 5 4 3 2 1

PRINTED IN THE UNITED STATES OF AMERICA

Series Introduction

Neuro-ophthalmology is an exceedingly important area of clinical neurology. Many patients present with ophthalmological disorders and most of the common neurological conditions also affect neuro-ophthalmological function. There has been an explosion in our knowledge of the pathophysiology of these disorders, many of which are now treatable. *Neuro-Ophthalmological Disorders: Diagnostic Work-Up and Management* is in keeping with our neurological series in providing practical, up-to-date information for the practicing clinician. Clinicians, including neurologists, ophthalmologists, and neurosurgeons who take care of patients with neuro-ophthalmological problems will find this book to be an important reference source, replete with the information they need to diagnose and treat such patients.

William C. Koller

Preface

The first papers published on clinical pathological correlates affecting the central nervous system were neuro-ophthalmological cases. Thus, neuro-ophthalmology is one of the oldest of the neurological specialties. The last two decades have witnessed a revolution in neuro-ophthalmology due to the development of improved imaging (CT and MRI scans) and a better understanding of the pathophysiology of disease. In addition, new insights in molecular genetics, immunology, pharmacology, anatomy, and physiology have resulted in therapies and approaches to several neuro-ophthalmological disorders that have been difficult to manage. Neuro-ophthalmologists no longer need to restrict themselves primarily to diagnostic issues, but can now take an active role in treatment and long-term management.

We have asked a variety of neurologists, ophthalmologists, and basic scientists, with particular interests and experiences in specific areas of neuro-ophthalmology, to write about their topic of interest. We have selected a wide variety of topics that form the frontiers of neuro-ophthalmology. In order to keep the topics clinically applicable, we asked the contributors to write their chapters in a practical, personal fashion that has clinical relevance to pathological problems encountered in daily practice.

The book is divided into sections tht cover functional, anatomical, technological, and pathological aspects of neuro-ophthalmology. It is written primarily for neurologists, ophthalmologists, and neurosurgeons with a clinical interest in neuro-ophthalmological problems.

We hope this book will provide an overview of some of the areas of progress in neuro-ophthalmology and serve as a reference source for practical information concerning the diagnosis and treatment of patients with neuro-ophthalmological disorders.

Ronald J. Tusa, M.D., Ph.D.
Steven A. Newman, M.D.

Contents

Part V PATHOLOGY

Contributors

Phil A. Aitken, M.D., F.A.C.S Chairman, Division of Ophthalmology; Associate Professor, Department of Surgery, University of Vermont College of Medicine, Burlington, Vermont

Robert W. Baloh, M.D. Professor, Department of Neurology, University of California School of Medicine, Los Angeles, California

Edward G. Buckley, M.D. Professor, Department of Ophthalmology, Duke University Medical Center, Durham, North Carolina

James J. Corbett, M.D. Professor and Chairman, Department of Neurology; Professor, Department of Ophthalmology, University of Mississippi School of Medicine, Jackson, Mississippi

Ian S. Curthoys, Ph.D. Reader, Department of Psychology, University of Sydney, Sydney, New South Wales, Australia

Robert B. Daroff, M.D. Professor, Department of Neurology, and Associate Dean, Case Western Reserve University School of Medicine; Chief of Staff, University Hospitals of Cleveland, Cleveland, Ohio

L. F. Dell'Osso, Ph.D. Professor, Departments of Neurology and Biomedical Engineering, Case Western Reserve University, Cleveland, Ohio

Joseph L. Demer, M.D., Ph.D. Associate Professor, Department of Ophthalmology, Jules Stein Eye Institute, Los Angeles, California

Kathleen B. Digre, M.D. Associate Professor, Departments of Neurology and Ophthalmology, University of Utah, Salt Lake City, Utah

Daniel B. Drachman, M.D. Professor, Departments of Neurology and Neuroscience, Johns Hopkins University School of Medicine, Baltimore, Maryland

Larry P. Frohman, M.D. Vice Chairman, Associate Professor, Departments of Ophthalmology and Neurosciences, University of Medicine and Dentistry of New Jersey, Newark, New Jersey

Karl C. Golnik, M.D. Assistant Professor, Department of Ophthalmology, Neurology, and Neurosurgery, The Storm Eye Institute and the Medical University of South Carolina, Charleston, South Carolina

John Guy, M.D. Associate Professor, Department of Ophthalmology and Neurology, University of Florida, Gainesville, Florida

G. M. Halmagyi, M.D. Clinical Associate Professor, Department of Neurology, Royal Prince Alfred Hospital, Sydney, New South Wales, Australia

William M. Hart, Jr., M.D., Ph.D. Professor, Department of Ophthalmology and Visual Sciences, Washington University School of Medicine, St. Louis, Missouri

Saunders L. Hupp, M.D. Associate Professor, Department of Ophthalmology, University of South Alabama College of Medicine, Mobile, Alabama

Donald R. Johns, M.D. Associate Professor, Departments of Neurology and Ophthalmology, Beth Israel Hospital, Massachusetts Eye and Ear Infirmary, and Harvard Medical School, Boston, Massachusetts

Randy H. Kardon, M.D. Department of Ophthalmology, University of Iowa and Department of Veterans Affairs, Iowa City, Iowa

David I. Kaufman, D.O. Associate Professor, Department of Internal Medicine, Division of Visual Science, College of Osteopathic Medicine, Michigan State University, East Lansing, Michigan

Shalom E. Kelman, M.D. Associate Professor, Department of Ophthalmology, University of Maryland Medical Systems, Baltimore, Maryland

Christopher Kennard, Ph.D., F.R.C.P. Professor and Chairman, Department of Clinical Neurology, Charing Cross and Westminster Medical School, London, England

Lanning B. Kline, M.D. Professor, Department of Ophthalmology, University of Alabama School of Medicine, Birmingham, Alabama

Gregory S. Kosmorsky, D.O. Department of Ophthalmology, Cleveland Clinic Foundation, Cleveland, Ohio

R. John Leigh, M.D. Professor, Department of Neurology, Case Western Reserve University and Veterans Affairs Medical Center, Cleveland, Ohio

Frederick E. Lepore, M.D. Professor, Department of Neurology, University of Medicine and Dentistry of New Jersey/Robert Wood Johnson Medical School, New Brunswick, New Jersey

Wolfgang E. Lieb, M.D. Assistant Professor, Department of Ophthalmology, Johannes Gutenberg-University, Mainz, Germany

Dennis C. Matzkin, M.D. Albert Einstein College of Medicine and Montefiore Medical Center, Bronx, New York

Joseph A. Mauriello, Jr., M.D. Associate Professor, Clinical Ophthalmology; Director, Oculoplastics and Ophthalmic Pathology, University of Medicine and Dentistry of New Jersey, Newark, New Jersey

John G. McHenry, M.D. Assistant Professor, Department of Ophthalmology, Wayne State University, Detroit, Michigan

Neil R. Miller, M.D. Professor, Departments of Ophthalmology, Neurology, and Neurosurgery, Johns Hopkins Medical Institutions, Baltimore, Maryland

Ramin Mostafavi, M.D. University of Medicine and Dentistry of New Jersey, Newark, New Jersey

Nancy J. Newman, M.D. Associate Professor, Department of Ophthalmology, Neurology, and Neurosurgery, Emory University School of Medicine, Atlanta, Georgia

Joseph R. Pernicone, Ph.D., D.O. Associate Professor, Department of Radiology, Michigan State University, East Lansing, Michigan

Robert D. Reinecke, M.D. Professor, Department of Ophthalmology, Jefferson Medical College; Director, Foerderer Eye Movement Center, Wills Eye Hospital, Philadelphia, Pennsylvania

Michael X. Repka, M.D. Associate Professor, Department of Ophthalmology and Pediatrics, Johns Hopkins University School of Medicine, Baltimore, Maryland

Norman J. Schatz, M.D. Professor, Department of Ophthalmology and Neurology, University of Miami, Miami, Florida

Robert C. Sergott, M.D. Attending Neuro-Ophthalmologist and Surgeon, Department of Neuro-Ophthalmology, Wills Eye Hospital, Philadelphia, Pennsylvania

Cherie J. Sewell, R.N., M.S., C.R.N.P. Adult Nurse Practitioner, Division of Neurology, Sinai Hospital, Baltimore, Maryland

James A. Sharpe, M.D., F.R.C.P.C. Professor and Chairman, Division of Neurology, University of Toronto; Director, Division of Neurology, The Toronto Hospital, Toronto, Ontario, Canada

James E. Siebert Chief Engineer and Senior Scientist, Department of Radiology, Michigan State University, East Lansing, Michigan

Thomas L. Slamovits, M.D. Albert Einstein College of Medicine and Montefiore Medical Center, Bronx, New York

Michael L. Slavin, M.D. Chief, Neuro-Ophthalmology, Long Island Jewish Medical Center, New Hyde Park; Associate Professor, Ophthalmology and Neurology, Albert Einstein College of Medicine, Bronx, New York

J. Lawton Smith, M.D. Professor of Ophthalmology (Emeritus), University of Miami School of Medicine, Bascom Palmer Eye Institute, Miami, Florida

Kyle H. Smith, M.D. Assistant Professor, Department of Surgery, Texas A&M University School of Medicine; and Division of Ophthalmology, Scott and White Clinic, Temple, Texas

Thomas C. Spoor, M.D., F.A.C.S. Professor, Departments of Ophthalmology and Neurosurgery, Kresge Eye Institute, Wayne State University, Detroit, Michigan

Barney J. Stern, M.D. Director, Division of Neurology, Department of Medicine, Sinai Hospital; Associate Professor, Department of Neurology, Johns Hopkins University, Baltimore, Maryland

B. Todd Troost, M.D. Professor and Chairman, Department of Neurology, Bowman Gray School of Medicine, Winston-Salem, North Carolina

Mary Lee Vance, M.D. Associate Professor, Department of Internal Medicine, University of Virginia Health Sciences Center, Charlottesville, Virginia

Rudolph S. Wagner, M.D. Clinical Associate Professor, Department of Ophthalmology, University of Medicine and Dentistry of New Jersey, Newark, New Jersey

Christina M. Whitney-Rainbolt, M.S.N., R.N. Adjunct Assistant Professor, Montana State University College of Nursing, Bozeman, Montana

W. Bruce Wilson, M.D. Clinical Professor, Department of Ophthalmology, University of Colorado Health Sciences Center, Denver, Colorado

Jacqueline M.S. Winterkorn, Ph.D., M.D. Associate Professor, Departments of Ophthalmology and Neurology and Neuroscience, Cornell University Medical College, New York; Chief, Division of Neuro-Ophthalmology, North Shore University Hospital–Cornell University Medical College, Manhasset, New York

Shirley H. Wray, M.D., Ph.D., F.R.C.P. Associate Professor, Department of Neurology, Harvard Medical School, Cambridge; Director, Unit for Neurovisual Disorders, Massachusetts General Hospital, Boston, Massachusetts

David S. Zee, M.D. Professor, Department of Neurology, Johns Hopkins Hospital, Baltimore, Maryland

I

AFFERENT SYSTEM

1

Amaurosis Fugax

Shirley H. Wray
Harvard Medical School, Cambridge, and Massachusetts General Hospital, Boston, Massachusetts

Amaurosis fugax, transient monocular loss of vision, is a major visual symptom that may herald stroke. A classification of monocular amaurosis fugax is presented here based on an analysis of 850 personal cases (1).

Type I amaurosis fugax is due to transient retinal ischemia, type II to retinal vascular insufficiency, type III to vasospasm, and type IV includes cases of amaurosis fugax associated with elevated anticardiolipid antibodies and cases of unknown etiology. Each of the four types is characterized by sporadic transient monocular loss of vision lasting a few seconds to several minutes. A meticulous history of the attack(s) together with a dilated fundoscopic examination of the retina are key to the diagnosis.

I. AMAUROSIS FUGAX TYPE I

A. Clinical History

Amaurosis fugax type I is a sudden attack of partial or complete transient monocular blindness (TMB) that lasts for seconds to minutes and is followed by total recovery (Table 1) (1–2). Partial visual impairment may also occur and is described by the patient as a grayout, as an ascending or descending curtain (altitudinal hemianopia, 20 of 35 cases), or as a blind moving sideways across

Table 1 Types of Amaurosis Fugax

	Type I	Type II	Type III	Type IV
Onset	Abrupt	Less rapid	Abrupt	Abrupt
Visual loss	All or partial	All or partial	Total or progressive contraction of visual fields	Partial
Length	Seconds or minutes	Minutes or hours	Minutes	Any length
Recovery	Complete	Complete	Usually complete	Complete
Pain	No	Yes	Often	No
Mechanism	Embolus to retinal vessel	Hypoperfused because of carotid occlusion	Angiospasm of the ophthalmic artery or central retinal artery	Unknown
Unusual features	Vision may black out completely	Peculiar visual aberrations	Visual loss may spare fixation	Anything goes

Source: Based on data in SH Wray. Extracranial internal carotid artery disease. In: Bernstein EF, ed. Amaurosis fugax. New York: Springer-Verlag, 1988: 72–80; and published by Burde RM. Amaurosis fugax, an overview. J Clin Neuro-ophthalmol 9(3):185–9.

the eye (hemianopia, 6 of 35 cases). Occasionally, the patient will describe moving tracks of light. Ipsilateral headache is rare (2 of 35 cases) (3).

In 1952, Fisher (4) drew attention to the association of amaurosis fugax of this brevity with contralateral hemiplegia. Since then amaurosis fugax has come to be regarded as one variety of carotid artery distribution transient ischemic attack (TIA). Like other TIAs, this symptom means the patient has an above-average risk of stroke. By extrapolation from data for TIAs in general, the risk of stroke and/or death is probably about 10% per annum (5), but death more often is due to ischemic heart disease than to stroke (6). In one study (7), cerebral vascular symptoms (TIA or stroke) occurred in 22 patients (43%) either before or after amaurosis fugax. Of 44 patients with no cerebral ischemic symptoms before the onset of amaurosis fugax, 15 (34%) subsequently had TIAs or strokes.

B. Clinical Signs

The majority of attacks of amaurosis fugax type I are due to embolism of fresh thrombus into the ophthalmic circulation from a source in the ipsilateral internal carotid artery in the neck or from the aorta or heart. Careful funduscopy in search of retinal emboli or other vascular changes, for example, a central retinal artery

(CRA) or branch retinal artery (BRA) occlusion, or anterior ischemic optic neuropathy (AION) or asymmetrical hypertensive retinopathy is the most important examination to perform next to auscultation of the neck and eye for a carotid artery bruit. To visualize the retinal microcirculation adequately, the pupil should be dilated with 10% phenylephrine (Neo-Synephrine) eye drops after the visual acuity has been measured and the pupillary reflexes recorded. The ophthalmoscopic appearance of a retinal embolus can provide specific information about the embolic material and its possible source (Table 2).

Bright yellowish, glinting lipid emboli (Hollenhorst plaques) are the most common emboli seen in the eye (Fig. 1). They are associated with atheromatous changes of the ipsilateral carotid artery or aortic arch disease (8,9). The embolic material has been confirmed to be cholesterol.

Calcific emboli are characteristically matte white, nonscintillating, and somewhat wider than the blood column. Calcific emboli may be dislodged by the surgical manipulation of calcified heart valves at the time of valvulotomy or

Table 2 Sources of Emboli

	Type	Patient age
Cardiac		
valves		
rheumatic disease	Platelet/calcium[a]	Any age
lupus	Platelet	Young woman
acute or subacute endocarditis	Marasmic	Damaged heart
floppy mitral valve	Platelet	Any age; mostly women
chamber		
myxoma	Myxoma	
mural thrombus	Platelet/clot	Older adult
Carotid artery		
ulcerated plaque	Platelet/cholesterol ester	Older adult
stenosis	Platelet	
fibromuscular dysplasia	Platelet	Young woman
Other		
amniotic fluid	Debirs?[a]	Young woman
long bone fractures	Fat[a]	Any age
chronic i.v. drug users	Talc[a]	Any age
disseminated intravascular coagulapathy[a]	?	?
Antiphospholipid antibody(s)	?	Young adult

Source: Modified from Burde RM. Amaurosis fugax, an overview. J Clin Neuro-ophthalmol 1989; 9(3): 185–9.

[a]Produces retinal infarction; no amaurosis fugax.

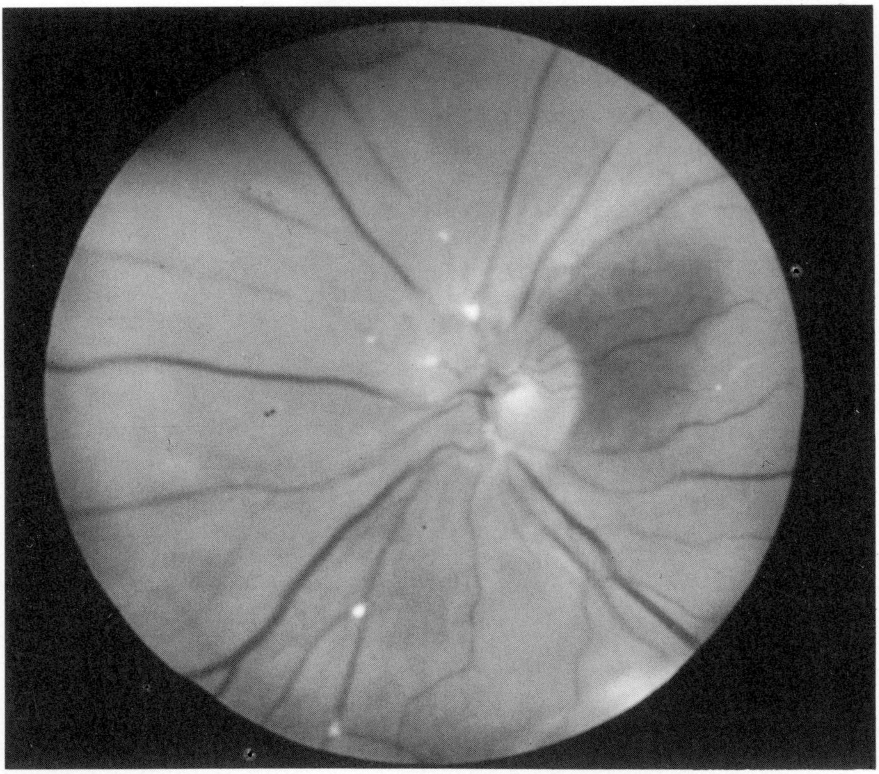

Figure 1 Fundus photograph showing multiple lipid emboli in the branches of the CRA.

may occur spontaneously from rheumatic valvular vegetation. Some of the circulating microemboli that pass through the retina, so-called migrant, pale emboli, are believed to be composed of platelets. Their occurrence is associated with thrombocytosis. The emboli that occur after myocardial infarction fall into the category of fibrin plugs. They are especially frequent in patients who have neurological complications after open heart surgery. The heart lesions traditionally associated with thromboembolism have been myocardial infarction producing mural thrombus; mitral stenosis, with or without atrial fibrillation; and bacterial or nonbacterial vegetative valvular lesions. Previously unrecognized potential sources of emboli have come to light: mitral-annulus calcification may be the origin of cerebral and retinal emboli in the elderly (10–12), and the prolapsing mitral valve may be the source in younger patients (13–15). In the case of embolic seeding from a myxoma of the heart, the histopathology of the embolus is like that of the original tumor (16).

Clinical experience has shown that the risk of permanent visual loss in patients with amaurosis fugax type I is relatively low; perhaps 3% per annum. In one series, only 11% of patients with CRA occlusion and 18% with occlusion of a BRA could remember a previous episode of amaurosis fugax (3). When complete monocular blindness occurs, it is due to a CRA occlusion. Partial blindness may be the sequelae to an occlusion of the CRA or BRA (see Fig. 1) or to ischemia of the optic nerve. There is no correlation, however, between multiple attacks of amaurosis fugax, defined as more than 20 before presentation, and subsequent permanent visual loss (7).

The results of carotid angiography in patients with amaurosis fugax type I has confirmed the high prevalence of ipsilateral carotid disease. A carotid bruit, a history of cerebral TIA, and hypertension all increase the yield of abnormal findings (7).

A clear association also is recognized between recurrent retinal ischemia causing amaurosis fugax and reversed ophthalmic artery flow ipsilateral to a complete internal carotid artery (ICA) occlusion (17–21). The pathogenic mechanisms believed to be responsible for recurrent amaurosis fugax and cerebral TIAs in such cases have differed. It has been suggested that the prominent retrograde ophthalmic artery flow seen in these circumstances may reflect a steal phenomenon from the ophthalmic artery–retinal circulation, and that when this happens, the orbital collateral channels are conscripted by the ipsilateral cerebral hemisphere at the expense of ocular perfusion needs. Surgical augmentation of intracranial blood flow by means of an ipsilateral external carotid–internal carotid bypass has been suggested as a beneficial procedure in these cases. However, other researchers (17) suggest that episodic ophthalmic artery hypotension and an ocular steal phenomenon are inadequate explanations for the recurrent intermittent attacks of acute transient ischemia of the retina or brain when robust orbital collaterals are evident angiographically. Their opinion is that microembolism from the stump of the occluded ICA to the symptomatic retina and hemisphere is the pathogenic mechanism, and ipsilateral external carotid endarterectomy with excision of the adjacent ICA stump is the procedure of choice.

Still further considerations arise when the ophthalmic artery has an anomalous origin. When ipsilateral amaurosis fugax occurred in a patient with stenosis of the external carotid artery, angiography showed that the ophthalmic artery originated from the middle meningeal artery. The retinal ischemic attacks ceased after the patient had an external carotid endarterectomy (21).

C. Associated Diseases

The importance of amaurosis fugax as a marker for generalized arteriosclerotic vascular disease should be noted. One study reported correlations with hypertension (18%), hyperlipidemia (61%), ischemic heart disease or peripheral vascular disease at presentation (25%), and at follow-up in an additional 18% of patients. A family history of ischemic heart disease, peripheral vascular disease, or stroke before the age of 60 years was present in 37% of the cases (7).

Amaurosis fugax type I may also occur in patients with nonarteriosclerotic vasculopathies: fibromuscular hyperplasia, granulomatous angiitis, congophilic angiopathy, systemic lupus erythematosus, Behçet's syndrome, and moyamoya disease. These rare angiopathies affect small-caliber arteries and, collectively, must be considered in any TIA.

States of altered coagulability and thrombocytosis such as the altered viscosity of the red blood cells in sickle cell disease and the altered blood viscosity in polycythemia are associated with a TIA. Amaurosis fugax type I associated with elevated levels of antiphospholipid antibody has recently been reported. This observation is discussed in a later section.

II. AMAUROSIS FUGAX TYPE II

A. Clinical History

Amaurosis fugax of type II may occur in patients with extensive, extracranial arterial occlusive disease involving both the ipsilateral internal and external carotid arteries. Amaurosis fugax type II is due to retinal vascular insufficiency. Temporary attacks of visual or cerebral disturbance that are hemodynamic occur before permanent structural changes develop in the eye and brain. In comparison with the brief transient attacks of amaurosis fugax type I, the temporary episodes of monocular visual loss characteristic of amaurosis fugax type II are less rapid in onset and longer in duration (the visual loss develops over minutes rather than seconds and lasts minutes up to 2 h). Recovery also takes place gradually (see Table 1) (1–2). Visual acuity may not be altered significantly during the attacks but contrast acuity is. Bright objects appear brighter, whereas dark objects may become difficult to see. The edges of bright objects can appear to flicker. When the bright, dazzling sensation is marked, the overall effect is one of overexposure and the patient may experience difficulty reading because of the glare of white paper. Yet although patients may not see to read, they can discern shapes and identify colors. When sight becomes fragmented and patchy, patients describe the appearance as a photographic negative. Occasionally, they note a transient closing in of the peripheral vision. Sometimes the attacks are accompanied by dull pain over the eye. Symptoms of generalized cerebral ischemia (faintness, fatigue, impaired concentration) often coexist but are mild compared with the visual symptoms.

Factors that provoke attacks of amaurosis fugax type II are systemic hypotension, venous hypertension, and extracerebral steal. The attacks occur on stooping or straining when venous pressure rises, on standing or during exercise, or on exposure to bright lights or a warm environment (22,23). This pattern suggests a temporary failure of retinal homeostasis. In the unique case of a man with amaurosis fugax type II provoked by facial heating with a hair dryer, the mechanism of the visual loss was believed to be diversion of blood to a dilated external carotid facial vascular bed resulting in temporary ocular oligemia on the affected side (23).

B. Clinical Signs

The unusual visual symptom(s) of amaurosis fugax type II are of retinal origin; however, investigations including retinal photostress tests have shown no indication of delayed retinal metabolism (23). Ophthalmodynamometry will show a low resting retinal perfusion pressure and further reduction during an attack of amaurosis is diagnostic. In addition, important venous changes in the retinal circulation accompany a progressive reduction in retinal arterial perfusion pressure. The retina will show stasis of blood in the veins and a low-pressure retinopathy and chronic ocular ischemia will develop. Early signs of a low-pressure retinopathy and hypoperfusion of the posterior vascular bed (including the retina, choroid, and optic disc) are delayed flow in the retinal arterioles (and secondarily in the venous circulation); the development of microaneurysms; multiple small blotlike intraretinal hemorrhages in the midperiphery of the retina and segmental narrowing and dilation of the major retinal veins; pulsating retinal arteries (if the intraocular pressure is about the level of the diastolic blood pressure in the retinal arteries); signs of optic disc ischemia (anterior ischemic optic neuropathy in acute ischemic insults, optic disc atrophy, and cupping in chronic cases); and choroidal infarcts (Table 3). Fundus fluorescein angiography can reveal marked circulatory abnormalities when routine ophthalmoscopy shows little change.

Low-pressure retinopathy may be seen in patients who have recently had a stroke (24,25) or who have ongoing transient monocular type II amaurosis fugax or cerebral ischemic attacks (24,26). It may also be seen in patients who have had cerebral vascular disease in the past but present no recent symptoms (25) or who have symptoms limited to mild visual loss (26,27). Occasionally, the retinopathy is an incidental finding (28). Low-pressure retinopathy has been detected in 20% of patients with ICA occlusion (18,29). Reconstructive surgery is sometimes possible in the proximal neck arteries, and external carotid–internal carotid bypass may be helpful if the external carotid is spared (29).

When both the external and internal carotid arteries are stenotic or occluded, the following signs of anterior segment ischemia also are present: rubeosis of the iris, sluggish reaction of the pupil to light because of sphincter ischemia or neovascular proliferation on the iris surface, and the development of secondary

Table 3 Ocular Signs of Low-Pressure (Venous Stasis) Retinopathy

Early signs	
	microaneurysms: small dot and blot
	intraretinal hemorrhages and nerve fiber layer hemorrhages which are most prominent within vascular arcades extending to midperiphery
Severe ischemia	
	dilation and darkening of retinal veins
	mild swelling of the optic disc
	retinal clouding
End stage	
	ocular ischemic syndrome

Source: From Burde RM. Amaurosis fugax, an overview. J Clin Neuro-ophthalmol 1989; 9(3):185–9.

neovascular glaucoma (Table 4) (30). At this stage, transcranial bypass is no longer practical nor is there evidence that laser treatment of the retina has a beneficial effect. Ischemic uveitis, present in 18% of the eyes with the ocular ischemic syndrome, is characteristically unresponsive to steroid medication and posterior synechiae can result. Spontaneous hyphema may also occur, and cataract can be a late complication.

Ischemic pain is a feature in some patients with amaurosis fugax type II. It is characterized by a constant ache over the orbit, upper face, and temple and aggravated when the patient is in an upright position (31,32). The pain is not related to glaucoma although glaucoma can cause eye pain in patients with ischemic oculopathy.

The differential diagnosis of unilateral low-pressure retinopathy is impending occlusion of the central retinal vein (CRV) and benign optic disc vasculitis (Table 5) (33). The most important determinant in distinguishing between an eye with chronic ocular ischemia and an eye with impending CRV occlusion is measurement of the retinal arterial and venous pressures. In ischemia, the CRA pressure is always extremely low and may be so low that spontaneous pulsation of the branches of the CRA at the disc head occur. Digital pressure on the globe may also be expected to collapse the veins at a very low pressure. When these tests indicate impending CRV occlusion, obstruction of the venous outflow, (e.g., caroticocavernous fistula or dural shunt) should be suspected.

Benign optic disc vasculitis is most often found in young, healthy adult patients who have no symptoms or signs of carotid artery disease and who are not diabetic. It is typically unilateral and self-limited with venous engorgement, retinal hemorrhage, and disc edema. The usual risk factors for vein occlusion are absent.

Table 4 Signs of Anterior Segment Ischemia

Conjunctiva and episclera
injection
ciliary flush
prominent large vessels
Pupil
sluggish reaction to light
relative afferent pupillary defect
Cornea
Edema (even with normal IOP)
Iris and anterior chamber angle
dilated vessels
rubeosis iridis
neovascular glaucoma
Anterior chamber
flare and cells
spontaneous hyphema
Lens
cataract

Source: From Mills RP. Anterior segment ischemia secondary to carotid occlusive disease. J Clin Neuro-ophthalmol 1989; 9(3):200–4.

The differential diagnosis of bilateral venous stasis retinopathy is diabetes mellitus and hyperviscosity syndromes (see Table 5) (33). Diabetes mellitus should affect the two eyes equally and produce bilateral retinopathy. When the retinopathy is strictly unilateral or markedly asymmetrical between the two eyes, with neovascular changes in the anterior segment of the eye, it is likely that this diabetic patient has associated severe ipsilateral carotid occlusive disease.

C. Associated Diseases

In the majority of patients suffering from extensive occlusion of the major arteries arising from the aortic arch, the cause is severe atherosclerosis. In young women, the cause may be inflammatory artertitis of a type similar to that reported in Takayasu's arteritis. Such cases may also have ischemic exercise pain in the jaw muscles from chewing. In the elderly, amaurosis fugax types I and II commonly occur in giant cell arteritis when a similar state of critical retinal perfusion exists (34), and every patient with amaurosis fugax over age 55 years requires an immediate sedimentation rate and fibrinogen level. When the index of suspicion

Table 5 Differential Diagnosis

	Venous stasis retinopathy	Diabetic retinopathy	Incomplete retinal vein occlusion	Benign optic disk vasculitis	Hyperviscosity syndromes[a]
Signs and symptoms of carotid artery disease	Yes	No	No	No	No
History of radiation treatment	No	No	No	No	No
Blood studies:	Normal	Elevated blood sugar	Normal	Normal	Possible abnormalities[b]
Laterality:	Unilateral	Bilateral	Usually unilateral	Unilateral	Bilateral
Area of retina	Midzonal region	Macular region	Periphery	Macula, disk, and peripapillary retina	Macular region
Optic disk edema	No	No	Yes	Yes	±
Ophthalmodynamometry	Abnormal	Normal	Normal	Normal	Normal

[a]These include polycythemia, macroglobulinemia, hemoglobinopathies, mylematosis, and lymphoma.
[b]The possible abnormalities involve the complete blood count, the differential count, the serum protein, and the hemoglobin electrophoresis.
Source: From McCrary JA III. Venous stasis retinopathy of stenotic or occlusive carotid origin. J Neuro-ophthalmol 1989; 9(3):195–9.

for temporal arteritis is high, immediate steroid treatment should be initiated pending a temporal artery biopsy.

Hyperviscosity syndromes also can cause amaurosis fugax type II. They can be diagnosed by appropriate laboratory studies, such as a complete blood count with differential serum protein and hemoglobin electrophoresis.

Amaurosis fugax type I or type II may also herald an ocular stroke due to a CRA or a BRA occlusion or due to arteritic, embolic, or nonarteritic atherosclerotic AION.

III. AMAUROSIS FUGAX TYPE III

A. Clinical History

The visual disturbance in amaurosis fugax type III is similar to that described for amaurosis fugax type II, but the affected eye shows no persistent or progressive signs of impaired retinal perfusion (see Table 1 [1,2]). Vasospasm is the mechanism suggested for amaurosis fugax type III. This mechanism may explain the transient monocular visual aura and visual loss in cases of ocular migraine. Migrainous amaurosis fugax is rare, however, and the diagnosis should be made only after all other causes of amaurosis fugax are excluded or when constriction of the retinal vessels is visualized funduscopically during an attack (35).

The following is a rare description of an episode of migrainous amaurosis fugax from a personal case:

> At the onset, floating bright, white lines were present, descending slowly from the top of the visual field over several seconds to involve the entire field. The lines slightly shimmered but neither pulsed nor flashed on and off. When the lines reached the bottom of the field, the pattern changed to a persistent gray-white, speckled pattern that impaired vision. The patient said this pattern resembled the background design of the Ishihara plates after being shown the test plate 12, and also mentioned that it resembled the interference pattern on a television screen. At the time, however, believing that her vision was impaired because the eye lid was shut, the patient inspected her eyes in the mirror. No accompanying symptoms occurred, in particular, no eye or head pain. The episode cleared abruptly over seconds, within 15 minutes of the onset and was described as being like "a lid being lifted off my vision." Sight returned to normal. Repeated stereotypic attacks occurred twice a day for nine days in spite of heparin treatment. A carotid angiogram, erythrocyte sedimentation rate, and other investigations showed no abnormality. The patient had a family history of migraine but was not known to experience migraines herself.

B. Clinical Signs

The clinical profile of 11 patients with vasospastic transient monocular blindness is shown in Table 6 (35–44); two patients were teenagers and three were

Table 6 Clinical Profile of Patients with Vasospastic Transient Monocular Blindness

Study	Patient's age/sex	Episode: Pattern of visual loss[a]	Episode: Duration	Episode: Frequency	Associated Condition
Ellenberger and Epstein (36)	?	?	5 min	?	?
Walsh and Hoyt (37)	17/M	Diffuse	Seconds	1 in 3 months	—
Newman et al. (38)	48/M	Constricting	5 min	3–12/day	Periarteritis nodosa
Kline and Kelly (39)	48/M[b]	Constricting	1–2 min	5 in 5 days	Cluster headaches
Schwartz et al. (40)	49/M	Diffuse	20 min	10 in 4 days	Eosinophilic vasculitis
Appleton et al. (41)	19/F	Miscellaneous	5–10 min	1 in 6 weeks	—
Burger et al. (35)	59/M[b]	Constricting	90 sec	30/day	—
	59/M	Diffuse	1–2 min	8 in 24 h	—
	65/F	Diffuse	15–20 min	12 in 11 months	Episodic headaches
	78/F[b]	Diffuse	3 min	5 in 4 days	Temporal arteritis
	78/F	Diffuse	30 sec	15 in 5 days	Temporal arteritis

[a]Classified according to the system of Bruno et al. (44).
[b]Photographic documentation of the episode.
Source: From Burger SK, Saul RF, Selhorst JB, Thurston SE. Transient monocular blindness caused by vasospasm. N Engl J Med 1991; 325:870–3.

middle-aged (48–49 years of age). This age distribution is consistent with the previous suggestion that nonembolic transient visual symptoms are not restricted to the young and the healthy (42). Eight of these patients had 1 to 12 brief (less than 5 mins) episodes of amaurosis fugax per day. Nine of the patients had a diffuse or constricting loss of visual field (44). One 78-year-old woman had an episode of monocular visual loss after she was asked to bend over and stand up. The subsequent ophthalmoscopic examination showed blanching of the CRA that lasted 3 min before suddenly clearing. Fundus photographs taken at the end of the attack showed dilatation of the arteries but persistent and segmental narrowing of the veins (35). The diagnosis in this case was temporal arteritis confirmed by a temporal artery biopsy. Visual loss after bending or exercising has been reported previously (43,45).

In other patients in whom the fundus has been observed during an amaurotic attack due to vasospasm, retinal arteriolar and venous narrowing, retinal edema, venous dilatation, and delayed fluorescein filling of retinal vessels has been noted (35,39,46). Vasospasm initially affects the retinal arteries and then the veins, and it is relieved first in the arterial bed and subsequently in the venous circulation. Infarction results if retinal ischemia is severe (47). In rare migrainous cases, vasospastic amaurosis fugax is complicated by CRA occlusion (48), anterior ischemic optic neuropathy, or retinal infarction (49).

C. Associated Diseases

Vasospastic amaurosis fugax may be associated with local or systemic inflammatory disorders and it has been reported in patients with pathologically confirmed temporal arteritis (35), periarteritis nodosa (38), and eosinophilic vasculitis (40). The connection between amaurosis fugax and migraine also is significant. In a review of 83 patients under age 45 years with sporadic amaurosis fugax, the investigator reports that episodic headache occurred in the majority of patients (50). Among another 24 patients with benign recurrent transient monocular blindness, half had a family history of migraine and nearly one third reported previous headaches. Tomsak et al. suggested that the recurrent visual symptoms were a variant of acephalgic migraine (43). The association of elevated levels of anticardiolipid antibodies in migrainers may, however, provide an alternative explanation.

IV. AMAUROSIS FUGAX TYPE IV

A. Clinical History

The classification of monocular amaurosis fugax into three different types led to the identification of a fourth group of patients with no clear etiology to explain the attack(s) of visual loss. The sporadic transient visual disturbance in this young group of patients resembled most closely type I amaurosis fugax except in the duration of the attack, which frequently is too long (30–60 min) or too short (for seconds only). Rarely do the episodes resemble the temporary loss of contrast vision typical of amaurosis fugax type II (see Table 1 [1,2]).

In a number of studies, including our own survey (1,4,51–56), between 5 and 40% of patients are regarded to have idiopathic amaurosis fugax, with all other causes having been ruled out. A 5-year study of 12 patients documented a benign outcome (54), and many investigators in fact regard amaurosis fugax in healthy children and young adults as benign events (41,43,54,56–59). However, a number of these patients may be experiencing sporadic attacks of vasospastic amaurosis fugax.

B. Clinical Signs

Patients with amaurosis fugax type IV have no clinical signs of cerebrovascular or retinal vascular disease. Rare cases, with elevated levels of antiphospholipid antibodies, may have fingernail splinter hemorrhages.

C. Associated Diseases

In one study, six patients (four women and two men) under the age of 34 years with episodic amaurosis fugax associated with elevated levels of antiphospholipid antibodies were reported (60). Patient 1, a 23-year-old woman 20 weeks into her first pregnancy, noted a uniocular total visual loss from the bottom up or the top down lasting approximately 2 min. She experienced 20–30 episodes of visual loss over 2 months. Patient 2, a 31-year-old woman in the postpartum period, reported episodic unilateral altitudinal visual loss occurring three to four times in one or other eye every day, with each episode lasting 1–5 min. Patient 3, a 25-year-old woman with a history of spontaneous abortion, experienced constriction of the visual field of the right eye at least 20 times each day. At other times, she also experienced a unilateral central migrating scotoma lasting seconds to minutes at least 20 times each day.

Splinter hemorrhages of the nail beds were present in four of the six patients. None had evidence of endocarditis. Some also had neurological symptoms such as spells of vertigo and diplopia, headache, or an episode of ataxia. Treatment with antiplatelet agents, or anticoagulants, or both led to a significant reduction in the incidence of spells of amaurosis fugax in five of the patients; however, no single therapeutic agent was generally effective. The clinical features and laboratory findings in the six patients are summarized in Tables 7 and 8.

Circulating antiphospholipid antibodies (lupus anticoagulant) (LA) and anticardiolipin antibody (ACLA) are immunoglobulins predominantly of the IgG or IgM class. Those of the IgG class appear to be most strongly implicated with clinical syndromes. Most investigators have found that individuals with ACLA also have LA, and over 90% of patients with LA have ACLA (61,62).

Table 7 Summary of Clinical Features of Patients

Patient no.	Age (yr)	Sex	Visual symptoms	Other neurological symptoms	Splinter hemorrhages (fingernail)	Other neurological findings	Echocardiography	CT/MRI findings
1	23	F	Unilateral total visual loss—2 min	R hand clumsiness; headaches; severe pre-eclampsia	Present	R upper extremity weakness	Thickened mitral valve without vegetation	Multiple infarctions on CT and MRI
2	31	F	Unilateral altitudinal visual loss—1–5 min	Vertigo; diplopia; headaches	Present	None	Mitral valve prolapse	Normal MRI
3	25	F	Constriction of visual field 20 times/day; central scotoma	None	Present	None	Normal	Normal CT
4	21	F	Unilateral total visual loss—5 min	Two episodes of transient amnesia; vertigo	Not examined	None	Normal	Normal CT
5	26	M	Altitudinal visual loss—30 s–20 min	Vertical diplopia; classic migraines	Present	None	Mild aortic regurgitation	Normal MRI
6	33	M	Central scotoma—5 min; oblique curtain to total visual loss	Diplopia; vertigo	Not examined	None	Mildly thickened mitral valve	Normal CT

Abbreviations: CT, computed tomography; MRI, magnetic resonance imaging; R, right.
Source: From Digre KB, Durcan FJ, Branch DW, Jacobson DM, Varner MW, Baringer JR. Amaurosis fugax associated with antiphospholipid antibodies. Ann Neurol 1989; 25:228–32.

Table 8 Laboratory Findings in Patients[a]

Patient no.	Platelet count cells × $10^3/\mu l$)	ANA	PTT (s)	PTT Correctible with 1:1 Mix	Anticardiolipin Antibodies IgG (GPL)	Anticardiolipin Antibodies IgM (MPL)	Treatment and results
1	129	Negative	52	No	243	16	Coumadin completely controlled spells
2	141	1:160	47	No	122	<4	Aspirin and coumadin failed to control spells Heparin controlled spells
3	349	Negative	36	Not done	18	<4	Aspirin and dipyridamole decreased incidence of spells to once every week
4	116	1:40	54	No	113	<4	Coumadin controlled spells
5	248	Negative	71	No	110	<4	Aspirin completely controlled spells
6	213	1:80	34.7 (control mean 25)	Partially corrected to 29.5	83	<4	Coumadin and aspirin failed to control spells

Abbreviations: ANA, antinuclear antibodies; PTT, activated partial thromboplastin time; Ig, immunoglobulin.

[a]Normal values: Platelet count, 140–400 × 10^3 cells/μl; ANA, <1:40; PTT, ≤35 sec, IgG, <8 GPL; IgM, <4 MPL

Source: From Digre KB, Durcan FJ, Branch DW, Jacobson DM, Varner MW, Baringer JR. Amaurosis fugax associated with antiphospholipid antibodies. Ann Neurol 1989; 25:228–32.

Nonetheless, there are reports of patients with one antibody or the other but not both (61,63,64). Only one of the six patients reported (patient 3) had ACLA and no LA. Worth noting is that until this report, the association of amaurosis fugax with elevated levels of circulating LA and/or ACLA had not been addressed even though amaurosis fugax had previously been observed in 11 cases (65–70). In fact, some investigators believed that these antibodies could only cause clinical disease (e.g., stroke, infarction) when other conditions (e.g., mitral valve prolapse, systemic lupus erythematosus, severe preeclampsia) were present (71). In keeping with this is the report that except for patient 3, five of the six patients with amaurosis fugax and elevated levels of antiphospholipid antibodies had, in addition, another associated disorder (60).

The pathophysiological mechanism by which these antibodies cause thromboembolic disease, including amaurosis fugax, is not yet adequately identified, but a suggested mechanism with considerable support is inhibition of prostacyclin production in vascular tissue. Prostacyclin, a prostaglandin product of vascular tissue, is both a vasodilator and an inhibitor of platelet aggregation (71). Prostacyclin's natural antagonist, thromboxane, appears to be a vasoconstrictor and promotor of platelet aggregation (72). Lupus anticoagulant inhibits prostacyclin production and allows thromboxane to work unopposed leading to vasoconstriction, platelet aggregation, and intravascular thrombosis (73). Still another theory proposes that LA inhibits protein C activation; thus counteracting its anticoagulant effect (74,75).

As a result of these observations, the evaluation of young patients with amaurosis fugax should include, as well as an ocular examination and echocardiogram, a search for splinter hemorrhages and a complete blood count, platelet count, activated partial thromboplastin time, and tests for antiphospholipid antibodies. Cerebral angiography is rarely necessary in this age group. Magnetic resonance or computed tomographic scanning of the brain should be performed only if there are findings suggestive of cerebral ischemia.

V. MANAGEMENT

Current management of amaurosis fugax is reviewed elsewhere (52). Selection of the diagnostic tests is straightforward, since atherosclerotic narrowing at the bifurcation of the common carotid artery is by far the most common problem. Often the carotid artery lesion(s) is identifiable by detection of a bruit. Bruits become audible when the residual lumen is narrowed by approximately 3 mm or less (about 50% stenosis). The higher the pitch of the bruit, the tighter the stenosis. Bruits with a particularly high pitch that fade into diastole are associated with a hemodynamically important stenosis of the internal carotid artery, with a residual lumen of less than 1.5 mm (75% stenosis or more) (76).

Kistler et al. (77) and Fisher (78) believe that retinal or cerebral ischemic symptoms are generally due to one of two pathophysiological mechanisms:

transient decreases in already low flow or embolism. Hemodynamic changes, however, leading to transient retinal ischemia occur less often than embolism. Sporadic monocular visual loss caused by low flow is associated with a hemodynamically important carotid stenosis (75% stenosis or more) (76). In the absence of stenosis of the origin of the internal carotid artery, a single embolic transient amaurotic attack suggests that the embolus had another origin; usually the heart.

A patient with transient ischemic attacks and a carotid bruit on the side appropriate to explain the symptoms should undergo selective carotid angiography. Angiography also is indicated in a patient suffering a typical attack of amaurosis fugax with no bruit (79). Crowell and Ojemann (79) emphasize that noninvasive tests of carotid circulation, including assessment of hemodynamic change and stenosis, are particularly important in studying patients with central retinal occlusion, evaluating patients with atypical or vague symptoms and possible carotid disease, and in assessing patients with established strokes. Among the most useful carotid tests are Doppler ultrasonography and oculoplethysmography, which indicates the presence of hemodynamic lesions; (80) phonoangiography, which analyzes the bruit to determine the residual lumen diameter; and B-scan ultrasonography, which images the artery with ultrasound. A battery of these tests has proven 90% effective in identifying carotid stenosis with a residual lumen of 2 mm or less (81). The false-positive rate is 3–5%.

Periorbital Doppler ultrasonography helps determine if there is a hemodynamically significant lesion, and the test reveals the direction of flow in external carotid branches in the forehead (82). Reversal of flow indicates reduced pressure in the internal carotid artery system. Periorbital Doppler ultrasonography requires careful positioning of the probes and a recognition that the test can be influenced by external carotid stenosis. Overall, it is the most effective test for studying the superficial orbital circulation. Oculoplethysmography (OPG) measures the relative arrival time of the ocular pulse in each eye (83) and a delay of greater than 20 ms is significant. This is the most useful test for studying the deep orbital circulation; however, results are difficult to interpret in 10–20% of patients because of technical artifacts. For internal carotid occlusion, OPG is 95% accurate (84).

Phonoangiography gives the most useful information in the evaluation of a carotid bruit (85–87). Quantitative phonoangiography can accurately estimate the residual lumen diameter at the point of stenosis in about 90% of patients (82,83). In addition, this test can be used to differentiate between bruits originating at the carotid bifurcation and those emanating from the thorax. Duplex studies with spectral phonoangiography and range-gated Doppler imaging can differentiate tight stenosis from occlusion (88,89).

In addition to the noninvasive studies of carotid circulation all patients with suspected carotid occlusive disease should have a medical evaluation with a complete blood count (90), sedimentation rate, fibrinogen level, measurement of blood sugar, blood urea nitrogen, serum electrolytes, clotting studies (prothrombin time, partial thromboplastin time, and platelet count), electrocardiogram, and chest radiography. Blood cholesterol and triglyceride levels should also be checked.

Medical evaluation can reveal significant medical risk factors, including symptomatic coronary artery disease, severe peripheral arterial disease, rheumatic heart disease, congestive heart failure, severe hypertension (blood pressure more than 180/110 mm Hg), and chronic obstructive pulmonary disease. Other risk factors include diabetes, hyperlipidemia, and obesity.

Because there has been no reliable medical therapy to reduce the extent of an atherosclerotic lesion once it has formed at the carotid bifurcation, surgical removal of the lesion has been the treatment of choice and the low morbidity reported among properly selected patients suggests that endarterectomy can be safe, particularly if it is performed by an experienced team of surgeons, physicians, cardiologists, anesthesiologists, and nursing personnel. The report of the North American Symptomatic Carotid Endarterectomy Trial Group published in the *New England Journal of Medicine* represents a notable affirmation of this point of view (91).

In patients whose risk of a cardiac event is deemed too high to warrant carotid endarterectomy, cerebral angiography can be replaced by magnetic resonance imaging (MRI) angiography. This is a noninvasive procedure that also avoids the risk of a lasting neurological complication. In this group of patients, the risk of subsequent stroke can be reduced with antiplatelet therapy (aspirin) or anticoagulation therapy (warfarin). The medical therapy used in the North American Trial was predominantly aspirin, usually at a dose of 13,000 mg/day. Kistler et al., in a recent editorial in the *New England Journal of Medicine* (76), report that the efficacy of the more commonly used dose of 325 mg/day is probably similar. But they suggest that given the high rate of stroke among patients treated with aspirin, low-intensity anticoagulation with warfarin (maintaining a normalized ratio of 1.5 to 2.5) may be more effective.

ACKNOWLEDGMENT

I wish to thank Fran Christie for typing this manuscript.

REFERENCES

1. Wray SH. Extracranial internal carotid artery disease. In: Bernstein EF, ed. Amaurosis fugax. New York: Springer-Verlag, 1988:72–80.
2. Burde RM. Amaurosis fugax, an overview. J Clin Neuro-ophthalmol 1989; 9(3):185–9.
3. Wilson IA, Warlow CP, Ross Russell RW. Cardiovascular disease in patients with retinal arterial occlusion. Lancet 1979; 1:1292–4.

4. Fisher CM. Transient monocular blindness associated with hemiplegia. Am Arch Ophthalmol 1952; 47:167–203.
5. Warlow CP. Transient ischemic attacks. In: Mattes WB, Glaser GH, eds. Recent advances in clinical neurology. Edinburgh: Churchill Livingstone, 1982: 191–214.
6. Cartlidge NEF, Whisnant JP, Elveback LR. Carotid and vertebral-basilar transient cerebral ischemic attacks: a community study. Mayo Clin Proc 1977; 52: 117–20.
7. Parkin PJ, Kendall BE, Marshall J, McDonald WI. Amaurosis fugax: some aspects of management. J Neurol Neurosurg Psychiatry 1982; 45:1–6.
8. Hollenhorst RW. The ocular manifestations of internal carotidarterial thrombosis. Med Clin N Am 1960; 44:897–908.
9. Hollenhorst RW. Significance of bright plaques in the retinal arterioles. JAMA 1961; 178:123–9.
10. D'Cruz IA, Cohen HC, Prabhu R, Bisla V, Glick G. Clinical manifestations of mitral-annulus calcification, with emphasis on its echocardiographic features. Am Heart J 1977; 94:367–77.
11. Guthrie J, Fairgrieve J. Aortic embolism due to myxoid tumor associated with myocardial calcification. Br Heart J 1963; 25:137–40.
12. diBono DP, Warlow CP. Mitral-annulus calcification and cerebral or retinal ischemia. Lancet 1979; 2:383–5.
13. Barnett HJM. Transient cerebral ischemia pathogenesis, prognosis and management. Ann R Coll Physicians Surg Can 1974; 7:153–73.
14. Barnett HJM. Delayed cerebral ischemic episodes distal to occlusion of major cerebral arteries. Neurology 1978; 28:769–74.
15. Barnett HJM, Boughner DR, Wayne Taylor D, Cooper PE, Kostuk WJ, Nichol PM. Further evidence relating mitral valve prolapse to cerebral ischemic events. N Engl J Med 1980; 302:139–44.
16. Cogan DG, Wray SH. Vascular occlusions in the eye from cardiac myxomas. Am J Ophthalmol 1975; 80:396–403.
17. Countee RW, Vijayanathan T, Chavis P. Recurrent retinal ischemia beyond cervical carotid occlusions. J Neurosurg 1981; 55:532–42.
18. Kearns TP, Siekert RG, Sundt TM Jr. The ocular aspects of bypass surgery of the carotid artery. Mayo Clin Proc 1979; 54:3–11.
19. Sundt TM Jr, Siekert RG, Piepgras DG, Sharbrough FW, Wayne Houser O. Bypass surgery for vascular disease of the carotid system. Mayo Clin Proc 1976; 51:677–92.
20. Whisnant JP. Extracranial-intracranial arterial bypass. Neurology 1978; 28:209–10.
21. Weinberg PE, Patronas NJ, Kim KS, Melen O. Anomalous origin of the ophthalmic artery in a patient with amaurosis fugax. Arch Neurol 1981; 38:315–7.
22. Furlan AJ, Whisnant JP, Kearns TP. Unilateral visual loss in bright light: an unusual symptom of carotid artery occlusive disease. Arch Neurol 1979; 36:675–6.
23. Ross Russell RW, Page NGR. Critical perfusion of brain and retina. Brain 1983; 106:419–34.
24. Kearns TP, Hollenhorst RW. Venous stasis retinopathy of occlusive disease of the carotid artery. Mayo Clin Proc 1963; 38:304–12.
25. Hedges TR. Ophthalmoscopic findings in internal carotid artery occlusion. Am J Ophthalmol 1963; 55:1007–12.

26. Bullock JD, Falter RT, Downing JE, Snyder, HE. Ischemic ophthalmia secondary to an ophthalmic artery occlusion. Am J Ophthalmol 1972; 74:486–93.
27. Carter JE. Panretinal photocoagulation for progressive ocular neovascularization secondary to occlusion of the common carotid artery. Ann Ophthalmol 1984; 16:572–6.
28. Grader J. Venous stasis retinopathy: a case report. Can J Ophthalmol 1975; 10: 107–10.
29. Edwards MS, Chater NL, Stanley JA. Reversal of chronic ocular ischemia by extracranial-intracranial arterial bypass: A case report. Neurosurgery 1980; 7:480–3.
30. Mills RP. Anterior segment ischemia secondary to carotid occlusive disease. J Clin Neuro-ophthalmol 1989; 9(3):200–204.
31. Kearns TP, Siekert RG, Sundt TM Jr. The ocular aspects of bypass surgery of the carotid artery. Mayo Clin Proc 1979; 54:3–11.
32. Campo RV, Aaberg TM. Digital subtraction angiography in the diagnosis of retinal vascular disease. Am J Ophthalmol 1983; 96:632–40.
33. McCray JA III. Venous stasis retinopathy of stenotic or occlusive carotid origin. J Clin Neuro-opthalmol 1989; 9(3):195–99.
34. Hollenhorst RW. Effects of posture on retinal ischemia from temporal arteritis. Trans Am Ophthalmol Soc 1967; 65:94–105.
35. Burger SK, Saul RF, Selhorst JB, Thurston SE. Transient monocular blindness caused by vasospasm. N Engl J Med 1991; 325:870–73.
36. Ellenberger, C Jr, Epstein AD. Ocular complications of atherosclerosis; what do they mean? Semin Neurol 1986; 6:185–93.
37. Walsh FB, Hoyt WF. Clinical neuro-ophthalmology. 3d ed. Baltimore: Williams & Wilkins, 1969:1671–3.
38. Newman NM, Hoyt WF, Spencer WH. Macula-sparing blackouts: clinical and pathologic investigations of intermittent choroidal vascular insufficiency in a case of periarteritis nodosa. Arch Ophthalmol 1974; 91:367–70.
39. Kline LB, Kelly CL. Ocular migraine in a patient with cluster headaches. Headache 1980; 20:253–7.
40. Schwartz ND, So YT, Hollander H, Allen S, Fye KH. Eosinophilic vasculitis leading to amaurosis fugax in a patient with acquired immunodeficiency syndrome. Arch Intern Med 1986; 146:2059–60.
41. Appleton R, Farrell K, Buncic JR, Hill A. Amaurosis fugax in teenagers: a migraine variant. Am J Dis Child 1988; 142:331–3.
42. Fisher CM. Late-life migraine accompaniments as a cause of unexplained transient ischemic attacks. Can J Neurol Sci 1980; 7:9–17.
43. Tomsak RL, Jergens PB. Benign recurrent transient monocular blindness: a possible variant of acephalgic migraine. Headache 1987; 27:66–9.
44. Bruno A, Corbett JJ, Biller J, Adams HP Jr, Qualls C. Transient monocular visual loss patterns and associated vascular abnormalities. Stroke 1990; 21:34–9.
45. Imes RK, Hoyt WF. Exercise-induced transient visual events in young healthy adults. J Clin Neuro-ophthalmol 1989; 9:178–80.
46. Troost BT. Migraine. In: Duane TD ed. Clinical ophthalmology. Vol. 2. Philadelphia: Harper Medical, 1976: 19:1–25.
47. Wolter JR, Burchfield WJ. Ocular migraine in a young man resulting in unilateral transient blindness and retinal edema. J Pediatr Ophthalmol 1971; 8:173–6.

48. Katz B. Migrainous central retinal artery occlusion. J Clin Neuro-ophthal 1986; 6:69–75.
49. Hupp SL, Kline LB, Corbett JJ. Visual disturbances of migraine. Surv Ophthalmol 1989; 33:221–36.
50. Tippin J, Corbett JJ, Kerber RE, Schroeder E, Thompson HS. Amaurosis fugax and ocular infarction in adolescents and young adults. Ann Neurol 1989; 26:69–77.
51. Fisher CM. Observations of the fundus oculi in transient monocular blindness. Neurology 1959; 9:333–47.
52. The Amaurosis Fugax Study Group. Current management of amaurosis fugax. Stroke 1990; 21:201–8.
53. Corbett JJ. Neuro-ophthalmic complications of migraine and cluster headaches. Neurol Clin 1983; 1:973–95.
54. Eadie MJ, Sutherland JM, Tyrer JH. Recurrent monocular blindness of uncertain cause. Lancet 1968; 1:319–21.
55. Marshall J, Meadows S. The natural history of amaurosis fugax. Brain 1976; 91:419–34.
56. Carroll D. Retinal migraine. Headache 1970; 10:9–13.
57. Longfellow DW, Davis FS Jr, Walsh FB. Unilateral intermittent blindness with dilatation of retinal veins. Arch Ophthalmol 1962; 67:554–5.
58. Poole CJM, Ross Russell RW, Harrison P, Savidge GF. Amaurosis fugax under the age of 40 years. J Neurol Neurosurg Psychiatry 1987; 50:81–4.
59. Sorensen PN. Amaurosis fugax. A unselected material. Acta Ophthalmol 1983; 61:583–8.
60. Digre KB, Durcan FJ, Branch DW, Jacobson DM, Varner MW, Baringer JR. Amaurosis fugax associated with antiphospholipid antibodies. Ann Neurol 1989; 25:228–32.
61. Harris EN, Gharavi AE, Boey ML, Patel BM, Mackworth-Young CG, Loizou S, Hughes GRV. Anticardiolipin antibodies: detection by radioimmunoassay and association with thrombosis in systemic lupus erythematosus. Lancet 1983; 3:1211–14.
62. Branch DW, Rote NS, Dostal DA, Scott JR. Association of lupus anticoagulant with antibodies against phosphatidyl-serine. Clin Immunol Immunopathol 1987; 42:63–75.
63. Branch DW, Rote NS, Scott JR. The demonstration of lupus anticoagulant by an enzyme-linked immunoadsorbent assay. Clin Immunol Immunopathol 1986; 39:298.
64. Triplett DA, Brandt JT, Musgrave KA, Orr CA. The relationship between lupus anticoagulants and antibodies to phospholipid. JAMA 1988; 295:550–4.
65. D'Alton JG, Preston DN, Bormanis J, Green MS, Kraag GR. Multiple transient ischemic attacks, lupus anticoagulant and verrucous endocarditis. Stroke 1985; 16:512–14.
66. Elias M, Eldor A. Thromboembolism in patients with the "lupus"-type circulating anticoagulant. Arch Intern Med 1984; 144:510–15.
67. Landi G, Calloni MV, Sabbadini MG, Mannucci, PM, Candelise L. Recurrent ischemic attacks in two young adults with lupus anticoagulant. Stroke 1983; 14:377–9.
68. Levine SR, Kieran S, Puzio K, Feit H, Patel SC, Welch KMA. Cerebral venous thrombosis with lupus anticoagulants. Report of two cases. Stroke 1987; 18:801–4.

69. Kushner M, Simonian N, Laposata M. The lupus inhibitor and brain ischemia. Ann Neurol 1987; 22:115.
70. Levine SR, Crofts JW, Lesser GR, Floberg J, Welch KMA. Visual symptoms associated with the presence of a lupus anticoagulant. Ophthalmology 1988; 95:686–92.
71. Levine SR, Welch KMA. The spectrum of neurologic disease associated with antiphospholipid antibodies. Arch Neurol 1987; 44:876–83.
72. Moncada S, Higgs EA, Vane JR. Human arterial and venous tissues generate prostacyclin (prostaglandin X), a potent inhibitor of platelet aggregation. Lancet 1977; 1:18–20.
73. Moncada S, Vane JR. Pharmacology and endogenous roles of prostaglandin endoperoxides, thromboxane A2, and prostacyclin. Pharmacol Rev 1979; 30:293–331.
74. Branch DW, Scott JR, Kochenour NK, Hershgold E. Obstetric complications associated with the lupus anticoagulant. N Engl J Med 1985; 313:1322–6.
75. Cariou R, Tobelem G, Soria C, et al. Inhibition or protein C with activation by endothelial cells in the presence of lupus anticoagulant. N Engl J Med 1986; 314:1193–4.
76. Kistler FP, Buonanno FS, Gress DR. Carotid endarterectomy—specific therapy based on pathophysiology. N Engl J Med 1991; 325:505–7 (editorial).
77. Kistler JP, Ropper AH, Heros RC. Therapy of ischemic cerebral vascular disease due to atherothrombosis. N Engl J Med 1984; 311:27–34.
78. Fisher CM. Concerning recurrent transient cerebral ischemic attacks. Can Med Assoc J 1962; 86:1091–9.
79. Crowell RM, Ojemann RG. Surgical management of extracranial occlusive disease. In: Barnett HM, Mohr JP, Stein BM, Yatsu FM, eds. Stroke pathophysiology, diagnosis, and management. Edinburgh: Churchill Livingstone, 1986:1003–58.
80. O'Leary DH, Persson AV, Clouse ME. Noninvasive testing for carotid artery stenosis: I. Prospective analysis of three methods. Am J Neuroroentgenol 1981; 137(6):1189–94.
81. Ackerman RH. The relative effectiveness of six noninvasive tests for carotid disease. Neurology 1976; 26:379–80.
82. Ginsberg MD, Greenwood SA, Goldberg HI. Noninvasive diagnosis of extracranial cerebrovascular disease: oculoplethysmography-phonoangiography and directional Doppler ultrasonography. Neurology 1979; 29:623–31.
83. Kartchner MM, McRae LP. Noninvasive evaluation and management of the "asymptomatic" carotid bruit. Surgery 1977; 82:840–7.
84. Ackerman RH. Noninvasive carotid evaluation. Stroke 1980; 11:675–8.
85. Duncan GW, Gruber JO, Forbes Dewey C Jr, Myers GS, Lees RS. Evaluation of carotid stenosis by phonoangiography. N Engl J Med 1975; 293:1124–8.
86. Kistler JP, Lees RS, Friedman J, Pressin M, Mohr JP, Roberson GS, Ojemann RG. The bruit of carotid stenosis versus radiated basal heart murmurs: differentiation by phonoangiography. Circulation 1978; 57:975–81.
87. Kistler JP, Lees RS, Miller A, Crowell RM, Roberson GS. Correlation of spectral phonoangiography and carotid angiography with gross pathology in carotid stenosis. N Engl J Med 1981; 305:417–9.

88. Fell G, Phillips DJ, Chikos PM, Harley JD, Thiele BL, Strandness DE. Ultrasonic duplex scanning for disease of the carotid artery. Circulation 1981; 64: 1191–5.
89. Zbornikova V, Akesson JA, Lassivik C. Diagnosis of carotid artery disease—comparison between directional Doppler, duplex scanner and angiography. Acta Neurol Scand 1982; 65:335–46.
90. Harrison MJH, Pollock S, Kendall BE, Marshall J. Effect of hematocrit on carotid stenosis and cerebral infarction. Lancet 1981; 2:114–5.
91. North American Symptomatic Carotid Endarterectomy Trial Collaborators. Beneficial effect of carotid endarterectomy in symptomatic patients with high-grade carotid stenosis. N Engl J Med 1991; 325:445–53.

2

Demyelinating Diseases: Optic Neuritis

Neil R. Miller
Johns Hopkins Medical Institutions, Baltimore, Maryland

The term *optic neuritis* describes a set of clinical signs and symptoms that are *assumed* to be produced by inflammation of the optic nerve.

I. CLINICAL MANIFESTATIONS

Optic neuritis usually occurs in patients between 15 and 45 years of age, with women being affected about four times as often as men (1,2). Most patients present with blurred vision in one eye preceded or accompanied by pain. The pain may be sharp or dull, and it is often exacerbated by movement of the affected eye. Visual acuity in an eye with optic neuritis varies considerably from a minimal decrease in central vision to no perception of light in about 4% of patients. Color vision is almost always impaired, even when central vision is normal or nearly so. Almost all patients with optic neuritis have a defect in the central visual field of the affected eye that occasionally may extend into the peripheral visual field. True central scotomas are rare, however, with many patients having arcuate, altitudinal, and even hemianopic defects in the central field. Patients with unilateral optic neuritis always have a relative afferent pupillary defect (Marcus Gunn pupil) on the affected side, as do many patients with asymmetric bilateral optic neuritis. However, some patients with bilateral optic neuritis have no evidence of a relative afferent pupillary defect despite clinically asymmetric disease, which indicates that pathological damage to both optic nerves is more symmetric than the clinical picture would suggest. The optic disc in an eye with optic neuritis may appear swollen, normal, or pale. If the disc is swollen, the optic neuritis is called *papillitis* or *anterior optic neuritis*, and it is assumed that the inflammation is occurring within the intraocular portion of the optic nerve. If the disc is normal in appearance, the disorder is called *retrobulbar optic neuritis* or simply *retrobulbar neuritis*. Retrobulbar neuritis occurs about twice as often as papillitis; however, whether the optic disc appears swollen or normal has no visual or systemic prognostic significance in a patient with optic neuritis. Optic atrophy in a patient with acute optic neuritis indicates previous damage to the optic nerve, since it takes at least 4–6 weeks to develop optic pallor after an acute optic neuropathy (3).

II. NATURAL HISTORY

The characteristic course for optic neuritis is one of maximum visual loss over about 2 weeks followed by some degree of recovery over the subsequent 2–6 months (4). Further recovery may occur 12 months or longer after onset of visual loss. Recovery may be complete in some patients, but many patients complain that visual function is not as good as it was before the attack. Even patients without any visual symptoms after an attack of optic neuritis often have some degree of optic nerve dysfunction that can be demonstrated by clinical, electrophysiological, or psychophysical testing (5).

III. DIAGNOSIS

Many patients who experience an attack of isolated optic neuritis will eventually develop multiple sclerosis (6,7), and it is thus believed that the majority of cases of optic neuritis are caused by demyelination. Although most patients with optic neuritis have no precursory illness, some patients develop signs and symptoms indicative of a nonspecific, viral illness several days or weeks before the onset of visual loss. Optic neuritis may also occur as the initial manifestation or in the setting of systemic inflammatory disorders other than multiple sclerosis, such as syphilis, sarcoidosis, systemic lupus erythematosus, and Lyme disease (Table 1) (1,5). Some patients, particularly men, have no evidence of systemic or neurological disease at the time that the optic neuritis occurs, nor do they ultimately develop such disease. In such cases, the condition is considered to be "idiopathic." Many physicians believe idiopathic optic neuritis is actually a limited form of multiple sclerosis.

Pathological processes other than inflammation may cause an acute optic neuropathy that mimics optic neuritis (Table 2) (1). These processes include compression, ischemia, infiltration, and toxic processes. In addition, Leber's hereditary optic neuropathy may present as initially unilateral visual loss that

Table 1 Causes of Optic Neuritis

Most common	Less common	Least common
Multiple sclerosis	Idiopathic Postviral	Granulomatous inflammation, especially syphilis or sacroidosis Collagen vascular (autoimmune) disorders Infectious mononucleosis Adjacent inflammation of paranasal sinuses or orbit

mimics optic neuritis, although such patients never complain of ocular or orbital pain, and the second eye always becomes affected sooner or later (8).

Because the diagnosis of optic neuritis is based entirely on clinical grounds, the responsibility of the physician with a patient with *presumed* optic neuritis is to eliminate the possibility of a process that is causing an optic neuropathy that is mimicking optic neuritis and, if no such lesion is present, to determine if there

Table 2 Differential Diagnosis of Optic Neuritis

- Other optic neuropathies
  - compressive
    - orbital
    - intracanalicular
    - intracranial
  - ischemic
  - toxic
  - nutritional (deficiency)
  - infiltrative
  - hereditary (particularly Leber's)
  - glaucoma
  - drusen of the optic disc
- Intraocular disease
  - retinal disease
  - retinal vascular disease
  - diseases of the ocular media
    - corneal disease
    - cataract
- Nonorganic visual loss
  - conversion reaction
  - malingering

is an underlying and potentially treatable cause for the optic neuritis. The minimum evaluation of such a patient includes a complete systemic and neurological history. If there is no history suggesting an underlying inflammatory disorder such as syphilis, sarcoid, systemic lupus erythematosus, or Lyme disease, it probably is not necessary to obtain any serologic studies. If the history is unreliable or suggestive of a systemic inflammatory disease, however, the physician may wish to obtain some or all of the following depending on the setting: a complete blood count, erythrocyte sedimentation rate, serum tests for syphilis, assay for antinuclear antibodies, assay for angiotensin converting enzyme, Lyme titers, assay for human immunodeficiency virus (HIV), and a chest radiograph. Patients with presumed optic neuritis that is painless, patients with bilateral presumed optic neuritis, and patients whose vision does not improve spontaneously or with treatment (see below) should undergo a blood test for the mitochondrial deoxyribonucleic acid (DNA) mutations that are associated with Leber's hereditary optic neuropathy (9–11).

There are two schools of thought regarding neuroimaging in patients with presumed optic neuritis. Many experts believe that one need not obtain any imaging studies in a "typical" case of optic neuritis and that neuroimaging should be performed only if the clinical presentation is atypical for optic neuritis (i.e., subacute, slowly progressive, painless) or if vision does not begin to improve spontaneously or with treatment (see below) within 3–6 weeks. Others, myself included, prefer to obtain magnetic resonance imaging (MRI) of the orbits and optic chiasmal region in patients with presumed *retrobulbar neuritis* to make certain that there is no evidence of a mass compressing the intracranial portion of the affected optic nerve, such as a pituitary adenoma, meningioma, or aneurysm, and to see if there are any periventricular hyperintense lesions that suggest underlying but asymptomatic demyelinating disease in the brain (12). Given the significant amount of information obtained from MRI scanning, there would seem to be little or no justification for obtaining a plain skull radiograph or polytomogram in any patient with an acute optic neuropathy, and computed tomographic scanning probably should be reserved for those patients who cannot for some reason undergo MRI.

Patients with optic neuritis whose history, examination, or both suggest the diagnosis of multiple sclerosis should undergo a complete neurological examination. Other tests that may be considered in such patients include testing of evoked potentials (visual, brainstem, somatosensory), MRI, and a lumbar puncture with cerebrospinal fluid (CSF) analyzed for protein, glucose, cellular, and immunoglobulin G (IgG) content as well as for oligoclonal bands and myelin basic protein.

IV. TREATMENT

Patients with demyelinating or idiopathic optic neuritis tend to recover spontaneously within weeks to months without treatment. The results of the Optic

Neuritis Treatment Trial (ONTT), sponsored by the National Institutes of Health, indicate that a 3-day course of high-dose intravenous methylprednisolone (1 g/day) followed by a 10-day course of oral prednisone begun within the first 8 days after onset of visual loss results in a more rapid improvement in all aspects of vision (e.g., acuity, contrast sensitivity, color field) by about 2–3 weeks compared with either oral prednisone alone or placebo (4). It does not, however, improve final visual outcome. High-dose systemic corticosteroids may also reduce the risk of multiple sclerosis in certain patients with isolated optic neuritis, particularly those with abnormal MRIs (13). Oral prednisone alone does not improve ultimate visual outcome, and its use is associated with an *increase* in episodes of both recurrent optic neuritis in the previously affected eye and optic neuritis in the opposite eye. I therefore recommend that the use of high-dose intravenous methylprednisolone followed by a short course of oral prednisone be considered in any patient with acute optic neuritis when a more rapid improvement in vision compared with the natural history of the condition is required or when the patient's initial visual acuity drops to less than 20/40 during the first week after onset of visual symptoms or when an MRI performed at the onset of visual loss shows significant periventricular lesions in the white matter. Although I cannot explain the apparent adverse effects of oral corticosteroids in patients with acute optic neuritis, I do not recommend their use for such patients, at least not at the usual dose of 1 mg/kg/day. There is no evidence that other anti-inflammatory agents have any effect on the degree or speed of recovery of visual acuity, color vision, contrast sensitivity, or visual field in patients with acute demyelinating or idiopathic optic neuritis.

Systemic corticosteroids may be extremely valuable in treating the rare cases of optic neuritis associated with certain systemic inflammatory disorders such as sarcoid and systemic lupus erythematosus (14–17). The early use of steroids in patients with these conditions may avert profound, irreversible visual loss. Similarly, patients with optic neuritis caused by syphilis or Lyme disease may benefit both visually and systemically from early and aggressive use of antibiotics (18–22).

REFERENCES

1. Miller NR. Walsh and Hoyt's clinical neuro-ophthalmology. 3d ed, Vol. 1. 227–248. Baltimore: Williams & Wilkins, 1982:227–48.
2. The Optic Neuritis Study Group. The clinical profile of optic neuritis: experience of the Optic Neuritis Treatment Trial. Arch Ophthalmol 1991; 109:1673–8.
3. Quigley HA, Davis EB, Anderson DR. Descending optic nerve degeneration in primates. Invest Ophthalmol Vis Sci 1977; 16:841–9.
4. Beck RW, et al. A randomized, controlled trial of corticosteroids in the treatment of acute optic neuritis. N Engl J Med 1992.

5. Perkin GD, Rose GC. Optic neuritis and its differential diagnosis. Oxford, England: Oxford University Press, 1979.
6. Francis DA, et al. A reassessment of the risk of multiple sclerosis developing in patients with optic neuritis after extended follow-up. J Neurol Neurosurg Psychiatry 1987; 50:758–65.
7. Rizzo JF III, Lessell S. Risk of developing multiple sclerosis after uncomplicated optic neuritis: A long-term prospective study. Neurology 1988; 38:185–90.
8. Newman NJ, et al. The clinical characteristics of pedigrees of Leber's hereditary optic neuropathy with the 11778 mutation. Am J Ophthalmol 1991; 111:750–62.
9. Johns DR et al. Leber's hereditary optic neuropathy: clinical manifestations of the 3460 mutation. Arch Ophthalmol 1992; 110:1577–81.
10. Johns DR et al. Leber's hereditary optic neuropathy: clinical manifestations of the 14484 mutation. Arch Ophthalmol 1993; 111:495–98.
11. Johns DR, et al. Leber's hereditary optic neuropathy: clinical manifestations of the 15257 mutation. Ophthalmology 1993; 100:981–6.
12. Beck RW et al. Brain magnetic resonance imaging in active optic neuritis. Arch Neurol 1993; 50:841–6.
13. Beck RW et al. The effect of corticosteroids for acute optic neuritis on the subsequent development of multiple sclerosis. N Engl J Med 1993; 329:1764–9.
14. Smith CA, Pinals RS. Optic neuritis in systemic lupus erythematosus. J Rheumatol 1982; 9:963–6.
15. Graham EM, et al. Optic neuropathy in sarcoidosis. J Neurol Neurosurg Psychiatry 1986; 49:756–63.
16. Jabs DA, et al. Optic neuropathy in systemic lupus erythematosus. Arch Ophthalmol 1986; 104:564–8.
17. Jordan DR, et al. Optic nerve involvement as the initial manifestation of sarcoidosis. Can J Ophthalmol 1988; 23:232–7.
18. Weinstein JM, et al. Acute syphilitic optic neuritis. Arch Ophthalmol 1981; 99:1392–5.
19. Farris BK, Webb RM. Lyme disease and optic neuritis. J Clin Neuro-ophthalmol 1988; 8:73–8.
20. Gustafson R, Svenungsson B. Optic neuropathy in Borrelia infection. J Infect 1988; 17:187–8.
21. Bialasiewicz AA, et al. Borrelia Burgdorferi infektion mit beidseitiger neuritis nervi optici und intrazerebalen demyelinisierungsherden. Klin Monatsbl Augenheilk 1989; 195:91–4.
22. Winward KE, et al. Ocular Lyme borreliosis. Am J Ophthalmol 1989; 108:651–7.

3

Low-Vision Rehabilitation in Neuro-Ophthalmology

Joseph L. Demer
Jules Stein Eye Institute, Los Angeles, California

I. EVALUATING LOW VISION

Most patients seen in a neuro-ophthalmology practice experience some degree of visual sensory impairment. Although diagnostic evaluation is of paramount importance and although many therapies are aimed at saving life or averting catastrophic total amaurosis, complete care of the patient requires that the neuro-ophthalmologist consider visual rehabilitation in a setting of irremediable but partial visual loss. *Low vision* is a term applied to the condition of significant visual loss where there nonetheless remains some functional, residual vision (1). Fortunately, the great majority of patients with visual loss in fact have low vision rather than no useful vision (2). There are three fundamental forms of visual impairment: loss of central acuity, which represents resolution; loss of sensitivity to contrast; and loss of visual field. In this chapter, the management of the fundamental forms of visual impairment is presented first followed by consideration of the effect of pathological nystagmus on visual function.

A. Visual Acuity

Loss of central visual acuity is one of the most obvious presenting complaints. It commonly persists after recovery from optic nerve disease, and it also may be due to inflammatory, compressive, ischemic, toxic, and nutritional causes, but acuity also may be reduced because of bilateral cortical lesions. Central acuity is usually quantified using a visual resolution task such as identification of Snellen letters (3). Since refractive error is a neurologically trivial cause of poor visual acuity, acuity should be tested with optimal refractive correction for both distance and near viewing. Distance vision is tested at a distance of 10–20 ft (3–6 m), whereas near vision is tested at the reading distance, usually 10–16 in. (25–40 cm). In either case, the patient is asked to make visual identification of a physical object or a figure on a chart or projection screen called an optotype. Objects and optotypes must be of calibrated size to quantitate acuity. Care must be taken to assure that the patient understands the task and is familiar with the objects or optotypes employed. Optotypes useful for literate patients may include English letters, Arabic numbers, or Oriental characters. For the illiterate, available charts include "E" or "C" characters in multiple orientations, as well as Allen pictures, which are stylized illustrations of everyday objects suitable for children.

Distance acuity is customarily recorded as the Snellen fraction. The Snellen fraction is the ratio of the actual viewing distance used in testing divided by the distance at which the optotype size at the patient's visual resolution threshold would be at the threshold of a normal observer. Thus, at a testing distance of 20 ft, standard vision represents threshold resolution of optotypes that a group of normal observers can, on average, just begin to resolve at a testing distance of 20 ft; this acuity would be recorded as "20/20." The metric equivalent, at 6 m, would be "6/6." At any testing distance, optotypes of standard 20/20 size are 5 min of arc in total height and contain individual features 1 min of arc in size. At 20 ft, 20/20–sized optotypes are 9 mm high. In fact, most healthy young normal subjects have corrected acuities of about 20/15, which corresponds to optotypes 3.75 min of arc in size and having features 0.75 min of arc in size.

Distance acuity reduced to the threshold level of legal blindness is recorded as "20/200"; this means that the patient can resolve at a testing of distance of 20 ft characters large enough that a group of normal subjects can just begin to resolve them at 200 ft. At any testing distance, optotypes of 20/200 size are 50 min of arc in total height and contain individual features 10 min of arc in size. At 20 ft, 20/200–sized optotypes are 9 cm high. The commonly accepted criterion for "low vision" is a corrected acuity of 20/70 or less in the better eye. At this level of vision and below, vision begins to limit functional activities, particularly reading.

Printed vision testing charts usually include multiple lines of optotypes having sizes corresponding to levels of acuity ranging from around 20/10 through around 20/200 at the testing distance for which they were designed. However, the range and precision of acuity testing can be extended by changing the testing distance. For example, profoundly reduced acuities of 10/200 (equivalent to 20/400) or 5/200 (equivalent to 20/800) can be measured by reducing the standard testing distance by a factor of two or four while employing the "20/200"–sized optotypes. Such efforts are prognostically valuable when evaluating patients with severe visual impairment. For visual impairment below the level of about 20/800, it is ideal to use specially designed low-vision charts that are available. In the absence of low-vision charts, acuity may be recorded as the maximum distance at which the patient can count the fingers of the examiner's hand. Thus, a severe level of visual impairment might be "finger counting at 3 ft." If fingers cannot be counted at any distance, but movement of the examiner's hand can be detected, acuity is specified as "hand motions." Visual acuity less than hand motions is recorded as the perception of light, with or without the ability to detect the direction of projection of a focal source such as a flashlight.

Many patients recovering from a neurological crisis have neglected or been unable to have a recent refraction or have lost their newest pair of spectacles. Older patients who have previously undergone cataract surgery may also require high-diopter power convex spectacle lenses or contact lenses for the correction of aphakia, which is the hyperopic refractive deficit caused by the absence of the crystalline lens. A thorough evaluation of visual function nearly always requires that refraction be performed by the examiner. Referral to a specialist for this purpose may be indicated.

For most literate patients, near visual function is of paramount importance. Near vision is measured using optotypes printed on a hand-held card or page, with optotype sizes correspondingly reduced for the viewing distance of 25–40 cm. Visual acuity at near is recorded using one of several print size scales, most commonly the Jaeger, "M," reduced Snellen, or typeface point scales. Even if acuity is normal at distance, vision may be impaired at the reading distance owing to a variety of causes, most commonly inadequate refractive correction. This is because patients over the age of about 45 years experience presbyopia, an age-related decline in the capacity for accommodation of the crystalline lens. By about 60 years of age, the average emmetropic patient has negligible accommodation and has become entirely reliant on convex lenses for reading. Opacities of the ocular media, particularly posterior subcapsular cataract, can selectively impair near vision, as can pathological forms of nystagmus exacerbated in the reading position.

B. Contrast Sensitivity

Contrast is the relative difference in the brightness of features in an image. Image *contrast intensity*, C, is defined by the following equation:

$$C = \frac{L_{max} - L_{min}}{L_{max} + L_{min}}$$

where L_{max} is the brightness of the bright part of the image (a letter, for example) and L_{min} is the brightness of the dark part of the image (the background, for example). A white letter against an absolutely black background has contrast of 1.0, or 100%; an absolutely black letter against a white background also has contrast of 100%, although the *contrast polarity* is opposite. Visual acuity is tested using high-contrast letters. Printed text, even employing black ink, has a contrast much lower than 100% owing to reflectance of the ink and imperfect whiteness of the paper. In a darkened room, projected acuity testing charts have contrast of 80–90%. Contrast is reduced when there are other sources of illumination besides the projector. Video displays produce higher levels of contrast—up to 96% (4). Visual situations encountered in everyday life involve far lower contrast than is employed in most clinical acuity testing, and neuro-ophthalmological disorders can selectively impair contrast sensitivity while sparing acuity for high-contrast optotypes.

The ability to detect threshold variations in contrast, in both the normally sighted and in patients with low vision, is in general a function of the *spatial frequency* content of the image. Stripes, called gratings, having sinusoidally varying brightness, are usually used to test contrast sensitivity at defined frequencies. Spatial frequency is defined to be the number of cycles of alternation of the bright and dim stripes per degree of visual angle. Printed grating charts clinically useful for the testing of contrast sensitivity have been developed by Arden (5) and Ginsberg (6); video display tests employing sinusoidal gratings are now available (7).

As seen in Figure 1, normal subjects exhibit maximal sensitivity to contrast for spatial frequencies of 2–4 cycles per degree (8), although spatial frequencies of over 25 cycles per degree can be detected when contrast is very high. The upper limit of spatial frequency detection corresponds roughly to threshold visual acuity for high-contrast Snellen letters (5). The reduced acuity of patients with low vision is reflected in a lower limit of maximum spatial frequency detection, but in these patients, the frequency of peak contrast sensitivity and absolute contrast sensitivity are usually reduced as well (9). It may be seen from Figure 1 that the shapes of contrast sensitivity functions of different patients may vary even though their Snellen acuities may be the same. A persistent loss of contrast sensitivity is frequently observed in patients who have recovered their Snellen visual acuity following optic neuritis (10,11). Although most patients are unable to describe the precise nature of their perceived visual deficit, some patients with unilateral decreased contrast sensitivity describe the sensation as images that are "faded" or "washed out."

C. Visual Field Loss

The visual field loss represents the horizontal and vertical extent of peripheral vision relative to central fixation. Threshold sensitivity to the size and brightness of objects normally exhibits a gradual decline toward the periphery, except for

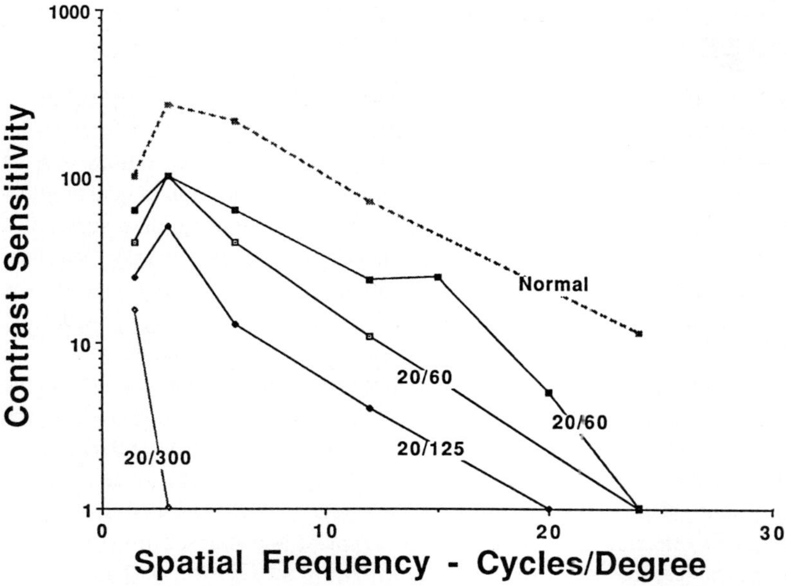

Figure 1 **Contrast sensitivity functions for normal subjects and for several patients with low vision. The abscissa represents spatial frequency in cycles of the sinusoidal grating per degree of visual angle. The ordinate indicates contrast sensitivity, the inverse of contrast threshold.**

an absolute scotoma, or blind spot, corresponding to the optic disc. Visual field deficits are commonly encountered in glaucoma, optic atrophy, and lesions of the posterior visual pathways.

The simplest clinical method of evaluating the visual field is by confrontation testing, with the patient facing the examiner at about arm's length. Confrontation testing is performed monocularly with fixation by the patient on a part of the examiner's face. The patient is then asked to count fingers held equidistant from the patient and examiner in each quadrant of the visual field. Moving fingers may also be moved centripitally from the periphery to identify the borders of the visual field, always using the visual field of the examiner as a reference.

Tangent screen testing, using test objects of calibrated size presented against a black screen, is an excellent method for evaluating the central visual field. Automated perimeters can systematically evaluate thresholds throughout the peripheral visual field but are of limited utility in patients who cannot fixate reliably.

II. LOW-VISION REHABILITATION—CENTRAL FUNCTION

Many patients facing the prospect of irreversible visual loss due to neurological disease are often greatly helped merely by being informed that low-vision rehabilitation services exist and that the patients have hope of making use of their residual vision. Depression and poor motivation are common in neurological patients with low vision, who are generally older people who have suffered a catastrophic sensory loss superimposed on other deficits. Consequently, complete management of such patients requires considerable effort and patience on the part of the clinician. Low-vision devices must be kept in inventory and demonstrated to the patient as a part of the evaluation procedure. Effective rehabilitation using low-vision aids often requires training, many times in the patient's home, school, or workplace. For many neuro-ophthalmologists, the optimal rehabilitation strategy may be to provide a supportive referral to a specialist in low vision, an optometrist or ophthalmologist working as a part of a rehabilitation team that includes an orientation and mobility instructor. Although such referrals are simple enough to make and may be invaluable for patients, these services have too often been overlooked in the past (12). This need not occur if the neuro-ophthalmologist considers fully the needs of the patient with low vision. Neuro-ophthalmologists should be familiar with the nature of available rehabilitation measures to refer effectively.

A. Simple Rehabilitation Measures

Before more complex visual rehabilitative measures are taken, most patients with deficits of central visual function can be advised to use high-intensity light for reading and other visual tasks. This is of particular help for patients with clear optical media and reduced contrast sensitivity. Large-print reading materials are now widely available. Also useful are high-visibility objects such as large-face clocks, telephone keypads, and shape-coded medicine bottles. Even those who lose all useful vision generally maintain the capability of handwriting. Cardboard masks and templates are available to assist in writing checks and formating letters for those who would otherwise lose their place on the page.

B. Optical Reading Aids

Optical reading aids are useful because they magnify the image of the page. By making the image larger, they in effect reduce the spatial frequency content of the printed page by a factor of their magnification. The required Snellen acuity for reading also is reduced in proportion to magnification.

The high-strength bifocal is a simple but very effective low-vision reading aid. Ordinary bifocals have a strength of about +2.50 diopters, which allow good focus up to a distance of 40 cm. Increasing the bifocal permits the reading material to remain in focus when moved much closer to the eye. Although the lens itself has only a minor effect as a magnifier, the greater proximity of the reading material to the eye increases its angular size at the retina providing most of the benefit (13). For example, a +5.00 reading aid allows good focus at reading distances a little closer than 20 cm making the image of the page on the retina about 100% larger that at the standard reading distance of 40 cm. Stronger reading aids generally must be provided in single-vision reading glasses and must additionally incorporate base-in prisms at powers above about +6.00 diopters to enable convergence of the visual axes at the short viewing distances required. High plus reading spectacles with prisms are sometimes termed microscopes (Fig. 2). A +12.00-diopter microscope enables reading at a distance of 8 cm from the page and is associated with a retinal image more than three times larger than at a reading distance of 25 cm. With such a device, a patient with best-corrected distance acuity of 20/60 could read text of 20/20 size. It is crucial to instruct patients that *it is not harmful to the eyes to read close to the page* (Fig. 3). Although this instruction probably contradicts the folk wisdom the patient has garnered through the years, it is crucial to the use of high plus reading

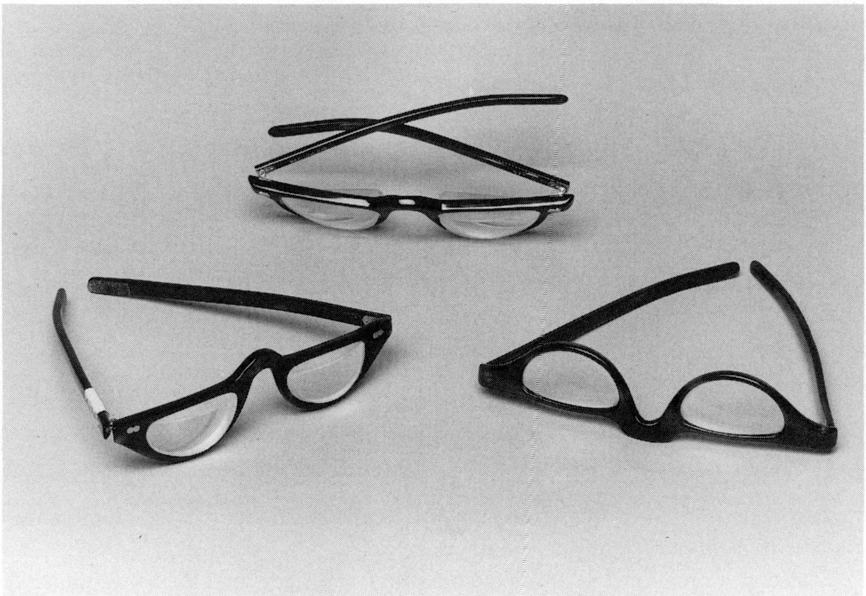

Figure 2 Microscope low-vision reading aids consist of convex (plus power) lenses and base-in prisms.

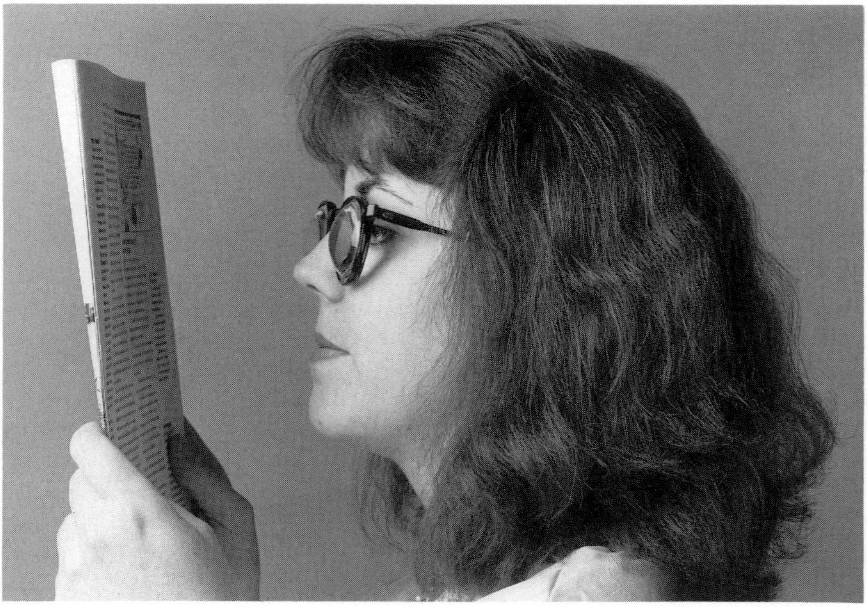

Figure 3 Low-vision patient reading with high plus reading lens. The reading material must be held close to the eyes.

aids and must be repeatedly emphasized. The patient's field of view on the page is necessarily reduced by proximity, so new scanning habits must also be learned.

Hand-held magnifiers are convex lenses mounted on handles as low-vision aids for reading; they are simple magnifying glasses (Fig. 4). In conjunction with ordinary reading spectacles, hand-held magnifiers can magnify severalfold while maintaining a relatively large field of view. Although the distance between lens and text must be maintained precisely, the distance from the eye to the magnifier is not critical. Although these devices are convenient for brief, intermittent use, many patients lack the manual dexterity to hold them for prolonged periods. This limitation is overcome by stand magnifiers, which incorporate structures to support the lens over the text at the optimal distance (Fig. 5). To scan the page, the reader with low vision either slides the magnifier stand over the text or slides the text under the magnifier. Stand magnifiers may also incorporate illuminating systems that produce a bright, enlarged image.

Telescopes are afocal magnifiers consisting of at least two lens elements and sometimes image-erecting prisms depending upon the design. Telescopic spectacles are telescopes mounted in spectacle frames. These devices produce angular magnification of images irrespective of object distance and are available as useful

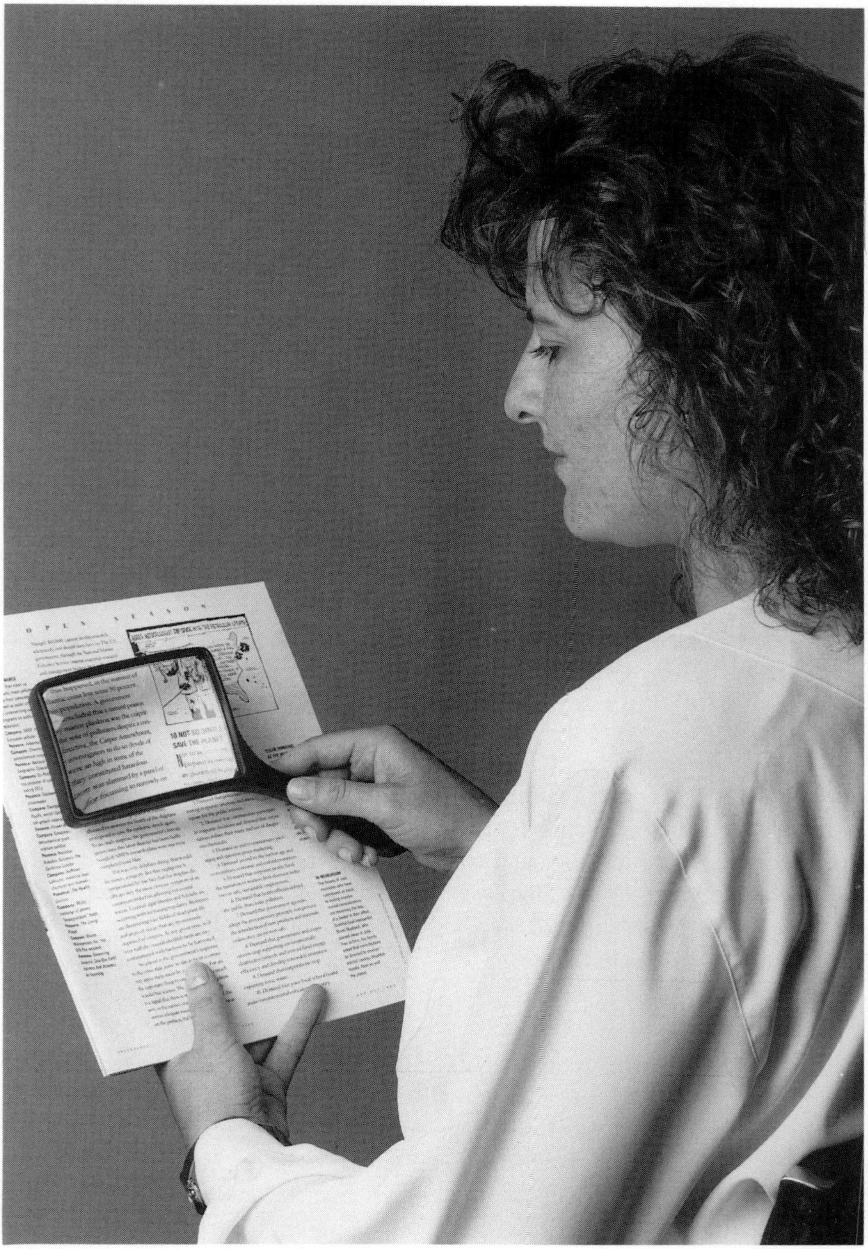

Figure 4 Hand-held magnifier low-vision aid.

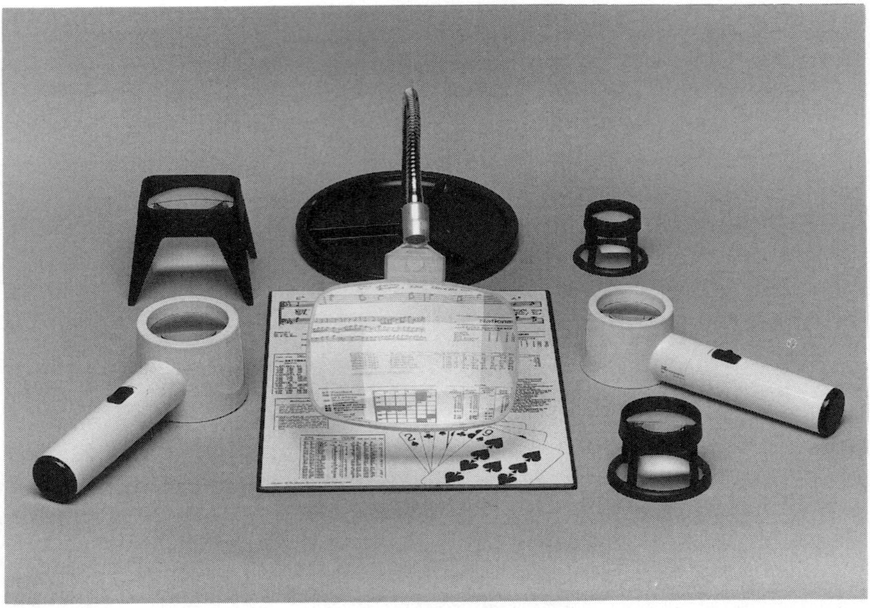

Figure 5 Stand magnifier low-vision aids. Some incorporate illumination.

low-vision aids in powers of 1.6× to 8×. "Close-focus" telescopic spectacles can be focused from optical infinity to near working distances and are also known as loupes or reading telescopes. The primary utility of reading telescopes is in situations where physical or social constraints prevent the patient from bringing the reading material close to the eyes. Reading telescopes may be particularly useful as adjuncts in the use of standard video display terminals.

C. Video-Based Low-Vision Aids

Optical magnifiers, such as loupes, telescopes, and convex lenses, achieve image enlargement at the expense of other image characteristics important for patients with low vision. Optical magnifiers inherently reduce image brightness, contrast, and useful visual field. In distinction to these devices, video-based image processing systems need not sacrifice other image characteristics to achieve magnification.

A closed-circuit television (CCTV) low-vision aid consists of a television camera, a two-axis positioner for either the camera or the text to be scanned, a light source to illuminate the material, and a video display monitor (Fig. 6) (14).

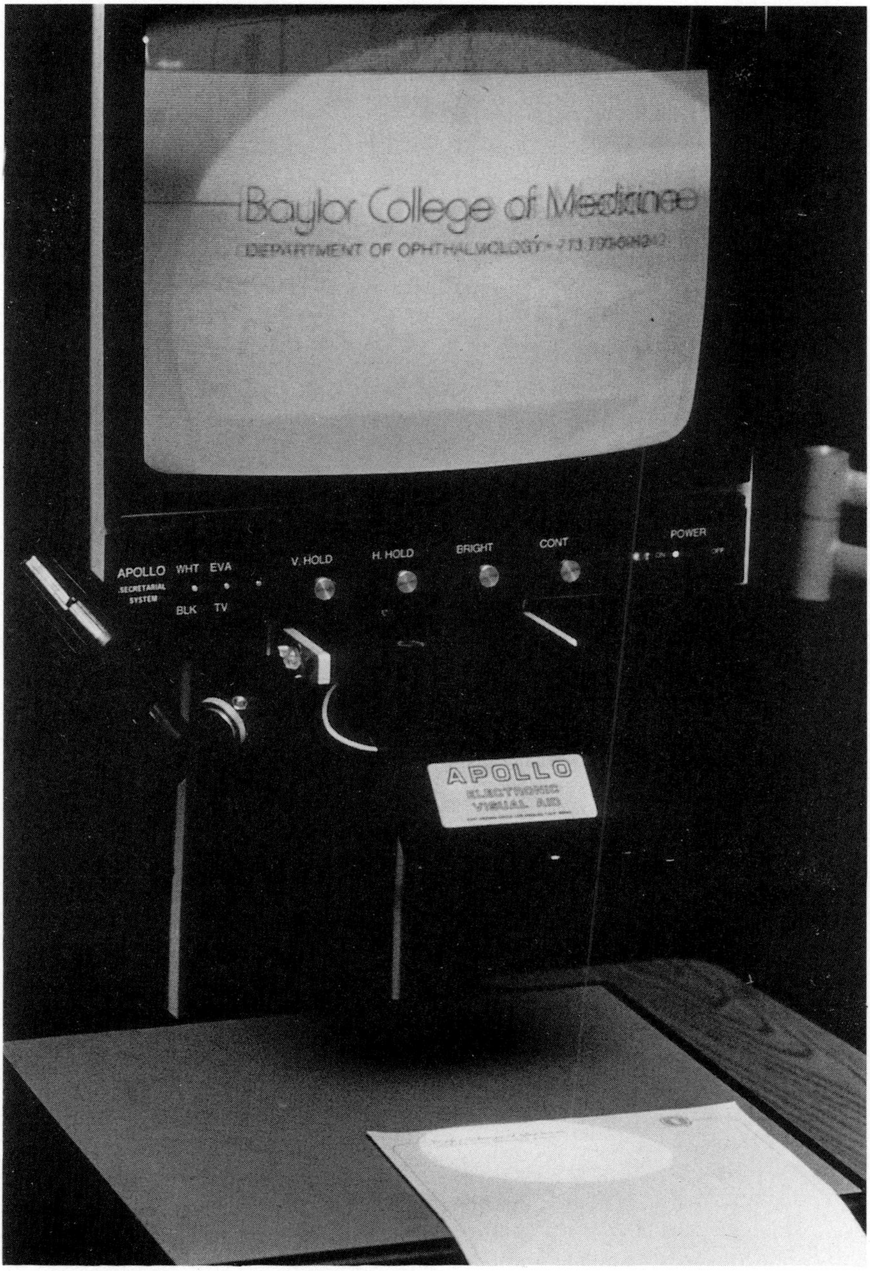

Figure 6 **Closed-circuit television (CCTV) low-vision aid. (Photo courtesy of Franklin I. Porter, M.S., O.D.)**

Magnification is achieved through use of a zoom lens on the camera, through the large size of the video monitor screen, and through reduction of the viewing distance of the patient. A total effective magnification of up to 140× is possible (14), although average magnification of about 8× is most commonly employed (15).

Since video image contrast is electronically controllable, video displays can be easily adjusted to produce any desired level of contrast intensity less than the maximum. This means that display contrast can usually be set to a level greater than that of the original subject matter. The reading rate of normal subjects declines markedly for contrast below 10%, as letters appear to fade into the background. Most readers with low vision exhibit a sensitivity to image contrast that resembles that of normal subjects reading faded text. In the majority of patients with low vision, the minimum image contrast required for fastest reading averages 3.9 times that required by normally sighted subjects (4). Most patients with low vision use all of the contrast available from a CCTV display (9).

In a video-based low-vision aid, character color only occasionally has a significant effect on reading. When there is an effect, reading performance is most likely to be impaired for red and to a lesser extent for blue characters (16). Reading performance is best for green or white characters on a dark background.

The primary limitations on the usefulness of CCTV low-vision aids are their high cost and physical size. These problems are likely to be mitigated by rapid and continuing improvements in consumer video technology, including small, portable cameras and hand-held video displays.

D. Computer Video Displays

Computer video terminals may be conveniently adapted as low-vision aids (17). In addition to the advantages of CCTV devices, computer video display terminals afford the opportunity to manipulate additional features of characters in order to increase readability. Enlarged characters should be smoothed for best readability (18). Character spacing should usually be increased to improve reading speed. This may be valuable for patients with central scotomata, who are forced to read using peripheral retinal loci where crowding effects may slow character recognition (19). Standard spacing between characters is 20% of character width for most printed text; in the peripheral visual field, this spacing has been found to increase the time required for recognition by 22–65% as compared with uncrowded characters.

The single most valuable computer video image enhancement is magnification. This can be achieved in many cases using general-purpose hardware and software (20). Most personal computer hardware and software includes built-in options permitting moderate character enlargement on the screen. Modern laser and ink jet printers produce large, high-contrast characters useful for patients with low vision. Special software also is available to enlarge computer video displays.

A costly but effective method of improving the readability of a computer video display is to increase the size of the monitor screen. Screen magnifiers are optical magnifiers that can be placed directly over video display screens providing magnification up to about 2× (20).

E. Telescopic Low-Vision Aids

Telescopic spectacles are particularly effective magnifiers for use at great distances. In theory, telescopes could be used to obtain unlimited magnification to correct nearly any degree of visual impairment. In practice, several factors limit the utility of telescopic low-vision aids, but they remain very useful in visual rehabilitation.

Being passive optical devices, telescopes do not create or increase light energy. Consequently, the magnified images produced by telescopes are less bright than images of the same object viewed directly. For some patients with low vision, reduction in brightness can more than offset the beneficial effect of magnification. Being inherently imperfect optical processors, telescopes degrade to some degree the contrast present in the unmagnified image (21). Better-quality telescopes, which are more costly, exhibit superior modulation transfer functions. Probably the most significant limitation of telescopic low-vision aids is their limited visual field. Because of practical limitations on the physical size and weight of telescopic visual aids, their useful fields of vision decrease with increasing magnification. A ×2 telescopic low-vision aid typically has a field of view of up to 23 degrees; a ×4 device typically has a field of view of up to 12 degrees; a ×6 telescopic low-vision aid typically has a field of view of about 7 degrees. Such limited fields of vision greatly complicate the problem of visual orientation and visual target search for the low vision patient and may present unacceptable risks for mobility tasks such as driving an automobile (22).

The simplest telescopic low-vision aids are hand-held monocular telescopes, as seen in Figure 7. These are useful for brief spotting tasks such as reading distant signs once the patient has determined the general location of the object of interest. The patient must be capable of holding the telescope with one or both hands, and the duration of each visual task must be brief enough so that the patient's ability to hold the telescope steadily is not impaired by fatigue. Monocular, hand-held telescopes are available in very compact form that will readily fit into a pocket or purse. Patients may obtain greater magnification and economical, high-quality optics with conventional opera glasses or sports binoculars.

Spectacle mounting of telescopes frees the patient's hands for other tasks and may improve targeting and visual search. Telescopic spectacles are used for a

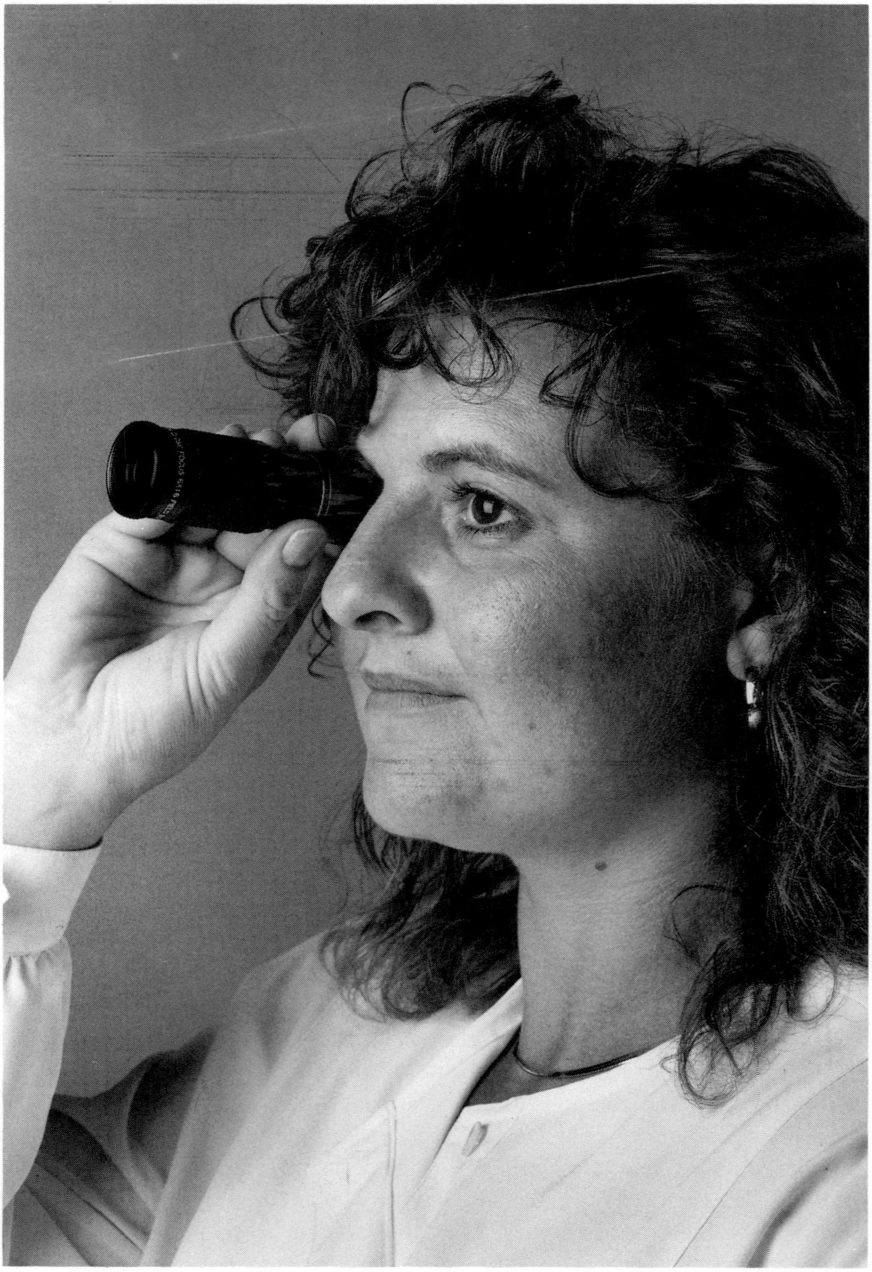

Figure 7 Hand-held monocular telescopic low-vision aid.

variety of tasks, principally for viewing distant objects as in educational or recreational settings (23). Some patients with best-corrected acuities of 20/125 or better employ telescopic spectacles for driving automobiles (24). In this application, telescopes are usually mounted monocularly, for use by one eye, to permit better peripheral vision by the fellow eye. Alternatively, in the *bioptic* configuration, a binocular set of telescopes is mounted in the upper part of the carrier lens so that there is both an unmagnified viewing path below the telescopes, and a magnified viewing path above through the telescopes (Fig. 8). The head is raised to view the periphery without magnification and the head is lowered to view centrally with telescopic magnification. Many motivated patients make successful use of telescopic spectacles for driving. The accident rate for automobile drivers with low vision using telescopic spectacles was 34% higher than normally sighted control subjects in one study, although drivers with low vision had fewer citations for moving violations (25). Despite apparently more cautious driving habits of drivers with low vision using telescopic spectacles, some specialists in low vision argue that the visual field limitation produced by bioptic spectacles is unacceptably hazardous for driving (22). Under appropriate conditions, such as familiar routes in the daylight, driving with telescopic spectacles can fill a critical transportation requirement at an acceptable level of risk.

Several factors limit rehabilitation success with telescopic spectacles and account for an approximately 33% failure rate when prescribed to motivated patients with low vision (26). The relatively great weight of telescopic spectacles may limit the duration of use. Owing to their conspicuous appearance, most telescopic spectacles present a cosmetic problem, particularly for adolescents. This problem has been reduced by the development of compact telescope designs incorporating prismatically folded optics that can be mounted behind a tinted spectacle lens (27). Typically, the mounting is bioptic and patients move their eyes down or to one side to view through the telescope.

Since they are supported by the head, telescopic spectacles necessarily magnify the visual effects of head movements. With telescopic spectacles powers of $\times 4$ or more, even involuntary head movements due to transmitted heartbeat and tremor are visually perceptible and may produce image motion sufficient to degrade visual acuity (28). Patients with low vision have greater head instability than normally sighted persons (29), but both head instability and the sensitivity to head motion of visual acuity with telescopic spectacles vary from patient to patient. Although the successful use of telescopic spectacles is negatively related to advanced age (30), the most effective means of predicting the successful use of telescopic spectacles in individual patients is based on laboratory measurements of head stability in the pitch (interaural) axis and the sensitivity of visual acuity with telescopic spectacles to imposed head motion in the yaw (vertical) axis (26,31). It has been recommended that telescopic spectacles be avoided in

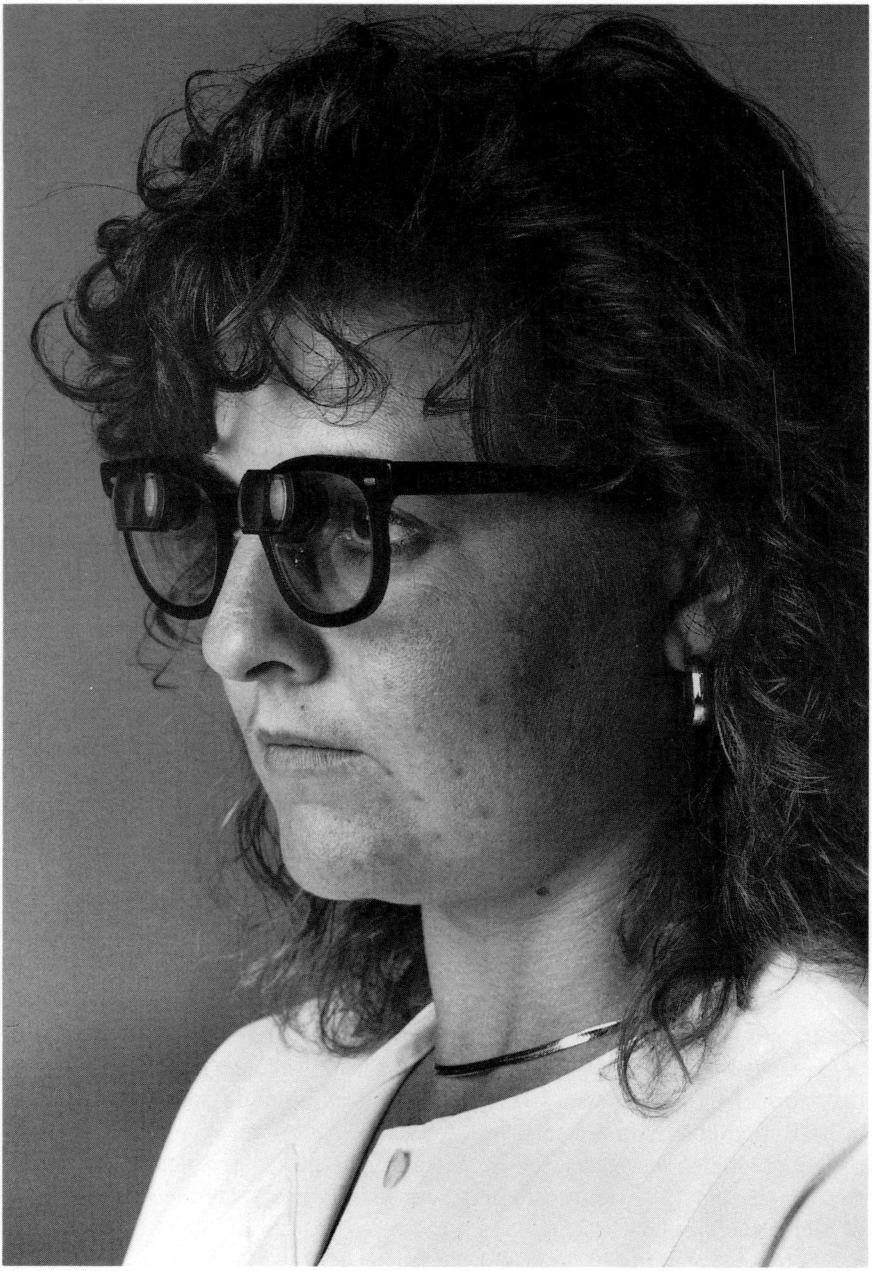

Figure 8 Bioptic telescopic spectacles.

Table 1 Some Sources of Materials for Low Vision

Sources	Materials
Designs for Vision, Inc. 760 Koehler Avenue Ronkonkoma, NY 11779 (800) 345-4009	Telescopic spectacles and accessories
Eschenbach Optik. 25 November Trail Weston, CT 06883 (203) 227-9409	Telescopic spectacles, stand and hand-held magnifiers, video low-vision aids, diagnostic sets for clinical use
Independent Living Aids, Inc. 27 East Mall Plainview, NY 11803 (800) 537-2118	High-visibility clocks, telephones, writing guides, templates, magnified insulin syringes, voice-synthesized devices, tactile kitchen devices, magnifiers, lamps, and video aids
Lighthouse Low-Vision Products 36-02 Northern Boulevard Long Island City, NY 11101 (800) 453-4923	Telescopic spectacles, stand and hand-held magnifiers, video low-vision aids, low-vision testing charts, diagnostic sets for clinical use
National Association for the Visually Handicapped 22 W. 21st Street New York, NY, 10010 (212) 889-3141	Large-print books, patient education materials, magnifiers, telescopic spectacles, high-visibility objects. Excellent referrals to large-print publishers
Royal Victorian Institute for the Blind 333 Burwood Highway, Burwood Victoria 3125, Australia (03) 808-6422, FAX (03) 808-2194	Educational software for patients with low vision, publications
Swift Instruments, Inc. 952 Dorchester Avenue Boston, MA 02125 P.O. Box 562 San Jose, CA 95106	"Bedspecs" 72° vertical angulated prism spectacles, useful for bedridden patients and down-gaze palsies
Telesensory Systems, Inc. 455 North Bernardo Avenue P.O. Box 7455 Mountain View, CA 94039-7455 (800) 227-8418, (414) 960-0920	Video low-vision aids, speech synthesizers, tactile aids
S. Walters, Inc. 30423 Canwood, Suite 126 Agoura Hills, CA 91301 (818) 706-2202 (800) 235-5666x4990 (outside California) (800) 331-5666x4990 (California only)	Telescopic spectacles and hand-held magnifiers, stand magnifiers, microscopes

patients with low vision with obvious head tremor (31), unless these patients can be taught to steady their heads against fixed objects when viewing with telescopic spectacles. Telescopic spectacles can be surprisingly successful in low-vision patients with nystagmus or optic atrophy.

Telescopic spectacles are relatively costly visual aids, ranging up to thousands of dollars for a pair. Unfortunately, the cost is seldom reimbursed by private insurance payors. If telescopic spectacles can be expected to restore productive employment potential, state rehabilitation agencies will sometimes provide reimbursement.

III. REHABILITATING PERIPHERAL VISUAL FIELD DEFECTS

Retrochiasmal lesions may produce large, congruous visual field defects such as hemianopsias. In such cases, the patient may be unaware of important parts of the visual environment, which places the patient at risk of collisions with objects or in other unsafe situations. Low-vision strategies have been suggested to optically move images from the scotomatous part of the field into closer proximity to the seeing field so that a small eye movement can bring the object into view. Mirrors mounted on spectacle frames have been suggested (32), but they have met with limited success, probably because of the reversed and moving mirror image (33).

A prism deviates gaze in the direction of its base, or thickest side. Smith et al. suggested the use of Fresnel paste-on prisms in hemianopic spectacles and avoiding reversed image motion (34). Fresnel prisms are thin prisms make of rows of wedge-shaped elements; for spectacle use they are fabricated as plastic membranes having one flat surface that will adhere to the rear surface of a spectacle lens. The 30-prism diopter power, which produces an image displacement of 15 degrees, is preferred. Owing to their plastic optics and multiple serrations, fresnel prisms reduce acuity by about one Snellen line (35).

Several strategies have been suggested for the placement of hemianopic prisms. Some practitioners advocate placement of the prism on only one spectacle lens (34), but this can produce diplopia (36). Most advocate placing the prisms far enough on the hemianopic side of the spectacle lenses that the prism edges are not observed by the patient unless an eye movement is made toward the hemianopic side (37,38). However, some advise placement of the prism edge at the midline and cutting a small circular hole out at the fixation point (34).

Patients generally require training in the proper use of hemianopic spectacles (39). An excellent discussion of such training is provided by Ferraro and Jose (38). Adequate motivation is important to success, and success is usually higher in patients with a history of sudden and stable visual field loss (39). Hemineglect often accompanies and greatly complicates hemianopias due to dominant hemisphere lesions (34). Patients with hemineglect have a poorer prognosis for rehabilitation using hemianopic spectacles.

IV. DISTURBANCES DUE TO PATHOLOGICAL NYSTAGMUS

Pathological nystagmus may produce disturbing symptoms of vertigo and oscillopsia, but it more commonly produces a reduction in visual clarity that most patients find difficult to describe. In normal subjects, retinal image motion of only a few degrees per second measurably degrades visual acuity (40) and movement of 15–25 degrees per second reduces acuity almost fivefold (41,42). Thus, during pathological nystagmus, the images of stationary objects are constantly in motion on the retina and are perceived at reduced acuity.

The most effective treatment of reduced acuity due to pathological nystagmus is directed at the cause of the nystagmus itself. For example, downbeat nystagmus associated with the Arnold-Chiari malformation may be treated neurosurgically. Other acquired forms of downbeat nystagmus can be treated with clonazepam. Periodic alternating nystagmus can sometimes be treated with baclofen (43).

Nystagmus intensity is usually defined to be the product of slow-phase eye velocity and nystagmus beating rate. Many forms of pathological nystagmus exhibit dampening of intensity by eye position in the orbit. This dependence can often be exploited therapeutically. Downbeat nystagmus commonly increases in intensity in down gaze, the habitual reading position for most patients. In patients with downbeat nystagmus, it is usually advisable to prescribe single-vision reading spectacles that can be used in primary position or up gaze rather than bifocals that force the patient to look down through the reading segment.

In other patients, nystagmus intensity is modulated by the state of convergence. If nystagmus is dampened on convergence, vision can often be improved through the use of base-out prisms in the spectacles, which force increased convergence effort. In prepresbyopic patients, nystagmus can often be reduced by stimulating the accommodative component of the near reflex through the additional use of concave lenses. Many patients exhibit a null in nystagmus intensity at a particular position of the eyes in the orbit. To view objects directly ahead of them, patients occasionally adopt a head turn to maintain the orbital null. If the head turn is extreme or cannot be maintained, prisms or surgery on the extraocular muscles can be performed effectively to move the null position close to primary (44).

ACKNOWLEDGMENTS

JLD is a Research to Prevent Blindness William and Mary Greve International Research Scholar, and was supported by National Eye Institute grant EY-08656 and a grant from the Karl Kirchgessner Foundation.

Franklin I. Porter, M.S., O.D., provided helpful criticism and suggestions for this chapter.

REFERENCES

1. Browning R, Jose R. The low vision triangle. Rehabilitative Optom 1984; 2:12–15.
2. National Society to Prevent Blindness. Visual Problems in the U.S.: A statistical analysis, prepared by Operations Research Department. New York: National Society to Prevent Blindness, 1980:19–20.
3. Strong G, Woo GC. A distance visual acuity chart incorporating some new design features. Arch Ophthalmol 1985; 103:44–6.
4. Rubin GS, Legge GE. Psychophysics of reading. VI—The role of contrast in low vision. Vision Res 1989; 29:79–91.
5. Arden GB. The importance of measuring contrast sensitivity in cases of visual disturbance. Br J Ophthalmol 1978; 62:198–209.
6. Ginsberg AP, Evans DW, Cannon MW, Owsley C, Mulvanny P. Large sample norms for contrast sensitivity. Am J Optom Physiol Optics 1984; 61:80–84.
7. Rubin GS. Reliability and sensitivity of clinical contrast sensitivity tests. Clin Vision Sci 1988; 2:169–177.
8. Lawton TB. Improved reading performance using individualized compensation filters for observers with losses in central fixation. Ophthalmology 1989; 96:115–26.
9. Brown B. Reading performance in low vision patients: relation to contrast and constrast sensitivity. Am J Optom Physiol Optics 1981; 58:218–26.
10. Dain SJ, Rammohan KV, Benes SC, King-Smith PE. Chromatic, spatial, and temporal losses of sensitivity in multiple sclerosis. Invest Ophthalmol Vis Sci 1990; 31:548–58.
11. Celesia GG, Kaufman DI, Brigell M, Toleikis S, Kokinakis D, Lorance R, Lizano B. Optic neuritis: a prospective study. Neurology 1990; 40:919–23.
12. Greenblatt SL. Training ophthalmology residents to treat patients with vision loss: results of a demonstration program. Ophthalmology 1990; 97:138–43.
13. Rubin ML. Optics for clinicians. Gainsville, FL: Triad Publishing, 1974.
14. Fonda GE, Thomas H, Schnur RN. Evaluation of closed-circuit television as an optical aid for the low vision patient. Trans Am Acad Ophthalmol Otol 1975; 79:OP468–OP482.
15. Goodrich GL, Apple LE, Frost A, Wood A, Ward R, Darling N. A preliminary report on experienced closed-circuit television users. Am J Optom Physiol Optics 1976; 53:7–15.
16. Legge GE, Rubin GS. Psychophysics of reading. IV. Wavelengths effects in normal and low vision. J Opt Soc Am 1986; 3:40–51.
17. Steele RD, Goodrich GL, Hennies D, McKinley JA. Reading aid technology for blind persons: responses to a questionnaire of experienced users. Assist Technol 1989; 1:23–30.
18. Legge GE, Rubin GS, Pelli DG, Schleske MM. Psychophysics of reading—II. Low vision. Vision Res 1985; 25:253–265.
19. Rohrkaste F, Whittaker S, Higgins K. Optimum letter spacing for word recognition in central and eccentric fields. Invest Ophthalmol Vis Sci 1989; 30(Suppl):397.

20. Goodrich GL, McKinley JI. A guide to large print computer access. J Vis Rehabil 1987; 1:29–40.
21. Katz M, Citek K, Arditi A. An instrument for measuring the modulation transfer functions of low power telescopes and telemicroscopes. Am J Optom Physiol Optics 1988; 65:190–7.
22. Fonda G. Bioptic telescopic spectacle is a hazard for operating a motor vehicle. Arch Ophthalmol 1983; 101:1907–8.
23. Hall A, Bailey IL, Kekelis LS, Raasch TW, Goodrich GL. Retrospective survey to investigate use of distance magnifiers for travel. J Visual Impair Blind 1987; 81:418–23.
24. Goodrich GL. Driving and telescopic aids: A bibliography. J Vis Rehabil 1988; 2:21–30.
25. Lippmann O, Corn AL, Lewis MC. Bioptic telescopic spectacles and driving performance: a study in Texas. J Vis Impair Blind 1988; 182–7.
26. Demer JL, Porter FI, Goldberg J, Jenkins HA, Schmidt K, Ulrich I. Predictors of functional success in telescopic spectacle use by low vision patients. Invest Ophthalmol Vis Sci 1989; 30:1652–65.
27. Spitzberg LA, Jose RT, Kuether CL. Behind the lens telescope: a new concept in biopics. Optom Vis Sci 1989; 66:616–20.
28. Porter FI, Goldberg J, Demer JL. Sensitivity of visual acuity to spontaneous head motion while wearing telescopic spectacle low vision aids. Invest Ophthalmol Vis Sci 1989; 30(Suppl):399.
29. Demer JL, Goldberg J, Porter FI. Effect of telescopic spectacles on head stability in normal and low vision. J Vestibular Res 1990; 1:109–22.
30. Porter FI, Goldberg J, White JM, Demer JL, Koval AV. Age-related and clinical factors in rehabilitative success with headborne telescopes. Invest Ophthalmol Vis Sci 1991; 32:816.
31. Demer JL, Porter FI, Goldberg J, Schmidt K. Validation of physiologic predictors of successful telescopic spectacle use in low vision. Invest Ophthalmol Vis Sci 1991; 32:2826–34.
32. Walsh TJ, Smith JL. Hemianopic spectacles. Am J Ophthalmol 1966; 61:914–5.
33. Bailey IL. Mirrors for visual field defects. Optom Mon 1982; 73:202–6.
34. Smith JL, Weiner IG, Lucero AJ. Hemianopic fresnel prisms. J Clin Neuro-ophthalmol 1982; 2:19–22.
35. Flom MC, Adams AJ. Fresnel optics. In: Tasman W, Jaeger EA, eds. Clinical Ophthalmology. Vol. 1. Hagerstown, MD: Harper & Row, 1990; 52:1–15.
36. Woo GC, Mandelman T. Fresnel prism therapy for right hemianopia. Am J Optom Physiol Optics 1983; 60:739–43.
37. Jose RT, Smith AJ. Increasing peripheral field awareness with fresnel prisms. Optical J Rev Optom 1976; 113:33–37.
38. Ferraro J, Jose RT. Training programs for individuals with restricted fields. In: Understanding Low Vision. New York: American Foundation for the Blind, 1983:363–73.
39. Gadbaw PD, Finn WA, Dolan MT, De L'aune WR. Parameters of success in the use of fresnel prisms. Optical J Rev Optom 1976; December:41–3.
40. Westheimer G, McKee SP. Visual acuity in the presence of retinal image motion. J Opt Soc Am 1975; 65:847–50.

41. Guedry RE, Lentz JM, Jell RM. Visual-vestibular interactions: 1. Influence of peripheral vision on suppression of the vestibulo-ocular reflex and visual acuity. Aviat Space Environ Med 1979; 50:205–11.
42. Benson AJ, Barnes GR. Vision during angular oscillation: The dynamic interaction of visual and vestibular mechanisms. Aviat Space Environ Med 1978; 49:340–5.
43. Halmagyi GM, Rudge P, Gresty MA, Leigh RJ, Zee DS. Treatment of periodic alternating nystagmus. Ann Neurol 1980; 8:609–11.
44. Dell'Osso LF, Flynn JT. Congenital nystagmus surgery: A quantitative evaluation of the effects. Arch Ophthalmol 1979; 97:462–9.

4

Diagnosis and Management of Idiopathic Intracranial Hypertension (Pseudotumor Cerebri)

Kathleen B. Digre
University of Utah, Salt Lake City, Utah

James J. Corbett
University of Mississippi School of Medicine, Jackson, Mississippi

Idiopathic intracranial hypertension (IIH) is a disorder that affects 0.9 per 100,000 of the general population but 19 of 100,000 obese women of child-bearing age. Women are preferentially affected 8:1 over men (1,2). Although IIH does not cause death, it poses a significant, and treatable, cause of visual loss in men and women (3). Optimum management requires a certain diagnosis.

I. CLINICAL PICTURE

Symptoms of IIH are often visual, including transient visual monocular and binocular obscurations (TVOs) or visual loss. TVOs last seconds and may or may not be postural. Headache also is a frequent accompaniment. Pain is described most commonly in the head and behind the eyes but neck, shoulder blade, and rarely arm and leg pain can occur. The increased cerebrospinal fluid (CSF) pressure may worsen previously existing migraine. Diplopia, usually horizontal, may be experienced. Even though there are reports of vertical diplopia, vertical diplopia should make the clinician rethink the diagnosis of IIH. It is well known that some individuals with IIH are totally asymptomatic and come to medical attention quite by accident.

On examination, the patient is usually obese. Disc swelling is present and occasionally asymmetrical. Papilledema, however, is a hallmark sign. Papilledema occasionally must be differentiated from pseudopapilledema including buried drusen or anomalous discs. True papilledema is recognized by seeing a cup, feathering of the nerve fiber layer, especially superiorly and inferiorly in mild cases. More advanced stages of papilledema will have hemorrhages (subretinal and splinter), both soft and hard exudate on the disc, and possibly choroidal folds. Papilledema is frequently graded mild, moderate, severe, and atrophic by its appearance. Asymmetrical—even unilateral—papilledema may at first confuse the diagnosis.

Increased spinal fluid pressure may occur without papilledema (4). This condition holds no risk for vision and is basically a headache management problem (5). Confrontation visual field abnormalities and relative afferent pupillary defects require even quicker evaluation and immediate treatment.

Historical features to note include the use of medications like vitamin A or recent systemic infections (Table 1). Although birth control pills and pregnancy were once thought to cause IIH, they are now merely thought to reflect the association of IIH with women of reproductive age (6). Other conditions that mimic IIH must be considered and excluded (Table 2).

In order to diagnose IIH correctly, a cranial computed tomography (CT)/magnetic resonance imaging (MRI) scan is mandatory. MR has the added advantage of sensitively assessing the venous sinuses. If only a CT scan is used, contrast must be given. MR and CT should be normal. Although "slit-like" ventricles are frequently mentioned, it has been convincingly shown that they are of no significance (7). An empty sella is reported in association with IIH, and IIH always should be sought when an empty sella is found.

Table 1 Causes of Symptomatic Intracranial Hypertension

Medication
- tetracycline
- nalidixic acid (usually in children)
- indomethacin and ketoprofen in Bartter's syndrome
- lithium
- steroid withdrawal
- danazol
- vitamin A and liver

Toxins
- heavy metals (especially lead in children)

Systemic illnesses
- systemic lupus erythematosus (SLE)
- uremia
- Cushing's disease and its treatment (possibly steroid withdrawal)
- hypoparathyroidism
- Behçet's disease

Table 2 Conditions That Mimic IIH

Dural venous thrombosis
Intracranial lesions (tumor, abscess)
Carcinomatous meningitis
Hydrocephalus
Guillain-Barré syndrome and other states of increased protein in the spinal fluid such as spinal cord tumors
Arteriovenous malformation (AVM)
Infectious disease: viral encephalitis and neurosyphilis
Pseudopapilledema (disc drusen and anomalous discs) and headache
Sarcoidosis of meninges

Cerebrospinal fluid always must be examined. Opening pressure should be measured in the lateral decubitus position. Careful pressure measurements are necessary, especially for borderline cases. The legs should be extended and the patient relaxed. Normal pressure is generally less than 200 mm H_2O, and abnormal pressure is considered to be greater than 250 mm H_2O. Pressures between 200 and 250 are nondiagnostic. Protein should be normal or slightly decreased and there should be no increase in cells. Cultures and cytology should be negative.

II. MANAGEMENT

Management of the patient with IIH begins with the correct diagnosis (see Table 3 for diagnostic criteria) (8).

Management of IIH requires special attention to the ophthalmological examination. Baseline assessments of best-corrected visual acuity (distance and near) should be obtained. Because the visual field is crucial for following the patient, a baseline must also be established as soon as possible.

Adequate visual fields in the management of IIH consist of automated Octopus (usually program 34), Humphrey (usually program 30-2), or Gold-

Table 3 Diagnostic Criteria for IIH

Disc elevation caused by increased intracranial pressure
Normal MR/CT
Carefully performed lumbar puncture with an opening pressure greater than 250 mm of water with normal CSF protein, glucose, and cells

mann perimetry using at least three isopters ($I_{2e}I_{4e}V_{4e}$). Enlargement of the blind spot is common and not particularly helpful in following a patient's visual function. Visual field constriction is often the result of chronic papilledema; central defects can occur when the papillomacular bundle is affected and frequently are associated with choroidal folds. Nasal visual field loss requires closer follow-up (9).

Photographs also are necessary to follow the disc appearance. Worsening or improving papilledema as well as new hemorrhages should raise concerns about changing vision and possibly visual loss. Relying on one's memory is sometimes hazardous.

Contrast sensitivity (Regan Plates or Pelli-Robson Charts) is helpful (9). Color vision testing by isochromatic plates occasionally is helpful. Intraocular pressure should also be assessed, since the combination on CSF pressure elevation and glaucoma together are very effective in damaging the optic disc.

Visual evoked potentials (VEP) and frequent lumbar punctures are not helpful in following a patient's vision or in making therapeutic changes (9).

If there are abnormalities in any part of the visual sensory system, treatment must begin. If the patient's visual sensory examination is normal, the patient can be reevaluated in 2–4 weeks. If the examination is then normal (aside from an enlarged blind spot), follow-up could be monthly for 6–12 months and then every 3–6 months as long as the vision is stable.

On return visits, visual acuity and visual field tests should be performed. Disc photos should also be taken especially if the disc or fundus has changed or the visual fields have worsened (Table 4).

Table 4 Visual Testing for IIH

Initial visit
visual acuity
pupillary check for relative afferent pupillary defect
visual field (automated or Goldmann perimetry)
color vision (color plate AO or HRR plates)
contrast sensitivity acuity
disc photos
Follow-up visit testing
visual acuity
pupil (RAPD)
visual field
color vision
disc photos if there has been a change
contrast sensitivity if there is any question of visual loss

III. TREATMENT

Medical management of IIH is necessary to treat frequent visual obscurations, headaches, and mild visual loss. No treatment is an option when the patient is asymptomatic, since 15% of patients spontaneously resolve (4).

Since obesity is the most common and proven factor associated with IIH, 90% in both men and women, weight loss should be encouraged (10,11). Success depends on the physician's approach and the dietician. Frequently, weight loss alone will be enough.

Repeated lumbar punctures are not encouraged except to reduce headache, because spinal fluid pressure returns to the previous level in 1.0–1.5 h and because frequent punctures can lead to chronic back pain.

Acetazolamide (Diamox), a carbonic anhydrase inhibitor, has been the drug of choice in the initial treatment of IIH. Although no study has shown the optimum dosage for treatment, usually 500 mg to 1 g, twice daily, is helpful (12). Side effects include a distaste for carbonated beverages, tingling of extremities, and depression. Kidney stones may develop.

Although oral glycerol has been used, caloric content, awkwardness of administration, and nausea make it a poor choice (Table 5). Furosemide, a loop diuretic and weak carbonic anhydrase inhibitor, has been used with varied success (4). Digoxin, a Na-K ATPase inhibitor, has anecdotally been reported to be useful.

Steroids can be used for the treatment of IIH but are a two-edged sword. There are reports of successful treatment of IIH, especially in children, but too often there are not only benefits but serious side effects, including acne, increased obesity, psychosis, and drug-induced diabetes. A short course may be beneficial but no extended long-term use is indicated. After steroids are stopped, papilledema frequently returns.

Failure of medical treatment, defined as visual loss, continued TVO, diplopia, or headache despite maximum medical therapy, leads one to consider surgical options (Table 6). The surgical procedure of choice has historically moved from subtemporal decompression to lumbar peritoneal shunts to optic nerve sheath fenestration (ONSF) (4). Several studies have shown that ONSF is safe, efficacious, and protects the optic nerve from further visual loss (Table 7). A small window or a series of linear incisions are made in the optic nerve sheath. The patient usually has an overnight in-hospital stay. Complications are rare and include pupil enlargement and bleeding. Visual loss after ONSF has been reported, including central retinal artery occlusion (CRAO) and loss of vision after cough-induced intraoptic nerve hemorrhage (13,14).

The crucial step in preserving vision in a patient with IIH is to act soon as visual loss is demonstrated and not to wait until little vision remains. Lumbar peritoneal shunts can be used if headaches appear to be the major portion of the

Table 5 Medications Used in Therapy for IIH

Medication	Dose	Action	Side effects	Precautions	Contraindications
Acetazolamide (Diamox)	1–2 g	carbonic anhydrase inhibitor	Tingling, distaste for carbonated beverages, renal stones, depression	Slight acidosis, may lose K; use cautiously with sulfa allergy	Kidney stones, allergy
Digoxin	.25 mg	Na-K ATPase pump	Cardiac	Monitor level	Sensitivity
Furosemide	.50 25 mg	loop diuretic	Metabolism	Monitor potassium	Sensitivity
Oral glycerol	1 g/kg 9 4–6°	diuretic	Hyperosmolar state, weight gain, nausea, pressure rebound; awkward to use	Monitor serum osmolality, rebound high pressure	
Steroids (see text)	80-mg burst and taper	unclear may decrease CSF production	Gastric intolerance, glucose intolerance, acne, weight gain, psychosis	Monitor glucose	Diabetes

Table 6 Indications for Surgical Treatment

Visual function
- progressive visual field loss
- decreased acuity not due to macular edema
- recent severe visual field loss

Uncontrollable headache (after medical treatment had been exhausted)
Anticipation of future hypotension (e.g., hemodialysis)
Psychiatric diseases which interfere with reasoning
Itinerant life-style with little hope of follow-up
Patients who cannot cooperate for visual sensory testing (especially children)

patient's problems (see Sec. IV). Lumbar peritoneal shunts can be put in as an outpatient. The correct valve must be chosen to ensure the correct cerebral spinal flow (low-resistant valves may give the patient low-pressure headaches). Complications are many, including occlusion of the shunt, shunt failure, a shunt that works too well, infections, and sciatica requiring multiple major surgical procedures.

IV. MANAGEMENT OF HEADACHE IN IIH

Headache management can be frustrating in these cases. If the vision is stable, headache management generally rests with migraine-like drugs and the basic principles of migraine headache (15) (Table 8).

If the headaches are continuous, frequent, or incapacitating in severity, prophylactic medication like nonsteroidal anti-inflammatory medication or beta blockers (propranolol, nadolol). Antidepressants (Prozac) are slightly more efficacious than tricyclics (amitriptyline) because of the weight gain associated

Table 7 Surgical Options for Treatment of IIH

Type	Advantage	Disadvantage	Complications
Optic nerve sheath decompression	Safe, easy, protects vision	No real help for headache (only about one half the time)	Rare Retrobulbar hemorrhage Tonic pupils
Lumbar peritoneal shunt	Helps headache	Frequent reoperation; shunt failure; replaces one headache with another	Infection, shunt failure, sciatica, low-pressure headache

Table 8 Medical Management of Headache with IIH

Prophylactic medications	
	beta blockers
	nonsteroidal anti-inflammatories (ibuprofen, naproxen sodium)
	fluoxetine hydrochloride (Prozac)
	Desipramine
Acute medications	
	nonsteroidal anti-inflammatories
	Midrin (isomepheptene, dichlorphenazone, acetaminophen)
	acetaminophen/aspirin with butalbitol (Fiorinal/Fioricet, Axotal, Esgic)

with tricyclics. Treatment of the acute headache with nonsteroidal anti-inflammatories, Midrin, and other headache medication (Fioricet, Esgic) can be helpful.

When headaches are refractory to these measures, some patients may require lumbar peritoneal shunt. Unfortunately, shunts may also cause headaches because of "hindbrain herniation," CSF leak, or a low-pressure syndrome due to a shunt that functions too well. ONSF has brought some headache relief.

V. SPECIAL CONSIDERATIONS IN TREATING IIH

Although the above-mentioned principles apply in treating all patients with IIH, some groups deserve special mention.

A. IIH in Children

IIH occurs in boys and girls with equal frequency. Children may lose vision just as adults (23%) (16). The same evaluation should be used as in adults. Sedation may be required for very young children in order to get an adequate MRI scan. A search for an offending agent should be made. Following children who are able to cooperate with testing can proceed as in the adult. When children are younger, and less cooperative, following the pupillary examination, and the appearance of the optic disc, becomes more important. Treatment of children with IIH can proceed as in adults. Pediatricians frequently use steroids to treat children with IIH. If vision stabilizes with 2 weeks of steroids, steroids can be tapered over 2 weeks. If no effect is seen after an initial 2-week trial, alternative therapy should be sought. Acetazolamide (60 mg/kg/day) can be used in children. Children who fail medical therapy (same criteria as adults) can undergo surgical therapy.

B. IIH in Men

Men are at reduced risk to develop IIH (2). When men present with papilledema, careful attention to detailed work-up is in order, since these cases may in fact have identifiable underlying conditions leading to IIH. Men may require more frequent follow-up, since it may be that they are at increased risk of visual loss. Black men in particular appear to be at increased risk of rapid visual loss and may require more expedient surgical treatment. Counseling for weight loss should occur, since, like women, men with IIH tend also to be obese. One should be judicious when lowering blood pressure in any hypertensive patient with IIH, since sudden drops in blood pressure may drop perfusion of the optic disc and lead to further visual loss.

C. IIH in Pregnancy

Pregnancy is not a risk factor for acquiring IIH, nor is pregnancy a special risk factor for visual loss (6). Termination of pregnancy is not a treatment for IIH. The pregnancy of a woman with IIH should be managed using standard obstetrical practice. Treatment of IIH should follow the general guidelines outlined as above. Weight loss and caloric restriction should not be recommended; however, weight gain can be limited to 20 lb. Medications such as acetazolamide may be used safely after 20 weeks (beyond the teratogenic period); usage before this has been associated in one case with a sacrococcygeal teratoma. Furosemide and thiazide diuretics can be used in the first trimester, but diuretic usage (including glycerol) in the second half of pregnancy can diminish placental blood flow and probably should be limited. Steroids have been safely used in pregnancy. Surgical management especially ONSF can be used safely during pregnancy.

REFERENCES

1. Durcan FJ, Corbett JJ, Wall M. The incidence of pseudotumor cerebri. Arch Neurol 1988; 45:875–77.
2. Digre KB, Corbett JJ. Pseudotumor cerebri in men. Arch Neurol 1988; 45:866–72.
3. Corbett JJ, Savino P, Thompson S, Kansu T, Schatz NJ, Orr LS, Hopson D. Visual loss in pseudotumor cerebri. Arch Neurol 1982; 39:461–74.
4. Corbett JJ. Problems in the diagnosis and treatment of pseudotumor cerebri. Can J Neurol 1983; 10:221–29.
5. Marcelis J, Silberstein SD. Idiopathic intracranial hypertension without papilledema. Arch Neurol 1991; 48:392–99.
6. Digre KB, Varner MW, Corbett JJ. Pseudotumor cerebri and pregnancy. Neurology 1984; 34:721–9.
7. Jacobson DM, Karanjia PN, Olson KA, Warner JJ. Computed tomography ventricular size has no predictive value in diagnosing pseudotumor cerebri. Neurology 1990; 40:1454–5.

8. Corbett JJ, Thompson HS. The rational management of idiopathic intracranial hypertension. Arch Neurol 1989; 46:1049–51.
9. Wall M. Sensory visual testing in idiopathic intracranial hypertension: measures sensitive to change. Neurology 1990; 40:1859–64.
10. Ireland B, Corbett JJ, Wallace RB. The search for causes of idiopathic intracranial hypertension. Arch Neurol 1990; 47:315–20.
11. Giuseffi V, Wall M, Siegel PZ, Rojas PB. Symptoms and disease associations in idiopathic intracranial hypertension (pseudotumor cerebri): a case-control study. Neurology 1991; 41:239–44.
12. Tomasak RL, Niffenegger AS, Remler BF. Treatment of pseudotumor cerebri with diamox (acetazolamide). J Clin Neuro-Ophthalmol 1988; 8:93–8.
13. Sergott RC, Savino PJ, Bosley TM. Modified optic nerve sheath decompression provides long-term visual improvement for pseudotumor cerebri. Arch Ophthalmol 1988; 106:1384–90.
14. Tse DT, Nerad JA, Anderson RL, Corbett JJ. Optic nerve sheath fenestration in pseudotumor cerebri. Arch Ophthalmol 1988; 106:1458–62.
15. Wall M. The headache profile of idiopathic intracranial hypertension. Cephalalgia 1990; 19:331–5.
16. Baker RS, Carter D, Hendrick EB, et al. Visual loss in pseudotumor cerebri of childhood. A follow-up study. Arch Ophthalmol 1985; 103:1681–6.

5

Syndromes of the Optic Chiasm

Saunders L. Hupp
University of South Alabama College of Medicine, Mobile, Alabama

Symptoms and signs of optic chiasm dysfunction are most often the result of extrinsic forces acting on the chiasm, but other traumatic, infectious, or inflammatory conditions may be present. The transition from recognition of these often specific signs to formulation of an efficient diagnostic and therapeutic plan requires knowledge of (1) the extrinsic and intrinsic anatomical relations of the chiasm; (2) a comprehensive differential diagnosis; and (3) current therapy of chiasmal disease.

The optic chiasm is composed of approximately 2.4 million axons and appears grossly as a flattened oblong structure formed by the union of the intracranial optic nerves at the base of the brain (1,2) (Fig. 1). It measures approximately 12 mm in transverse diameter, 8 mm in anteroposterior diameter, and 4 mm in thickness. The intracranial optic nerves do not lie on a horizontal plane but rather rise upward from the optic canals in a plane inclined, on an average, 45 degrees from the horizontal. The chiasm also is oriented in this upward sloping plane with its anterior notch directed downward and forward toward the anterior clinoid processes and its posterior notch posteriorly and superiorly. Because of its relationship to the third ventricle and subarachnoid basal cisterns, the optic chiasm is virtually surrounded by cerebrospinal fluid.

The unique anatomical relations of the afferent visual axons as they traverse the chiasm produces a characteristic spectrum of symptoms and signs composing what we will describe as the chiasmal syndrome (3). Axonal fibers

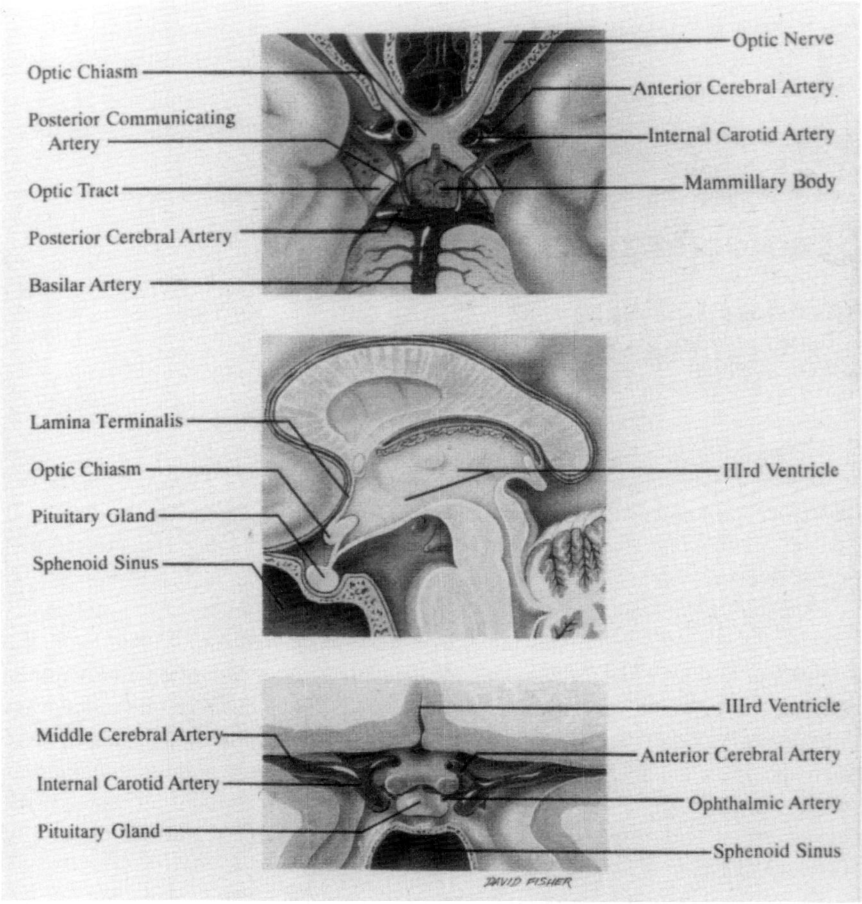

Figure 1 The optic chiasm viewed axially (top), sagittally (middle), and coronally (bottom). (Adapted from Ref. 5.)

are segregated into nonoverlapping groups dividing each visual field vertically through the center of vision (the vertical meridian) into temporal and nasal fields. Each nasal field is projected to the contralateral visual cortex through axons that cross in the chiasm. Conversely, each temporal visual field is projected to the ipsilateral visual cortex via axons that travel directly through the chiasm.

Painless, progressive visual loss is the most common feature associated with chiasmal dysfunction and may involve peripheral or central visual function in very characteristic patterns to be described below. Along with visual disturbances, other nearby structures such as the pituitary gland, cavernous sinus, hypothalamus, olfactory nerves, and frontal lobes may be involved and pro- duce pain, ptosis, oculomotor paralysis, endocrine dysfunction, and loss of smell.

I. CLINICAL FEATURES

The optic chiasm is exclusively involved in the transmission of afferent visual information and therefore the majority of symptomatology from chiasmal disease affects central and peripheral vision. Two configurations of visual field loss are the "signatures" of chiasmal involvement (4). The first characteristic pattern of visual field loss is a bitemporal hemianopia (Fig. 2). This is often produced by an extrinsic lesion compressing the crossing nasal fibers in the optic chiasm. This classic bitemporal hemianopia may involve only the superior visual fields if the lesion produces extrinsic compression initially from below. Conversely, superior chiasmatic compression may cause only an inferior hemianopic field loss. The second characteristic pattern of visual field loss is termed a "junctional scotoma" and is caused by extrinsic compression at the termination of the optic nerve and anterior chiasm by involving the crossing nasal fibers of the contralateral optic nerve (Fig. 3).

Visual field testing may be performed using automated static or kinetic techniques. I find that confrontation testing on either side of the vertical meridian superiorly, centrally, and inferiorly with a red object (swizzle stick, eye-drop bottle top) is extremely sensitive for the detection of hemianopic defects.

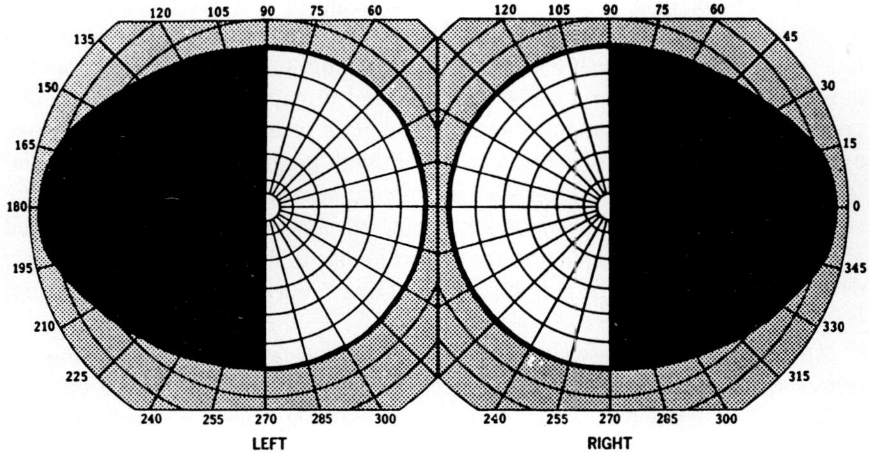

Figure 2 Complete bitemporal hemianopia from damage of nasal crossing fibers of the chiasm. Note abrupt border at the 90-degree vertical meridian. (Adapted from Ref. 4.)

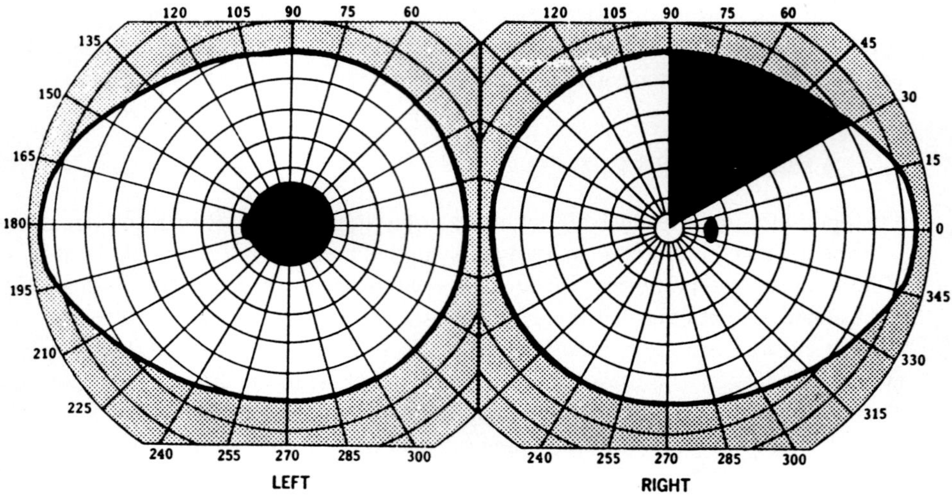

Figure 3 Junctional scotoma indicating a lesion at the anterior junction of the left optic nerve and chiasm. (Adapted from Ref. 4.)

The symptoms of visual loss from a chiasmal syndrome are often insidious and the patient may not perceive that the peripheral vision is affected. Instead, the patient may complain of an inability to perform various fine motor tasks requiring careful depth perception or binocular vision. Binocularity may be impaired owing to a lack of the normal overlap of the visual fields and be associated with diplopia from visual field "slip." Convergence for near visual tasks may create a confusing scotoma, "postfixation blindness," directly behind the point of fixation from loss of both temporal visual fields. Especially with a postfixed chiasm, the patient may only complain of central visual loss in one eye. The critical clinical finding in a patient with progressive monocular visual loss is the finding of an asymptomatic temporal hemianopic visual defect in the seemingly "normal" eye. This is the diagnostic junctional scotoma mentioned above and localizes the lesion to the anterior chiasm. The temporal hemianopic defects need not always be peripheral and, at times, may be central or paracentral (Fig. 4).

Although visual symptomatology (acuity, color, and visual field) may be pronounced, an afferent pupillary defect or optic nerve pallor may be difficult to detect. The afferent pupillary defect may be absent if there is involvement of the body of the chiasm with symmetrical nerve fiber damage. Optic nerve pallor can accompany the chiasmal syndrome and has been said to take on a characteristic "bow tie" appearance. This may not be particularly obvious and the nerves can appear almost normal. Certainly, if a junctional syndrome is

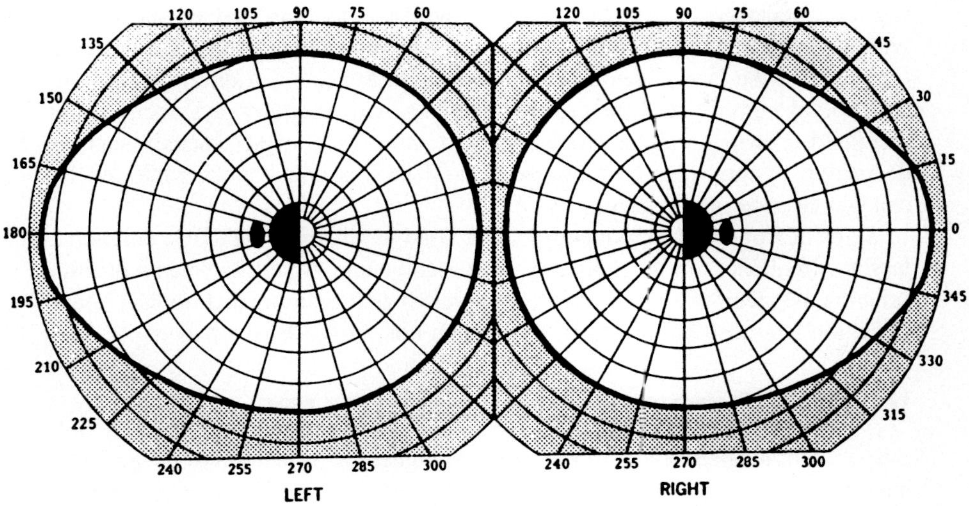

Figure 4 Central bitemporal hemianopia from damage limited to the crossing nasal central macular fibers. (Adapted from Ref. 4.)

advanced, one would expect marked pallor of the ipsilateral optic nerve and very little change in appearance on the contralateral side.

The optic nerve may appear swollen or excavated in a chiasmal syndrome. Papilledema accompanies a chiasmal syndrome most often when an intracranial mass is suprasellar or rarely if the tumor is remote producing anterior third ventricular enlargement. The clinician should not be deterred from consideration of a chiasmal syndrome by the presence of optic nerve cupping more typical of glaucoma. Progressive axonal damage from compression may be accompanied by increasing nerve head excavation.

Complaints of diplopia, pain, or ptosis may be found in patients with chiasmal syndromes due to involvement of cranial nerves III, IV, V, and VI as they traverse the cavernous sinus. These symptoms often appear late in a chiasmal syndrome, because an enlarging pituitary mass can expand superiorly through the diaphragm sellae more easily than laterally. Rarely, interruption of the fibers of the third-order neuron of the oculosympathetic pathway can produce a Horner's syndrome causing ipsilateral ptosis and miosis.

Endocrine abnormalities are not infrequent accompaniments of visual complaints due to the involvement of the hypothalamic pituitary axis. These endocrinological abnormalities are more easily detected in women because of interruption of the normal menstrual cycle. Galactorrhea may be noted in both men and women. It is important to ask about sexual function, and often there will be impotence or loss of libido that will not be expressed by the patient without specific questioning. Symptoms and signs of Cushing's syndrome (adiposity of the face, amenorrhea, impotence, dusty complexion, hypertension, and polycythemia) may be present. Patients with pituitary dysfunction and increased growth hormone production will show signs of acromegaly such as deepening of the voice and enlargement of the extremities, as evidenced by changes in shoe or ring size.

Signs of frontal lobe dysfunction (decreased psychomotor activity, emotional lability, frequency, or incontinence) may accompany visual loss when a planum sphenoidale meningioma expands to compress both the chiasm and frontal cortex. Olfaction may also be impaired and is often not noticed by the patient.

II. EVALUATION OF CHIASMAL DISEASE

Suspicion of localization by examination combined with elements of the patient's history as described above should be followed by an efficient algorithm of diagnostic tests. The initial evaluation of chiasmal disease should be imaging of the chiasm and perichiasmal structures.

Magnetic resonance imaging (MRI) has now replaced computed tomography (CT) as the initial procedure of choice in imaging of the optic chiasm (5). Soft tissue resolution is enhanced without interference of bone artifact. Direct multiplaner imaging in the axial, coronal, and sagittal planes without patient repositioning or the need for reconstructed views is now standard technique. MRI more accurately detects tissue composition (e.g., hemorrhage, fat, cerebrospinal fluid) with identifying characteristics on T_1- and T_2-weighted images. These capabilities of MRI allow more accurate distinction between intrinsic and extrinsic lesions of the chiasm. Although MRI is usually the best technique for chiasmal imaging, there may be a complementary role for CT when it becomes important to detect bone changes and/or small amounts of calcification.

One recent development in MRI that holds great promise as a noninvasive method of studying the cerebral circulation including the perisellar vasculature, is MR angiography. Several different techniques are available that result in blood appearing as increased signal intensity without injection of contrast medium. Computer reconstruction results in three-dimensional images that can be viewed in multiple projections. Because giant aneurysms and arteriovenous malformations may cause chiasmal disease, this evolving MR technique may also assist in chiasmal evaluation. With continued improvements, MR angiography may replace invasive cerebral angiography in many cases.

Neuroradiological investigation is often followed by hematological testing. The various infectious, inflammatory, and hormonal studies are listed in Table 1. Infectious and inflammatory chiasmal disease may be identified by results of a complete blood count, erythrocyte sedimentation rate, and immunological tests

Table 1 Diagnostic Evaluation of Chiasmal Disease

Imaging
magnetic resonance imaging
computed tomography
magnetic resonance angiography
cerebral angiography
chest x-ray
bone scan
Hematology
complete blood count
erythrocyte sedimentation rate
serum prolactin
serum cortisol
somatomedin C
serum chemistry (e.g., calcium, liver enzymes)
serum angiotensin-converting enzyme
FTA
HIV
lupus cell preparation
serum protein electrophoresis
Cerebrospinal fluid
opening pressure
cell count and differential
protein
glucose
cytology
culture (bacterial, fungal, TB)
multiple sclerosis immunologic panel
VDRL

directed at specific infectious or inflammatory markers. Also, other diagnostic studies such as a chest radiography (TB, sarcoidosis) and/or an evaluation of the cerebrospinal fluid may be indicated.

Endocrinological evaluation is often necessary when a pituitary mass is identified. If the patient has no symptoms of endocrine dysfunction, I usually start with only a serum prolactin and cortisol evaluation. Serum prolactin is normally raised with hypoglycemia, so it is best to obtain a postprandial serum sampling. Most prolactin-secreting tumors elevate the serum prolactin above 100 ng/ml (normal <20 ng/ml). Serum cortisol has a diurnal fluctuation and it is necessary to sample both morning and night serum. Even more reliable in the evaluation of cortisol production is a 24-h urine collection for free cortisol. Elevated cortisol values need to be correlated with adrenocorticotropin (ACTH) production, including a dexamethasone-suppression test. Excessive secretion of growth hormone resulting in acromegaly is best evaluated by a serum somatomedin C analysis.

III. DIFFERENTIAL DIAGNOSIS OF SYNDROMES OF THE OPTIC CHIASM

Chiasmal disease is most often the result of extrinsic compression, although infection, inflammation, intrinsic tumors, and trauma can be found. Table 2 lists these various causes.

Several disease states that may imitate a chiasmal syndrome are listed in Table 3. These diseases of the anterior optic nerve or retina may at times produce progressive visual loss, optic nerve pallor, and visual field changes (such as enlarged blind spots) that may be suggestive of chiasmal disease.

IV. TREATMENT

Some mode of therapy, either medical, surgical, or radiological, is almost always indicated in chiasmal syndromes. This therapy often requires a combined team of specialists (ophthalmologist, endocrinologist, radiologist, neurosurgeon, oncologist).

Treatment of endocrine tumors of the pituitary gland has been enhanced with the development of drugs with specific hormonal activity (6,7). Prolactin-secreting adenomas may be treated primarily with bromocriptine if they are either difficult to resect completely owing to invasion of the cavernous sinus or the lesion is small and not associated with significant visual dysfunction. Bromocriptine and somatostatin are used to modulate the hormonal effects of growth hormone–secreting pituitary adenomas, but surgery remains the primary modality to control these tumors (8,9). Growth hormone–secreting adenomas are more invasive than prolactinomas, with a higher incidence of cavernous sinus extension.

Meningiomas of the parasellar region are usually benign, slow-growing tumors that are poorly responsive to either chemotherapy or traditional radiotherapy. Furthermore, even though it is well known that meningiomas increase their growth during pregnancy, hormonal modulation of meningioma growth has not been particularly successful. Thus, they are treated with surgical resection when they become symptomatic. Recently, an antiprogesterone compound, mifepristone (RU486), has demonstrated positive results in a group of patients with meningiomas that were not totally resectable (10).

Stereotactic radiosurgery, or the "gamma knife," is a new technique designed

Table 2 Etiology of Chiasmal Disease

Tumors
pituitary
craniopharyngioma
meningioma
glioma
dysgerminoma
ependymoma
metastatic carcinoma
angioma
plasmacytoma
myoblastoma
remote tumor with enlarged third ventricle
Vascular
ophthalmic artery aneurysm
dolichoectatic internal carotid
ischemia
Inflammatory
demyelinating disease
sarcoidosis
histocytosis X
"arachnoiditis"
Infectious
syphilis
TB
"anything" with HIV^+
Trauma
direct or indirect
Other
empty sella
midline cysts
radiation necrosis
pituitary hyperplasia or apoplexy
pneumosinus dilitans

to cause tumor necrosis with a single intense dose of carefully aimed radiation (11,12). The radiation exposure to adjacent tissue has such a steep fall-off that structures 1–2 mm from the treatment zone receive virtually no irradiation. Exact localization of the area to be treated requires three-dimensional imaging techniques whose coordinates are correlated with the focused delivery system of the radiation. Unfortunately, the optic nerves and chiasm are neural tissues that are exquisitely radiosensitive, which limits the gamma knife to lesions approx-

Table 3 Imitators of Chiasmal Disease

Big blind spot syndrome
Low-tension glaucoma
Hereditary optic atrophy
Toxic or metabolic optic neuropathy
Optic nerve drusen
Tilted optic nerves
Anterior optic nerve trauma
Prior papilledema
Retinal disease/trauma

imately 3–5 mm from these structures. The gamma knife has been applied to pituitary adenomas, meningiomas, and craniopharyngiomas.

Surgical removal remains the most frequent therapy for sellar and parasellar tumors (7). The surgical approach may either be transbasal (transnasal, transsphenoidal, or transethmoidal) or via a transcranial incision. The transnasal transsphenoidal approach has become one of the most popular surgical techniques because of improvements in microsurgical instruments and neuroanesthesia. It is limited by the inability to extend laterally beyond midline structures such as the sella or cribriform plate. Most vascular lesions as well as tumors that extend beyond the midline limits mentioned above require the direct and more extensive visualization provided by a transcranial approach.

Whatever the treatment, the ophthalmologist is an integral part of the therapeutic and diagnostic team directing the diagnostic evaluation of the visual system and evaluating the response to therapy.

REFERENCES

1. Hoyt WF. The human optic chiasm. In: Smith JL, ed. Neuro-ophthalmology, Symposium of the University of Miami. Springfield, IL: Charles C Thomas, 1964:64–111.
2. Miller NR. Walsh and Hoyt's clinical neuro-ophthalmology. Vol. 1. 4th ed. Baltimore: Williams & Wilkins, 1982:60–8.
3. Miller NR. Walsh and Hoyt's clinical neuro-ophthalmology. Vol. 1. 4th ed. Baltimore: Williams & Wilkins, 1982:123–7.
4. Bajandas FJ, Kline LB. Neuro-ophthalmology review manual. 2d ed. Thorofare, NJ: Slack, 1987:1–10.
5. Hupp SL, Kline LB. Magnetic resonance imaging of the optic chiasm. Surv Ophthalmol 1991; 36:207–16.
6. Blackwell RE. Hyperprolactinemia. Evaluation and management. Endocrinol Metab Clin N Am 1992; 21(1):105–24.

7. Wilson CB. Role of surgery in the management of pituitary tumors. Neurosurg Clin N Am 1990; 1(1):139–59.
8. Lamberts SW, Reubi JC, Krenning EP. Somatostatin analogs in the treatment of acromegaly. Endocrinol Metab Clin N Am 1992; 21(3):737–52.
9. Fahlbusch R, Honegger J, Buchfelder M. Surgical management of acromegaly. Endocrinol Metab Clin N Am 1992; 21(3):669–92.
10. Grunberg SM, Weiss MH, Spitz IM, Ahmadi J, Sadun AA, Russell CA, Lucci L, Stevenson LL. Treatment of unresectable meningiomas with the anti-progesterone agent mifepristone. J Neurosurg 1991; 74:861–6.
11. Bakay RA. Stereotactic radiosurgery in the treatment of brain tumors. Clin Neurosurg 1992; 39:292–313.
12. Fabrikant JI, Levy RP, Steinberg GK, Phillips MH, et al. Stereotactic charged-partical radiosurgery: clinical results of treatment of 1200 patients with intracranial arteriovenous malformations and pituitary disorders. Clin Neurosurg 1992; 38:472–92.

6

Color Vision Testing in Clinical Neuro-Ophthalmology

William M. Hart, Jr.
Washington University School of Medicine, St. Louis, Missouri

Color vision testing in the clinical evaluation of patients with neuro-ophthalmic disease has traditionally been confined to its use in the detection of signs and symptoms of damage to the afferent visual system anterior to the lateral geniculate nucleus. Such testing is usually limited to the use of interocular comparisons of brightly colored objects and of pseudoisochromatic plates to detect the presence of significant defects in hue discrimination. Findings of acquired color deficits are hallmark characteristics of diseases affecting the central visual field representation within the papillomacular bundle of retinal ganglion cell axons and serve as a crude proxy for determining the health of the central 10 degrees of the visual field. Beyond this, however, more revealing color vision tests are both complex and difficult to interpret, which makes their clinical use difficult.

For this reason, time-consuming tests, such as the color sorting tests, as represented by the Farnsworth Munsell 100-hue test, and more exacting tests of hue discrimination, such as the various forms of anomaloscopy, have for the most part been confined to use in experimental laboratories and clinical research projects. However, it has long been known that certain patterns of damage to hue discrimination do occur preferentially in some forms of anterior afferent visual system disease, and clinicians have long sought a means of using this information to better understand the problems of their patients.

Early in this century, Köllner, working in Berlin, published a monograph in which he observed empirically that patients with primary optic nerve disease frequently showed a preponderance for hue discrimination difficulties between reds and greens, whereas patients with primary retinochoroidal disorders more frequently showed evidence of hue discrimination difficulties between blues and yellows (8). This general phenomenon has come to be known as "Köllner's rule."

However, Köllner's rule is not at all absolute, there being numerous well-known exceptions. A common exception is primary open-angle glaucoma, which preferentially damages the optic nerve and yet is characterized by a blue-yellow pattern of color deficit. Thus, although optic nerve diseases have a tendency toward producing a preferential defect in red-green discrimination, some primary neuropathies can on occasion do exactly the opposite.

Corresponding exceptions to Köllner's rule can be found for retinochoroidal diseases as well. Although many retinal diseases (e.g., the various forms of retinitis pigmentosa) affect the peripheral visual field with sparing of central vision until late in their courses and produce predominantly blue-yellow color deficits, there are other retinal diseases (e.g., primary cone dystrophies and Stargardt's disease) that can produce preferential deficits for red-green discrimination.

Understanding the pathophysiological basis for these various patterns, and the ability to detect them quickly and efficiently during the clinical examination, can give the neuro-ophthalmologist an advantage in better understanding the pathophysiology of disease and to allow more precise topographic localization of disease.

I. CLINICAL TESTS OF COLOR VISION

To be useful, a clinical test of color vision should be relatively quick and simple and be of sufficient sensitivity and specificity to allow the examiner to use the results in a clinically meaningful way. The use of small, brightly colored test objects to perform interocular comparisons and to map areas of defective visual field by confrontation testing has been widely practiced for decades. The use of pseudoisochromatic plates, such as the American Optical Hardy-Rand-Rittler series or the Ishihara album, have likewise been used routinely for many years as screening tools for clinical detection of anterior visual system disease. Beyond their role as simple detecting devices, however, these tests have been of limited additional value in differential diagnosis.

A brief review of the methods used in designing these tests is useful for understanding how they may be applied in a logical way to exploring a patient's color vision problems more completely.

The historical development of color vision theories and the derivation of testing methods to confirm or deny these theories have been exhaustively reviewed and readers should refer to such work for further information (7,13). Suffice it to say that the normal color vison experience covers a gamut of sensation that can be matched by suitable mixing of a minimum of three primary "sensations," which can in turn be represented by three suitably chosen spectral (monochromatic) lights. Given a reference light of any given spectral composition and intensity, its appearance can be exactly matched by suitable mixing of the three monochromatic "primaries." The subject being tested must be given full control of the brightnesses and proportions of the three elements being mixed. This trivariant phenomenon underlies the basis for the graphic format in which the gamut of color perception is routinely graphed and is commonly referred to as a color triangle.

The color triangle shown in Figure 1 was established early in this century as an international standard for the graphical representation of normal human color perception. It was based on extensive testing of a selected series of "normal" observers. It serves to condense onto a single two-dimensional plane, a simplified representation of a complex sensory phenomenon; it is referred to as the CIE chromaticity diagram. Within the diagram is a curvilinear line segment called the spectrum locus curve, which represents the various sensations for each of a series of monochromatic lights in the visible spectrum. A straight line segment at the bottom of the triangle, connecting the two ends of the spectrum locus curve, represents sensations obtained by proportional mixing of monochromatic lights from the two ends of the curve. The area within the diagram bounded by these line segments represents the total gamut of human color perception. Any point inside this boundary represents a color sensation that can be matched by suitable mixing of any three lights along the spectrum locus curve defining the apices of a triangle that completely surrounds the point in question.

All systems that have been devised for categorizing colors have required three variables to establish a system of exact definition, and the CIE color vision triangle is no exception. Such trivariant systems can also be represented by volumetric coordinate systems. In the case of the CIE diagram, a volumetric representation has been flattened into a plane by imposing a constraint on the trivariance: that the sum of all three variables will always be unity.

This tripartite feature of color organization systems can be expressed in linguistically familiar terms such as hue, saturation, and brightness. In the CIE diagram, hues are represented by the various loci around the perimeter of the triangle (the spectrum locus curve and its straight line segment at the bottom), whereas saturation or color purity is represented by points along a line between the hue locus in question and the center of the triangle, where colors fade through increasingly pastel shades into a neutral appearance indistinguishable from white. The third variable, brightness or intensity, varies roughly with vertical (Y-axis) position within the diagram and is equal to the sum of intensities of all three "primary" sensations.

The color vision defects that have been most extensively studied are the congenital dyschromatopsias. These disorders, inherited in a sex-linked recessive

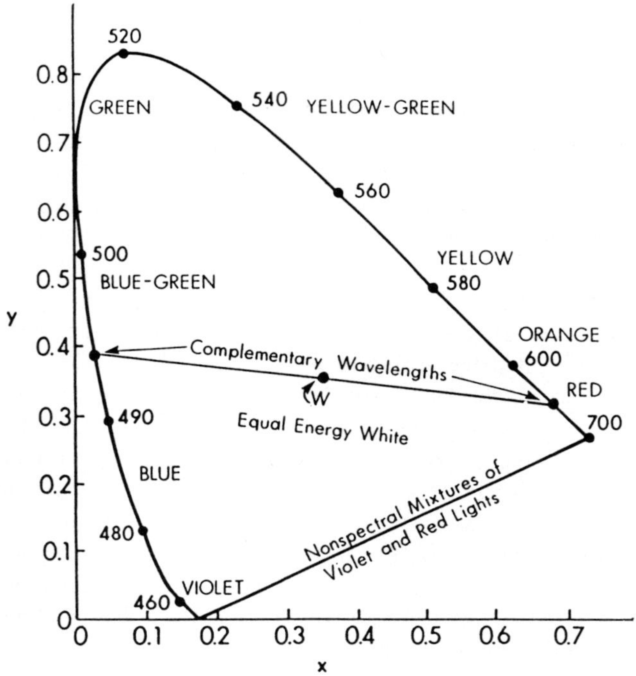

Figure 1 The CIE chromaticity diagram. Color representation is spatially arranged, although not strictly proportionally in all directions. Proportionality does hold, however, for any given straight line segment, and any straight line segment within the diagram represents a series of color sensations that can be produced by proportional mixing of the colors found at either end of the segment. Point "W" represents the mixture of equal energies of the three primary sensations and produces a white appearance. Complementary wavelengths are pairs of monochromatic lights that when mixed in suitable proportion with one another yield an appearance indistinguishable from "W." The curved line labeled with the positions of the various visible monochromatic lights is the spectrum locus curve. The color names are those associated with the various sensations produced by the monochromatic stimuli. Notice that the straight line segment produced by mixing monochromatic stimuli of 540 and 700 nm lies almost directly atop the corresponding segment of the spectrum locus curve, and that mixing of lights that are green and red in appearance will yield colors that are variably yellow. Further, mixing of yellow and blue lights will yield colors that vary across the white region at the center of the diagram. (From Ref. 6.)

pattern, produce characteristic defects in hue discrimination when mapped within the CIE chromaticity diagram. Affected individuals have defective color vision in which whole families of related colors, falling along linear profiles within the chromaticity diagram, are indistinguishable from one another. These profiles are referred to as isochromatic lines of color confusion. Figure 2 diagrams the isochromatic lines of confusion for each of the three principal varieties of congenital dyschromatopsia: *protan*, *deutan*, and *tritan* (so named because they represent the first, second, and third forms discovered). A protanoptic individual lacks the ability to sense purely red light, and as a consequence, colored mixtures that vary only in their content of redness all *appear* identically the same, as long as the intensities of complementary lights being used to produce the color mixtures are suitably varied.

The testing method called anomaloscopy is used to quantify this phenomenon. A comparison reference light is given consisting, for instance, of a mixture of red and green lights that produce a yellow stimulus. The subject is then required to vary the intensities of red and green components of a light mixture to establish a "match" with the reference stimulus. A trichromatic individual will always choose within a very narrow range the same proportion of red and green components to match the yellow reference light. However, a protan individual will be able to form a satisfactory match with a range of intensities of green light only, using little of the red light. In practice, there are varying degrees of protanomaly present in the human population, including mild to moderately severe forms, through total red blindness or protanopia. The molecular genetics of the congenital dyschromatopsias are now fairly well understood for the red and green (protan and deutan) deficient forms. The reader is referred to other sources for a more complete description (10–12).

Hue discrimination tests of color vision are best understood by appreciating the way in which they exploit the isochromatic phenomena. Pseudoisochromatic plates, for instance, contain isoluminant object/background boundaries formed by varying sizes of blobs that differ from one another in color along isochromatic confusion lines. Since red-green congenital dyschromatopsias constitute a large majority of congenital color vision defects, the majority of pseudoisochromatic tests have been designed for the detection of protan and deutan types of congenital color vision deficiency. Although one published album was intended to detect varying degrees of tritan dyschromatopsia, it has been unfortunately lacking in several respects and does not appear to be clinically useful.

So while pseudoisochromatic plates may be helpful for the detection of red-green deficiencies in hue discrimination, they are not useful for detecting blue-yellow patterns of defects, nor are they helpful for discriminating between various patterns of dyschromatopsias in their differential diagnosis.

Color sorting tests for hue discrimination, however, are more or less ideally suited to differentiating between red versus green or blue versus yellow color

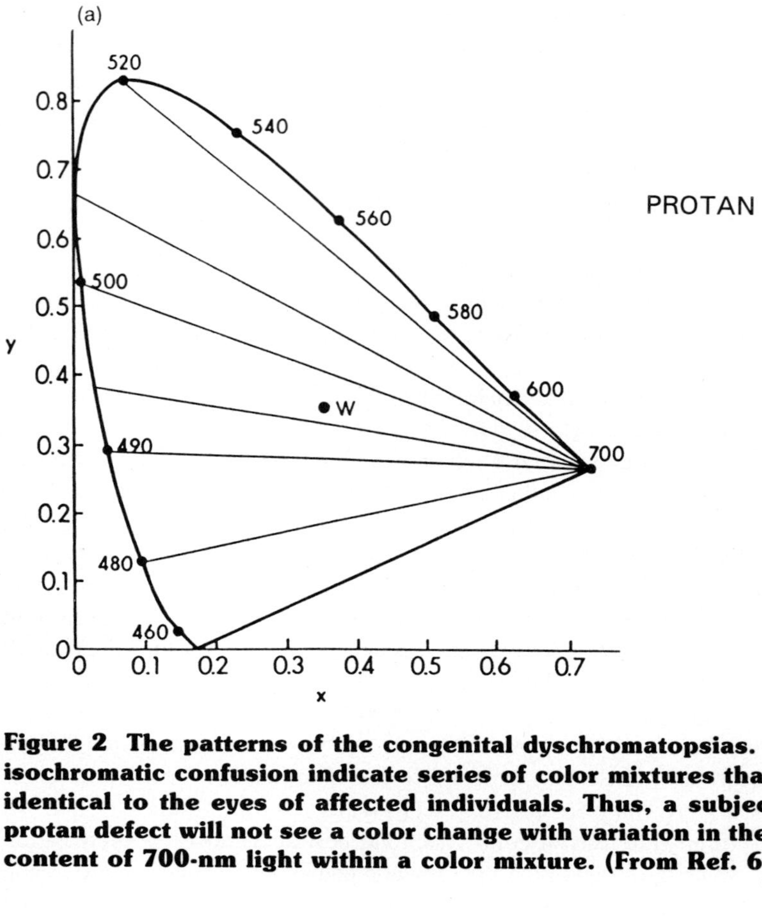

Figure 2 The patterns of the congenital dyschromatopsias. Lines of isochromatic confusion indicate series of color mixtures that appear identical to the eyes of affected individuals. Thus, a subject with a protan defect will not see a color change with variation in the relative content of 700-nm light within a color mixture. (From Ref. 6.)

discrimination deficiencies. The best known of these tests are the Farnsworth-Munsell 100-hue, the Farnsworth D-15, and the Lanthony New Color Test (3,9). Figure 3 diagrams the positions of the various colored caps of the 100-hue test within the CIE chromaticity triangle. The positions of the cap colors form an oval near the center of the diagram. If one compares the position and borders of this oval to the diagrams of pseudoisochromatic lines shown in Figure 2, it can be appreciated that some caps along the circumference of this oval would be more difficult to distinguish from one another than would caps within other sectors of the oval. For instance, whereas a normal trichromat would be able to distinguish caps from one another with equal facility in all sectors of the oval, an individual with a protan color deficiency would have greater difficulty distinguishing caps falling between numbers 10 and 30 and between numbers 50

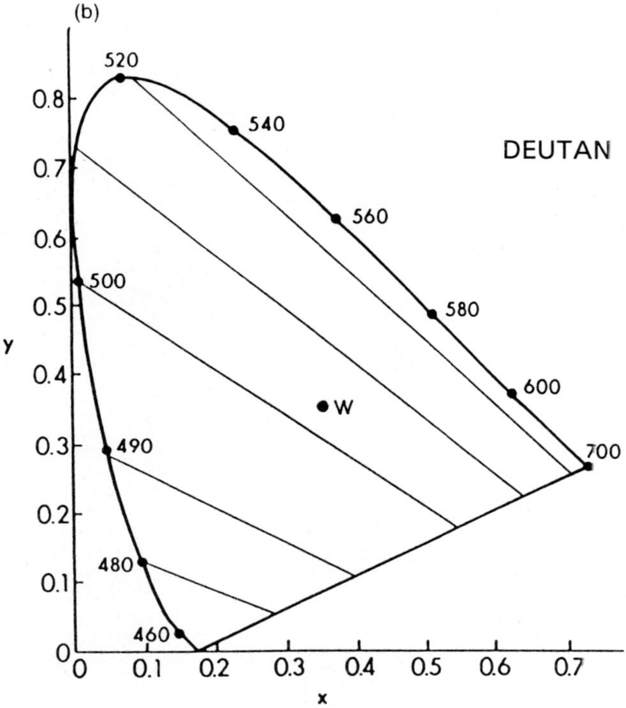
(b)
DEUTAN
520
540
560
580
600
700
500
490
480
460
W
y
x
0
0.1
0.2
0.3
0.4
0.5
0.6
0.7
0.8

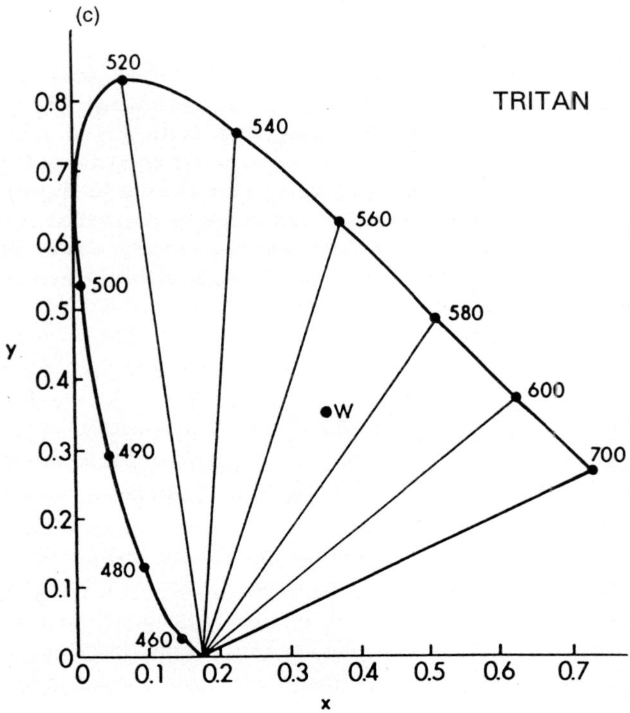
(c)
TRITAN
520
540
560
580
600
700
500
490
480
460
W
y
x
0
0.1
0.2
0.3
0.4
0.5
0.6
0.7
0.8

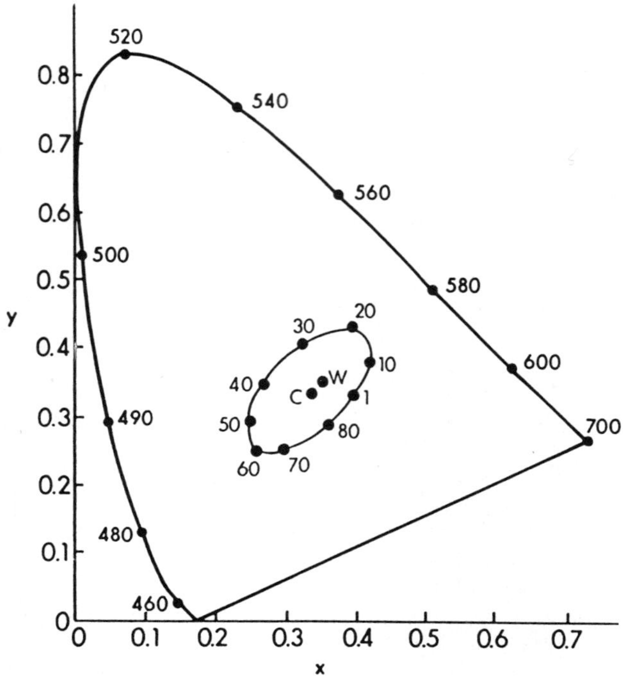

Figure 3 Color caps of the Farnsworth Munsell 100-hue test, as plotted within the CIE chromaticity diagram. "W," equal energy white; "C," standard illuminant C (light from a tungsten bulb fitted with specified blue filter). Compare the lines of isochromatic confusion for each of the three types of acquired dyschromatopsias shown in Figure 2 to the oval pattern of the 100-hue caps. Sequences of caps that are generally tangent to isochromatic lines are approximately equal in appearance to affected individuals leading to transpositional errors in colored cap ordering. (From Ref. 6.)

and 75. Figure 4 shows the various patterns for the typical congenital dyschromatopsias, as mapped by the Farnsworth-Munsell test. (Note that there are only 85 caps represented, 15 of the original 100 caps having been eliminated from the test as redundant.)

The standard graphical representation of results of the 100-hue test is a polar diagram in which the various radii represent the caps and the eccentricity along each radius is proportional to the extent of confusion (transpositional error in ordering) between the cap and its associated neighbors. Thus, a tight circle toward the center of the diagram is characteristic of normal trichromatic color discrim-

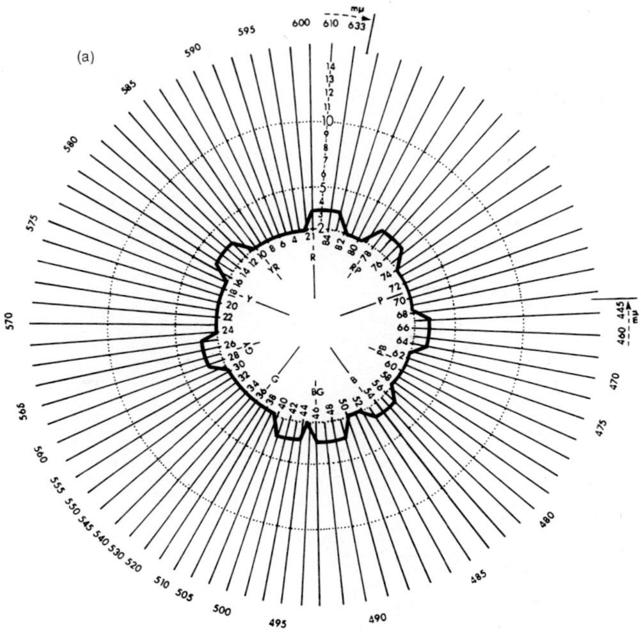

Figure 4 Typical results of Farnsworth Munsell 100-hue test for (a) normal trichromats for each of the three types of congenital dyschromatopsias. Opposing zones of transpositional errors produce axes of symmetry in the dyschromatopsia plots. (b) Protan and (c) deutan patterns (confusion of red/green mixtures) have oblique axes of symmetry from upper left to lower right. These two axes are very nearly the same and are difficult to differentiate from one another. (d) The axis for tritan individuals is nearly vertical. (From Ref. 6.)

ination, whereas points falling farther away from the center of the circle represent varying degrees of defective hue discrimination.

Looking at the geometrical representation given in Figures 2 and 3, it can be appreciated that for an individual with a dyschromatopsia characterized by a family of isochromatic lines of confusion there should be two regions of cap confusion on opposite sides of the 100-hue oval; and when the resulting errors are plotted on the polar coordinate form, they should appear as opposing sectors in which values lie farther away from the center of the diagram roughly forming an axis of symmetry. In the case of tritan defects, this axis of symmetry is nearly vertical, whereas in the case of protan and deutan defects, these axes are oblique (from upper left to lower right) and differ from one another by only a relatively

(b)

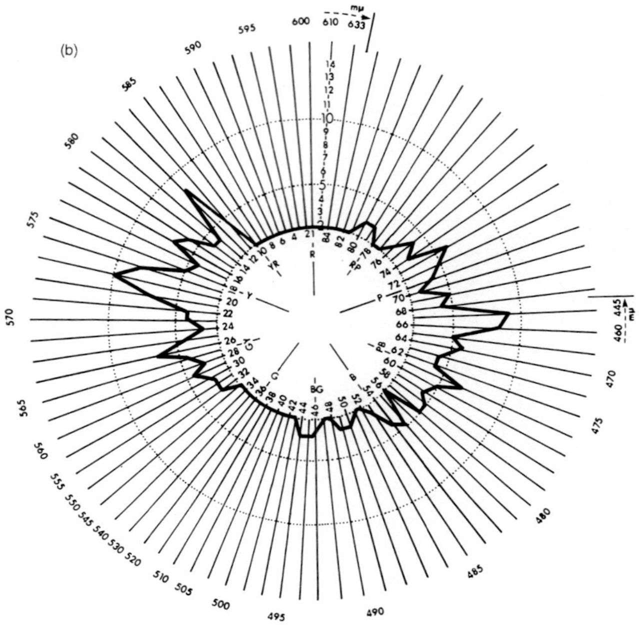

(c)

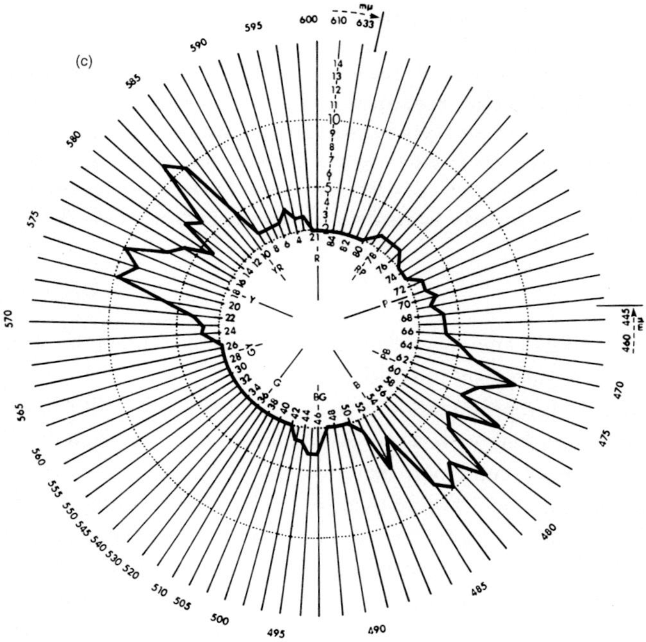

Figure 4 (*Continued*)

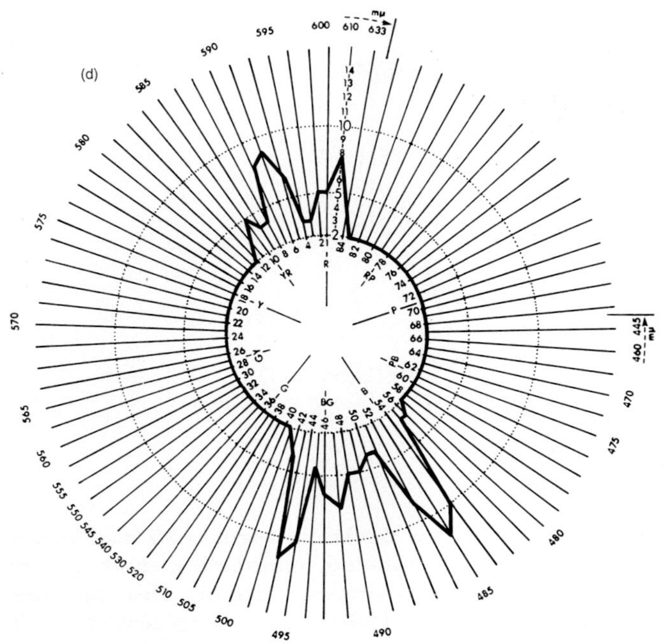

narrow angle. This is a reflection of the fact that the isochromatic lines for protan and deutan defects in the CIE diagram are nearly parallel with one another.

A shorter and faster clinical test of hue discrimination is the Farnsworth D-15. It is more of a screening test that the 100-hue, but often yields valuable information. It consists of 15 movable and 1 fixed caps in a single box. The various hues of the caps from a color sequence around the periphery of about the same hue circle as in the 100-hue test (Fig. 5). The subject is asked to sort the caps by color progression, and the results are plotted on the chart by connecting with straight line segments the various cap numbers as ordered by the test subject. The resulting patterns found in dyschromatopsia differ from the normal circumferential plot of Figure 5 as shown in the examples of Figure 6.

II. ANATOMICAL DETAILS OF IMPORTANCE IN COLOR VISION

Color discrimination, like visual acuity, is directly proportional to the density of cone photoreceptors in the retina. The anatomical distribution of cones as a function of eccentricity within the retina is densest at the fovea, where color discrimination reaches its peak. Both color discrimination and cone density

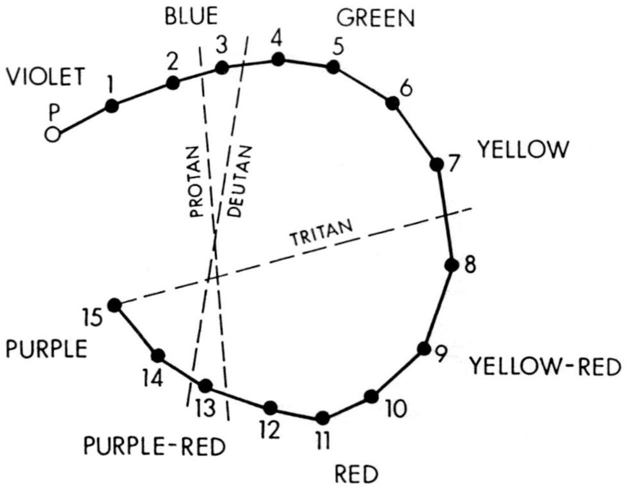

Figure 5 Standard recording form for the Farnsworth D-15 test. When all 15 caps have been correctly sequenced, connecting their points with straight line segments draws a reversed C shape. The caps are a reduced subset of those used in the 100-hue test. This test is much more quickly administered but gives a correspondingly reduced sensitivity and specificity for detecting and defining the axes of a dyschromatopsia. When several connecting line segments parallel one of the dotted lines on the chart, one can conclude that a dyschromatopsia of the type indicated is present. (From Ref. 6.)

decrease sharply at locations away from the center of the fovea, although some remnants of color perception persist all the way out into the far periphery of the visual field. Although the peripheral visual field is not truly "color blind," the colors of perimetric test objects must subtend large visual angles in order to be reliably differentiated in the periphery. This is a reflection of the need for spatial summation from a sparse population of photoreceptors spread over a large area and is precisely analogous to the lower levels of luminance sensitivity and spatial acuity found in the peripheral visual field of the light-adapted eye.

There are, however, some notable peculiarities in the distribution of cones in the fovea and perifoveal retina. These peculiarities account for some of the phenomena of color perception found in the acquired diseases of the retina and optic nerve. The first peculiarity of importance is the fact that close to 95% of cones belong either to the red- or green-sensitive class, whereas only about 5% of the cone population is devoted to short wavelength–sensitive (blue) receptors. This means that the sensitivity for detection of changes in color is much higher

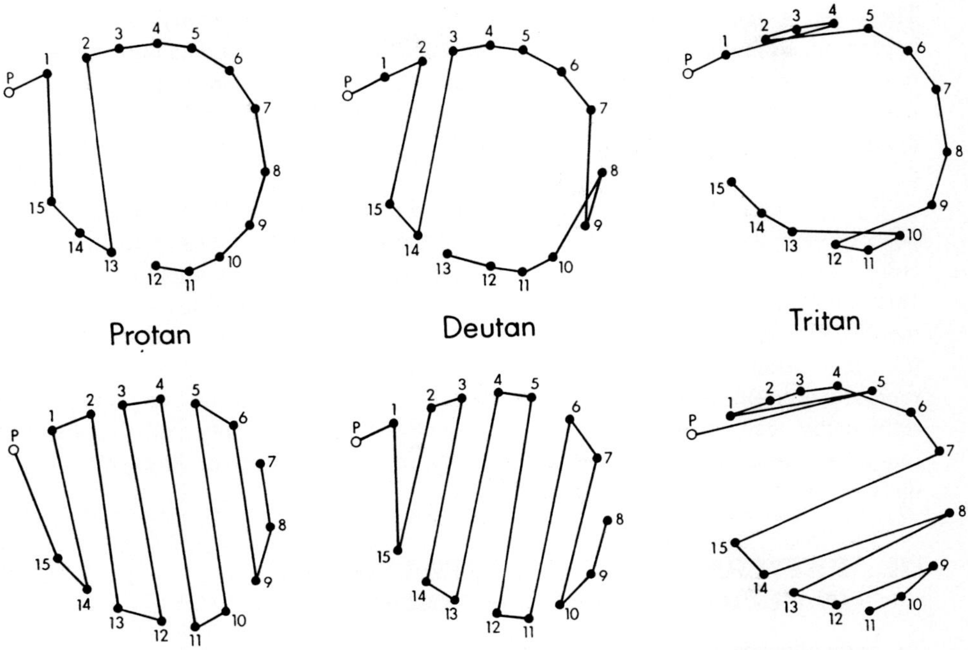

Figure 6 D-15 test results for various dyschromatopsias. Upper patterns typical for mildly affected subjects and lower patterns for the more severely affected. (From Ref. 6.)

in the red-green dimension of color space than in the blue-yellow. This is another way of saying that the "color acuity" of blue-yellow discrimination is lower than that for red-green discrimination and consequently requires test objects of larger size and of longer duration to be reliably discriminated. The second peculiarity of retinal cone anatomy is that blue cones, much like the distribution of rods in the retina, are entirely excluded from the foveal cone matrix (1,2,17). Blue cones are found in their highest numbers and spatial densities in the perifoveal macula, approximately 2–3 degrees away from fixation, and their density profile then falls off into the periphery in a manner more or less parallel to that for red and green cones. This exclusion from the foveal cone matrix means that there is actually a small physiological scotoma for blue detection that is approximately 0.5 degrees in angular size, a phenomenon called small-field tritanopia (15,16). Thus, very small but brightly colored test objects, which vary in the blue-yellow dimension, are virtually indistinguishable from one another when viewed centrally by the human eye. Test objects must actually be larger than 0.5 degrees in diameter to be reliably distinguishable in the blue-yellow color dimension.

The caps of the Farnsworth-Munsell 100-hue test were originally sized to approximate the diameter of the test objects used for the original data collection in establishing the CIE chromaticity diagram. At a reading distance of approximately 13–15 in, these caps subtend an angle a little larger than 2 degrees in diameter. They are thus large enough to overlap the high density areas for blue cone distribution in the perifoveal retina.

What the cone distributions in the fovea and parafovea mean from a practical point of view is that perifoveal depression of the visual field can take place with considerable reduction in blue-yellow discrimination ability but without causing very much change in foveal visual acuity. (Recall that a Snellen test object in the 20/20 to 20/15 range falls well within the foveal cone matrix.) Conversely, this also means that small, focal areas of damage confined to the foveal representation in the visual field, such as is seen in solar or sun gazing retinopathy, can result in substantial reductions of visual acuity and loss of red-green discrimination but with relatively little impairment of blue-yellow discrimination.

III. PATTERNS OF DYSCHROMATOPSIA IN NEURO-OPHTHALMIC DISEASE

As originally observed by Köllner (8), primary diseases of the retina and optic nerve commonly produce dyschromatopsias that fall into patterns that are generally predictable. It is important, however, to understand that these generalizations are only relative and that there are frequent exceptions to the rules. Verriest further classified acquired dyschromatopsias and then compared them with patterns of the congenital dyschromatopsias (14). He recognized three principal types, designated by their roman numerals as I, II, and III. Type I was said to be protanlike, Type II was said to be deutanlike, and type III tritanlike. The type III, or tritanlike, acquired dyschromatopsia is one in which blue and yellow hues are confused with one another and is the pattern most commonly found in acquired diseases of the retina and choroid. Thus, retinal detachments with the macula on, cystoid macular edema, toxic retinopathies, central serous retinopathy, widespread chorioretinitis, benign concentric annular macular dystrophy, diabetic retinopathy, retinal vein occlusion, and juvenile hereditary retinoschisis have all been reported as being associated with acquired blue-yellow hue discrimination deficits (6).

It should be noted parenthetically that what most of these entities have in common is that they frequently cause damage to the peripheral portions of the central visual field with relative preservation of foveal function. The phenomenon of foveal preservation in retinal disease and especially in primary disorders of the macula has been previously noted (4,5). For a variety of reasons, both anatomical and pathophysiological damage to the macular portion of the retina, whether by primary degenerative, toxic, ischemic, or inflammatory disease, will commonly result in a perifoveal depression of the macular representation of the visual field with relative preservation of visual acuity and foveal cone function.

An example of this phenomenon is shown in Figure 7. Automated static perimetry of the central 10 degrees of the visual field (Humphrey visual field analyzer, program 10-2) in a woman with a history of prolonged use of hydroxychloroquine to treat systemic lupus erythematosus demonstrates an annular depression of the visual field at approximately 3–7 degrees of eccentricity with complete preservation of foveal sensitivity. Visual acuity recorded at the time of the field shown in Figure 7 was 20/20. Since the retinal distribution of blue cones is known to be richest in those regions most heavily damaged in such a perifoveal annular depression of the visual field, one can naturally expect that the hue discrimination ability for blue-yellow performance would be preferentially impaired in an eye with such damage. Figure 8 shows a typical type III acquired dyschromatopsia by Farnsworth-Munsell testing in a patient with hydroxychloroquine retinopathy.

By Verriest's classification, types I and II acquired dyschromatopsias are those in which an acquired protanlike or deutanlike color discrimination deficit is found. Optic nerve diseases reportedly causing typical type I and type II acquired

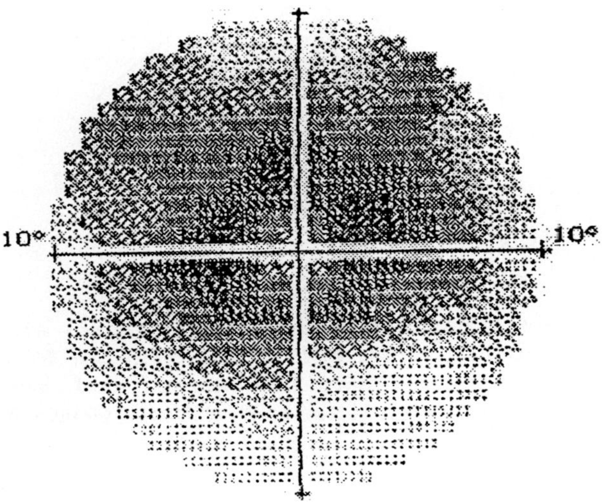

Figure 7 Static perimetry of central 10° of visual field in a patient with early hydroxychloroquine retinopathy. Notice annular extrafoveal depression of central field with relative sparing of fixation. Visual acuity 20/20, 10-2 program of Humphrey visual field analyzer with "fovea option" on. (Data courtesy of Dr. Barry Milder, St. Louis, MO.)

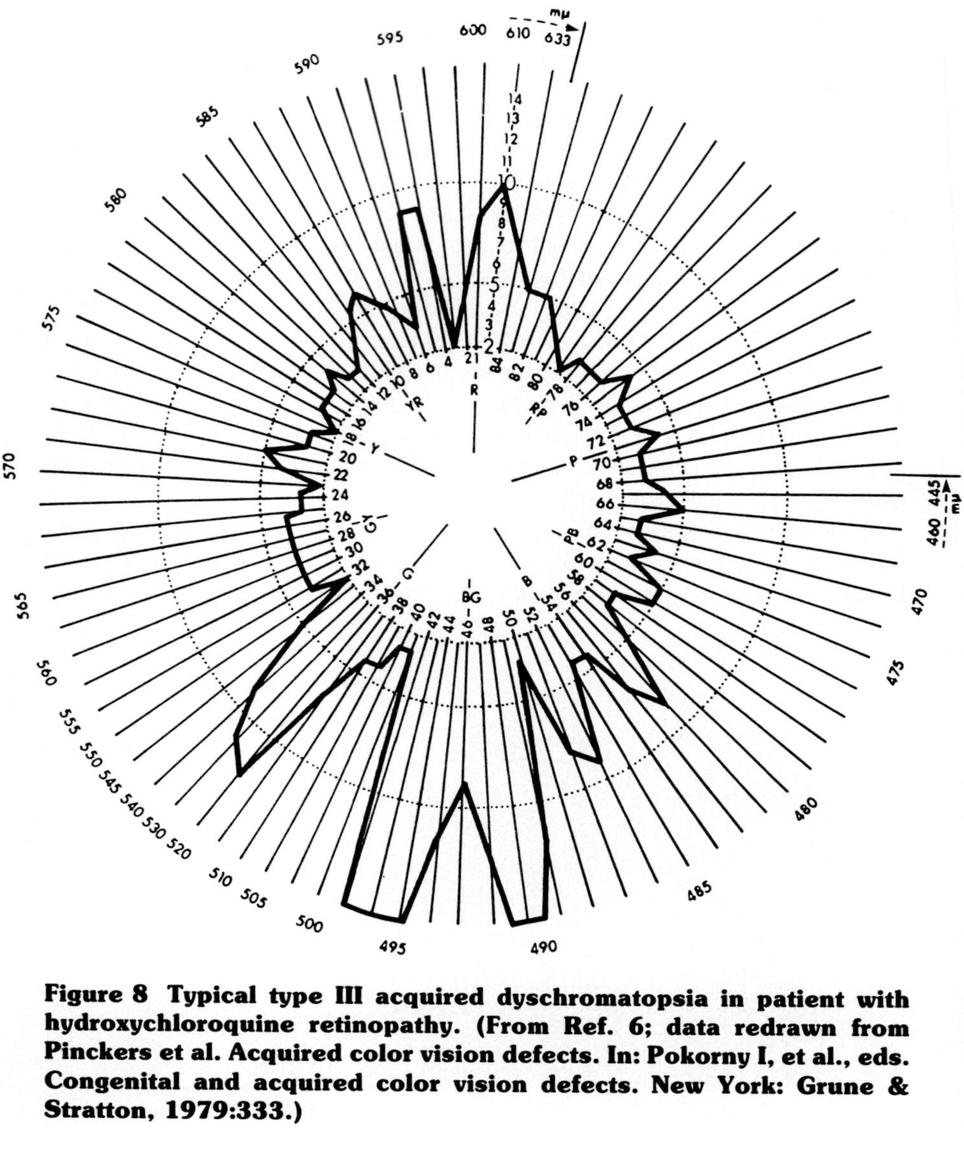

Figure 8 Typical type III acquired dyschromatopsia in patient with hydroxychloroquine retinopathy. (From Ref. 6; data redrawn from Pinckers et al. Acquired color vision defects. In: Pokorny I, et al., eds. Congenital and acquired color vision defects. New York: Grune & Stratton, 1979:333.)

dyschromatopsias include retrobulbar optic neuritis, toxic optic neuropathies, Leber's hereditary optic atrophy, and compressive and truamatic optic neuropathies. Note that these are all disorders that usually produce reductions in visual sensitivity in localized regions in the central visual field. Such central scotomas are often confined to small areas at and very close to fixation while preserving more peripheral portions of the central visual field. Figure 9 illustrates a type II, or deutanlike, acquired dyschromatopsia in a patient with the early phase of Leber's hereditary optic atophy. (Remember that both types I and II should be thought of as showing a predominance of color confusion in the red-green dimension.) In another example of acquired red-green dyschromatopsia, Figure 10 illustrates the pattern of visual field damage and color deficiency found in a patient with a macular photocoagulation scar. A central scotoma with relative preservation of extrafoveal visual field is commonly associated with an oblique axis of predominantly red-green dyschromatopsia.

Conversely, there are optic nerve diseases that are commonly associated with type III (blue-yellow or tritanlike) acquired dyschromatopsias. Such neuropathies include dominantly inherited optic atrophy, the various glaucomas and ocular hypertension, chronic papilledema, and anterior ischemic optic neuropathy. These are all conditions that also are commonly associated with relative preservation of visual acuity, which means that foveal function with its superior red-green discrimination is often spared leaving an apparent predominance of damage to blue-yellow discrimination.

IV. RATIONAL INTERPRETATION OF COLOR VISION AND VISUAL FIELD TEST RESULTS

It is necessary to put these observations into a conceptual framework that will provide a logical basis for the clinical evaluation of patients with known or suspected retinopathies or optic neuropathies. The first point to be made is that in comparing visual field and color vision test results, only the central 10 degrees of the visual field are of practical importance. For this reason, if perimetric tests are to be used in helping to sort out the problems, the conventional use of automated static perimetry in the central 30 degrees of the visual field is not ideal. Preferably, the clinician will want to use a test program that confines attention to the central 10 degrees of the visual field, such as in the 10-2 program of the Humphrey instrument.

The second point is that simple color comparison testing, confrontation perimetry with colored test objects, and pseudoisochromatic plates, although helpful for *detection* of dyschromatopsias, do not help with their classification. To sort out the relative presence or absence of a type I or II versus a type III

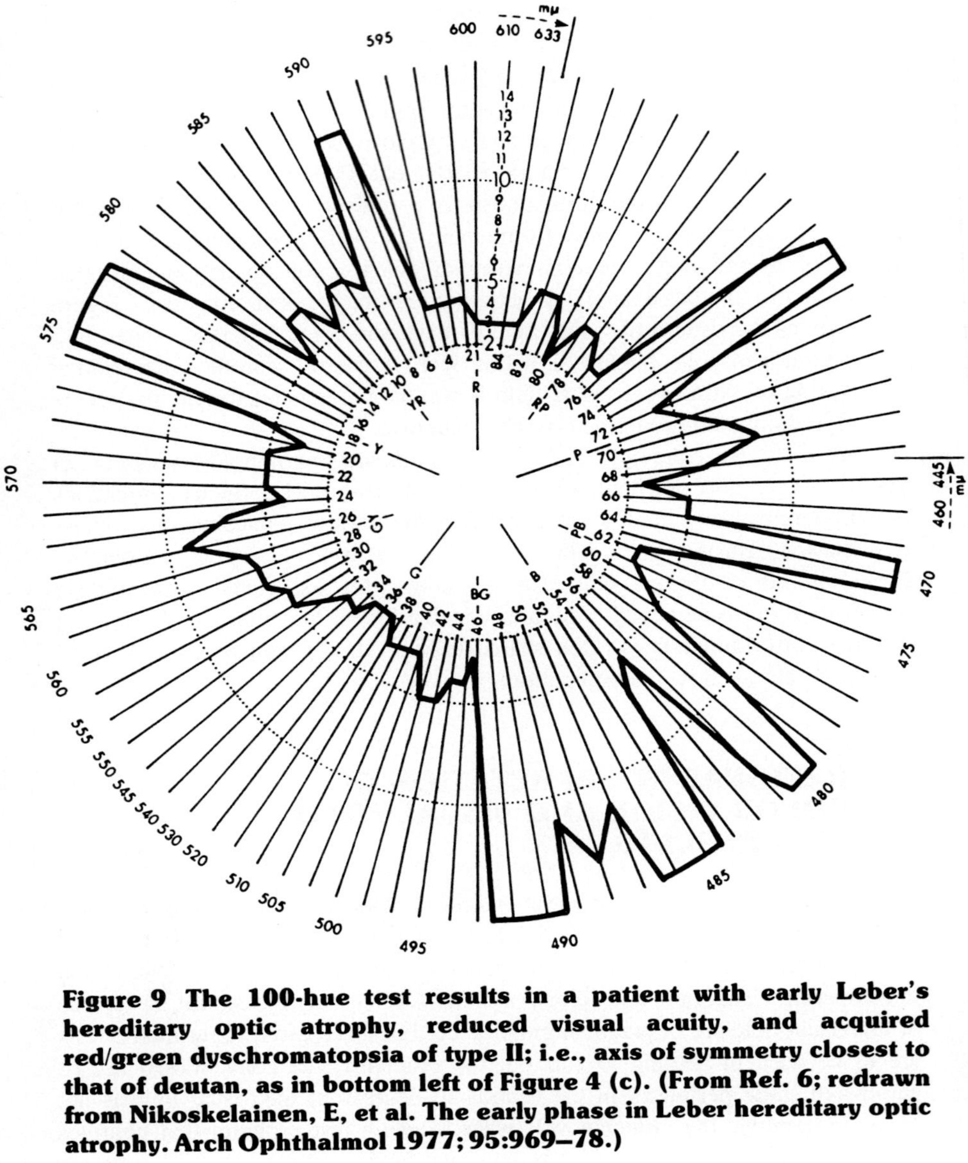

Figure 9 The 100-hue test results in a patient with early Leber's hereditary optic atrophy, reduced visual acuity, and acquired red/green dyschromatopsia of type II; i.e., axis of symmetry closest to that of deutan, as in bottom left of Figure 4 (c). (From Ref. 6; redrawn from Nikoskelainen, E, et al. The early phase in Leber hereditary optic atrophy. Arch Ophthalmol 1977; 95:969–78.)

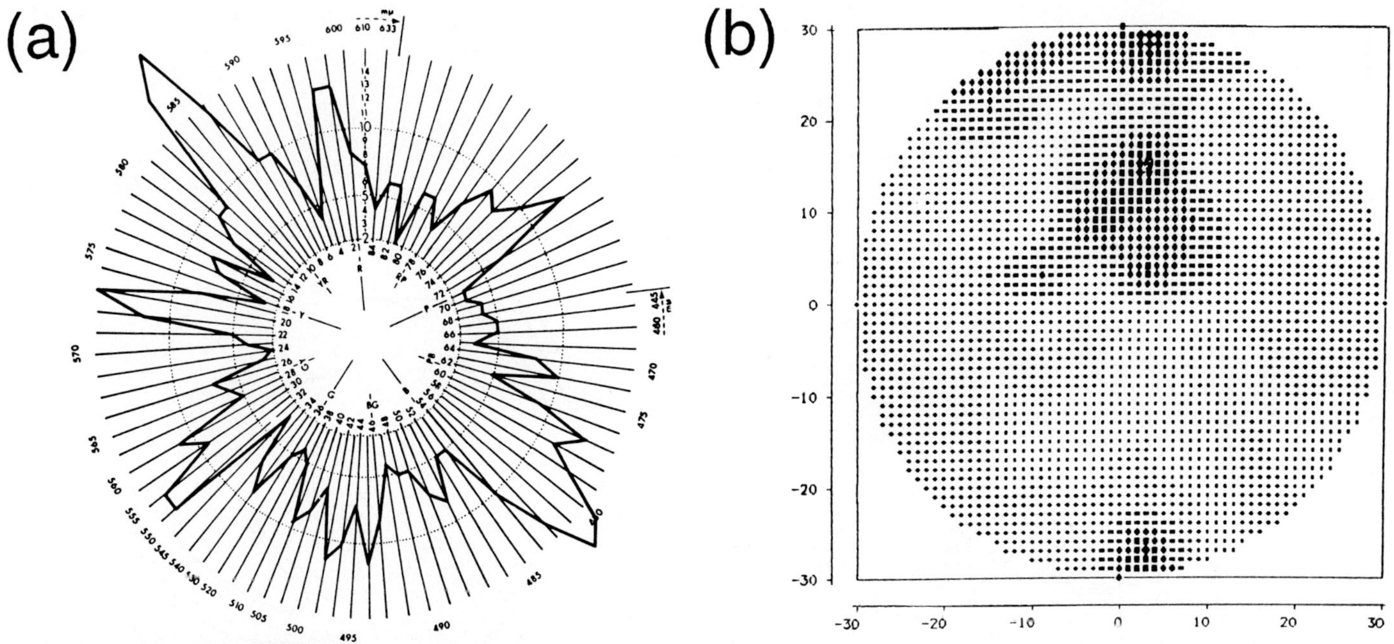

Figure 10 Acquired red/green dyschromatopsia in patient with macular photocoagulation scar and visual acuity reduced to 20/200. (a) Axis of symmetry in 100-hue test mimics that of deutan congenital dyschromatopsia. (b) Static perimetry shows central and paracentral scotoma in superior quadrant with sparing of extrafoveal macular function in other three quadrants. (c,d) Kinetic color contrast perimetry with both red and blue variant test objects shows pattern of visual field defect in central 30 degrees identical to that of threshold static luminance perimetry. (From Ref. 5.)

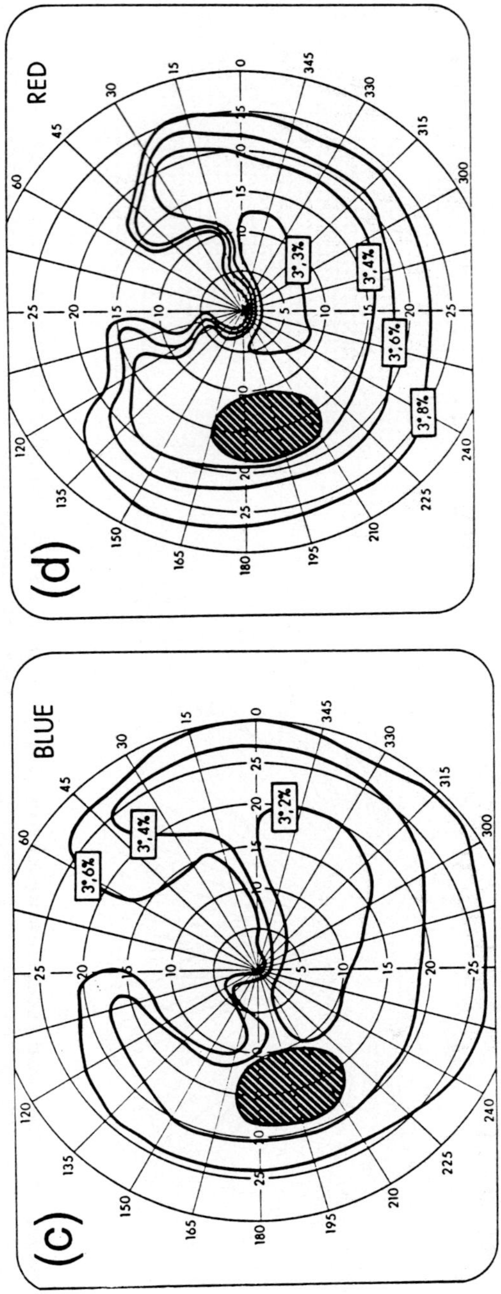

Figure 10 ***(Continued)***

acquired dyschromatopsia requires at least the use of a color sorting test such as the Farnsworth-Munsell 100-hue or the Farnsworth D-15 test.

The third point of practical importance is that the use of color testing to discriminate between retinal and neural diseases is most likely to be of practical value when one is dealing with relatively subtle disorders that do not permit an ophthalmoscopic differentiation. It is not uncommon in the early stages of neural diseases to have a largely normal appearing fundus at a time when the patient reports very distinct, characteristic changes in vision, and which changes can be reliably measured by a combination of visual acuity testing, pupillary testing, hue discrimination testing, and central static perimetry.

The fourth point to be stressed is that color vision testing is only likely to be of genuine value when it gives clearly interpretable results. In the later stages of acquired diseases, color discrimination patterns are frequently anarchic and are so poorly defined as to be virtually useless, other than to say that there is a widespread retinal or neural disorder of some sort.

Using the results of a combination of hue discrimination testing and static perimetry of the central 10 degrees of the visual field, one should be able to decide whether there has been a preferential impairment of the foveal versus the perifoveal projection of the visual field. If one has disease of the foveal projection and the retina appears normal, there is a greater likelihood that one is dealing with a primary optic neuropathy of some sort and one can concentrate attention in that direction. If on the other hand, one is dealing with greater impairment of the perifoveal projection of the visual field, and the retina appears ophthalmoscopically to be normal, one cannot assume that retinal function is normal and should investigate retinal function more carefully, such as with fluorescein angiography or maculoscopic electroretinography of macular cone function, for instance. On the other hand, if a blue-yellow defect of color vision is found in the presence of relatively good visual acuity (20/60 or better) and retinal function is normal, there is likely to be an optic neuropathy of the sort that usually spares acuity in its early stages, such as glaucoma. In this instance, one can concentrate more attention on finding supporting evidence of primary neuropathic disease.

REFERENCES

1. de Monasterio F, Schein S, McCrane E. Staining of blue-sensitive cones of the macaque retina by a fluorescent dye. Science 1981; 213:1278–81.
2. de Monasterio F, McCrane E, Newlander J, Schein S. Density profile of blue-sensitive cones along the horizontal meridian of macaque retina. Invest Ophthalmol Vis Sci 1985; 26:289–302.
3. Farnsworth D: The Farnsworth-Munsell 100-Hue Test for the examination of color discrimination. A manual. Baltimore: Munsell Color, 1949:7.
4. Hart WM Jr: Three-dimensional topography of the central visual field: Sparing of

foveal sensitivity in macular disease. Acta: XXIV International Congress of Ophthalmology. Philadelphia: Lippincott, 1983:184–9.
5. Hart WM Jr, Burde RM. Color contrast perimetry. The spatial distribution of color defects in optic nerve and retinal diseases. Ophthalmology 1985; 92:768–76.
6. Hart WM Jr. Acquired dyschromatopsias. Survey of ophthalmology 1987; 32:10–31.
7. Hurvich L: Color vision deficiencies. In: Jameson D, Hurvich L, eds. Visual psychophysics. Berlin: Springer-Verlag, 1972:582–624.
8. Köllner H: Die Störungen des Farbensinnes. Ihre klinische Bedeutung und ihre Diagnose. Berlin: Karger, 1912.
9. Lanthony P. The new color test. Doc Ophthal 1978; 46:191–9.
10. Nathans J, Thomas D, Hogness D. Molecular genetics of human color vision: the genes encoding blue, green, and red pigments. Science 1986; 232:193–202.
11. Nathans J, Piantanida T, Eddy R, Shows T, Hogness D. Molecular genetics of inherited variation in human color vision. Science 1986; 232:203–10.
12. Nathans J, Davenport C, Maumenee I, Lewis R, Hejtmancik J, Litt M, Lovrien E, Weleber R, Bachynski B, Zwas F, Klingaman R, Fishman G. Molecular genetics of human blue cone monochromancy. 1989; 245:831–838.
13. Sherman P: Colour vision in the 19th century. The Young-Helmholtz-Maxwell theory. Bristol, England: Adam Hilger, 1981.
14. Verriest G. Further studies on acquired deficiency of color discrimination. J Opt Soc Am 1963; 53:185–95.
15. Williams D, MacLeod D, Hayhoe M. Foveal tritanopia. Vision Res 1981; 21:1341–56.
16. Williams D, MacLeod D, Hayhoe M. Punctate sensitivity of the blue-sensitive mechanism. Vision Res 1981; 21:1357–75.
17. Williams D. Topography of the foveal cone mosaic in the living human eye. Vision Res 1988; 28:433–54.

7

Traumatic Optic Neuropathies

Thomas C. Spoor and John G. McHenry
Wayne State University, Detroit, Michigan

The optic nerve may be divided into four sections: intraocular, intraorbital, intracanalicular, and intracranial (Fig. 1). The optic nerve may be injured anywhere along its course by contussive or penetrating oribitocranial injuries.

I. OPTIC NERVE COMPRESSION: Orbital Hemorrhage

Evaluating patients with traumatic optic neuropathies first entails detection and treatment of reversible causes of optic nerve dysfunction. Subperiosteal and intraorbital hemorrhages, if detected, are readily treatable causes of traumatic optic neuropathies. Subperiosteal hemorrhages in the orbit may resolve spontaneously; however, if optic nerve function is compromised, the hemorrhage may be surgically evacuated. This is particularly indicated in the face of worsening optic nerve function or failure to show spontaneous improvement.

A. Case 1

A 10-year-old boy was injured in a motor vehicle accident and rendered unconscious. On regaining consciousness, he complained of decreased vision in the left eye (Fig. 2). Examination revealed visual acuity decreased to 20/40, an afferent pupillary defect, and a swollen left optic disc. Computed tomography

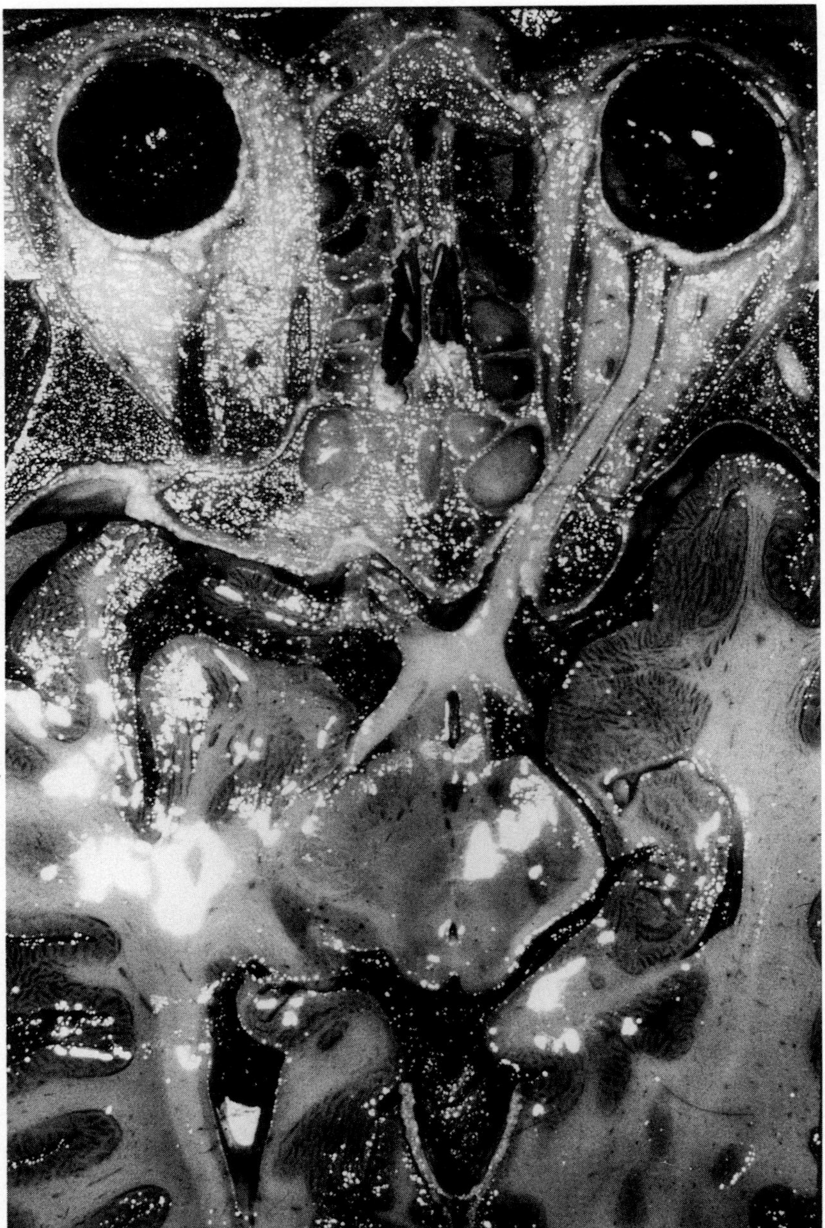

Figure 1 Axial cadaver section demonstrating course and sections of optic nerve.

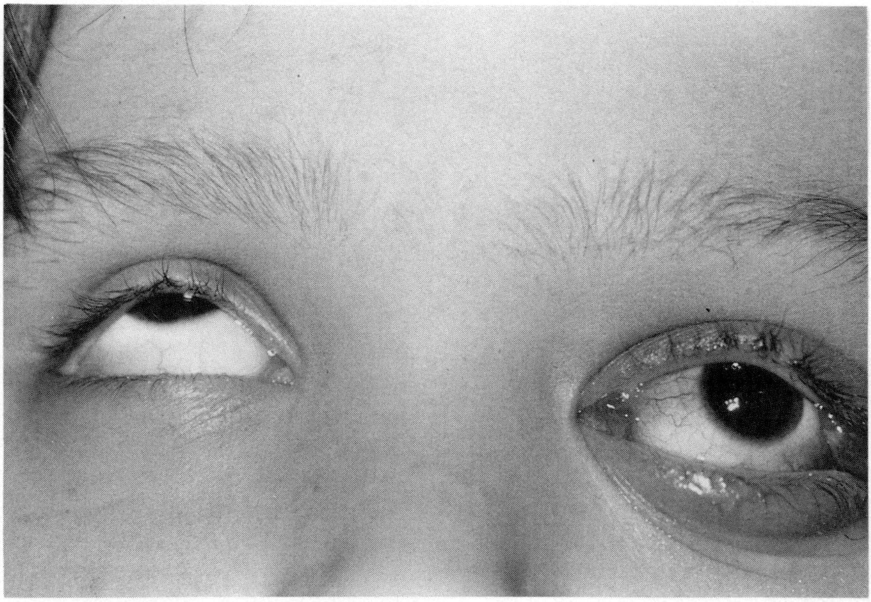

Figure 2 Subperiosteal hemorrhage in left superior orbit.

(CT) of the orbits demonstrated a large subperiosteal mass in the superior orbit (Fig. 3). Surgical exploration confirmed a subperiosteal hematoma, which was evacuated. Visual acuity returned to normal postoperatively, and the optic disc swelling regressed.

Subperiosteal hemorrhages are easy to treat surgically, and since they are confined to the subperiosteal space, morbidity is minimal. In a case like that described, a subbrow incision is made in the superotemporal orbit. The periosteum is incised and reflected over the orbital rim. The hemorrhage is located and evacuated with suction (Fig. 4). The bony surface is then inspected for bleeding or cerebrospinal fluid (CSF) leaks and bleeding. Both may be repaired by applications of surgical and bone wax. The periosteum is closed with absorbable sutures. A Penrose drain may be placed but usually is not necessary if adequate hemostasis is obtained. The subcutaneous tissue is closed with a buried 5-0 absorbable suture, and the skin is closed in a cosmetically acceptable fashion.

Intraorbital hemorrhages may be more difficult to manage. If there is no significant elevation of orbital pressure and no evidence for optic nerve compression or impending central retinal artery occlusion, patients may be observed and the hemorrhages allowed to resolve spontaneously. If visual function is threatened or compromised, however, intraorbital pressure must be

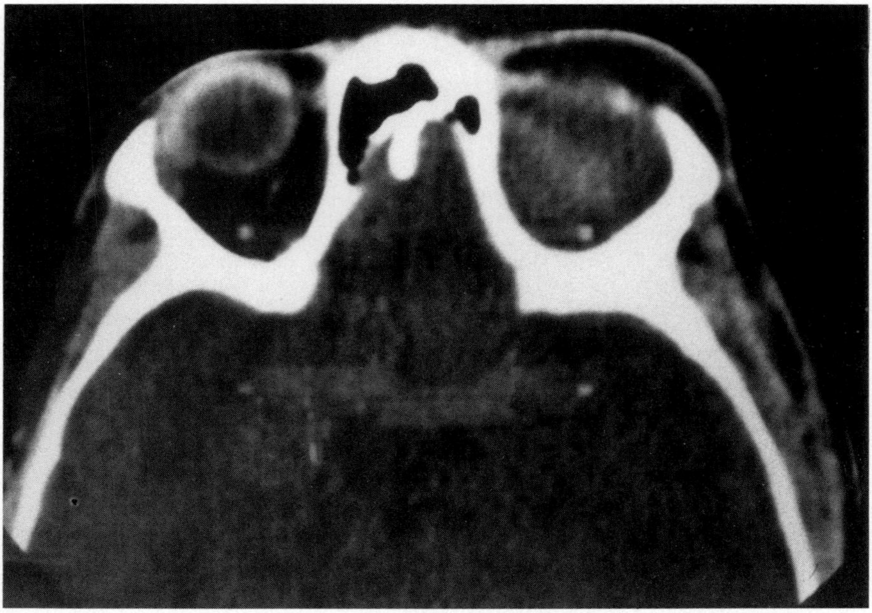

(a)

Figure 3 CT scan demonstrating subperiosteal hemorrhage left orbit. (a) Axial. (b) Coronal.

lowered expeditiously. A lateral canthotomy and cantholysis may be easily accomplished at the bedside. After infiltration of the lateral aspects of the upper and lower eyelids and lateral canthus with local anesthetic, the lateral canthus is crushed with a hemostat and incised with scissors. The lower eyelid is reflected, and the inferior crus of the lateral canthal tendon is incised with scissors. This usually markedly reduces intraorbital pressure and restores visual function. If this is unsuccessful, the superior crus of the lateral canthal tendon may be incised in a similar fashion.

After performing a lateral canthotomy with or without cantholysis, it is necessary to follow the patient diligently to detect recurrent hemorrhage.

B. Case 2

A 30-year-old man received multiple blows to the face with a baseball bat. Visual acuity was counting fingers in the right eye and 20/30 in the left eye. Intraocular pressures were 70 and 36. There was massive proptosis in both eyes. No hyphema, vitreous hemorrhage, or choroidal rupture was noted. The CT scan showed no fractures. Lateral canthotomies with inferior cantholysis were performed in both eyes, with a diminution of intraocular pressure to 28 and 20, respectively. Visual

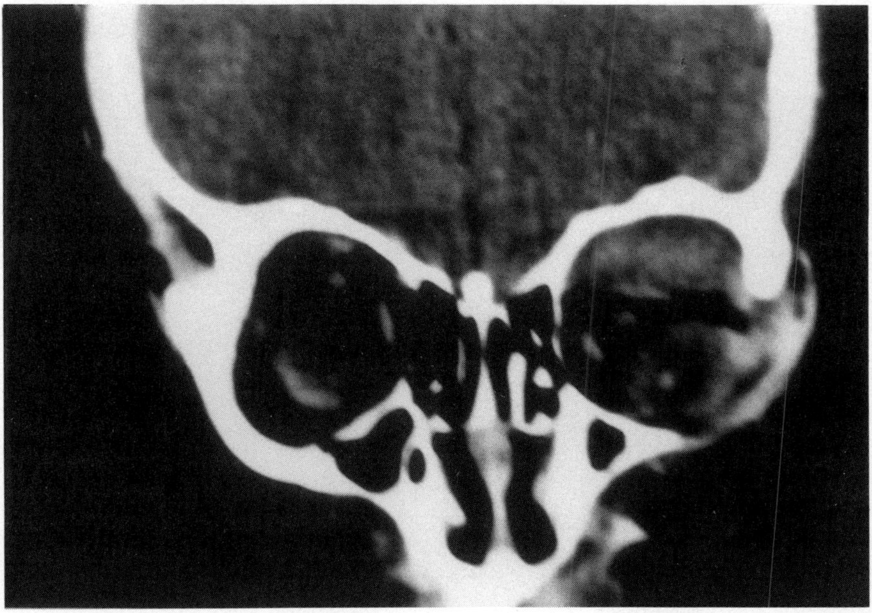

(b)

acuity improved to 20/200, and the proptosis was reduced. Forty-eight hours after the canthotomy, hemorrhage recurred in the right orbital causing a return of the proptosis and a decrease in the visual acuity to counting fingers. Cantholysis was again performed. Two days later, visual acuity was 20/80.

Recurrent retrobulbar hemorrhages may be a sign of systemic blood clotting abnormality, and a hemorrhage evaluation might be helpful.

C. Case 3

A 38-year-old man with a history of alcohol abuse was struck in the face with a 2 × 4 board. He had a retrobulbar hemorrhage with counting fingers vision and an afferent pupillary defect. A lateral canthotomy with cantholysis was performed. Bleeding continued for 36 h. Twelve hours after the bleeding stopped, the patient blew his nose and the retrobulbar hemorrhage reaccumulated. The patient's prothrombin time was 18. Lateral canthotomy with cantholysis was again performed. Vitamin K improved his coagulation time, and the patient had no further bleeding.

Rarely, if canthotomy and cantholysis are unsuccessful, bony orbital decompression, as done for dysthyroid orbitopathy, may be performed emergently. This may be accomplished transiently or via a cul-de-sac and direct external ethmoidectomy approach.

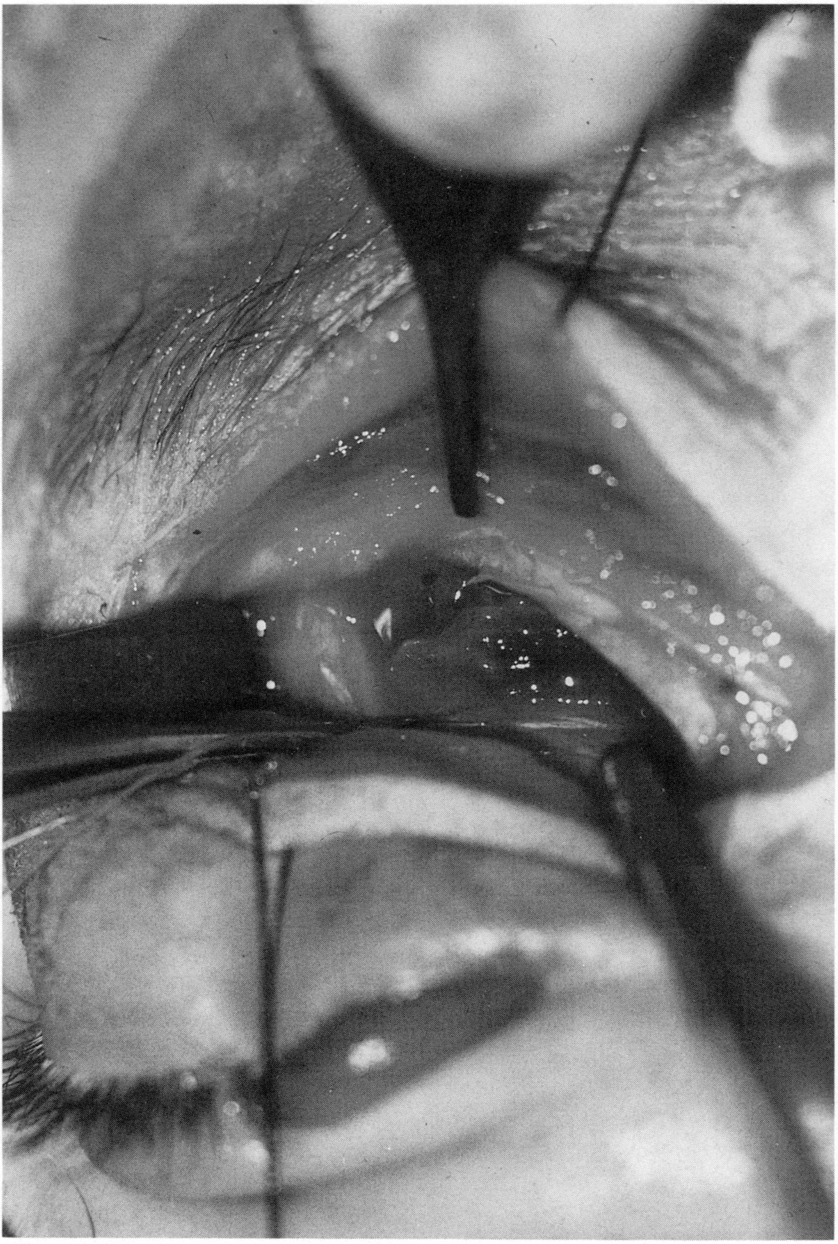

Figure 4 Evacuation of subperiosteal hemorrhage.

II. OPTIC NERVE SHEATH HEMORRHAGES

The optic nerve may be compressed by an accumulation of blood within the optic nerve sheath. Patients may have slowly progressive visual loss with a fundus resembling a central retinal vein occlusion (1) or marked visual loss and an optic nerve that appears swollen or normal. CT demonstrates a mildly enlarged optic nerve (Fig. 5). Even if the optic nerve appears mildly enlarged on CT, this is significant. Standardized echography of the optic nerve will demonstrate a positive 30-degree test indicating fluid accumulation between the optic nerve and its meningeal sheaths (Fig. 6). Prompt optic nerve sheath fenestration allows evacuation of blood and restoration of visual function.

III. DIRECT OPTIC NERVE INJURY

Direct injuries to the optic nerve by penetrating foreign bodies are rarely treatable. Visual loss is sudden and irreversible and result from total or partial transection of the nerve (Fig. 7). The fundus is initially normal with posterior optic nerve injuries. Patients with anterior optic nerve injuries have signs of optic nerve

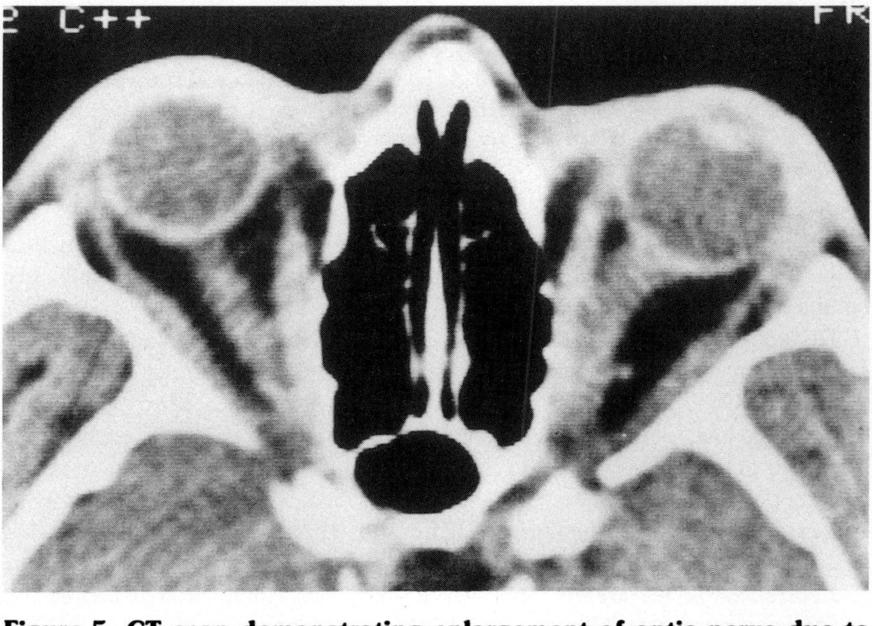

Figure 5 CT scan demonstrating enlargement of optic nerve due to hemorrhage within optic nerve sheath.

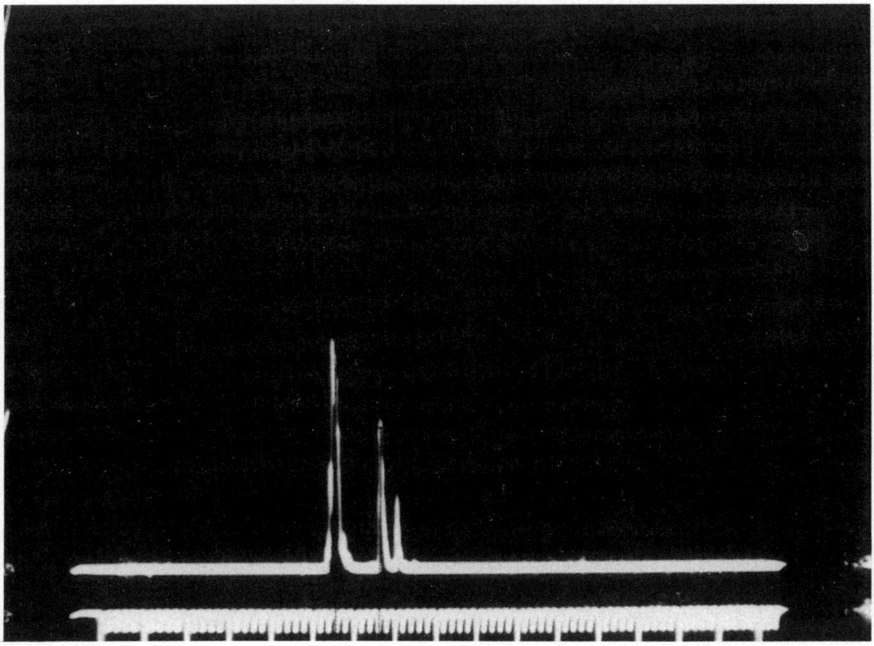

(a)

Figure 6 (a) Standardized echography demonstrates enlargement of left optic nerve. (b) Positive 30-degree test. Repeat echography with eye in 30 degrees of abduction demonstrates significantly smaller optic nerve sheath diameter as a result of fluid shift.

dysfunction and an abnormal-appearing fundus (Fig. 8). This is particularly true if the injury is to the intraocular optic nerve or to the optic nerve immediately behind the globe.

Disruption of the central retinal artery has a distinctive clinical picture of retinal edema, venous sludging, a cherry red spot, and arteriolar attenuation. Disruption of the posterior ciliary circulation may be evidenced by peripapillary hemorrhage and edema at the posterior pole or optic disc swelling secondary to traumatic anterior ischemic optic neuropathy (Fig. 8). Partial avulsion of the optic nerve from the globe appears as an anterior marginal tear and is initially evident as a peripapillary hemorrhage that resolves after several weeks and leaves a doubly pigmented scar and mild optic dystrophy. Visual loss is usually severe and correlated to the area of optic nerve injury (2). Complete avulsion of the optic nerve causes total blindness and a distinctive fundus appearance of a round hole in sclera that fills in with gliotic tissue over several months.

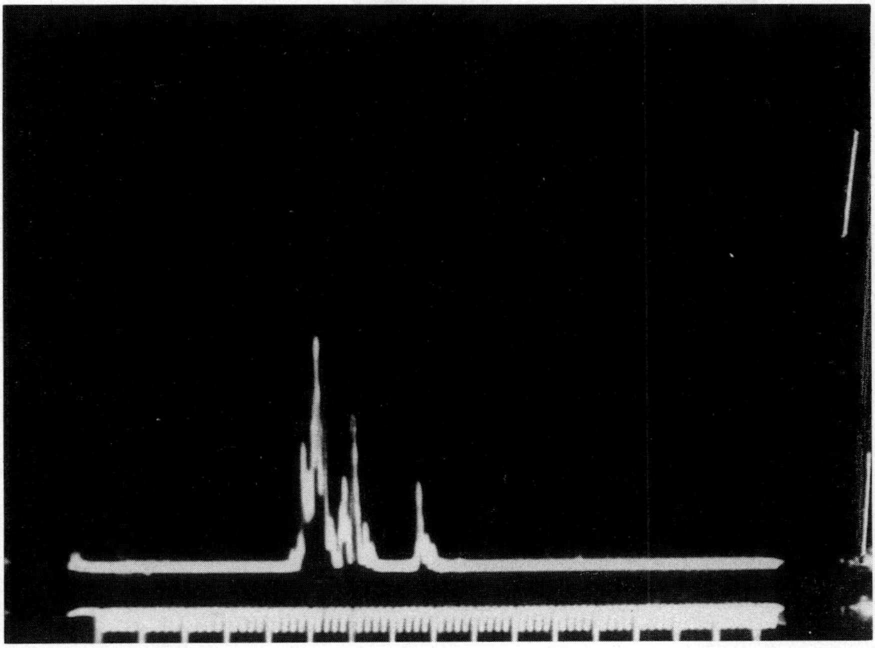

(b)

Patients with posterior optic nerve injuries have evidence for optic nerve dysfunction (decreased vision, visual field defects, and an afferent pupillary defect) in spite of a normal-appearing fundus. Optic atrophy and nerve fiber layer dropout will become evident in 4–8 h. One of the most tragic types of optic nerve avulsion is iatrogenic and may occur during sinus surgery.

A. Case 4

A 48-year-old physician was undergoing removal of a maxillary sinus polyp. Profuse bleeding occurred, obscuring the landmarks. At the conclusion of the procedure, the left pupil was fixed and dilated. Ophthalmological consultation was requested and the patient evaluated in the operating room. There was pallid edema of the optic nerve and a nonperfused ischemic fundus (Fig. 9). Pathological examination revealed optic nerve, orbital fat, and extraocular muscle in the specimen. Although the patient was placed on intravenous megadose steroids, there was no improvement in vision from NLP. Postoperative CT demonstrated total optic nerve transection (Fig. 10).

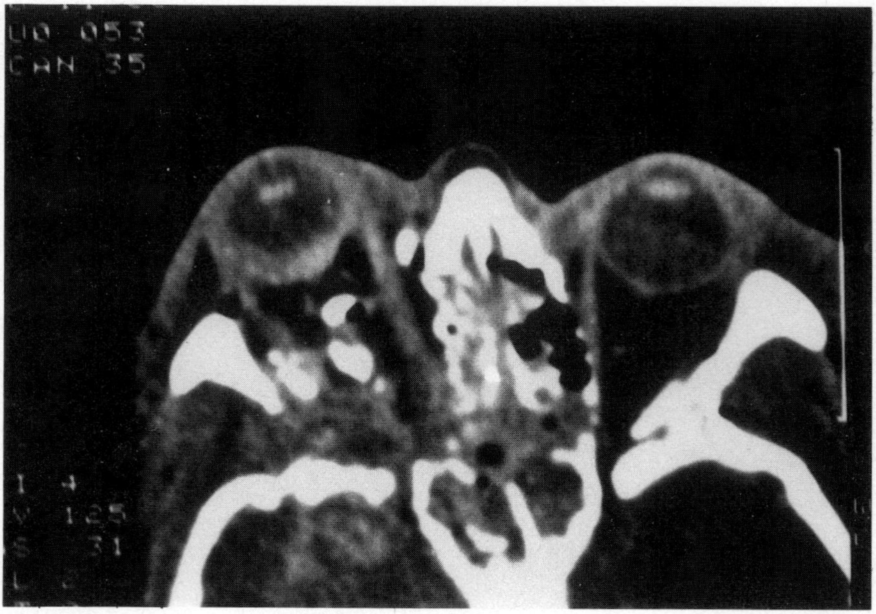

(a)

Figure 7 CT scan demonstrating transection of optic nerve by bullet fragment. (a) Axial. (b) Coronal.

IV. INDIRECT OPTIC NERVE INJURY

No consensus exists as to the appropriate treatment for patients with indirect optic nerve trauma secondary to blunt facial or cranial injury. Optic nerve injury occurs in 4% of patients sustaining midfacial, supraorbital, or frontal sinus fractures (3). Multiple pathophysiological mechanisms may cause indirect injury to the optic nerve, but some may be evident only at autopsy.

After studying the optic nerves from 70 patients dying from head trauma, Walsh (4) differentiated primary from secondary optic nerve injuries. Primary injury mechanisms include hemorrhage in the optic nerve or its sheath, lacerations of the nerve or sheaths, and contusion necrosis of the optic nerve. Secondary mechanisms of injury include optic nerve edema and necrosis or infarction resulting from vascular obstruction, local compression of vessels, or circulatory failure. Shearing injury of individual examinations may also produce secondary edema, further compromising the undamaged nerve fiber.

Imachi and coworkers (5) found intraneural and nerve sheath hemorrhages in a large percentage of patients with indirect optic nerve injury. Other mechanisms

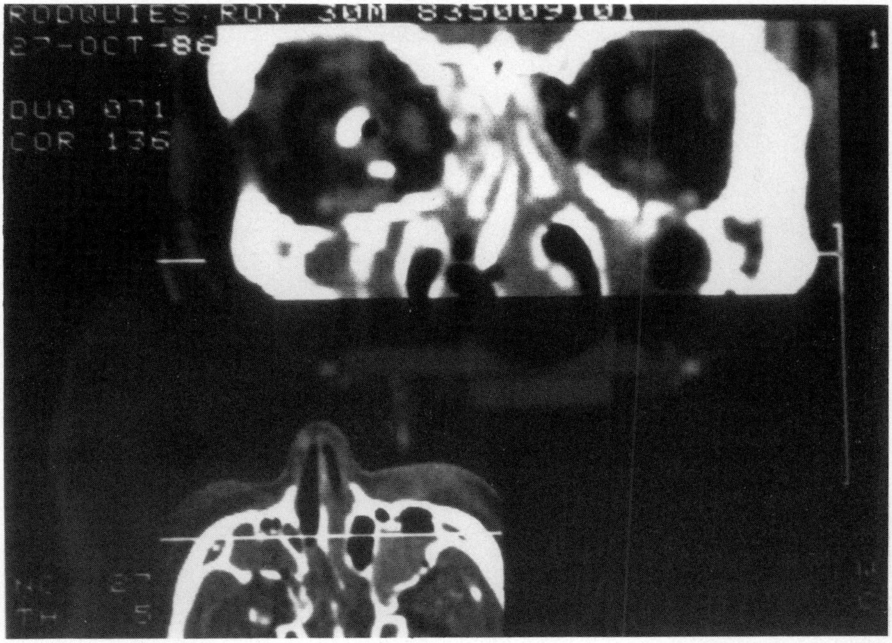

(b)

included partial or complete tears in the nerve and optic canal features, both with and without optic nerve compression.

In some cases, the mechanism of injury is obvious. CT demonstrates an orbital or canalicular fracture compressing or lacerating the optic nerve or disrupting its blood supply (Fig. 11). Visual loss may be sudden and total or slow and progressive. Most agree that patients with progressive visual loss and a demonstrable optic canal fracture should be treated with corticosteroids and offered surgical decompression of their optic canal by a transethmoidal or transcranial approach (6). Documented delayed progressive visual loss caused by indirect optic nerve injury is a definite indication for optic canal decompression (2).

There is no consensus regarding appropriate treatment for patients sustaining sudden severe visual loss at the time of injury with or without a demonstrable optic canal feature. We can only speculate as to the mechanism of injury in patients sustaining traumatic optic neuropathies with no evidence for canalicular fracture. One theory suggests that the optic nerve or its blood supply is torn at the canalicular entrance to the orbit because of continued momentum of the eye and optic nerve as the head suddenly decelerates on impact (6). A recent case report describes a traumatic optic neuropathy secondary to a static force applied

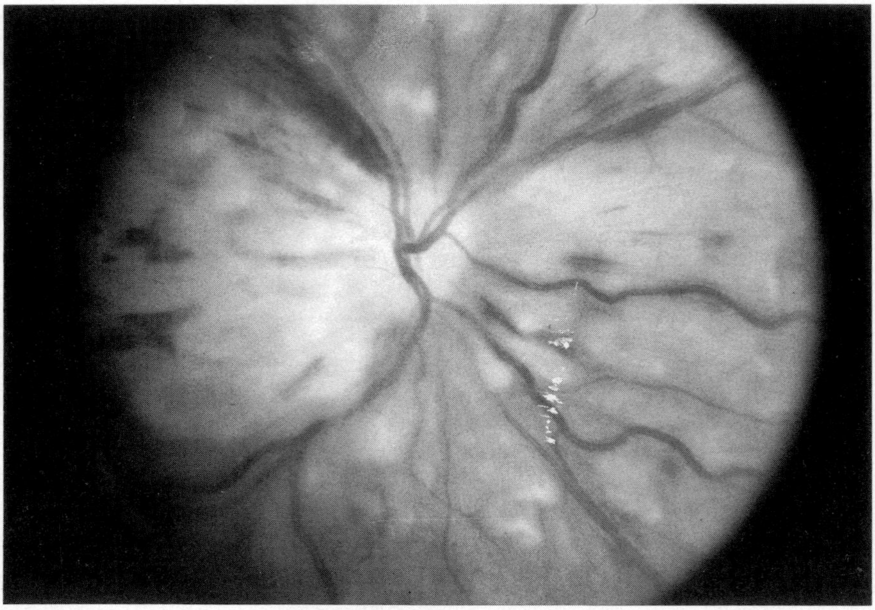

Figure 8 Injury to anterior optic nerve compromising blood supply to posterior globe.

to the supraorbital region (barbell) (7). In most cases, the mechanism of indirect injury to the optic nerve is probably secondary to a combination of both sudden deceleration and orbital bone deformation (6).

In the past, a patient with a history of immediate visual loss following trauma was presumed to have an optic nerve avulsion or infarction, and no treatment was instituted. However, a patient with slowly progressive visual loss following blunt orbitocranial trauma was suspected to have a compressive injury to the optic nerve that was possibly amenable to treatment, with a potential recovery of some or all of the visual deficit. Therefore, a much more aggressive diagnostic and therapeutic regimen was instituted. Neuroradiological search for optic canal fractures was performed, and the patient was treated with intravenous corticosteroids in the interim. If an optic canal fracture was present, surgical decompression was often attempted.

Accurate description of the temporal course of visual loss is often unavailable. Many patients are unconscious, intoxicated with drugs or alcohol, or otherwise uncooperative. We treat all patients with traumatic optic neuropathies with a course of intravenous megadose corticosteroids while they undergo neuroradiological evaluation and stabilization.

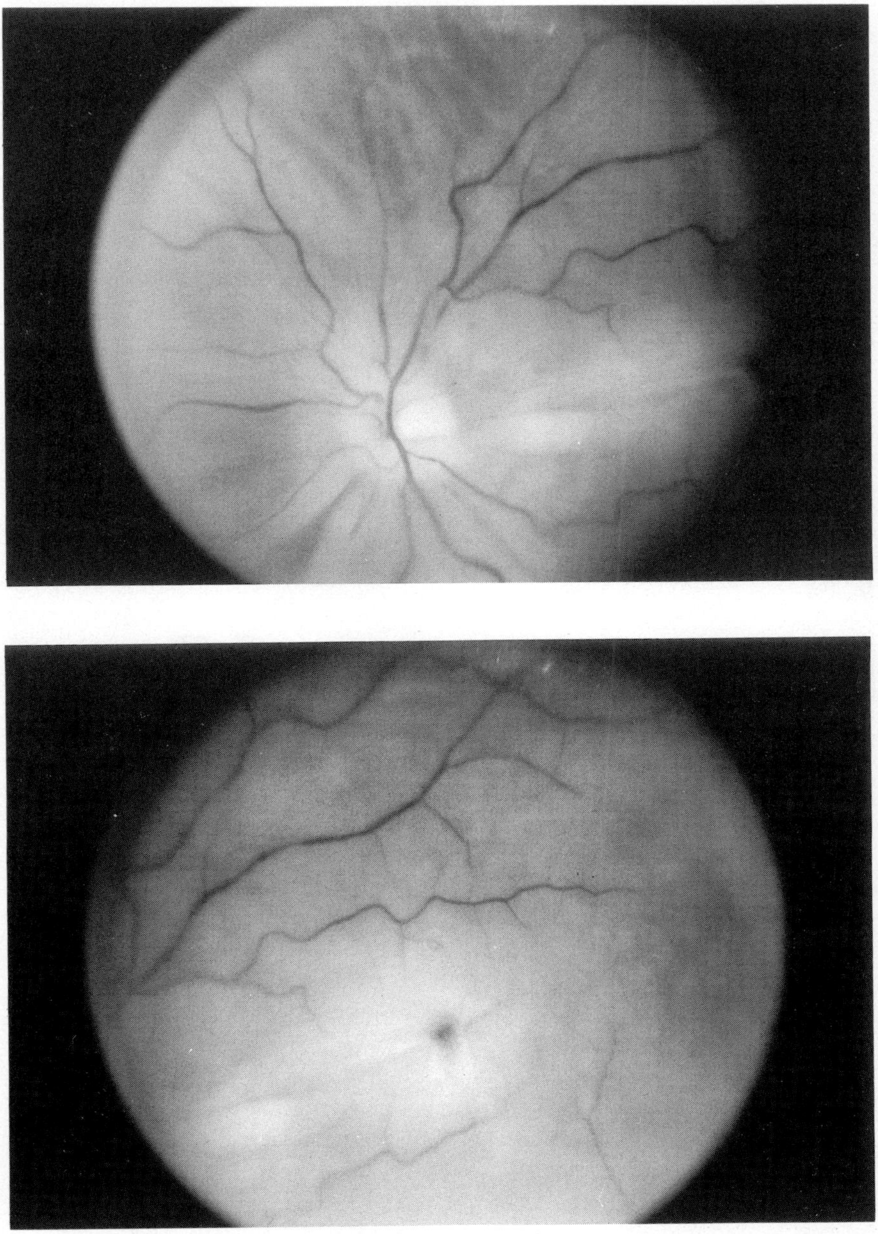

Figure 9 Fundus appearance 48 h after iatrogenic transection of intraorbital optic nerve.

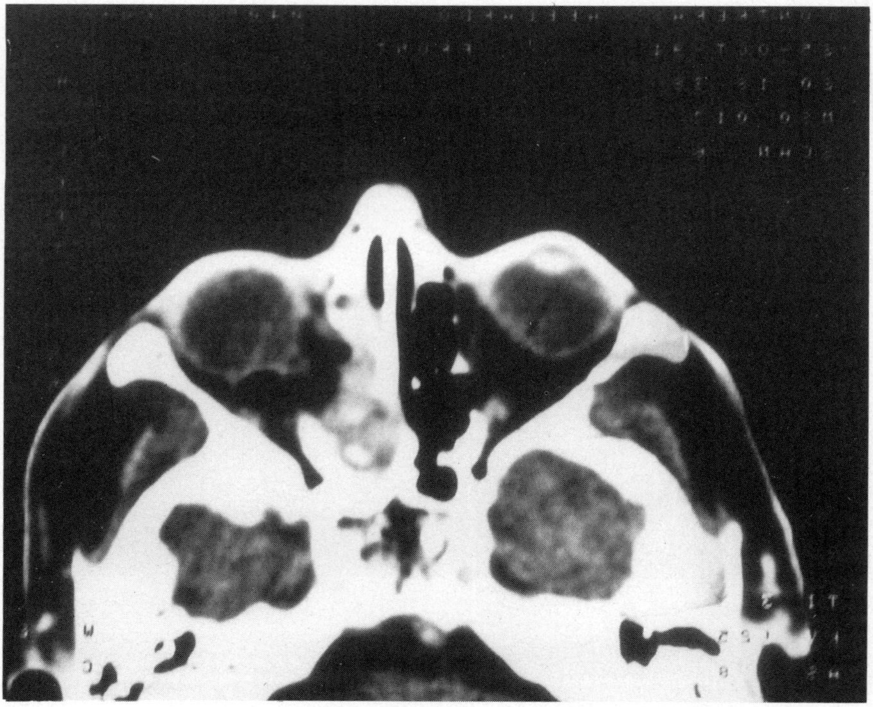

Figure 10 CT scan demonstrates transection of intraorbital optic nerve.

No good data are available to guide the clinician to the proper treatment regimen, nor is there consensus as to the proper treatment of traumatic optic neuropathies. A recent review of indirect optic nerve injury again documents improvement in both treated and untreated patients and return of vision in some eyes that showed no light perception (8). Multiple anecdotal cases described return of vision in initially blind eyes untreated, treated with megadose corticosteroids, and treated with decompression of the optic canal. Total blindness immediately after injury does not negate possible return of vision and should not be a contraindication to aggressive medical and surgical management (8–10).

A review by Joseph et al. indicates that patients treated with corticosteroids and transethmoidal optic canal decompression had better visual recovery than patients treated with corticosteroids alone or left untreated (10). Unfortunately, there is no controlled, double-blind study comparing these treatment modalities. These injuries are sufficiently uncommon that there is unlikely to be such a study. Consequently, we treat most traumatic optic neuropathies in otherwise healthy

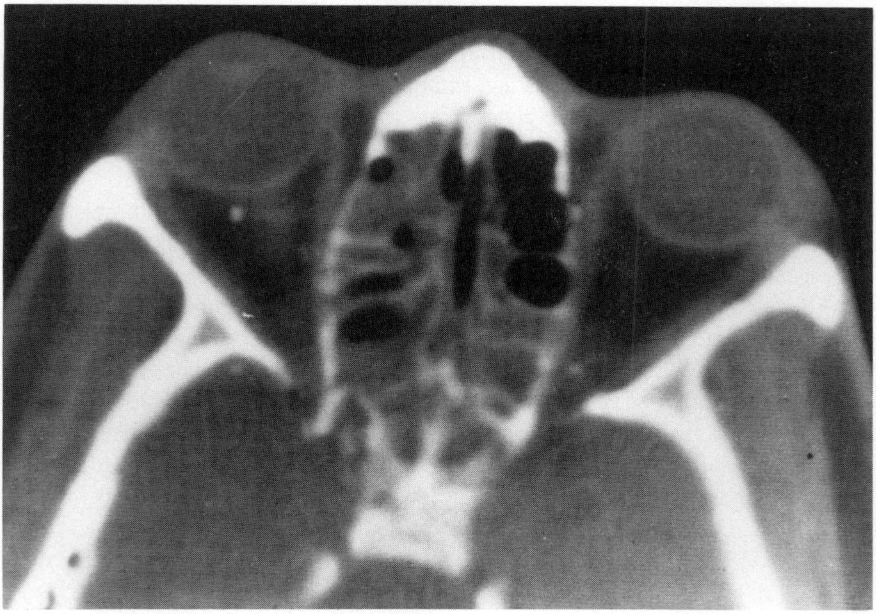

Figure 11 CT scan demonstrating fracture of medial wall of optic canal.

patients realizing that some spontaneous recovery of vision may occur in 29–50% of cases (11–13). Some patients with compressive optic neuropathy are responsive to medical and/or surgical treatment, and identifying this subset of traumatic optic neuropathy is difficult. Most patients with traumatic optic neuropathy should be treated in the hope that they will attain their maximum visual potential. Patients with obvious anterior optic nerve injuries (i.e., avulsion, infarction, or retinal artery occlusion) will not benefit from treatment (see Figs. 7 and 8).

Patients with negative neuroradiological studies and traumatic optic neuropathies are given a trial of intravenous high-dose corticosteroids immediately after the injury. A loading dose of 30 mg/kg intravenous dose is given 2 h later, followed by 15 mg/kg every 6 h. Rigorous maintenance dosing is required to maintain the pharmacological effect on the injured central nervous system (CNS) (14). Megadose corticosteroids have a different mechanism of action from pharmacological doses. By normalizing calcium transport and preventing phospholipase production, they reduce CNS edema, microcirculatory spasm, and neural necrosis and thereby allow the small nutrient vessels that feed the nerve to regain patency (9,14,15). If no subjective or objective visual improvement is seen within 48 h, therapy is discontinued. When a positive response occurs, the regimen is continued for a total of 3 days and then rapidly tapered. Our experience indicates that megadose corticosteroids benefit patients with indirect optic nerve injury secondary to blunt trauma and sometimes benefit patients with direct optic nerve injury resulting from penetrating trauma. We have had no serious complications treating these acutely injured patients with a short course of megadose methylprednisolone (9).

To prevent possible gastrointestinal bleeding, we concurrently administer H_2 blockers (ranitidine 150 mg twice a day), especially in at-risk patients taking aspirin or nonsteroidal anti-inflammatory agents. Traumatic optic neuropathy may coexist with ocular injuries, including hyphemas and traumatic cataracts. Patients who have afferent pupillary defects along with other ocular injuries may be considered for treatment of their traumatic optic neuropathy, with intravenous megadose corticosteroids, optic nerve sheath decompression, or optic canal decompression.

In unconscious and semiconscious patients with traumatic optic neuropathy, the regimen delineated above is initiated and the patient followed with frequent repeat examinations and the appropriate neuroradiological examinations as soon as possible. Unchanged quantitative relative afferent pupillary defect (measured with neutral density filters), visual evoked potential (VEP), or visual acuity (if obtainable) after 24–48 h of treatment is an indication to discontinue the therapy. If improvement occurs, therapy is continued for a total of 3 days. Citing experience with acute spinal cord injuries, a case can be made to use megadose corticosteroids for only 24 h (16). This maximizes these metabolic effects and minimizes their immunosuppressive activity. Visual acuity will usually stabilize by this time if treatment is successful. Visual function may continue to improve for weeks after cessation of corticosteroids therapy. Deterioration of vision after cessation of therapy warrants reinstitution of corticosteroids followed by optic canal decompression.

A. Case 5

A 32-year-old man was struck with a board across the right orbit. Visual acuity was 20/800 in the right eye with an afferent pupillary defect and a normal-appearing fundus. Computed tomography was normal.

After 48 h of megadose corticosteroids, visual acuity improved to 20/30 and automated perimetry was performed (Fig. 12). Twenty-four hours later, while receiving 250 mg intravenous methylprednisolone every 6 h, visual acuity in the right eye deteriorated to counting fingers, and the visual field deteriorated (Fig. 13). An expeditious extracranial optic canal decompression was performed with marked improvement in visual function (Fig. 14).

Traumatic optic neuropathies with neuroradiological signs of injury to the nerve (i.e., canalicular fracture or bone spicule impinging on the nerve itself) (see Fig. 11) warrant surgical decompression with a perioperative course of

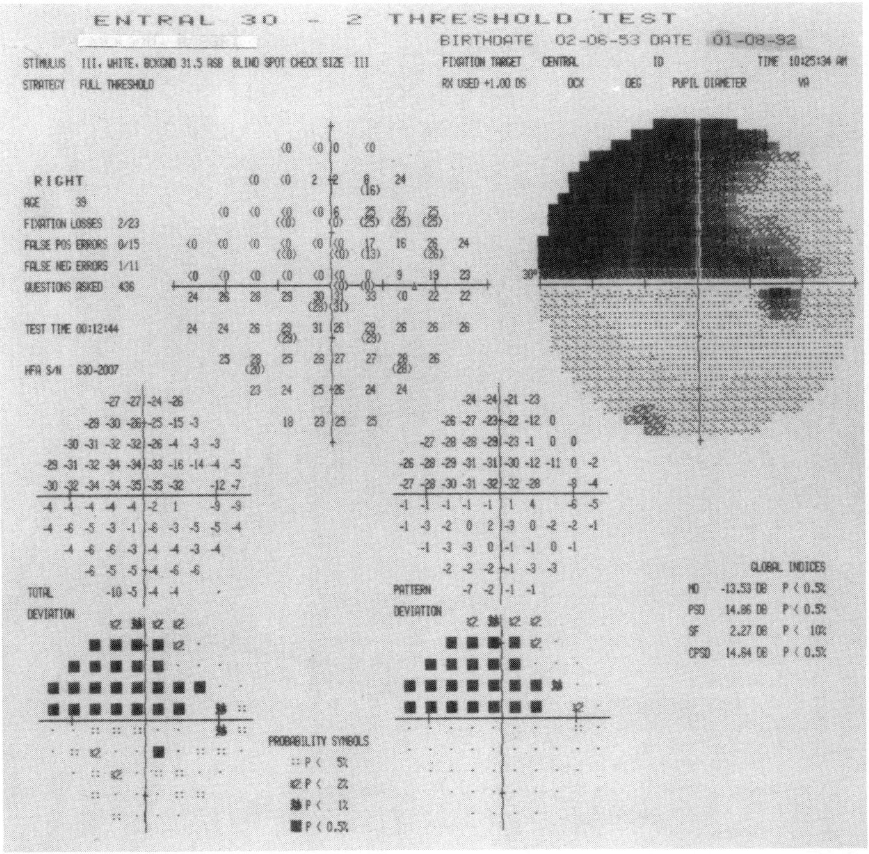

Figure 12 Automated perimetry (Humphrey 30-2) demonstrating superior altitudinal defect secondary to traumatic optic neuropathy.

intravenous corticosteroids. A narrowing of the optic foramen in the presence of a traumatic optic neuropathy with a medical orbital wall fracture that is unresponsive to intravenous steroids should also be surgically explored. Patients with traumatic optic neuropathies with delayed or progressive visual loss unresponsive to intravenous steroids may also be surgically explored and decompressed. In traumatic optic neuropathies with delayed or progressive visual loss unresponsive to steroids or deteriorating during treatment with or after the withdrawal of steroids, optic canal decompression is indicated.

Optic canal decompression involves removal of the roof or medial wall of the optic canal. In the past, this was performed via frontal craniotomy. This approach to optic canal decompression requires a neurosurgeon, and early consultation

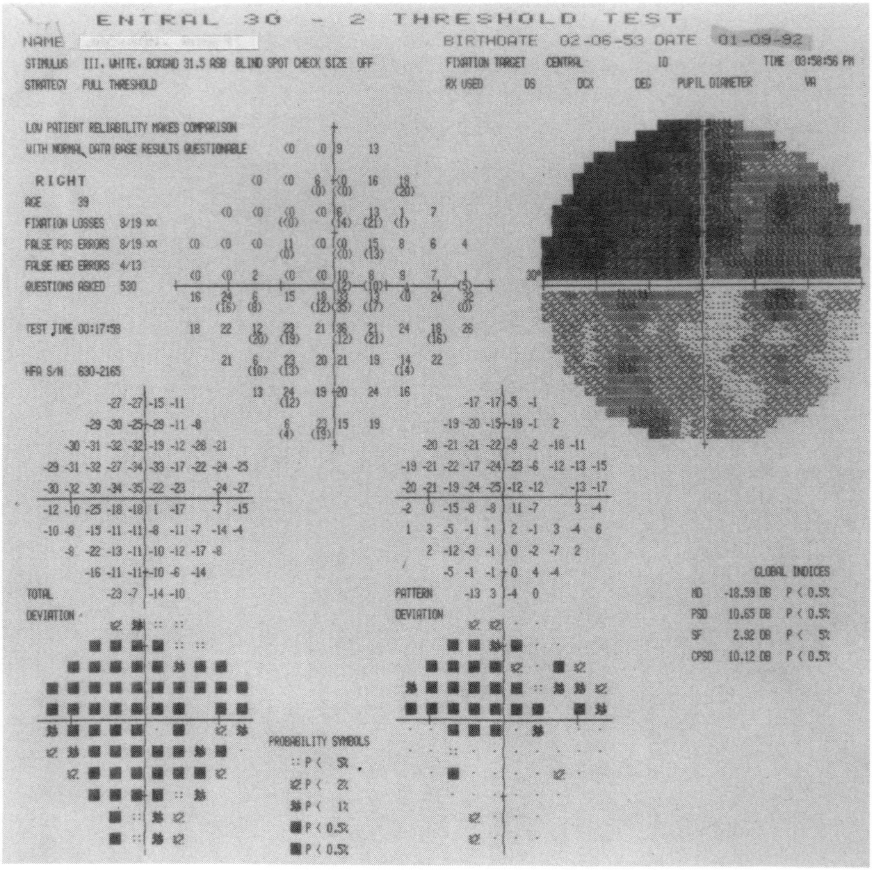

Figure 13 Deterioration of visual field after tapering megadose corticosteroids.

should be sought to expedite this therapy if needed. Neurosurgeons are often reticent to perform transcranial optic canal decompression in patients with closed head injury, elevated intracranial pressure, and cerebral edema. Retraction on a contused frontal lobe may produce infarction. Extracranial optic canal decompression may be accomplished via a transantral, transnasal, or external ethmoidectomy approach. We advocate external ethmoidectomy with removal of the medial wall of the optic canal. This procedure can be performed by a surgeon familiar with ethmoid and sphenoid sinus anatomy. This approach affords good exposure and permits visualization of the involved anatomy (10,17). We have anecdotal cases where decompression has been performed in eyes unresponsive to megadose corticosteroids with resultant recovery of vision (18).

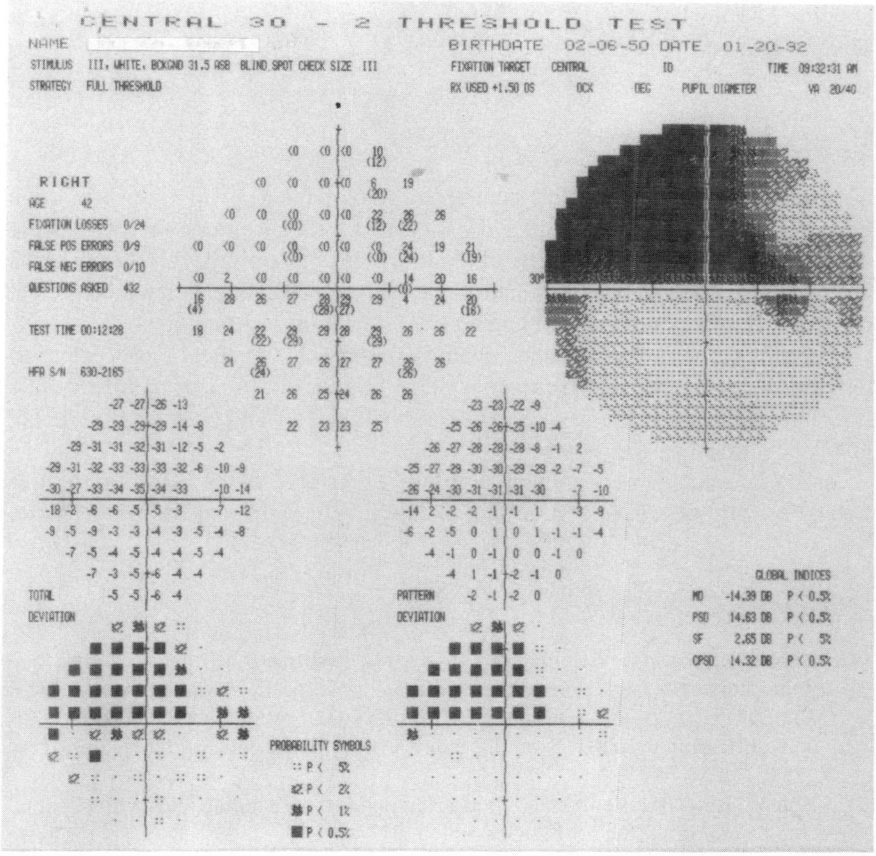

Figure 14 Improvement in visual field following optic canal decompression.

Three studies reinforce and/or alter our approach to traumatic optic neuropathies. In a double-blind study, megadose corticosteroids positively altered the clinical course of patients with spinal cord injuries compared with untreated controls (16). These data were so convincing that the study was terminated and the data published in the *New York Times* (3) months before its formal publication in the medical literature. This successful use of megadose corticosteroids for spinal cord trauma lends credence to our experience using megadose steroids to treat traumatic optic neuropathies. We found that patients treated with high-dose and megadose corticosteroids had significant improvement in visual acuity and visual field (9). Additionally, 11 of 14 patients treated with extracranial optic nerve decompression had significantly improved visual function. Three of five patients had no light perception before treatment (10). All were treated with preoperative and postoperative corticosteroids.

V. CONCLUSIONS

The diagnosis and appropriate management of patients with traumatic optic neuropathies remains challenging. First, detect treatable causes of optic nerve compression—orbital, subperiosteal, and intrasheath hemorrhage. These should be treated expeditiously. Computed tomography and examination should detect concurrent injuries requiring neurosurgical evaluation and treatment.

There is no consensus or documented evidence that medical (corticosteroid) or surgical optic nerve decompression alters the natural course of traumatic optic neuropathies. This warrants support of a randomized trial comparing treatment and no treatment of the patients.

In the interim, there is enough anecdotal experience in the literature to offer treatment with megadose corticosteroids and timely optic canal decompression.

REFERENCES

1. Hupp SL, Buckley EG, Byrne ST, et al. Post-traumatic venous obstruction retinopathy associated with an enlarged optic nerve sheath. Arch Ophthalmol 1984; 102:254–6.
2. Kline LB, Morawetz RB, Swaid S. Indirect injury of the optic nerve. Neurosurgery 1984; 14:756–64.
3. Holt JE, Holt GR, Blodgett JM. Ocular injuries sustained during blunt facial trauma. Ophthalmology 1983; 90:14–8.
4. Walsh FB. Pathological-clinical correlations: indirect trauma to the optic nerves and chiasm. Invest Ophthalmol 1966; 5:433–49.
5. Imachi J, Ione K, Takahashi T. Clinical and pathohistologic investigations of optic nerve lesions in cases of head injuries. Jpn J Ophthalmol 1968; 12:70–85.
6. Anderson RL, Pange WR, Gross CE. Optic nerve blindness following blunt forehead trauma. Ophthalmology 1982; 89:445–55.
7. Pavin V. Evidence of orbital deformation in indirect optic nerve injury. J Clin Neuro Ophthalmol 1988; 8:9–11.
8. Lessell S. Indirect optic nerve trauma. Arch Ophthalmol 1989; 107:382–6.
9. Spoor TC, Hartel W, Lensink DB, et al. Treatment of traumatic optic neuropathies with high-dose and megadose corticosteroids. Am J Ophthalmol 1990; 110:665–9.
10. Joseph MP, Lessell S, Rizzo J, Momose J. Extracranial optic nerve decompression for traumatic optic neuropathy. Arch Ophthalmol 1990; 108:1091–3.
11. Hughes B. Indirect injury to the optic nerves and chiasm. Bull Johns Hopkins Hosp 1963; 111:98–126.
12. Fujitani T, Inoue K, Takahashi T, et al. Indirect traumatic optic neuropathy: visual outcome of operated and non-operated cases. Jpn J Ophthalmol 1986; 30:125–34.

13. Gjerris F. Traumatic lesions of the visual pathways. In: Vinken PJ, Bruyn GW, eds. Injuries of the brain and skull, part II. New York: Elsevier, 1976:27–56.
14. Braughler JM, Hall ED. Current application of "high-dose" steroid therapy for CNS injury. J Neurosurg 1985; 62:805–10.
15. Maxwell RE, Long DM, French LA. The clinical effects of a synthetic glucocorticoid used for brain edema in the practice of neurosurgery. In: Reulen JH, Schumann K, eds. Steroids and brain edema. New York: Springer-Verlag, 1972:219–32.
16. Bracken MB, Shepard MJ, Collins WF, et al. A randomized, controlled trial of methylprednisolone or naloxone in the treatment of acute spinal-cord injury. N Engl J Med 1990; 322:1405.
17. Osguthorpe JD. Transethmoidal decompression of the optic nerve. Otolaryngol Clin N Am 1985; 18:125–37.
18. Spoor TC, Mathog R. Restoration of vision after optic canal decompression following five days of total blindness and megadose corticosteroid therapy. Arch Ophthalmol 1986; 104:804–6.

8

Nonarteritic Anterior Ischemic Optic Neuropathy

Shalom E. Kelman
University of Maryland Medical Systems, Baltimore, Maryland

I. SIGNIFICANCE AND BACKGROUND

Nonarteritic ischemic optic neuropathy (NAION), the most common cause of acute nerve disease in the elderly (1–3). Usually causes permanent and often severe visual loss. Visual function can be impaired either through (1) decreased central visual acuity, (2) peripheral visual field loss, or (3) both.

No proven treatment currently exists to reverse or arrest this loss. NAION strikes both eyes in up to 40% of affected patients (4) and takes a devastating toll on independence and quality of life. To date, incidence and prevalence data have not been available; however, data collected from us from a sample of U.S. neuro-ophthalmologists (unpublished data) has allowed us to estimate that 6100 new cases are seen each year in the United States, or an annual incidence of 2.44 per 100,000.

Final visual acuity in patients with NAION declines to 20/200 or worse (legal blindness) in 45% of affected eyes (5,6). Decreased central visual acuity correlates with impaired performance of daily activities deemed important for quality of life (e.g., reading, driving, working, sewing).

Even when patients with NAION have vision better than 20/64, visual function can be severely compromised because of visual field defects, particularly if defects are present bilaterally. For example, many patients with NAION would be prohibited from driving under the guidelines established by the Low Vision

Committee of the American Academy of Ophthalmology and approved by the Board of Directors of the American Academy of Ophthalmology on February 25, 1989. NAION classically presents with an altitudinal defect that compromises far and midperipheral vision and paracentral vision. Far peripheral vision, for example, is needed to see cars in adjacent lanes while driving or steps while walking. Midperipheral vision is needed to see a pedestrian leaving the sidewalk or detect another car approaching an intersection. Other common presenting visual field defects are cecocentral scotomas and arcuate scotomas that affect midperipheral and paracentral vision. Blind spots in the paracentral area can hide small objects such as children or traffic lights.

II. ETIOLOGY

Lieberman et al. (13), Hayreh (1), and Quigley et al. (10) hypothesize that NAION is caused by vascular insufficiency leading to optic nerve head ischemia. This hypothesis is supported by several observations: abrupt onset of vision loss typical for vascular disease; clinical pathological evidence of small blood vessel closure (7); lack of ocular inflammation clinically and histopathologically (8–10); and experimental production of an NAION-like picture in monkeys from occlusion of the posterior ciliary arteries (11).

There is general agreement that NAION results from transient nonperfusion of nutrient vessels. Lieberman et al. (7) have proposed that NAION is caused by diffuse small vessel disease leading to hypoperfusion. Perfusion drops below a critical threshold causing infarction of a segment of the optic nerve (12). The wide range of visual field defects and visual loss with NAION can be explained by the extent and number of the blood vessels involved. A more precise etiology is difficult to define in light of the general disagreement over the exact blood supply to the anterior optic nerve (13,14). Specific occlusion of the posterior ciliary arteries does not appear to be absolutely necessary for NAION (15,16). Indeed, experimental occlusion of the posterior ciliary arteries does not always produce NAION (12).

Anatomical factors appear to contribute to the vascular event initiating NAION (15). Clinically, the number of discs congenitally lacking a physiological cup in the eyes with NAION is higher than expected. When a cup is present, it is almost always small (17). Presumably, in eyes with NAION, these discs have small scleral openings that crowd the nerve fibers as they pass through the restricted space in the optic disc and lamina cribrosa, and thereby predispose to an ischemia spiral.

Current theory holds that NAION begins as a minor ischemic event that later progresses to a major infarction due to congenitally anomalous optic nerves (18). The inciting ischemia event leads to local anterior nerve edema, and this causes further ischemia. The nerve edema compromises both intracellular edema (intra-axonal swelling) and extracellular edema (interneural fluid from extravasation).

Axonal swelling, resulting from axoplasmic flow stasis, compresses interaxonal capillaries in a restricted space, and thus secondarily compromises vascular flow (15). The compact arrangement of nerves and blood vessels within the tight scleral canal contributes to an ischemic spiral. In this case, local infarction with edema leads to more ischemia and further edema.

In addition to intra-axonal swelling, there is interaxonal edema from extravasation of fluid between axons, which further increases intraoptic nerve pressure and decreases blood flow to the optic nerve head (2,19). Clinopathological studies have indicated that this extracellular edema involves not only the anterior optic nerve head but also the retrolaminar portion of the optic nerve (9).

Thus, although NAION begins as a local sectoral change, it progresses because the localized infarct edema raises tissue pressure causing further capillary embarrassment (1,13). The local increase in the tissue pressure affects nerve fibers untouched by the initial ischemia event through capillary strangulation and perhaps through direct mechanical effects (18). Thus, the most damaging event is not the initial ischemic episode but rather an ischemic spiral produced by the secondary edema in a closed space. The clinical observation that visual loss progresses in a subgroup of patients with NAION within 1–4 weeks after the onset of symptoms (18,20–22) supports the ischemic spiral hypothesis.

III. REVIEW OF THE LITERATURE OF THE NATURAL HISTORY OF NAION

Table 1 reviews the available English-language literature on the natural history of NAION prior to 1990. Visual acuity of patients presenting with NAION is reported to be especially poor: About one quarter to two thirds (27–64%) of presenting patients have an initial visual acuity worse than 20/200 (6,23–26).

Unfortunately, only about half of the articles reporting on the natural history of NAION present data on change in visual acuity over time. Furthermore, in some of the studies reported, various treatments, such as phenytoin (Dilantin) and corticosteroids, were employed in an unknown number of eyes (22,27–29). In reports that present data on both initial and final visual acuities, no data are available regarding change in visual acuity over time for individual patients; rather distributions of initial and final visions are presented; the reported rates of improvement are low, ranging from 0 to 33% for untreated eyes. Given the limitations of the data, it is impossible to evaluate prognostic factors for improvement in vision in patients with NAION. For example, are patients with the worst initial visual acuity more likely to improve, or is improvement more likely in those patients whose initial vision was only moderately impaired?

The literature on the incidents of bilateral NAION has been summarized by

Table 1 Literature Summary of NAION Case Reports with VA Data

Article	Year	Patients	Eyes	VA < 20/80[a]	Improvement in VA	Length of F/U	Treatment	Bilateral
Kelman	1991	7	7	100%	100%	7 mos.	ONDS	14%
Sergott	1989							
Treated		17	24	94%	76%	12.5 mos.	ONDS	41%
Untreated		26	27	100%	7%	14.5 mos.	None	4%
Kline	1988	6	6	100%	0%	4 mos.	None	0%
Borchert, Bessell	1988	10	17	17%	0%	Not available	3-steroids	Not available
Repka et al.	1983	169	184	42%	0% (F/U on 83 patients)	8–13 yrs. Mean = 5 yrs.	None	24%
Hayreh	1981a	3	5	0%	80%	2.3 mos.	Steroids	Not available
Hayreh	1981b	4	8	25%	Not available	10 mos.–3 yrs.	Prednisone	Not available
Hayreh	1980	11	13	30%	Not available	Not available	None	Not available
Barr et al.	1980	12	21	19%	Not available	Not available	None	Not available
Pavan et al.	1980	8	16	0%	Not available	3.5 yrs.	3-panretinal photocoagulation	Not available

Hayreh, Pokhajsky	1979	133	97	30% (<20/200)	Not available	Not available	None	37%
Boghen, Glaser	1975	29	37	46% (<20/200)	5%	Mean 6.4 yrs. 3 yrs. for 93%	None	38%
Ellenberger et al.	1974	19	28	29%	0%	Minimum of 3 mos.	Dilantin Placebo	48%
Eagling et al.	1974	33	47	27% (<20/200)	Not available	Not available	Some patients received steroids	42%
Ellenberger et al.	1973	48	60	42%	33% (for initial VA < 20/30)	Mean 29 yrs. Median 1 yr.	None	48%
Keltner et al.	1972	7	10	70%	Not available	6 mos.	Dilantin	Not available
Cullen	1967	19	21	Not available	No change			10.5%
Miller, Smith	1966	11	19	42% (<20/200)	Not available	Variable		75%
Skillern, Lockhart	1959	14	22	64% (<20/200)	14%	Variable	None	57%
Carroll	1952	14		Not available	Not available	Not available	None	Not available

[a]Where VA levels not given in terms of 20/80 or worse, the VA level used is in parenthesis

Beri et al. (4). The incidence of bilateral disease has been reported at rates ranging from 10 to 74%, perhaps because it is a function of length of patient follow-up. They found that at 1 and 5 years of follow-up, 17.5 and 34.5%, respectively, of all patients with AION had developed bilateral disease.

Visual field defects are often noted in association with NAION—63 to 1000% of the time (24,26,30,31). They include altitudinal scotomas, central scotomas, arcuate defects and quadrantic defects (6,25). Repka et al. (6) tabulated the location and type of visual field defect on Goldman perimetry. Forty-six percent of patients had inferior altitudinal defect, and isolated central scotomas were reported in 20%. Hayreh and Podhajsky (25) reported inferior nasal or inferior altitudinal defects in 57% of patients with NAION and central scotoma in 26%.

Data on changes in the visual field over time are even more limited than data on visual acuity (32). Ellenberger (30) noted improvement in the central scotomas in six of eight patients, whereas the arcuate defects in 43 eyes did not change.

There are a few reports in the literature noting what appears to be progressive and recurrent forms of NAION. Boghen and Glaser (5) were the first to report evidence of progression, which they saw in 11 of 39 patients over a 4-week period. Most of these cases occurred within 9 days of initial onset. Sergott (33) described 24 patients who experienced progressive loss of vision with NAION; however, he did not describe the detailed time course of the visual progression. Borchert and Lessell (22) describe five patients with progression over a month or longer in NAION and four patients with recurrence in the same eye after a longer interval. Beck et al. (20) described four cases of recurrent NAION in the same eye, three of which recurred within 3 weeks of initial onset. Kline (21) described six patients with NAION who experienced worsening of visual acuity and field loss during the 6-week period after the onset of NAION.

Several reports indicate associations of systemic disease with NAION, including hypertension and diabetes (16,34). Beri et al. (4), in a study of the incidence of bilateral NAION, found a statistically significant association between bilateral NAION and the presence of diabetes in younger patients. No controlled studies looking at these relationships have been performed.

There are several problems with the literature cited concerning NAION. First, all studies are based on patient data, collected in the past, and selected specifically for publication. Second, because these reports are based on patient data and do not represent planned research studies, there is no evidence of standardized data measurement or collection either within or between studies. Third, most reports are based on a small number of patients. Fourth, follow-up is variable and generally poor. Finally, in a number of studies, arteritic and nonarteritic AION cases have been lumped together. Thus, the available information regarding the incidence and natural history of NAION cannot be relied on and must be interpreted cautiously.

IV. TREATMENT

Until recently, the clinician's main task in managing NAION had been to exclude temporal arteritis (which is treatable with corticosteroids) and to bring under control other factors, such as elevated blood pressure, which might impact on the final visual outcome (35). Although various nonsurgical treatments, such as corticosteroids and Dilantin, have been tried, no therapy for NAION has been proven effective and universally accepted (28,36,37). In 1989, Sergott and colleagues (33) suggested that optic nerve sheath decompression surgery (ONDS) may improve visual function in the progressive form of anterior ischemic optic neuropathy, which is characterized by progressive worsening of vision over several weeks (22). These investigators (33) and others (38–40) demonstrated improvement in either visual acuity of visual field following ONDS. Some, but not all, of the surgical reports, claim that "progressive" patients may have a higher probability of achieving improvement in vision following ONDS. More recently, the favorable results of the initial studies have been challenged; for example, Glaser and colleagues (41) reported only a 26% rate of improvement following surgery. Because this falls within the range of spontaneous improvement from NAION described in the natural history literature (28,42), it implies no treatment effect.

A. Why Should ONDS Work in NAION?

The presumed mechanism of action in ONDS revolves around restoration of impaired blood flow to the optic nerve through reduction of the pressure around the nerve. ONDS decreases pressure on the nerve by removing surrounding cerebrospinal fluid (CSF); this releases secondary edema and thereby improves perfusion and prevents or restores visual loss by salvaging functional neurons (18). Improved blood flow velocity in the ophthalmic and posterior ciliary arteries following ONDS, as measured using color Doppler techniques, supports this hypothesis (43). Observations in similar conditions (e.g., pseudotumor cerebri, optic neuropathy with acute retinal necrosis) provides a theoretical basis for ONDS in the treatment of NAION.

In the normal eye, glial columns serve as pressure barriers betwen the retrolaminar nerve (that portion of the optic nerve posterior to the lamina cribrosa) and the anterior optic nerve (anterior to the lamina cribrosa). ONDS releases the pressure in the retrolaminar nerve. Thus, in the normal eye, the glial columns would prevent an effect of ONDS to alter pressure in the anterior optic nerve. Experimental studies (44,45), however, demonstrate that anterior optic disc swelling, such as occurs in NAION and pseudotumor cerebri, disrupts this pressure barrier at the lamina. Optic nerve swelling breaks the glial columns permitting pressure communication between the anterior nerve and the intrasheath CSF. Because of this communication, reduction in the local retrolaminar CSF pressure brought about through ONDS permits reduced edema in the swollen anterior prelaminar nerve. ONDS also serves to decrease the pressure on the swollen retrolaminar nerve by relieving surrounding CSF pressure. This allows the swollen, confined nerve to expand into the surrounding nerve sheath space thereby approving perfusion.

In pseudotumor cerebri, pressure on the optic nerve originates outside the optic nerve; this is in contrast to the intraneural origin of pressure in NAION. Nevertheless, these two conditions are similar in terms of swelling and pressure buildup. In pseudotumor cerebri, ONDS corrects pressure-induced optic nerve ischemia and reverses visual loss from optic nerve swelling (46–50). Release of pressure on the optic nerve through ONDS restores the pressure balance in the optic nerve capillaries and reverses hypoperfusion (51). A similar mechanical relief of pressure in patients with NAION could result in improvement of visual function.

Although some of the studies cited above suggest that ONDS may be an effective therapy in the treatment of NAION, none of the surgical studies allow firm conclusions to be drawn. All of these surgical reports lack to some degree (1) suitable, randomized control groups, (2) uniform testing procedures, (3) standardized definitions of "progressive" NAION, and (4) sufficient numbers for adequate statistical power. For these same reasons, claims of improved outcome in "progressive" patients, although intriguing, are at best hypothesis generating and at worst meaningless. Therefore, at present, no firm recommendation can be made regarding the efficacy and safety of ONDS for the treatment of NAION whether "progressive" or "nonprogressive."

Clearly no reasonable clinician would want to withhold a new, promising, low-risk treatment for a blinding disease of the elderly where there is a uniformly poor prognosis. In the present context, however, there is no consensus on either the promise of the new treatment or the prognosis of patients with NAION without treatment. In addition, the potential treatment for NAION, ONDS, is not without some risk. In a review of past cases of ONDS, Sergott and colleagues (18) found that 26 of 200 (13%) cases had ocular complications, including permanent visual loss in three patients. Higher rates of complications have been described by Plotnik and Kosmorsky at the American Academy of Ophthalmology Annual Meeting (Dallas, TX, November 1992).

When a new treatment for any condition is introduced, the "gold standard" for testing safety and efficacy is the randomized, clinical trial (RCT). By definition, the RCT is controlled; that is, there are at least two study groups: one in which patients receive the new treatment (e.g., ONDS) and the other in which they receive a placebo or the standard care administered to patients with the condition of interest. The RTC is the appropriate methodology for testing any new intervention and, especially for problems with great public health and economic implications, should be used to test all new treatments prior to general use.

B. The Ischemic Optic Neuropathy Decompression Trial (IONDT)

The IONDT is a multicenter randomized clinical trial funded by the National Eye Institute to study the effects of ONDS on patients with NAION. The IONDT is being conducted at 26 U.S. clinical sites and includes a Chairman's Office, Coordinating Center, and Reading Center. Patients diagnosed with NAION within 10 days of the onset of visual symptoms are randomized to either ONDS or careful follow-up. Follow-up is for at least 12 months and the primary outcome is a change in visual acuity of at least three lines at 6 months. The following questions will be specifically addressed by the trial: (1) What is the natural history of NAION? (2) Is treatment with ONDS more effective in restoring and maintaining visual acuity and visual field than careful follow-up without treatment? (3) Are there adverse effects associated with ONDS?

To be eligible for participation in the study, patients must meet the following criteria: be age 50 years or older, have best corrected visual acuity of 20/64 or worse in the affected eye, disc edema, and a relative afferent pupillary defect. Patients with simultaneous bilateral NAION or no light perception are not eligible.

Eligibility is determined at a Baseline Eligibility Visit, which is scheduled within 10 days of onset of symptoms of NAION. The Baseline Eligibility Visit consists of a medical history, neuro-ophthalmic examination, measurement of visual acuity using New York Lighthouse charts, visual fields using a Humphrey Field Analyzer (Zeiss-Allergan, San Leandro, CA), and a medical examination designed to determine the ability of the patient to undergo surgery should that be the treatment assigned. Eligible participants must be randomized and receive surgery, if so assigned, within 14 days from the onset of symptoms. The criterion that patients must be randomized and receive treatment within 14 days of the onset of visual symptoms was established to optimize the timing of treatment of NAION. Use of this approach alone, however, may fail to identify patients whose vision is better than 20/64 initially but who progress to poorer vision over the next few weeks. In order to include these patients, the IONDT study design includes two groups of patients; those who are eligible in all respects at the Baseline Eligibility Visit and those who are eligible in all respects except that their visual acuity is better than 20/64. Any patient falling into this latter group will be followed weekly. Should vision decline to 200/64 or worse within 30 days from the onset of symptoms, these patients will become eligible for enrollment. These late-entry patients will be defined as having "progressive NAION" for the purposes of the study.

Follow-up visits are scheduled for 1 week, 1 month, 3 months, 6 months, and every 6 months thereafter following randomization. Visual acuity will be measured and a neuro-ophthalmic examination conducted at each visit. Visual fields will be measured at the 3- and 6-month follow-up visits.

In addition to the randomized, controlled study design, the IONDT utilizes defined, standardized techniques and quality assurance mechanisms typical of National Eye Institute sponsored clinical trials. In addition, innovative programs for surgeon training, certification, supervision, and quality assurance have been instituted. This will standardize the surgical approach and assure a high level of surgical expertise.

The study plans to enroll a total of 300 patients at the 26 participating clinical centers. Recruitment began in November 1992 and will continue through May 1994.

It is hoped that the IONDT will answer many of the questions related to the natural history and management of NAION.

REFERENCES

1. Hayreh SS. Anterior ischemic optic neuropathy. New York: Springer-Verlag, 1975.
2. Hayreh SS. Anterior ischemic optic neuropathy. Arch Neurol 1981; 38(11):675–8.
3. Hayreh SS. Anterior ischemic optic neuropathy. Differentiation of arteritic from non-arteritic type and its management. Eye 1990; 4 (Pt.1):25–41.
4. Beri M, et al. Anterior ischemic optic neuropathy. VII. Incidence of bilaterality and various influencing factors. Ophthalmology 1987; 94(10):1258–71.
5. Boghen DR, Glasner JS. Ischemic optic neuropathy. The clinical profile and history. Brain 1975; 98(4):689–708.
6. Repka MX, et al. Clinical profile and long-term implications of anterior ischemic optic neuropathy. Am J Ophthalmol 1983; 96(4):478–83.
7. Lieberman MF, Shahi A, Green WR. Embolic ischemic optic neuropathy. Am J Ophthalmol 1978; 86:206–10.
8. Henkind P, Charles NC, Pearson J. Histopathology of ischemic optic neuropathy. Arch Ophthal 1970; 69:78–90.
9. Knox DL, Duke JR. Slowly progressive ischemic optic neuropathy: a clinicopathologic case report. Trans Am Acad Ophthalmol Otolaryngol 1971; 75:1065–8.
10. Quigley HA, Addicks EM, and Green WR. Optic nerve damage in human glaucoma III. Quantitative correlation of nerve fiber loss and visual field defect in glaucoma, ischemic neuropathy, papilledema, and toxic neuropathy. Arch Ophthalmol 1981; 100:135–46.
11. Hayreh SS, Baines JA. Occlusion of the posterior ciliary artery. II. Chorio-retinal lesions. Br J Ophthalmol 1972; 56(10):736–53.
12. Anderson DR, Davis EB. Retina and optic nerve after posterior ciliary artery occlusion. Arch Ophthalmol 1974; 92:422–6.
13. Lieberman MF, Maumenee AE, Green WR. Histologic studies of the vasculature of the anterior optic nerve. Am J Ophthalmol 1976; 82:405–23.
14. Olver JM, Spalton DJ, MACE. Microvascular study of retrolaminar optic nerve in man: the possible significance in anterior ischemic optic neuropathy. Eye 1990; 4:7–24.
15. Beck RW, et al. Structural factors in the pathogenesis of ischemic optic neuropathy. Am J Ophthalmol 1984; 98(5):649–50 (letter).

16. Ellenberger C. Ischemic optic neuropathy as possible early complication of vascular hypertension. Am J Ophthalmol 1979; 88:1045–51.
17. Beck RW, Servais GE, Hayreh SS. Anterior ischemic optic neuropathy. IX. Cup-to-disc ratio and its role in pathogenesis. Ophthalmology 1987; 94(9):1180–8.
18. Sergott RC, Savino PJ, Bosley TM. Optic nerve sheath decompression: a clinical review and proposed pathophysiologic mechanism. Aust NZ J Ophthalmol 1990; 18(e):365–73.
19. Wirtschafter JD, Rizzo JF, Smiley BC. Optic nerve axoplasm and papilledema. Surv Ophthalmol 1975; 20:157–89.
20. Beck RW, et al. Anterior ischemic optic neuropathy: recurrent episodes in the same eye. Br J Ophthalmol 1983; 67:705–9.
21. Kline LB. Progression of visual defects in ischemic optic neuropathy. Am J Ophthalmol 1988; 106:199–203.
22. Borchert M, Lessell S. Progressive and recurrent nonarteritic anterior ischemic optic neuropathy. Am J Ophthalmol 1988; 106(4):443–9.
23. Skillern PG, Lockhart G. Optic neuritis and uncontrolled diabetes mellitus in 14 patients. Ann Intern Med 1959; 51:468–75.
24. Miller GR, Smith JL. Ischemic optic neuropathy. Am J Ophthalmol 1966; 62:103–55.
25. Hayreh SS, Podhajsky P. Visual field defect in anterior ischemic optic neuropathy. Doc Ophthalmol Proc Ser 1979; 19:53–71.
26. Eagling EM, Sander MD. Miller SJH. Ischemic papillopathy: clinical and fluorescein angiographic review of forty cases. Br J Ophthalmol, 1974; 58:990–1008.
27. Keltner JL, et al. Effect of diphenylhydantoin in ischemic optic neuritis. Trans Am Ophthalmol Soc 1972; 70:113–30.
28. Ellenberger CJ, Burde RM, Keltner JL. Acute optic neuropathy. Treatment with diphenylhydantoin. Arch Ophthalmol 1974; 91(6):435–8.
29. Hayreh SS, and Zahoruk RM. Anterior ischemic optic neuropathy. VI. In Juvenile diabetics. Ophthalmologica 1981; 182(1):29–41.
30. Ellenberger CJ, Keltner JL, Burde RM. Acute optic neuropathy in older patients. Arch Neurol 1973; 28(3):182–5.
31. Cullen JF. Ischemic optic neuropathy. Trans Ophthalmol Soc UK, 1967; 87:182–5.
32. Cho MH. Remission of visual field loss in non arteritic anterior ischemia optic neuropathy. Am J Optom Physiol Optics 1986; 63:472–6.
33. Sergott RC, et al. Optic nerve decompression may improve the progressive form of nonarteritic ischemic optic neuropathy. Arch Ophthalmol 1989; 107(12):1743–54 (see comments).
34. Guyer DR, et al. The risk of cerebrovascular and cardiovascular disease in patients with anterior ischemic optic neuropathy. Arch Ophthalmol 1985; 103:1136–42.
35. Miller NR. Walsh and Hoyt's Clinical Neuro-Ophthalmology. Vol. 1. 4th ed. Baltimore: Williams & Wilkins 1982:212–26.
36. Glaser, JS, ed. Prechiasmal visual pathways. 2d ed. Neuro-Ophthalmology, Topical Diagnosis. Philadelphia: Lippincott, 1990:83–170.
37. Hayreh SS, Anterior ischemic optic neuropathy. III. Treatment, prophylaxis, and differential diagnosis. Br J Ophthalmol 1974; 58(12):981–9.

38. Kelman SE, Elman MJ. Optic nerve sheath decompression for nonarteritic optic neuropathy improves multiple visual function measurements. Arch Ophthalmol 1991; 109(5):667–71.
39. Spoor TC, Wilkinson MJ, Ramocki JM. Optic nerve sheath decompression for the treatment of progressive nonarteritic ischemic optic neuropathy. Am J Ophthalmol 1991; 111(6):724–8 (see comments).
40. Spoor TC, McHenry JG, Lau-Sickon L. Progressive and static nonarteritic ischemic optic neuropathy treated by optic nerve sheath decompression. Ophthalmology 1993; 100(3):306–11.
41. Jablons MM, et al. Optic nerve sheath fenestration for treatment of progressive ischemic optic neuropathy: results in 26 patients. Arch Ophthalmol 1993; 111(1):84–7.
42. Movsas TZ, et al. The natural course of non-arteritic ischemic optic neuropathy. Invest Ophthalmol Vis Sci 1991; 42:951.
43. Flaharty PM, et al. Optic nerve sheath decompression may improve blood flow in anterior ischemic optic neuropathy. Ophthalmology 1993; 100(3):297–302.
44. Tso MO, Hayreh SS. Optic disc edema in raised intracranial pressure. IV. Axoplasmic transport in experimental papilledema. Arch Ophthalmol 1977; 95(8):1458–62.
45. Tso MO, Hayreh SS. Optic disc edema in raised intracranial pressure. III. A pathologic study of experimental papilledema. Arch Ophthalmol 1977; 95(8):1448–57.
46. Smith JL, Hoyt WF, Newton TH. Optic nerve sheath decompression for relief of chronic monocular choked disc. Am J Ophthalmol 1969; 68:633–639.
47. Galbraith JEK, Sullivan JH. Decompression of the perioptic meninges for relief of papilledema. Am J Ophthalmol 1973; 76:687–92.
48. Brourman ND, Spoor TC, Ramocki JM. Optic nerve sheath decompression for pseudotumor cerebri. Arch Ophthalmol 1988; 106(10):1378–83.
49. Corbett JJ, et al. Results of optic nerve sheath fenestration for pseudotumor cerebri. The lateral orbitotomy approach. Arch Ophthalmol 1988; 106(10):1391–7 (see comments).
50. Sergott RC, Savino PJ, Bosley TM. Modified optic nerve sheath decompression provides long-term visual improvement for pseudotumor cerebri. Arch Ophthalmol 1988; 106(10):1384–90.
51. Hayreh SS, Pathogenesis of oedema of the optic disc. Doc Ophthalmol 1968; 24(2):289–411.
52. Hayreh SS. Anterior ischemic optic neuropathy. V. Optic disc edema an early sign. Arch Ophthalmol 1981; 99(6):1030–40.
53. Hayreh SS. Anterior ischemic optic neuropathy. IV. Occurrence after cataract extraction. Arch Ophthalmol 1980; 98(8):1410–6.
54. Barr CC, Glaser JS, Blankenship G. Acute disc swelling in juvenile diabetes. Clinical profile and natural history of 12 cases. Arch Ophthalmol 1980; 98(12):2185–92.
55. Pavan PR, et al. Optic disc edema in juvenile-onset diabetes. Arch Ophthalmol 1980; 98:2193–5.
56. Carroll FD. Optic neuritis: A 15 year study. Am J Ophthalmol 1952; 35:75–82.

9

Optic Nerve Sheath Decompression

Robert C. Sergott
Wills Eye Hospital, Philadelphia, Pennsylvania

Optic nerve sheath decompression (ONSD), also known as optic nerve sheath fenestration, releases the cerebrospinal fluid surrounding the anterior intraorbital optic nerve by incising its meningeal sheath. Despite being developed by Louis de Wecker and Robert Carter, two of the nineteenth century's most prominent ophthalmologists, no surgical procedure in neuro-ophthalmology, and perhaps in all of ophthalmology, has been so ridiculed and questioned in twentieth century academic and clinical practice. Yet, as this century rapidly draws to a close, ONSD has reemerged as the treatment of choice for vision-threatening papilledema and may have promise for other optic neuropathies. In this chapter, we examine the techniques for ONSD, the indication for the procedure, and the postoperative care as well as potential complications.

I. SURGICAL TECHNIQUE

The intraorbital optic nerve may be approached surgically by a medial or lateral orbitotomy. Although each technique has outspoken advocates, the method employed depends largely on the surgeon's experience and "comfort level." No convincing data exist to recommend one approach versus the other.

A. Medial Approach

In our opinion, ONSD is best performed under general anesthesia, because potential intraoperative problems, pain control, and hemorrhaging may be handled in a safer manner. Following the induction of general endotracheal anesthesia, the area around the eye and orbit is prepared in a sterile fashion. The unoperated eye is covered with a plastic shield to avoid inadvertent direct pressure on the globe. A wire Barraquer's lid speculum is inserted into the lids of the operated eye, and a lateral canthotomy is performed.

Three and a half millimeters posterior to the medial limbus, the conjunctiva is incised with blunt Westcott scissors. A perimetry is then performed for 180 degrees and sparing the temporal conjunctiva. The 3.5-mm incision point is measured with calipers so that the medial rectus muscle is not detached.

Using curved Stephen's scissors, the quadrants between the medial and vertical recti are opened with sharp and blunt dissection. The surgeon first sharply opens Tenon's capsule between the muscles and then the scissors are used to spread the tissue open so that bare sclera is exposed. A Gass' muscle hook is used to place 4-0 black silk traction sutures beneath the vertical recti.

Attention is then directed to the medial rectus muscle that is dissected free of its attachments. A 6-0 Vicryl suture, double-armed with S-29 needles, is then weaved through the medial rectus, near its insertion to the globe, in a manner identical to a muscle recession procedure. The medial rectus is then disinserted from the globe leaving approximately 1 mm of muscle on the globe.

At this point, the operating microscope is moved into position. Hemostasis is achieved with light, wetfield bipolar cautery anterior to the previous muscle insertion. Cautery directly on the remaining medial rectus will shrink this tissue and make placing the next suture quite difficult.

Under operating microscope control, the globe is stabilized with 0.12-mm toothed forceps and a "baseball stitch" traction suture is placed at the previous insertion of the medial rectus muscle. The suture is called a baseball stitch because the bites are close together resembling the laces on a baseball. The belly of the needle is placed directly behind the muscle insertion on the thinnest part of the sclera (0.3 mm), and then the needle is advanced through the sclera. In this way, the needle never encounters the thinnest part of the sclera.

The eye is then elevated and abducted using the traction sutures and baseball stitch. The next critical landmark is the intrascleral course of the medial long posterior ciliary artery. Appearing as a slightly elevated ridge in the mid equatorial region, this structure is identified in approximately 80% of patients.

During traction on the globe, the size of the pupil is monitored continuously. If the pupil dilates 2 mm more than its original diameter, the eye is returned to normal anatomical position. Failure to observe and act on pupillary changes increases the risk of a central retinal artery occlusion. Since the patient is in a monocular situation with the contralateral eye occluded, pupillary dilation may reflect amaurotic status due to retinal and/or optic nerve hypoperfusion.

A Fischer malleable restriction is used to open the posterior reflection of Tenon's capsule. In younger patients, this tissue is thicker and scissors must be used to open this structure.

After the reflection of Tenon's capsule is opened, the orbital fat is mobilized and migrates anteriorly. The fat is maneuvered with the Fischer retractor and cotton-tipped applicators to expose the ciliary vessels coursing over the optic nerve. Compared with the yellow orbital fat, the dura of the optic nerve has a grayish–pearl white color. The optic nerve is isolated between two cotton-tipped applicators (or neurosurgical cottonoids). The applicators are rotated gently to retract the ciliary vessels and expose a relatively avascular area of optic nerve meninges.

The surgical assistant seated temporally elevates and abducts the eye with the traction sutures, and the assistant seated medially holds the malleable retractor and one or both cotton-tipped applicators. The operating surgeon then uses a long-handled corneoscleral V-lance (#20 Alcon blade or tympanic membrane blade) to incise the dura approximately 1–2 mm posterior to the junction of the optic nerve and globe. After the subarachnoid space is entered, a gush of cerebrospinal fluid (CSF) occurs. The incision is then extended with long-handled neurosurgical transsphenoidal scissors (Codman). The scissors have blunt tips and only the top blade is mobile. Therefore, the lower blade may enter the subarachnoid space without fear of lacerating the optic nerve. The lower blade then elevates the dura, permitting a full-thickness cut to be made without endangering the underlying optic nerve.

A Stephens' tenotomy hook then is placed in the subarachnoid space and moved anteriorly and posteriorly to break the adhesions and trabeculations in this area. This maneuver allows for drainage of CSF that is loculated within regions of the subarachnoid space. We recommend placing two additional linear incisions in other areas of the meningeal sheath to insure complete decompression of the entire nerve (1). Likewise, the subarachnoid adhesions are lysed for 360 degrees around the entire circumference of the nerve. Some surgeons prefer to excise a 3 $\times$ 5 mm rectangular window of dura. We believe that the multiple incision technique allows for a more complete decompression of the nerve and prevents the orbital fat from adhering directly to the nerve and thereby interfering with CSF drainage. In addition, removing a window requires a transverse cut at 90 degrees to the path of the ciliary vessels, a technique that potentially could interfere more with blood supply to the anterior optical nerve.

The traction sutures are then removed, and the medial rectus is reattached in the standard manner 5.5 mm from the limbus.

A light patch and shield is applied to the operated eye, and the shield is removed from the contralateral eye.

B. Lateral Approach

Compared with the medial, somewhat more ophthalmic approach, the lateral exposure of the optic nerve is a much more "oculoplastic" surgical approach. A lateral or Kronlein's orbitotomy is performed, and the intraconal space is opened with Sewell's retractors to expose the optic nerve.

The lateral approach allows for a longer segment of the intraorbital optic nerve to be exposed but slightly more manipulation of the nerve is required, since the nerve is traveling medially away from the region of surgical incision.

In the traditional orbitotomy, bone must be removed (2); however, the technique has now been modified to avoid removal of the lateral orbital wall (3). The intraorbital part of the procedure involving manipulation of the optic nerve and its meninges is the same for both the lateral and medial approaches.

C. Intraoperative Complications

Vaso-occlusive events to the optic nerve and retina constitute the major source of morbidity for ONSD. Such developments doom the eye to visual function between counting fingers and bare light perception. The incidence of these disastrous complications ranges from 1 to 11% depending upon the series (4,5).

We believe that an intraoperative or immediate postoperative (within the first 24 h after surgery), central retinal artery occlusion or ischemic optic neuropathy depends on the degree of surgical manipulation and how carefully the pupillary diameter is monitored intraoperatively. The differential diagnosis of intraoperative pupillary dilation is listed in Table 1. When this event occurs, we immediately return the globe to normal anatomical position and touch the globe with a cotton-tipped applicator. If the globe is very firm (and usually it is soft from the traction), we become concerned about angle-closure glaucoma due to forward rotation of the iris-lens or choroidal detachments. If the eye is soft, the differential diagnosis is between a blind amaurotic eye due to vascular hypoperfusion and an intraoperative Adie's pupil due to ciliary nerve traction. The Adie's-like pupil situation will often produce eccentric pupillary dilation, the residual effects of which can be transient or permanent postoperative complications.

Hemorrhaging due to laceration of a ciliary artery is the most anxiety-provoking intraoperative complication. It is absolutely critical not to plunge the suction apparatus into the orbit. Such a reckless maneuver can cause the ciliary vessels to be pulled into the suction tip and thereby worsening the situation. The blood should be absorbed using cotton-tipped applicators. Invariably the bleeding stops spontaneously and any residual oozing can be stopped by bovine thrombin applied topically with cotton-tipped applicators for only 30 s. Longer exposure to bovine thrombin could occlude the vasculature to the optic nerve and retina. We avoid

Table 1 Differential Diagnosis of Intraoperative Pupillary Dilation

Condition	Shape of pupil	Intraocular pressure	Management
1. Occlusion of perfusion to optic nerve and retina	Usually round	Normal to Low	Return eye to normal anatomic position and wait at least one minute before resuming surgery
2. Adie's-like pupil and stretched ciliary nerves	Usually eccentric	Normal to Low	Relieve pressure on globe
3. Angle-closure glaucoma	Round	High	1. Intraoperative mannitol, acetazolamide (Diamox), beta blocker
a. Forward rotation of lens-iris diaphragm			
b. Choroidal detachment			2. Consider peripheral iridectomy intraoperatively if medical means do not reduce pressure
			3. Vigorous dilation for choroidal detachment

electrical cautery near the optic nerve unless absolutely necessary because of the risk of optic nerve injury because of the electricity and associated heat energy.

Scleral perforations also are possible, and these situations must be managed with precise localization and cryotherapy of the opening. Obviously, thorough peripheral retinal examination is required in the event of this complication.

II. ABSOLUTE INDICATIONS FOR ONSD

A. Pseudotumor Cerebri

Once referred to as "benign" intracranial hypertension, pseudotumor cerebri (PTC) is certainly *not* benign in terms of visual function. The now classic work of Corbett and colleagues illustrated how chronic papilledema may have devastating consequences on both visual acuity and visual field (6).

Occurring most commonly, but certainly not exclusively in obese, young women, PTC may present with headache, visual loss, diplopia, or be detected on routine ophthalmological examination. The diagnosis is established for the following criteria: (1) normal neuro-ophthalmological examination except for papilledema and double vision; (2) normal computerized tomographic (CT) or magnetic resonance imaging (MRI) scans except for enlarged optic nerves and an empty sella; and (3) increased intracranial pressure as measured by lumbar puncture but an otherwise normal cerebrospinal fluid analysis.

CT scanning in PTC not only served as an important diagnostic approach but also focused neuro-ophthalmology's attention on the enlarged optic nerves and ONSD. Moreover, Corbett, based upon his unsatisfactory experience at Wills Eye Hospital and the University of Iowa with medical management and lumboperitoneal shunts, strongly advocated ONSD for patients with deteriorating visual function. ONSD had a lot to overcome, since in 1977 members of the Frank Walsh Neuro-Ophthalmology Society had almost unanimously condemned ONSD as an operation looking for an indication.

Despite the widespread and sometimes harsh, opposition to ONSD, Corbett and the late Henry Van Dyke remained convinced that ONSD was a necessary and often singular therapeutic option for many patients with ONSD. Then in 1988, in one issue of the *Archives of Ophthalmology*, three institutions published independent studies describing the successful treatment of vision-threatening papilledema with ONSD (1,2,7). All three reports showed remarkably similar results with resolution of the papilledema and improvement and/or stabilization of visual acuity and field. Although some controversy has arisen regarding the long-term efficacy of ONSD, as one group has reported a relatively frequent reoperation rate (8), but other investigators have observed a good long-term prognosis (1,2,4). ONSD appears to have supplanted lumboperitoneal shunting as the surgical procedure of choice for vision-threatening papilledema associated with PTC.

Since the exact mechanism(s) for loss of vision due to papilledema still remains undefined, but it probably involves both direct pressure on axons and ischemia, the perfect timing of ONSD is not established. However, as more clinical experience has been accumulated, criteria for ONSD have evolved and these are summarized in Table 2. It now appears as more surgeons become more familiar with the surgery, ONSD is being performed sooner in the patient's course.

Table 2 Indications for ONSD for Pseudotumor Cerebri

1. Severe visual acuity loss (20/40 $\leq$) at presentation
2. Severe visual field loss at presentation
3. Worsening visual function depite maximal medical therapy
4. Inability to tolerate diuretics and/or corticosteroids
5. Anticipated hypotension and/or anemia (such as hemodialysis)
6. Anticipated poor compliance with medication and follow-up visits
7. Progressive visual loss despite functioning lumboperitoneal shunt
8. Multiple shunt failures and revisions
9. Intractable transient visual observations

Therefore, with earlier intervention, the chances for a "surgical cure" are greater. But, on the other hand, the chances for disastrous surgical complications also are greater. Therefore, the exact timing of surgery depends on both the degree of visual loss as well as the surgeon's skill and expertise.

Fueling the controversy surrounding ONSD is tremendous uncertainty about how the operation actually relieves papilledema for both the short and long term. Three theories for the mechanism of action for ONSD exist: (1) filtration of CSF; (2) scarring and obliteration of the subarachnoid space so that the optic disc no longer is exposed to increased pressure; or (3) some combination of the first two hypotheses (9,10). Although clinical and neuroradiological data offer some support for the filtration theory for the short-term effect of ONSD, the available histopathological material appears to be more consistent with the subarachnoid space obliteration concept. Therefore, both mechanisms may be important. However, regardless of this pathophysiological uncertainty, ONSD has emerged as an important means to preserve and restore vision for patients with PTC.

B. Nonresectable Central Nervous System Mass

Although most central nervous system (CNS) mass lesions may be resected neurosurgically, some lesions such as meningiomas adjacent to the saggital sinus and arteriovenous malformation of the vein of Galen cannot be removed without excessive risk of life-threatening hemorrhage. In this clinical scenario, the patients have unrelenting increased intracranial or impaired cerebral venous drainage and their papilledema continues to worsen (11).

Diuretics and corticosteroids offer only temporary relief for this clinical syndrome. In our experience, we have found that these patients are referred too late in their course for ONSD to save usable vision. We believe that the same principles that governs the management of PTC should be applied to this condition. Again, this syndrome emphasizes that papilledema is more than a physical finding of neuro-ophthalmological disease but a disease process unto itself in terms of its possible adverse effects upon optic nerve function.

C. Postdecompression Blindness

Another rare neuro-ophthalmological condition for which ONSD has rationale is the entity termed postdecompression blindness (12). In this situation, patients with severe papilledema due to CNS mass lesions lose vision following uncomplicated craniotomies.

It has been postulated that in some way the sudden decrease in intracranial pressure causes the papilledema to decompensate. Alternatively, the worsening visual function could be the natural history of such severe chronic papilledema and the postoperative worsening has nothing to do with removal of the mass lesion.

In our experience, ONSD is the only treatment that can improve the visual function of these patients. Unfortunately, owing to the unavoidable altered mental status of craniotomy patients in the immediate postoperative period, the decreased visual function is often not recognized for some time.

D. Posttraumatic Central Retinal Vein Occlusion

Although once reported to be helpful for central retinal vein occlusions (CRVO) (13,14), ONSD currently has no role in the spontaneous variety of this disease, which is usually associated with hypertension, diabetes mellitus, and/or glaucoma. However, on rare occasions, head and orbital trauma, either accidentally or associated with a retrobulbar injection, may lead to a CRVO often combined with a central retinal artery occlusion (5,16).

In these traumatic cases, the CRVO is caused by a hemorrhage within the subarachnoid space of the intraorbital optic nerve. ONSD is the only way to deal with this rare type of CRVO. The most common setting for this problem is with retrobulbar anesthesia. In the circumstance, the anesthetic itself could have an additional adverse effect on retinal and optic nerve perfusion. Neuroimaging studies often will not show an enlarged optic nerve sheath complex, perhaps because of nonclotted arteriovenous blood is less expansile compared with CSF.

The prognosis for these patients is related to their degree of retinal ischemia at the time of surgery. Therefore, prompt diagnosis and action are required.

III. POSSIBLE INDICATIONS FOR ONSD

A. Progressive Nonarteritic Ischemic Optic Neuropathy

Based on the progressive nature of the visual loss in approximately 25% of patients with progressive nonarteritic ischemic optic neuropathy (P-NAION) and the predisposing small anatomical configuration of the optic disc, ONSD was performed on a series of patients and the results were better than the previous natural history of this disorder (16). Although two independent studies verified these results (17,18), this work has produced tremendous controversy (19).

More recently, another institution produced less favorable results (20), but in both of these studies there was a statistically significant delay in surgery compared with patients obtaining a favorable outcome (21). A national trial is now in progress to attempt to resolve these questions. In addition, the natural history of NAION is now under critical reexamination, especially in terms of the rate of spontaneous improvement that previously was agreed to be virtually nonexistent (22,23).

B. Optic Neuropathy Associated with the Acute Retinal Necrosis Syndrome

Some patients with the acute retinal necrosis (ARN) syndrome develop visual loss that is not totally accounted for by their retinal findings. In these individuals, optic nerve involvement appears to be responsible for the loss of visual function and neuroimaging studies will demonstrate enlarged optic nerve silhouettes (4).

IV. POSTOPERATIVE CARE AND COMPLICATIONS

Because of the definite risk of orbital, subarachnoid, and optic nerve hemorrhage in the immediate postoperative period, we advocate a regimen of strict bedrest for the first 12–18 h after surgery. Topical antibiotic ointment is sufficient infection prophylaxis, and systemic antibiotics are required only if the patients have had prior nasolacrimal procedures or are at risk for endocarditis.

Intramuscular meperidine (Demerol) is usually required to alleviate the postoperative pain. Topical ice compresses applied to the operated eye also are beneficial not only for pain control but also for reduction of postoperative soft tissue swelling.

The medial cornea must be monitored carefully for dellen formation. If undetected, the dellen can become secondarily infected. Double vision is usually a transient postoperative complication; presumably due to trauma to the medial rectus muscle and its neural supply.

Central retinal artery occlusion and traumatic optic neuropathy are the most devastating post-operative complication. Treatment is to no avail, and the patients remain permanently blind in the operated eye. The frequency of minor and major complications varies from institution to institution, as with any highly technical surgical procedure.

REFERENCES

1. Sergott RC, Savino PJ, Bosley TM. Modified optic nerve decompression provides long-term visual improvement in pseudotumor cerebri. Arch Ophthalmol 1988; 106:1384–90.
2. Corbett JJ, Nerad JA, Tse, DT, et al. Results of optic nerve sheath fenestration for pseudotumor cerebri: the lateral approach. Arch Ophthalmol 1988; 106:1391–7.
3. Flaharty PM, Sergott RC. Optic nerve sheath decompression. Ophthalmol Clin N Am 1992; 5:395–404.
4. Sergott RC. Optic nerve sheath decompression: neuropathologic, clinical, and hemodynamic results and rationale. Trans Am Ophthalmol Soc 1991; 89:675–720.
5. Plotnik JL, Kosmorsky GS. Operative complications of ONSD. Ophthalmology 1993; 100:683–90.

6. Corbett JJ, Savino PJ, Thompson HS, et al. Visual loss in pseudotumor cerebri. Arch Neurol 1982; 38:461–74.
7. Brourman ND, Spoor TC, Ramocki JM. Optic nerve sheath decompression, for pseudotumor cerebri. Arch Ophthalmol 1988; 106:1378–83.
8. Spoor TC, Ramocki JM, Madeon MP, et al. Treatment of pseudotumor cerebri by primary and secondary optic nerve sheath decompression. Am J Ophthalmol 1991; 112:177–85.
9. Keltner JL. Optic nerve sheath decompression: how does it work? Has its time come? Arch Ophthalmol 1988; 106:1365–9 (editorial).
10. Seif SL, Shah LA: A model for the mechanism of optic nerve sheath fenestration. Arch Ophthalmol 1990; 108:1326–9.
11. Horton JC, Seiff SR, Pitts LH, et al. Decompression of the optic nerve sheath for vision-threatening papilledema caused by dural sinus occlusion. Neurosurgery 1992; 31:203–12.
12. Beck RW, Greenberg HS. Post-decompression optic neuropathy. J Neurosurg 1985; 63:196–9.
13. Vasco-Posado J. Modification of the circulation in the posterior pole of the eye. Am Ophthalmol 1972; 10:48–59.
14. Arciniegas A. Treatment of the occlusion of the central retinal vein by section of the posterior ring. Ann Ophthalmol 1984; 16:1081–6.
15. Sullivan KL, Brown GC, Forman AR, et al. Retrobulbar anesthesia and retinal vascular obstruction. Ophthalmology 1983; 90:373–7.
16. Sergott RC, Cohen MS, Bosley TM, Savino PJ. Optic nerve decompression may improve the progressive form of nonarteritic ischemic optic neuropathy. Arch Ophthalmol 1989; 107:1743–54.
17. Kelman SE, Elman MJ. Optic nerve decompression for nonarteritic ischemic optic neuropathy improves multiple visual function measurements. Arch Ophthalmol 1991; 109:667–71.
18. Spoor TC. Optic nerve sheath decompression for the treatment of progressive non-arteritic ischemic optic neuropathy. Am J Ophthalmol 1991; 111:724–8.
19. Hayreh SS: The role of optic nerve sheath fenestration in management of anterior ischemic optic neuropathy. Arch Ophthalmol 1990; 108:1063–4 (letter).
20. Jablons MM, Glaser JS, Schatz NJ, et al. Optic nerve sheath decompression for treatment of progressive ischemic optic neuropathy. Arch Ophthalmol 1993; 111:84–7.
21. Sergott RC: Discussion of manuscript by Yee, et al. Trans Am Ophthalmol Soc 91: (in press).
22. Boghen DR, Glaser JS. Ischemic optic neuropathy: the clinical profile and natural history. Brain 1975; 98:689–708.
23. Repka M, Savino PJ, Schatz NJ, et al. Clinical profile and long-term implications of anterior ischemic optic neuropathy. Am J Ophthalmol 1983; 96:478–83.
24. Sergott RC, Belmont JB, Savino PJ, et al. Optic nerve involvement in the acute retinal necrosis syndrome. Arch Ophthalmol 1985; 103:1160–2.
25. Sergott, RC, Anand R, Belmont JB, et al. Acute retinal necrosis neuropathy. Arch Ophthalmol 1989; 107:692–6.

10

Hereditary Optic Neuropathies

Nancy J. Newman
Emory University School of Medicine, Atlanta, Georgia

The hereditary optic neuropathies are a heterogeneous group of disorders that are primarily manifested by bilateral optic atrophy and have hereditable etiologies suggested by familial expression or demonstrated by genetic analysis. Their classification has traditionally relied on the grouping of similar clinical characteristics and similar patterns of transmission. However, there is evidence for significant intrafamilial and interfamilial variability of expression in all these disorders.

Commonly, optic neuropathies will manifest with central visual loss, dyschromatopsia, and central visual field defects. There is eventually pallor of the optic discs and loss of nerve fiber layer. The inherited optic neuropathies are characteristically bilateral and symmetrical. The exact location of initial pathology and the underlying pathophysiological mechanisms of optic nerve injury in these disorders remain unknown. Visual evoked responses are typically abnormal and flash electroretinography is usually normal. Since the optic nerves are part of the central nervous system, they share this system's poor capacity for regeneration and healing after injury. The hereditary optic neuropathies are unlikely to respond to therapies instituted after the appearance of optic atrophy.

Some of the hereditary optic neuropathies are regularly associated with systemic or neurological abnormalities, and others have visual loss as their only manifestation. As a group, the hereditary optic neuropathies are generally distinguished from those disorders in which optic atrophy occurs secondary to abnormalities in lysosomal storage or as a result of primary retinal degeneration. This distinction becomes difficult, however, when assessing the familial neurological combined systems degeneration in which optic atrophy may be a variable component. Still other, primarily skeletal, diseases may exhibit bilateral optic atrophy secondary to optic nerve compression.

This chapter continues the traditional classification of the hereditary optic neuropathies by inheritance pattern. A better understanding of the underlying genetic etiologies will depend on accurate definition of the modes of transmission. As such, I have divided the optic neuropathies into those of autosomal dominant, autosomal recessive, and mitochondrial (maternal) inheritance. As more specific genetic defects are elucidated, our idea of what constitutes a specific phenotype will necessarily change. It is becoming clear that different genotypes can result in similar or identical clinical profiles. Alternatively, the same genetic defect may result in different phenotypes. An extension of the last concept is the individual who carries the genetic cause of a disorder but never expresses the disease.

Management of the hereditary optic neuropathies has by necessity been limited to familial genetic counseling. More accurate definition of the underlying genetic abnormalities will certainly aid in counseling. Additionally, identification of the abnormal genes and their abnormal products may allow for more directed therapy to replace or bypass the metabolic deficiencies.

I. DOMINANT OPTIC NEUROPATHY

Autosomal dominant inheritance characterizes a simple form of familial optic neuropathy comprehensively described by Paul Kjer. Given the significant interfamilial and intrafamilial clinical variability of this disorder, separation of this disease into an infantile and a juvenile form is probably not warranted. Onset of visual loss is insidious and usually first noted between the ages of 4 and 8 years. The degree of visual impairment is moderate, typically ranging from 20/40 to 20/200, with 40% of patients having vision 20/60 or better. There is some evidence for mild progression in that children rarely exhibit acuities of less than 20/200, whereas 10% of patients 15–44 years of age and 25% of those older will have visual function below this level. Spontaneous recovery of vision has not been reported. Symmetrical visual loss is the rule, but occasional cases of even dramatic asymmetry can occur.

Defects in color vision are a constant finding, especially a characteristic blue-yellow dyschromatopsia. It is this tritanopia that accounts for the so-called "inverted" peripheral visual fields to color in this disorder in which the isopter tested with the blue test object falls within the isopter plotted with the red object. This is the reverse of the color fields predicted in normal subjects and in patients with other acquired optic neuropathies reflecting the tritanopic preferential diminution of blue perception. Visual fields typically reveal centrocecal defects. With vertical extension of the blind spots, bitemporal hemianopic depression may be simulated, falsely suggesting pathology at the chiasm.

The classic ophthalmoscopic appearance of dominant optic atrophy is temporal pallor of the optic discs, frequently with associated sectoral temporal excavation. Less commonly there is diffuse pallor of the optic nerve heads. Nonglaucomatous cupping of the optic discs may also be seen. Loss of the papillomacular nerve fiber bundle is frequently dramatic.

Most patients with dominant optic neuropathy do not have other associated systemic or neurological abnormalities. The presence of nystagmus may reflect an earlier onset of the disorder and more severe visual dysfunction. Associated sensorineural hearing loss and mild mental retardation have been reported.

With the exception of very rare cases of profound visual deterioration, progression of visual loss in this disorder is mild and the majority of affected individuals enjoy relatively normal lives. Indeed, the symptoms and signs of visual dysfunction may be so subtle as to go unrecognized until a relative presents with more significant clinical features. Diagnosis in seemingly isolated cases necessitates examination of family members. Despite reports of possible visual improvement following lysis of chiasmal arachnoid adhesions, therapy in this disorder is essentially limited to genetic counseling. Although a specific genetic defect has yet to be established, there is evidence linking dominant optic atrophy to a locus on chromosome 2 of the nuclear genome.

II. RECESSIVE OPTIC NEUROPATHIES

As a group, the autosomal recessively inherited optic atrophies are less commonly encountered than those inherited in a dominant fashion and tend to cause more severe visual dysfunction. They also are more frequently associated with a wide variety of neurological and systemic abnormalities. This has led to some difficulties in the classification of some of these disorders; that is, whether they should be considered primary optic nerve degenerations with concomitant neurological abnormalities or simply clinical variants of familial neurological disorders such as the hereditary ataxias. Complicating this issue is the possibility that some of these cases may not actually reflect autosomal recessive inheritance but rather may be examples of unrecognized dominant inheritance or mitochondrial disease. Until the underlying genetic defects are better defined, these questions remain unresolved.

Rarely, an uncomplicated recessively inherited optic neuropathy is seen in children under the age of 4 years. This has been termed "congenital" optic atrophy, but the presence of visual dysfunction in infancy is difficult to assess. Severe visual loss with acuities worse than 20/200 is characteristic. There is typically achromatopsia or severe dyschromatopsia. The ophthalmoscopic appearance is that of diffuse disc pallor, sometimes accompanied by arteriolar attenuation. Electroretinography is normal. Nystagmus is common, reflecting the early and severe visual loss, but other neurological abnormalities are characteristically absent. Consanguinity between parents has been reported in over 50% of cases.

A more complicated form of recessively inherited optic neuropathy is the so-called "infantile" optic atrophy, or Behr's syndrome. In these patients, optic atrophy with moderate to severe visual loss is acquired usually prior to age 10 years. Nystagmus may be present and there is dyschromatopsia and temporal pallor of the optic discs. Associated neurological abnormalities include ataxia, spasticity, hypertonia, and mental retardation.

The specific association of autosomal recessively inherited optic atrophy and juvenile-onset diabetes mellitus, Wolfram's syndrome, has been considered a distinct clinical entity. The visual loss typically has its onset between the ages of 5 and 21 years and is characteristically slowly progressive. Ultimate acuities are usually worse than 20/400. There is severe dyschromatopsia and marked diffuse disc pallor, sometimes with nonglaucomatous optic disc cupping. Glucose intolerance is usually but not invariably noted prior to visual loss. Diabetes insipidus and sensorineural hearing loss are also common associations. Other neurological and systemic manifestations include ataxia, seizures, ptosis, mental retardation, nystagmus, short stature, anosmia, abnormal electroretinography, and elevated cerebrospinal fluid protein. Interestingly, many of these abnormalities are commonly encountered in patients with mitochondrial diseases. It remains to be seen whether individuals with Wolfram's syndrome may actually reflect a variety of different causative genetic defects. Management is necessarily limited to metabolic control of diabetes mellitus and diabetes insipidus and recognition of visual and hearing deficits early enough to institute appropriate aids.

III. MITOCHONDRIAL OPTIC NEUROPATHIES

It has long been recognized that some hereditary optic neuropathies are not inherited in a classic mendelian fashion. More recently, true maternal inheritance has been demonstrated in some of these pedigrees. This observation directed attention to the mitochondrion, the only extranuclear site of genetic material.

Mitochondria are small cytoplasmic organelles that provide most of the energy required for cell maintenance and growth. There are hundreds of mitochondria per cell, with more being present in those tissues particularly reliant on mitochondrial energy production. The central nervous system, including the eyes, has especially high energy requirements. Consequently, mitochondrial diseases frequently have neurological and ophthalmic manifestations.

Located within each mitochondrion are between 2 and 10 circles of deoxyribonucleic acid (DNA) similar but not identical to the nuclear genetic material. The mitochondrial DNA encodes for 13 proteins essential to the mitochondrial energy-production system, oxidative phosphorylation. These particular proteins are produced within the mitochondria and are joined by other nuclear-encoded proteins and cofactors that must be transported into the mitochondria from the cytoplasm. Hence, diseases of mitochondrial energy production could conceivably result from either nuclear or mitochondrial genetic defects.

Abnormalities in mitochondrial DNA are inherited in a strictly maternal fashion. During sexual reproduction, the cytoplasmic contents of the zygote are derived entirely from the mother's ovum. Every offspring, male or female, will inherit the mother's mitochondrial DNA. However, only the daughters will pass on their mitochondrial DNA to their children. If a nonlethal defect is present in a woman's mitochondrial DNA, this will be inherited by all her children and transmitted by her daughters.

Leber's hereditary optic neuropathy is characterized by subacute bilateral central visual loss and ultimately optic atrophy. When initially affected, patients are typically between the ages of 15 and 30 years, but examples of younger and older onset are common. There is a male predominance of between 60 and 90%.

Central vision progressively deteriorates usually over months. In classic descriptions, there is an interval of weeks to months between sequential eye involvement. However, in one review, over 50% of patients reported simultaneous onset. Rarely, involvement of the second eye may be delayed for years or the disease may remain symptomatically monocular. There are typically no other symptoms at the time of visual loss, although Uhthoff's symptom, a transient worsening of vision with exercise or temperature elevation, has been described.

Although visual acuities may range from 20/20 to no light perception, most patients will deteriorate to ultimate acuities of 20/200 or worse. Color vision is affected early and often severely. Visual fields show central or cecocentral defects. Spontaneous recovery of vision may occur even years after initial loss. Typically, this recovery assumes the configuration of a small island of vision of a few degrees within a dense central scotoma.

Much has been made of the characteristic funduscopic appearance of patients with Leber's hereditary optic neuropathy. In some patients with acute visual loss, one may see striking hyperemia of the optic disc, dilation and tortuosity of vessels, circumpapillary telangiectatic microangiopathy, and swelling of the nerve fiber layer around the disc ("pseudoedema"). Despite the edematous appearance of the disc, there is absence of disc leakage on fluorescein angiography. Asymptomatic maternal relatives at risk for the disease may exhibit an identical ophthalmoscopic picture. However, many patients never demonstrate features of the classic Leber's fundus even when examined at the time of acute visual loss. In all Leber's patients, the discs eventually become pale and there is nerve fiber layer loss, especially of the papillomacular bundle. Nonglaucomatous cupping may be seen.

Ancillary testing in the diagnosis of Leber's hereditary optic neuropathy is in general unrevealing. The exception, as noted above, is fluorescein angiography that can help distinguish Leber's disc changes from those of other optic neuropathies with disc edema by the former's lack of disc leakage. Visual evoked responses are predictably abnormal and electroretinograms are typically normal. In one study, brainstem auditory evoked potentials were nonspecifically abnormal in 7 of 11 patients. Cerebrospinal fluid analysis and electroencephalograms are typically normal. Brain neuroimaging with computed tomography or magnetic resonance imaging is usually unremarkable. However, lesions have been demonstrated in the optic nerves of affected individuals on magnetic resonance imaging of the orbits with fat-suppression techniques.

The majority of patients with maternally inherited optic neuropathy have only visual symptoms and signs. Some families, especially in Finland, have members with cardiac conduction abnormalities, specifically the preexcitation syndromes. Electrocardiograms should be obtained on all patients with suspected mitochondrial disease. Neurological abnormalities when present are usually minor. However, there are individual pedigrees with optic neuropathy plus more severe neurological deficits, including movement disorders, dystonia, basal gangliar lesions, spasticity, psychiatric disturbances, or acute encephalopathy.

The maternal inheritance pattern recognized in pedigrees with Leber's hereditary optic neuropathy prompted examination of the mitochondrial genome and the discovery of point mutations linked to this disease. Between 40 and 60% of Leber's families worldwide demonstrate a single nucleotide replacement mutation at position 11778 in the mitochondrial DNA (the so-called Wallace mutation). The mutation changes the coding for a highly conserved amino acid in one of the proteins essential to oxidative phosphorylation. Restriction endonucleases can test for the presence and quantity of this mutation in samples of blood and other tissues. Several other mitochondrial DNA point mutations have since been identified as causative in Leber's hereditary optic neuropathy. These mutations occur at different positions in the mitochondrial genome coding for different proteins involved in mitochondrial energy production. Some mutations are more pathogenic for the disease (so-called primary mutations) than others (so-called secondary mutations). Diagnostic centers specializing in mitochondrial disease provide a panel of tests screening for the presence of any of these mutations.

Genetic analysis has expanded our view of what constitutes the mitochondrial optic neuropathies. Patients and families somewhat atypical for the classic Leber's profile have tested positive for the mitochondrial DNA mutations. In a review of the clinical characteristics of patients with optic neuropathy and the Wallace mutation, 18% of the patients were older than 37 years, 14% younger than 16 years. Features of the characteristic Leber's fundus were observed in only 58% of patients. A family history of Leber's was absent in 57% of probands. Some of these singleton cases were outside the typical age range for Leber's hereditary optic neuropathy, some were women, and some did not exhibit the classic ophthalmoscopic abnormalities. Genetic analysis established the diagnosis of Leber's hereditary optic neuropathy in clinical situations that might not have otherwise suggested the disease. Mitochondrial optic neuropathy should be considered in the differential diagnosis of any unexplained bilateral optic neuropathy regardless of age of onset, patient gender, funduscopic appearance, or family history.

What genetic analysis has yet to fully explain are the determinants of expression of this disorder. The underlying causative mutation obviously plays a role in phenotypic expression. For example, the 11778 mutation has the worst prognosis for visual recovery. However, many of the mutations are at present clinically indistinguishable. Furthermore, individuals who carry the same mutation may present differently, and some will never exhibit clinical evidence of the disorder. The relative quantity of mutant mitochondrial DNA versus normal mitochondrial DNA in individuals and in various tissues may play some role in expression. Other contributing genetic factors could include other mitochondrial or nuclear DNA abnormalities that modify expression of the causative mutation. A factor located on the nuclear X chromosome might help explain the male predominance for phenotypic expression. Features of the patient's internal and external environment may also play a role. Systemic illnesses, nutritional deficiencies, or toxins that typically stress the mitochondrial energy production system might be particularly detrimental to an already genetically taxed mitochondrial apparatus.

Attempts at therapy in this disorder have generally been disappointing. Steroids, hydroxycobalamin, or cyanide antagonists have not proved useful during the acute phase of visual loss. Despite reports of visual improvement after the lysis of chiasmal arachnoid adhesions in patients with Leber's hereditary optic neuropathy, it is unlikely that surgical therapy will provide the answer in this disorder. At least two attempts at optic nerve sheath fenestration for this disease were ineffectual. To prevent potential stress on mitochondrial energy production, we recommend that patients at risk for Leber's hereditary optic neuropathy avoid tobacco, alcohol, and environmental toxins.

Identification of the specific genetic defects in this disorder may allow for a more directed approach to therapy. Succinate and coenzyme Q are naturally occurring cofactors necessary for normal mitochondrial energy production. There has been some anecdotal success in using these agents to treat other mitochondrial diseases such as the mitochondrial myopathies. Their efficacy in the treatment of acute mitochondrial optic neuropathy, in the prophylaxis against visual loss in the second eye, and in the prevention of visual loss in family members at risk remains to be demonstrated.

SELECTED READINGS

Dominant Optic Neuropathy

Hoyt CS: Autosomal dominant optic atrophy: a spectrum of disability. Ophthalmology 1980; 87:245.

Kivlin JD, Lovrien EW, Bishop DT, Maumenee IH. Linkage analysis in dominant optic atrophy. Am J Hum Genet 1983; 35:1190.

Kjer P. Infantile optic atrophy with dominant mode of inheritance: a clinical and genetic study of nineteen Danish families. Acta Ophthalmol (Copenh) 1959; Suppl. 54:1.

Kline LB, Glaser JS. Dominant optic atrophy: the clinical profile. Arch Ophthalmol 1979; 97:1680.

Smith DP. diagnostic criteria in dominantly inherited juvenile optic atrophy: a report of three new families. Am J Optom 1972; 49:183.

Recessive Optic Neuropathy

Behr C. Die komplizierte, Hereditar-familare optikusatrophie des kindesalters: En bisher nicht beschriebener synptomkomplex. Klin Monatsbl Augenheilkb 1909; 47:138.

Francois J. Mode d'heredite des heredo-degenerescences du nerf optique. J Genet Hum 1966; 15:147.

Lessell S, Rossman NP. Juvenile diabetes mellitus and optic atrophy. Arch Neurol 1977; 34:759.

Waardenburg PJ. Different types of hereditary optic atrophy. Acta Genet Statist Med 1957; 7:287.

Wolfram DJ. diabetes mellitus and simple optic atrophy among siblings. Mayo Clinic Proc 1938; 13:715.

Mitochondrial Optic Neuropathy

Leber T. Ueber hereditare and congenitalangelegte sehnervenleiden. Graefes Arch Ophthalmol 1871; 17:249.

Newman NJ. Leber's hereditary optic neuropathy. New genetic considerations. Arch Neurol 1993; 50:540.

Newman NJ, Lott MT, Wallace DC. The clinical characteristics of pedigrees of Leber's hereditary optic neuropathy with the 11778 mutation. Am J Ophthalmol 1991; 111:750.

Newman NJ. Mitochondrial disease and the eye. Ophthalmol Clin North Am 1992; 5:405.

Nikoskelainen E, Hoyt WF, Nummelin K. Ophthalmoscopic findings in Leber's hereditary optic neuropathy. I. Fundus findings in asymptomatic family members. Arch Ophthalmol 1982; 100:1597.

Nikoskelainen E, Hoyt WF, Numelin K. Ophthalmoscopic findings in Leber's hereditary optic neuropathy. II. The fundus findings in the affected family members. Arch Ophthalmol 1983; 101:1059.

Nikoskelainen E, Hoyt WF, Nummelin K, et al. Fundus findings in hereditary optic neuroretinopathy. III. Fluorescein angiographic studies. Arch Ophthalmol 1984; 102:981.

Nikoskelainen EK, Savontaus M-L, Wanne OP, et al. Leber's hereditary optic neuroretinopathy, a maternally inherited disease. A genealogic study in four pedigrees. Arch Ophthalmol 1987; 105:665.

Smith JL, Hoyt WF, Susac JO. Ocular fundus in acute Leber optic neuropathy. Arch Ophthalmol 1973; 90:349.

van Senus AHC. Leber's disease in the Netherlands. Doc Ophthalmol 1963; 17:1.

Wallace DC, Singh G, Lott MT, et al. Mitochondrial DNA mutation associated with Leber's hereditary optic neuropathy. Science 1988; 242:1427.

11

Evaluation and Treatment of Pituitary Tumor

Mary Lee Vance
University of Virginia Health Sciences Center, Charlottesville, Virginia

The diagnosis of a patient with a pituitary tumor has become straightforward with the advent of hormone assays and precise imaging techniques. Appropriate treatment most often requires the closely coordinated efforts of the primary care physician, endocrinologist, ophthalmologist, neurosurgeon, and, in some instances, radiotherapist. Once a tumor is discovered, the following questions must be addressed before embarking on therapy:

1. Is there visual compromise?
2. Is there significant hypopituitarism (secondary adrenal insufficiency, secondary hypothyroidism) requiring immediate replacement?
3. Is the tumor secretory?
4. Is the tumor a prolactinoma?
5. Is there a role for medical therapy (dopamine agonist drug for prolactinoma)?
6. Is there a role for surgery?

Enlargement of the pituitary is common and is usually the result of a pituitary adenoma. The prevalence of an asymptomatic pituitary microadenoma (<10 mm) in unselected autopsy studies is approximately 26%. Immunocytochemical staining reveals that the most common tumor type is prolactin-secreting (40%) (1,2). The prevalence of a pituitary macroadenoma (>10 mm) is not known but occurs less commonly than the smaller lesions. With improved imaging techniques (high-resolution computed tomography [CT], magnetic resonance imaging [MRI]), the incidentally discovered adenoma is now a common event. The diagnosis of a pituitary mass occurs either because of symptoms of a mass lesion (headache, visual disturbance), an endocrine syndrome (excessive or deficient hormone production), or incidentally. Regardless of how the patient comes to diagnosis, the evaluation remains the same and encompasses the efforts of the primary care physician, the ophthalmologist, endocrinologist, and neurosurgeon. This discussion includes a description of clinical manifestations of a pituitary tumor, appropriate evaluations, and currently recommended treatments.

I. CLINICAL PRESENTATION

If the pituitary mass is sufficiently large to impinge on the optic chiasm or invade the cavernous sinus and impair cranial nerve function, the initial manifestation of disease is either loss of vision or disturbance of ocular motility. Although this may be the symptom that prompts the patient to seek medical care, on thorough questioning, it is often evident that the patient has symptoms of endocrine dysfunction, the most common being hypogonadism in men and menstrual disturbance in premenopausal women.

Symptoms of endocrine dysfunction vary according to which hormone or hormones are produced in excess or which hormone or hormones are deficient. Pituitary insufficiency of one or more hormones is more common in patients with a macroadenoma (>10 mm) and is thought to result from compression of normal gland or destruction of normal gland from spontaneous hemorrhage of the tumor. The prevalence of one or more pituitary hormone deficiencies in patients with a macroadenoma ranges from 30 to 100%, with growth hormone (GH) deficiency being 100% in some series (3). Although gonadotropin (luteinizing hormone [LH], follicle-stimulating hormone [FSH]) or GH deficiency is a problem, it does not constitute an emergency. Deficiency of adrenocorticotropin (ACTH) or thyroid-stimulating hormone resulting in secondary adrenal insufficiency and hypothyroidism, respectively, requires immediate diagnosis and treatment. Symptoms of target hormone deficiency are listed in Table 1. It is important to recall that many of these symptoms are rather nonspecific, but in the setting of a pituitary tumor, they may be the only indication of endocrinopathy. The symptoms and signs of patients with excessive hormone production are listed in Table 2. Some patients have obvious evidence of hormone hypersecretion as in the case of florid Cushing's syndrome or long-standing acromegaly. However, by the time a patient develops these obvious clinical manifestations, it is likely that the disease has been present for years, particularly in acromegaly. Hopefully, with increased physician awareness of symptoms and signs of endocrine disturbance and with readily available and inexpensive

Table 1 Symptoms of Hormone Deficiency in Patients with Pituitary Disease

Pituitary hormone deficiency	Target hormone deficiency	Symptoms
ACTH	Cortisol	Fatigue, weight loss, anorexia, nausea, abdominal pain, decreased memory, headache
TSH	Thyroxine (T_4), Triiodothyronine (T_3)	Fatigue, weight gain, cold intolerance, constipation, decreased memory
LH, FSH	Women: estrogen, progesterone	Women: menstrual irregularity, amenorrhea, infertility, hot flashes, decreased libido, dyspareunia
	Men: testosterone	Men: decreased libido, impotence, infertility
Growth hormone	IGF-1	Children: growth retardation
Prolactin	—	Women: inability to nurse
		Men: no known syndrome
Vasopressin (ADH)	—	Polyuria, polydipsia, nocturia

hormone assays, the diagnosis can be made before significant morbidity and irreversible changes occur.

II. ENDOCRINE EVALUATION

All of the hormone tests needed to diagnose hormone hypersecretion or deficiency can be made in the outpatient setting, with either a single blood test or a 24-h urine collection. Most patients who present to an ophthalmologist because of visual problems as the initial manifestation of a pituitary tumor will have a large tumor and thus be at greater risk for adrenal and thyroid deficiency. These hormone deficiencies may be a medical emergency. The other urgent diagnostic test is to determine if the pituitary tumor is prolactin-secreting, since prompt institution of medical therapy can result in rapid tumor shrinkage and improvement of visual abnormalities.

The recommended screening hormone measurements are listed in Table 3. Although it is important to exclude significant hormone deficiency and hormone excess, the tests should be ordered according to clinical features. For example, in a patient with no symptoms or signs of excessive cortisol production, a 24-h urine collection to measure free cortisol as a screening test for Cushing's is unnecessary. Since symptoms of hypothyroidism and adrenal insufficiency may be nonspecific, serum thyroxine (T_4) and morning cortisol must be measured in all patients. Dynamic endocrine tests (stimulatory, suppressive) are often

Table 2 Symptoms and Signs of Hormone Hypersecretion in Patients with a Pituitary Adenoma

Pituitary hormone	Target hormone excess	Symptoms and signs
ACTH	Cortisol	Symptoms: fatigue, muscle weakness, depression, weight gain Signs: Adults: hypertension, central obesity, dorsal and supraclavicular fat, violaceous striae, acne, hirsutism (women), proximal muscle weakness Children: growth retardation
TSH	T_4, T_3	Symptoms: nervousness, palpitations, heat intolerance, sleep disturbance, weight loss. Signs: tachycardia, sweating, tremor, goiter (no exophthalmos)
LH, FSH	None	Symptoms: Women: menstrual disturbance, infertility, decreased libido, hot flashes, dyspareunia. Men: decreased libido, impotence. Signs: Men: decreased facial, axillary, pubic hair (long-standing disease), fine facial wrinkles Excessive LH, FSH secretion rarely associated with increased testosterone in men.
Growth hormone	IGF-1	Symptoms: Adults: joint pain, excessive sweating, dental malocclusion, enlargement face, hands, feet Children: excessive growth rate Signs: frontal bossing, prominent ocular ridge/ prognathism, large hands, feet, hyperhidrosis, hypertension, excessive skin tags, cystic acne
Prolactin	—	Symptoms: Women: menstrual disturbance, amenorrhea, infertility, decreased libido, hot flashes, dyspareunia. Men: decreased libido, hot flashes, impotence, breast enlargement, tenderness. Signs: Women: galactorrhea; Men: gynecomastia, galactorrhea, soft testes, decreased facial, axillary, pubic hair (testicular and hair changes only with long-standing gonadal failure)

performed in order to confirm the impression from the screening test. In a patient with suspected acromegaly and an elevated serum insulinlike growth factor-1 (IGF-1) level, the definitive test is the oral administration of glucose with measurement of growth hormone and glucose. Similarly, in a patient with an elevated 24-h urinary free cortisol, measurement of the plasma ACTH concen-

Table 3 Screening Endocrine Studies in a Patient with a Pituitary Mass

Hormone deficiency	Thyroxine (T_4)
	Morning cortisol
	Testosterone (men)
Hormone excess	Prolactin
	LH, FSH, Alpha subunit
	IGF-1
	24-h urine free cortisol

tration and suppressive tests with dexamethasone are necessary. If there is any question about the need for glucocorticoid replacement, this should be given and stimulatory tests can be performed at a later time. One important caveat is that thyroid hormone should never be given until adrenal insufficiency is excluded. Administration of thyroid hormone in the setting of adrenal insufficiency will precipitate an adrenal crisis because of the increase in metabolic rate from thyroid hormone administration.

III. MEDICAL TREATMENT OF PITUITARY TUMORS

The preferred treatment for a prolactin-secreting pituitary tumor is a dopamine agonist such as bromocriptine or pergolide. Numerous studies have documented the beneficial effects of medical therapy on reduction of tumor size, improvement of visual abnormalities, suppression of prolactin, and reversal of compromised pituitary function, most commonly hypogonadism (4–8). Over 90% of patients treated with a dopamine agonist have a good clinical and biochemical response. A few patients do not respond despite administration of adequate doses. This failure to respond to a dopamine agonist is related to the number of dopamine receptors on adenoma cells (9). Therefore, increasing the dose above the recommended amount (bromocriptine, 2.5 mg three times a day) is usually ineffective. If a tumor is unresponsive to dopamine agonist therapy, surgical resection is required.

Medical therapies for a growth hormone–secreting tumor include a somatostatin analogue, octreotide, and in some patients, a dopamine agonist. Hyopthalamic somatostatin inhibits GH secretion and the somatostatin analogue, an 8–amino acid peptide, octreotide, reduces GH secretion in over 90% of patients (10,11). Reduction of GH and IGF-1 to normal occurs in approximately 42% of patients (10). Although some patients have a decrease in tumor size, the magnitude of reduction is not as great as that observed with prolactin-secreting tumors treated with a dopamine agonist. Thus, the primary therapy for a GH-secreting tumor is surgical resection. Medical therapy is used most commonly for patients who have residual GH hypersecretion. Some patients have been treated with octreotide prior to surgery with variable results regarding reduction in tumor size. Octreotide must be given by subcutaneous injection, usually every 8 h. Prior to development of octreotide, the dopamine agonist drugs bromocriptine and pergolide were the only medical treatments available. Dopamine agonist drugs often reduce GH and IFG-1 concentrations but rarely to normal.

The preferred choice of treatment for a nonsecretory or gonadotropin-secreting tumor is surgical resection. If the patient cannot undergo surgery or refuses an operation, a dopamine agonist should be given, since a few patients have had improvement in visual abnormalities with this therapy. Visual improvement usually occurs without significant change in overall tumor size on MRI or CT scan. However, some decrease, albeit undetectable with current imaging techniques, has occurred since visual field abnormalities improved (12).

IV. WHEN IS SURGERY INDICATED?

Surgery is indicated as primary therapy for all pituitary tumors except prolactinomas. Surgical resection of a pituitary tumor is most often carried out via a transsphe- noidal approach. This method is associated with less morbidity than is craniotomy and may result in complete removal of the adenoma. The most important factors in assuring a successful outcome are the experience of the neurosurgeon and the size of the tumor (13–16). In centers of excellence in transsphenoidal surgery, complete resection of a macroadenoma ($\geq$10 mm) may be accomplished, particularly if there is no tumor invasion of the dura, cavernous sinus, or bone. Despite presumed complete removal, the recurrence rate is approximately 16% (13,14). Other important factors influencing surgical "cure" is the presence of bone, dural, or cavernous sinus invasion. If pathological examination of the tissue reveals dural or bone invasion by the tumor, it is quite probable that the tumor will recur. This may be quite delayed with recurrence after 10 years, requiring additional treatment of 6% in one series (14). This feature requires that any patient with a pituitary tumor receive regular evaluations and life-long medical follow-up.

V. WHEN IS RADIATION THERAPY INDICATED?

Radiation therapy, either conventional or focused (gamma knife, proton beam), is most commonly used as adjunctive therapy when the patient has residual disease after surgical resection. The primary limitations of pituitary radiation are the delay in effectiveness and high probability of permanent hypopituitarism. Prompt reduction in tumor size with improvement in visual abnormalities or suppression of hormone hypersecretion does not occur with radiation therapy. For example, in acromegaly, reduction of growth hormone to normal rarely occurs within the first 5 years and may require 10–20 years. During this time of GH hypersecretion, patients continue to experience the effects of excessive GH and the risk of permanent morbidity and premature mortality persists.

Development of pituitary hormone deficiency after radiotherapy is a certainty, but the timing is highly variable (17–21). In one study, 50% of patients had one or more hormone deficiencies within 2 years of radiation (18). Endocrine evaluation is necessary before and at regular intervals after radiotherapy to determine which, if any, hormone deficiency has developed and to institute appropriate replacement therapy. As noted above, development of ACTH or TSH deficiency requires prompt detection and treatment. An important factor in recommending pituitary radiation is the age of the patient and the desire for fertility, since the onset of pituitary deficiency or the particular hormone deficiency cannot be predicted. Thus, all patients must be informed of the likelihood of requiring hormone replacement therapy and the potential for infertility must be explained to a woman of childbearing age or a man who may wish to father a child. Damage to the visual system with pituitary radiation has been reported, which emphasizes the need for an experienced radiotherapist to administer this treatment.

Focused radiation (gamma knife, linac, proton beam), usually administered in one treatment in contrast to 20 treatments of fractionated doses of conventional radiation, is certainly more convenient for a patient. Focused radiotherapy is restricted to patients with a small intrasellar lesion (<10 mm) that does not approach or approximate the optic chiasm. Radiation scatter from a concentrated dose of radiation carries a significant risk of damage to the chiasm. It is not yet known if focused radiation with the gamma knife results in more rapid control of hormone hypersecretion, since this is a recently developed method of delivering radiotherapy.

Occasionally, a patient refuses surgery or cannot undergo the procedure. In this situation, pituitary radiation may be the only definitive treatment for a non-prolactinoma. As noted earlier, a trial of bromocriptine for a nonsecretory tumor or octreotide for a GH- or TSH-secreting tumor should be given. If radiation treatment is given to a patient with a macroadenoma with suprasellar extension, there is some risk of chiasmal compression from radiation-induced edema; this may respond to a brief course of pharmacological doses of dexamethasone.

VI. OPHTHALMOLOGICAL EVALUATIONS

Specific ophthalmological studies will not be discussed. All patients with a pituitary tumor of >10 mm at the time of diagnosis should undergo a full ophthalmological examination, including automated perimetry. If visual abnormalities are present, immediate therapy is required to preserve remaining function and, hopefully, reverse the abnormalities. If a patient has a prolactinoma and visual abnormalities, it is prudent to repeat the examination after 2 weeks of dopamine agonist treatment. The visual examination is more sensitive than is an imaging study, since improvement in visual fields and acuity may occur before demonstrable change in the MRI scan. If the serum prolactin declines significantly and the tumor decreases in size with dopamine agonist therapy and there is no improvement in visual abnormalities, it may be presumed that the chiasm (or optic nerve) has been damaged permanently. Late improvement, however, is possible. All patients with an abnormal preoperative ophthalmological examination require a postoperative evaluation. One caveat is that some patients, particularly the elderly, may have difficulty concentrating on automated perimetry study immediately after surgery. These patients should be retested when more stable, usually 2 to 3 weeks after discharge. If pituitary radiation is recommended, a pretreatment ophthalmological examination should be performed in the event of later visual deterioration.

VII. CONCLUSIONS

Once a patient has the diagnosis of a pituitary tumor, there is a need for life-long monitoring. These patients are at risk for tumor recurrence with subsequent development of visual impairment or development of hypopituitarism. They are also at risk for spontaneous hemorrhage into a tumor (pituitary apoplexy) with acute resulting visual compromise and/or hormone deficiency. As noted, optimal care of the patient with a pituitary tumor requires the expertise of and interaction among physicians of several medical specialties.

REFERENCES

1. Costello RT. Subclinical adenoma of the pituitary gland. Am J Pathol 1936; 12:205–15.
2. Burows GN, Wortzman G, Rewcastle NB, Holgate RC, Kovacs K. Microadenomas of the pituitary and abnormal sellar tomograms in an unselected autopsy series. N Engl J Med 1981; 304:156–8.
3. Arafah BM, Harrington JF, Madhoun ZT, Selman WR. Improvement of pituitary function after surgical decompression for pituitary tumor apoplexy. J Clin Endocrinol Metab 1990; 71:323–8.
4. Vance ML, Evans WS, Thorner MO. Drugs five years later: bromocriptine. Ann Intern Med 1984; 100:78–91.
5. Molitch ME, Elton RL, Blackwell RE, et al. Bromocriptine as primary therapy for prolactin-secreting macroadenomas: results of a prospective multicenter study. J Clin Endocrinol Metab 1985; 60:698–705.

6. Liuzzi A, Dallabonzana D, Oppizzi G, et al. Low doses of dopamine agonists in the long-term treatment of macroprolactinomas. N Engl J Med 1985; 313:656–9.
7. Kendall-Taylor P, Hall K, Johnston DG, et al. Reduction in size of prolactin-secreting tumors in men treated with pergolide. Br Med J 1982; 285:465–467.
8. Kleinberg DL, Boyd AE, Wardlaw S, et al. Pergolide for the treatment of pituitary tumors secreting prolactin or growth hormone. N Engl J Med 1983; 309:704–9.
9. Pellegrini I, Rasolonjanahary R, Gunz G, et al. Resistance to bromocriptine in prolactinomas. J Clin Endocrinol Metab 1989; 69:500–9.
10. Vance ML, Harris AG. Long term treatment of 189 acromegalic patients with the somatostatin analog octreotide. Arch Intern Med 1991; 151:1573–8.
11. Ezzat S, Snyder PJ, Young WF, Boyajy LD, Newman C, Klibanski A, Molitch ME, Boyd AE, Sheeler L, Cook DM, Malarkey WB, Jackson I, Vance ML, Thorner MO, Barkan A, Frohman LA, Melmed S. Octreotide treatment of acromegaly. A randomized, multicenter study. Ann Intern Med 1992; 117:711–18.
12. Vance ML, Ridgway EC, Thorner MO. FSH and alpha subunit secreting pituitary tumor treated with bromocriptine. J Clin Endocrinol Metab 1985; 61:580–4.
13. Laws ER Jr. Pituitary surgery. Endocrinol Metab Clin North America 1987; 16:647–65.
14. Ebersold MJ, Quast LM, Laws ER Jr, et al. Long-term results in transsphenoidal removal of nonfunctioning pituitary adenomas. J Neurosurg 1986;64:713–9.
15. Nelson PB, Goodman ML, Flickenger JC, Richardson DW, Robinson AG. Endocrine function in patients with large pituitary tumors treated with operative decompression and radiation therapy. Neurosurgery 1989; 24:398–400.
16. Harris PE, Afshar F, Coates P, Doniach I, Wass JAH, Besser GM, Grossman A. The effects of transsphenoidal surgery on endocrine function and visual fields in patients with functionless pituitary tumours. Q J Med 1989; 71:417–27.
17. Constine LS, Woolf PD, Cann D, et al. Hypothalamic-pituitary dysfunction after radiation for brain tumors. N Engl J Med 1993; 328:87–94.
18. Snyder PJ, Fowble BF, Schatz NJ, Savino PJ, Gennarelli TA. Hypopituitarism following radiation therapy of pituitary adenomas. Am J Med 1986; 81:457–62.
19. Littley MD, Shalet SM, Beardwell CG, Ahmed SR, Applegate G, Sutton ML. Hypopituitarism following external radiotherapy for pituitary tumours in adults. Q J Med 1989; 70:145–60.
20. Kliman B, Kjellberg RN, Swisher B, Butler W. Proton beam therapy of acromegaly: a 20-year experience. In: Black PMcL, et al., eds. Secretory tumors of the pituitary gland. New York: Raven Press, 1984:191–211.
21. Linfoot JA. Alpha particle pituitary irradiation in the primary and post-surgical management of pituitary microadenomas. In: Faglia G, Giovanelli MA, MacLeod RM, eds. Pituitary microadenomas. Vol 29. London: Academic Press, 1980:514–29.

12

Optic Nerve Gliomas: Treatment Differences for the Benign and Malignant Varieties

W. Bruce Wilson
University of Colorado Health Sciences Center, Denver, Colorado

Optic nerve gliomas (optic gliomas) are tumors of the optic nerve, chiasm, and optic tracts. They may occur in isolation or in combination with other diseases. They are found in association with neurofibromatosis 1 (NF-1) and possibly in association with NF-2, although the latter association is not clear (1). It is probable that the highest incidence of optic gliomas is found either in association with NF-1 or as a sporadic expression. The ones that are thought to be due to a sporadic mutation are rarely associated with other stigmata of disease. Most optic gliomas then occur in association with NF-1 or are sporadic. Less common are the rare optic gliomas found in association with the diencephalic syndrome or the rare malignant adult glioma. These two types, one common and relatively benign and the other rare and clinically malignant, suggest there may be two types of natural history and treatment: "benign" ones that grow slowly, invade rarely, and may not need radical therapy and "malignant" ones that may grow rapidly, invade early, and may not respond in spite of radical therapy.

Optic gliomas make up approximately 1% of all intracranial tumors (2). The age at diagnosis for the benign type of optic gliomas ranges from birth through old age, although the initial clinical expression of this type of optic glioma is rare after age 10 years (3–5). Although the benign type of childhood optic glioma can occur at birth, these younger cases, while usually relatively benign histologically, more often are large tumors that involve both the diencephalon and the chiasm and behave in an aggressive, invasive manner. The adult malignant gliomas usually occur in early adult life.

The sex distribution for optic gliomas is fairly equal. There has never been any documented racial predilection, although these tumors may be more common in the Caucasian race.

I. ETIOLOGY AND ASSOCIATED DISEASE

The only etiology for optic nerve glioma that has been clearly worked out is its association with NF-1. This is a 17 Q 11.2 locus abnormality. It has been said that probably 20–30% of optic gliomas are associated with NF-1. The reverse association is similar; that is, in all cases of NF-1, probably 15% have optic glioma (6). These figures may be subject to correction as time goes on, because many factors, such as long-term follow-up, may not have been used in all of these cases. Increased use of magnetic resonance imaging (MRI) in long-term follow-up is likely to increase both the frequency of associated glioma and the incidence of NF-1 in patients with an optic glioma. There are some studies that have reported a higher incidence of optic glioma in NF-1—up to 50 or 60% (6). Since it is somewhat problematic as to whether optic gliomas occur in association with NF-2, no real etiological determination can be made in that case. There has been a suggestion that meningiomas have a higher than chance association with optic gliomas. This may be tainted by a diagnosis of meningioma in patients with meningieal reaction to an underlying glioma. Certainly other gliomas are much more common in association with optic gliomas, but this is probably related to their association with the entire complex of NF-1.

Hypothalamic gliomas do have an association with chiasmal glioma, but it is usually not possible to tell clinically or radiographically whether the tumor started in the chiasm and spread to the hypothalamus or started in the hypothalamus and spread to the chiasm or whether there were two separate gliomas (7–9). There are a few cases where it seems relatively clear that a hypothalamic tumor spread to the chiasm, such as the case reported by Davis et al. (10). There also are less convincing cases where the tumors seemed to start in the chiasm and spread to the hypothalamus (5,11).

II. NATURAL HISTORY

As mentioned above, the natural history of optic gliomas can probably be divided into two types. When one speaks of "optic glioma," one is usually talking about the fairly benign childhood pilocytic type of glioma that occurs as a sporadic expression or occurs with NF-1. Even so, this type of glioma can probably be divided into two types; those that have fairly stable, benign course and do not threaten function or life and those that are infiltrative, destroy vision, and cause other neurological problems (2,3,7,12,13). Specific illustrations of those that seem to be the "benign of the benign," which grow locally to a certain point then stop are noted by Wilson (5) and Borit (14). This tumor usually starts in the optic nerve and there is a reasonably short course of growth in these patients, so that by the time symptoms and signs are noted by the family or a physician and the patient is referred, the tumor has come to a relatively stable position and may not grow much beyond that point. Others, although in the distinct minority, grow posteriorly from one nerve or more likely from the chiasm, and their spread may cause blindness or death. Even though the chiasmal type of the fairly benign glioma group may cause death, it is unusual. In fact, in one series only two of nine patients could be determined to have died as a result of the infiltration of the chiasmal glioma itself (13).

In both those that remain stable and do not cause major neurological problems, which are more likely to occur in one optic nerve, or optic gliomas that infiltrate and cause problems, which are more likely to start in the chiasm, delayed degeneration within the tumor can cause clinical changes without tumor growth. Proptosis or further reduction in vision can be observed (13). It may be difficult to differentiate local degeneration with an increase in the size of the tumor from local growth of the tumor without further infiltration (5,9).

Origination of optic gliomas may potentially be unicentric, multicentric, or diffuse centric. It would seem that most tumors are unicentric in that they tend to grow from one spot and spread over time as they are followed clinically and by MRI scans (5). Further support for the concept that these tumors are unicentric is found in cases where the tumor has been only partially resected and where some tumor remains at the proximal cut end of one optic nerve. These tumors generally do not show a tendency for further growth over many years, which suggests that most of the tumors do not represent diffuse centricity or multiple centricity. In one series studying the issue of multicentricity, no examples were found of tumors starting in more than one location and finally fusing into one tumor; for example, a tumor starting in each optic nerve and finally growing in the optic chiasm (5). Chiasmal gliomas may occasionally undergo malignant evolution (15).

The natural history of hypothalamic gliomas shows that they are much more aggressive. Although they are usually not cytologically malignant, they often lead to death (10). The same can be said for the malignant adult gliomas (7).

III. CLINICAL MANIFESTATIONS

Most of our clinical information about optic gliomas comes from the more benign-acting pilocytic cell type occurring in childhood and probably more commonly known as childhood optic glioma. Whether they occur in one nerve or involve the optic chiasm determines whether clinical signs occur in one eye or both. A loss in visual acuity is an almost constant finding at presentation. There usually is some accompanying compromise of color vision and visual field. However, some of these tumors occur in infancy, so these determinations are difficult. If there is loss of vision, more often than not there will be a relative afferent pupil defect on the side of the optic glioma. Examination may show pallor or edema of the optic nerve depending on the stage of tumor development (5). Proptosis without measurable visual loss may also be the presenting sign, although this is much less common. Shunt vessels may be seen on the optic nerve head (16). The eye itself may have congenital abnormalities: coloboma, microphthalmos, or macrophthalmos, usually associated with NF-1 (6). Lisch's nodules, hamartomas of the iris, may be seen. As mentioned above, if optic gliomas occur in association with NF-2, they certainly are very rare. Even so, patients with NF-2 uncommonly have congenital abnormalities in the optic disc or have choroidal hamartomas or lens opacities.

Ocular motility is frequently affected if the glioma is in the orbit but otherwise is rarely abnormal, since the ocular motor nerves III–VI are almost always spared with chiasmal involvement. Ocular motility changes usually represent a mechanical difficulty with movement due to tumor size and position. Nystagmus may be seen in one or both eyes and is usually associated with decreased vision. This is almost uniformly seen if the chiasm is involved. In hypothalamic chiasmal gliomas, involvement of the upper brain stem may produce nystagmus.

Neurological signs such as precocious puberty, epilepsy, hemiparesis, delayed development, and the diencephalic syndrome may be seen with large hypothalamic tumors. Hydrocephalus may also occur if the tumor is large enough to block the third ventricle or foramina of Monro. In these cases, headache is a common symptom as well (8).

IV. PATHOLOGY

The so-called benign childhood optic gliomas are almost all a relatively low-grade form of astrocytoma commonly referred to as a pilocytic astrocytoma. In some cases, the designation grade I is used, but it is problematic as to whether this is a semantic difference or a real one. In any case, these are relatively benign histologically (5,9,14). It has been suggested that at least some of these represent choristomas of the anterior visual system (17).

It is difficult to tell in some cases of optic glioma, particularly those occurring in NF-1, whether the tumor is surrounded by a neoplastic process outside the optic nerve or whether there is simply hyperplasia of the arachnoidal tissues. In either case, striking radiographic changes can be seen where tissue surrounds the optic glioma. Often there is well-preserved visual function (6).

The extent of involvement of the visual system in childhood optic gliomas varies. It may be localized in one optic nerve or it may run from one end of the visual system, that is, adjacent to the eye, to the other. It may include the geniculate body, so that there may be tumor infiltration of the entire course of the ganglion cell that starts in the retina and ends in the lateral geniculate body (3,9).

The malignant adult gliomas are of a higher grade of malignancy than those we have discussed in the section just completed. Diencephalic gliomas, although behaving aggressively, are generally cytologically benign.

V. DIAGNOSTIC PROCEDURES

The computed tomographic (CT) scan has been the standard for diagnosing optic gliomas for the last two decades but is being replaced by MRI. There is not much calcific material in optic gliomas and tissue differentiation and characterization is better with MRI, particularly in those that occur intracranially. It is reported that the usual configuration for an optic glioma that involves one optic nerve is a large fusiform optic nerve without the polar expansions at either end in the orbit that are more characteristic of meningioma (16). Cysts and rare calcific changes may occur in optic gliomas. It is quite common for the optic canal to be enlarged (5,16), which is often the diagnostic finding on pre-CT plain films.

When the MRI scan became the standard imaging technique for evaluating optic glioma, it had been hoped that this might help us differentiate the proximal end of the tumor and therefore determine whether or not the optic glioma was invading the chiasm (Fig. 1). It was hoped that possible progression of a glioma toward the chiasm could be followed permitting surgery in a timely fashion before invasion of the chiasm occurred. However, it has been very difficult to differentiate the edge of the optic glioma even with gadolinium-enhanced MRI. Many optic gliomas do not light up on T_2 images and demonstrate little or no enhancement with gadolinium. Difficulty defining the proximal end of the optic glioma persists. The enlargement of the nerve still seems to be as good as any to define the proximal end of the glioma (5). Elongation and kinking of the nerve also is characteristic (18). The double density that is seen in regard to optic nerve glioma also is characteristic and probably almost pathognomonic for NF-1. What one sees is a high T_2 signal around the optic nerve. This surround tissue signal is approximately the consistency of water arising from the gliomatosis that surrounds the optic nerve in the case of an optic glioma (18). Bilateral involvement of the anterior visual system, that is, both optic nerves affected by the glioma, also is essentially pathognomonic for NF-1 (18). Occasionally, large cysts of optic gliomas are seen on MRI scanning, and some of these can occur in the chiasmal area and increase to such a degree that they may compromise the brain adjacent to the cyst and do need surgical attention (19). There are a

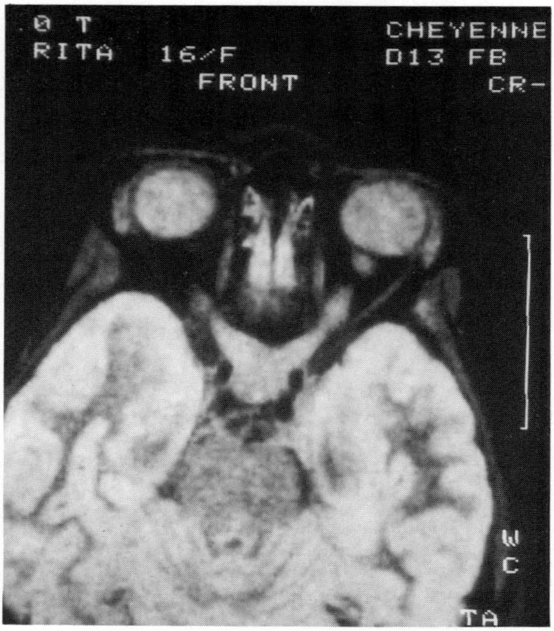

Figure 1 Axial and coronal MRI sections of a glioma of the chiasm and optic nerves in a 16-year-old girl with NF-1.

number of associated hamartomas that occur with optic gliomas but this is mostly in the setting of NF-1. In other words, one can get high signal intensity spots within the peduncles, pons, globus pallidus, midbrain, thalamus, and cerebrum (6). Better-known findings are café au lait spots and neurofibromas characteristic of NF-1.

It is becoming clearer with time that when one has a characteristic appearance of intrinsic optic nerve and/or chiasmal enlargement on MRI that a diagnosis can usually be made on the MRI scan alone without biopsy. Cerebrospinal fluid (CSF) analysis is rarely helpful in the diagnosis of optic glioma. Biopsy of hypothalamic gliomas may be needed.

VI. DIFFERENTIAL DIAGNOSIS

Any lesion of the optic nerve and chiasm may masquerade as an optic nerve or chiasmal glioma. The two lesions that are probably the most difficult to differentiate from optic glioma on MRI imaging are germinoma of the visual system and optic nerve choristoma, since these may be intrinsic to the visual

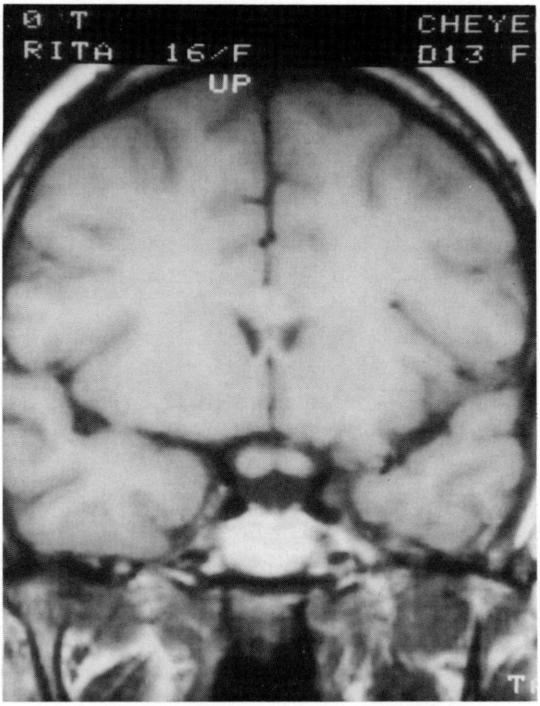

system without an exophytic component. However, the latter is very rare and the former also is fairly uncommon, so that the search for other signs of NF-1 might clinch the diagnosis without having to resort to a biopsy.

Craniopharyngiomas usually have characteristic sellar enlargement, pituitary hypofunction, and calcium within the tumor that would differentiate these from an optic glioma. They also do not appear to be intrinsic to the visual system on careful MRI scanning. Optic nerve sheath meningioma limited to the orbit might be difficult to tell from an optic glioma in the orbit, but an increase in signal on T_2 with MRI scanning generally indicates a meningioma. Also, meningiomas enhance strongly with gadolinium. This is especially well seen with fat-suppression sequences. Rarely do optic gliomas increase much in signal on T_2 imaging or with gadolinium. In addition, a meningioma is almost always going to surround the nerve rather than cause a diffuse enlargement of the optic nerve. It tends to have polar enlargement of the tumor in the orbital apex and next to the globe with some calcium deposited and does not adhere to the nerve or seem intrinsic to it as soon as the nerve passes through the canal and enters the intracranial space.

Metastatic tumors of the nerve are quite rare, although they may occur. One then needs to search for a primary tumor. The three types of tumors that seem to have the most frequent metastatic involvement of the optic nerve are breast, oat cell of the lung, and melanoma. The general physical examination, laboratory evaluation, and appropriate imaging will usually clarify this issue.

Occasionally, pituitary tumors can be confused with optic glioma, particularly if the studies are not of high quality. The sella again is involved, as it is with the craniopharyngioma, and often two densities can be seen on the MRI in the sella. One density is the gland and the other is the tumor surrounding the gland. Again, these tumors do not seem to be intrinsic to the optic nerve or chiasm and endocrine studies indicating pituitary dysfunction are helpful in making the diagnosis.

Rarely do aneurysms in the area of the sella or suprasellar space adhere closely enough to the visual system to appear intrinsic and be confused with an optic glioma after imaging studies. The MRA scanning technique should settle this issue. Infiltration of the visual system by sarcoidosis or some other infectious or inflammatory pathophysiology can, in some cases, come close to mimicking optic glioma, but generally the outside of the optic nerve is shaggy. The cerebrospinal fluid space about the optic nerve and chiasm may show evidence of inflammation.

VII. TREATMENT

A rational approach to therapy of each variety of optic glioma can only be made when the natural history is carefully considered. For years, many investigators have suggested that surgery is the preferred mode of treatment. This goes back to the report of Hudson in 1912 (20).

If a tumor involves the chiasm, it is obvious that surgery, although it may occasionally be helpful (19), almost certainly cannot effect a cure without inducing blindness and possibly other complications. If a tumor affects one nerve, an excision at the anterior border of chiasm may affect a cure, since most of these tumors appear to be unicentric (21,22). Of course, this will not resolve the problem if the tumor is multicentric or diffusely centric or if the chiasm is already involved. Additionally, one must realize that unilateral (one optic nerve) gliomas rarely invade the central nervous system when they originate intraorbitally and even in those rare cases vision may be good for years. Death from this extension is even rarer.

Occasionally, a debulking procedure of a large exophytic chiasmal glioma, with or without a cystic component, is helpful (19). This can relieve additional compression of the anterior visual pathways.

Others have felt that observation of these tumors is proper, since the chance of infiltration is so rare. Even if they involve the chiasm, the chance of blindness, death, or major dysfunction of the brain or endocrine system is rare (23,24). This aspect of natural history certainly suggests careful consideration of the risk/benefit ratio before surgery is undertaken.

Numerous references suggest conventional radiotherapy is beneficial in these tumors. A 4 to 8 million electron volt linear accelerator is used and doses vary from 2000 to 5000 cGy. The concern with radiotherapy is that a number of cases have complications as a result of the procedure (9,25). The endocrine problems include short stature associated with decreased growth hormone and neuropsychological dysfunction. Many examples of radionecrosis of the medial temporal lobes, which are usually within the ports of the radiation therapy, are given in the literature (12,19,26–28). In spite of these potential complications of radiotherapy, an occasional patient has had a marked improvement in visual function after radiotherapy. There doesn't seem to be any literature that favorably reports that particle radiation plays a part in treatment of optic gliomas at this time. There are no current reports on the use of focused radiation therapy (gamma knife) and the risk of radiation-induced necrosis suggests this will not be a useful mode of therapy.

Although studies of chemotherapy are relatively limited, there are those who suggest that vincristine and actinomycin D used in a small number of patients may be of benefit in either reducing the size of the tumor or at least in stabilizing it (12). Other therapeutic regimens have also been advocated (28).

Until more benefit can be shown from either radiation therapy or chemotherapy, excision of the unilateral optic glioma that has not involved the chiasm is probably the most practical way of treating this tumor. The exception is the patient with a chiasmal glioma who is facing blindness. Then radiotherapy is a logical consideration. In the case of almost all of the optic gliomas, at least of the fairly benign childhood type, the deoxyribonucleic acid (DNA) replication and cell growth is so slow that the response from either method of therapy would be expected to be limited. Fortunately, it also suggests that most patients may do very well without treatment at all.

REFERENCES

1. Michels VV, Whistnant JP, Garrity JA, et al. Neurofibromatosis Type 1 with bilateral acoustic neuromas. Neurofibromatosis 1989; 2:213–7.
2. Lloyd LA. Gliomas of the optic nerve and chiasm in childhood. Trans Am Ophthalmol Soc 1973; 71:488–535.
3. Miller NR, et al. Evaluation and management of gliomas of anterior visual pathways. Brain 1974; 97:743–54.
4. Chutorian AM, et al. Optic gliomas in children. Neurology 1964; 14:83–95.
5. Wilson WB. Tumor spread in unilateral optic glioma-II. Neurofibromatosis 1989; 2:195–203.
6. Hoyt WF, Imes RI. Optic gliomas of neurofibromatosis 1. In: Ishibashi Y, Hori Y, eds. Tuberous sclerosis and neurofibromatosis. Elsevier, 1990:

7. Hoyt WF, Meshel LG, Lesser S. Malignant optic glioma of adulthood. Brain 1973; 96:121–32.
8. Russell DS, Rubinstein LJ. Pathology of tumors of the nervous system. Baltimore: Williams & Wilkins, 1977.
9. Wong JYC, Uhl V, Wara W, et al. Optic glioma. Cancer 1987; 60:1847–51.
10. Davis PC, Hoffman JC, Weidenheim KM. Large hypothalamic gland optic chiasm gliomas in infants. AJNR 1984; 5:529–85.
11. Wong IG, Lubow M. Management of optic glioma of childhood-A review of 42 cases. Neuro-Ophthalmol Symposium of University of Miami Bascom Palmer Eye Institute 1972; 6:51–60.
12. Rosenstock JG, Packer RJ, Bilaniuk L, et al. Chiasmatic optic glioma treated with chemotherapy. J Neurosurg 1985; 63:862–66.
13. Imes RK, Hoyt WF. Childhood chiasmal gliomas: update on the fate of the patients in the 1969 San Fran study. Br J Ophthalmol 1982; 70:179–82.
14. Borit A, Richardson EP Jr. Biological and clinical behavior of pilocystic astrocytomas of the optic pathways. Brain 1982; 105:161–87.
15. Wilson WB, Feinsod M, Hoyt WF, et al. Malignant evolution of childhood chiasmal pilocytic astrocytoma. Neurology 1976; 26:322–5.
16. Jakobiec FA, Depot MJ, Kennerdell JS, et al. Combined clinical and CT diagnosis of orbital gliomas and meningiomas. Ophthalmology 1984; 91:137–55.
17. Kazim M, Kennerdell JS, Maroon J, et al. Choristoma of the optic nerve and chiasm. Arch Ophthalmol 1992; 110:236–8.
18. Imes RK, Hoyt WF. MRI signs of optic nerve glioma in NF1. Am J Ophthalmol 1991; 111:729–34.
19. Wilson WB, Finkel RS, McCleary L, et al. Large cystic optic glioma. Neurology 1990; 40:1898–1900.
20. Hudson AC. Primary tumors of the optic nerve. R Lond Ophthalmol Hosp R 1912; 18:317–439.
21. Wright JE, McNab AA, McDonald WI. Optic nerve glioma and the management of optic nerve tumors in the young. Br J Ophthalmol 1989; 73:962–74.
22. Rush JA, Younge BR, Campbell RJ, et al. Optic glioma: long term follow up of 85 histopathologically verified cases. Ophthalmology 1982; 89:1213–9.
23. Hoyt WF, Baghdassarian S. Optic glioma of childhood: natural history and rationale for conservative management. Br J Ophthalmol 1969; 53:793–8.
24. Glaser JS, Hoyt WF, Corbett J. Visual morbidity with chiasmal glioma. Arch Ophthalmol 1971; 85:3–12.
25. Traveras JM, Mount LA, Wood EJ. The value of radiation therapy in the management of glioma of the optic nerves and chiasm. Radiology 1956; 66:518.
26. Horwick A, Bloom HJG. Optic gliomas: radiation therapies and prognosis. Int J Radiat Oncol Biol Phys 1985; 11:1067–79.
27. Brauner R, Malandry F, Rappaport R, et al. Growth and endocrine disorders in optic glioma. Eur J Pediatr 1990; 149:825–8.
28. Petronio J, Edwards MSB, Prados M, et al. Management of chiasmal and hypothalamic gliomas of infancy and childhood with chemotherapy. J Neurosurg 1991; 74:701–8.

II

EFFERENT SYSTEM

13

Development of Congenital and Infantile Nystagmus

Robert D. Reinecke
Jefferson Medical College; and Foerderer Eye Movement Center for Children, Wills Eye Hospital, Philadelphia, Pennsylvania

Almost 20 years ago, the grandmother of a 1-month-old infant was present as the mother asked, "Does my child have nystagmus?" The grandmother interrupted,

> I should warn you doctor, that when we have asked that question of doctors before when a grandchild was this young, the doctor often gave what turned out to be a wrong answer. That is, some of my grandchildren were thought to have no nystagmus and within a few months nystagmus became apparent. So, please take your time before you answer.

I took my time. I saw family members who had nystagmus. They gave a history of developing nystagmus at about 4 months of age. Several of these infants were feared to be blind at the time their nystagmus was first noticed. No blindness evolved, but the consideration of blindness enhanced the family's skepticism of physicians' advice. Our patient developed wide sweeping nystagmus at the age of 4 months. The grandmother remarked, "This large nystagmus was present in the children when the doctors thought them to be blind, but the nystagmus lessened to that found in the adults of our family." The adult nystagmus in this family was the jerk type with a null point. As we followed the child, the grandmother's caution proved appropriate. The wide sweeping nystagmus at age 4 months gave way at about age 8 months to fine pendular nystagmus, and finally at 14 months, jerk nystagmus developed. By about age

6 years, almost all of the nystagmus was jerk type with a null point and the child showed a head turn appropriate to the eccentric null point.

This family evidenced another typical finding. The children were all quite blond and the irides showed mild transillumination. The blondness changed at puberty to dark brunette hair and the skin started to tan moderately.

I. INFANTILE NYSTAGMUS

As more infants were observed who did not have nystagmus until about 4 months of age, we came to understand the similarity of the development of nystagmus to that of developing infantile esotropia. In the early 1970s, emphasis was placed on using the term *congenital* esotropia only if the esotropia actually was present at birth rather than developing during the first year of life. The more appropriate term was thought to be *infantile* esotropia. We reasoned that the term *congenital* nystagmus was usually not accurate as most children developed their nystagmus at about age 4 months. We suggested the term *infantile* nystagmus be used for children who did not have the nystagmus develop until this later time. Seventeen years elapsed before sufficient data allowed reasonable proof of the chronological development and evolution of the nystagmus in infants, children, young adults, and older adults.

A. Development of Nystagmus

For the past 15 years, eye movement recordings have been obtained on most of the patients with nystagmus whom I have seen. Sufficient nystagmus recordings done at different ages enabled extrapolation to a meaningful development scheme of nystagmus types and confirmed our earlier suspicion of the correctness of that grandmother's observations. The review (1) of our patient histories showed that at about age 4–5 months, the child with nystagmus is often referred to us by a pediatrician or an ophthalmologist with a tentative diagnosis of blindness. Eye movement recordings show what we have come to call triangular waveforms. The eyes swing from side to side at about one to two cycles per second at amplitudes of 20–40 degrees. The recordings show a waveform of each eye that appears schematically as in Figure 1.

Although the waveforms are called triangular, because of their shape, a subtlety at one peak escaped our attention until recently. Near the right or left peak of each triangular wave a small *foveation* period is seen (Fig. 2). Foveation means that flat portion of a waveform that would allow the fovea to be precisely on target during that plateau. This plateau is typically a sign for future good vision. Unfortunately, waveform analysis is in its infancy and current computer software is only beginning to yield meaningful analysis of these nystagmus waveform subtleties.

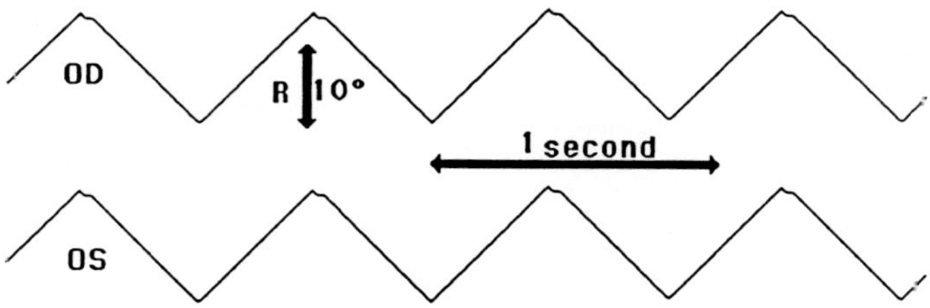

Figure 1 Diagram of triangular eye movements to the right and to the left of a 5-month-old child that represent the first phase of infantile nystagmus.

During the period where the principal waveform is triangular, the eyes are oscillating horizontally to the extent that the observers often fail to see any meaningful horizontal fixations and thus have severe concerns about the child's vision. The examiner can point out that, although the patient is not making meaningful horizontal eye movements, the infant is able to fixate superiorly and inferiorly. This is best demonstrated by the examiner moving in such a fashion that his or her head is above the infant's head so that the infant has to look up to see the examiner's face. Another helpful sign is the presence of vertical optokinetic nystagmus (OKN). About 90% of the children showing triangular nystagmus can be demonstrated to respond to a vertically moving target with vertical OKN. The OKN demonstrates vision and may assure parents that their child has vision. Television tape recordings are often helpful to demonstrate the OKN to the parents. Upward rotation of the OKN drum demonstrates the OKN slightly easier than downward rotation, since the slow following movement of the eyes upward keeps the eyes open wider and thus shows the vertical OKN movement of the corneas. As the drum is rotated downward, the eyelids follow

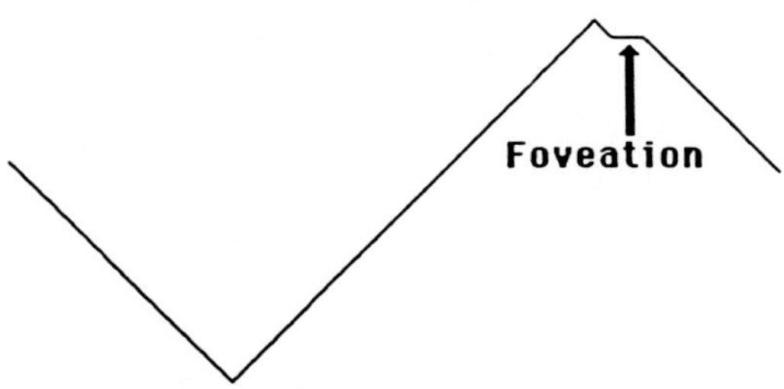

Figure 2 Magnified diagram of triangular eye movements to show the foveation portion close to the peak of the triangular eye movements. This foveation may or may not be present.

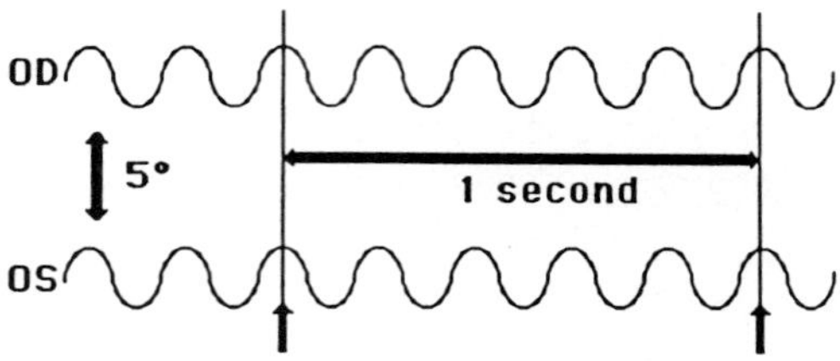

Figure 3 Diagram of pendular nystagmus typically found as a significant waveform at about age 8 months. Note the right and left eyes' symmetry at the arrows.

the eyes and the corneas are harder to see, although the jerking of the lids as they follow the eye can demonstrate the downward OKN.

At about age 8 months, the triangular eye movements give way to pendular nystagmus (Fig. 3). The pendular movements typical of the second phase of infantile nystagmus are regular and symmetrical. They oscillate at about five to eight cycles per second and about 2 degrees of amplitude. The small oscillations are interrupted by the retained triangular eye movements and occasional saccades.

If the infant is seen initially at this age while the pendular eye movements constitute a significant portion of the waveforms, the pendular eye movements can be confused with spasmus nutans. Since spasmus nutans often occurs at about 6–8 months of age, and since the spasmus nutans eye movements are similar to the pendular eye movements of infantile nystagmus in that they are about the same amplitude of 1–2 degrees and at a frequency of five to nine cycles per second, the distinguishing factor of asymmetries of the eyes' movements are important. The head nodding may or may not be present when the spasmus nutans is first suspected. Contrast the following diagram of spasmus nutans (Fig. 4) with the pendular eye movements of infantile nystagmus (see Fig. 3).

At age 5–8 months when the onset of small pendular infantile nystagmus begins, the parents often report that the nystagmus is improving and that the

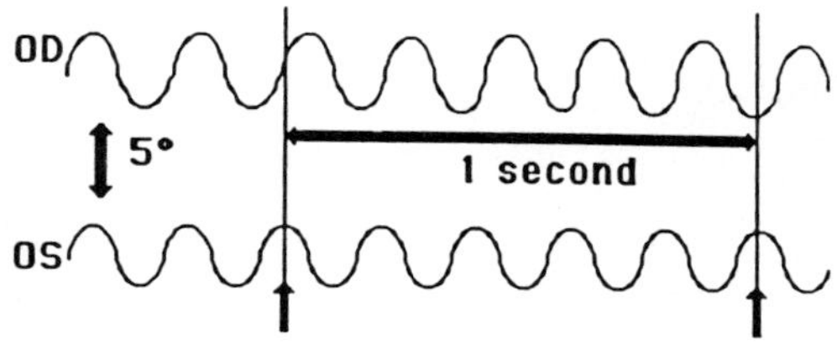

Figure 4 Diagram of the asymmetrical pendular nystagmus typically found as a hallmark of spasmus nutans. Note the right and left eyes' asymmetry at the arrows.

child is beginning to see. As the large triangular waveforms decrease in number and are replaced by the higher frequency pendular waveforms, the latter are less noticeable and the child can be seen to move the eyes horizontally in fixational patterns. The vertical following movements are usually easy to demonstrate at this stage.

From age 6–8 months, symmetrical horizontal and vertical saccades typically can be seen on the eye movement recordings. At about age 12–14 months, jerk nystagmus gradually becomes the dominant waveform. The slow phase of the waveform has a pattern of increasing velocity as described by Dell'Osso (2). The eyes' slow and fast phases of the jerk nystagmus will tend to be symmetrical on each side of the null point and will gradually replace the triangular and pendular waveforms that dominated earlier. Throughout the patient's life, the two other waveforms can be seen briefly from time to time in eye movement recordings.

As the jerk waveforms come into prominence, the null point gradually becomes discernible. Considerable individual differences in the onset of the identifiable null point and the resultant preferred head position are found. Occasionally, the preferred head position will be noted by the parents prior to a demonstrable null point and the changing direction of the jerk nystagmus on each side of the null point (Fig. 5).

Since the jerk waveform of infantile nystagmus appears at about age 1 year, it can be confused with latent or manifest latent nystagmus that becomes evident at about the same age. Occasionally, the pediatrician or referring ophthalmologist will note the latent nystagmus on covering one eye. Since latent and manifest latent nystagmus may be asymmetrical as dependent on which eye is covered or

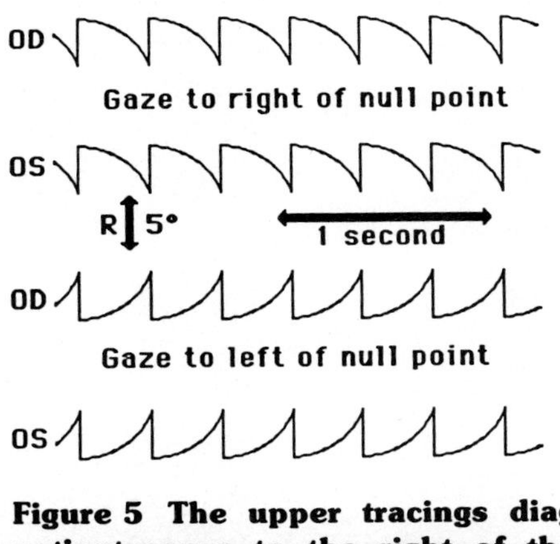

Figure 5 The upper tracings diagram the jerk nystagmus as the patient gazes to the right of the null point. The lower tracings represent the nystagmus during gaze to the left of the null point. Note the increasing velocity of the slow phase.

used for fixation, this may cause some confusion. The problem can be solved easily with eye movement recordings and identifying the decreasing velocity of the slow phase of latent or manifest latent nystagmus as contrasted with the diagnostic increasing velocity of the slow phase in infantile nystagmus (Fig. 6).

Although the jerk of latent and infantile nystagmus can be in the same direction, given the appropriate conditions, the latent form can be distinguished from infantile nystagmus by several characteristics (see Fig. 6). The jerk changes direction in respect to the null point in infantile nystagmus, that is, when the patient looks to the right of the null point the nystagmus beats to the right, and when looking to the left of the null point, the nystagmus beats to the left. When the gaze is precisely on the null point, the nystagmus is minimal for that patient. A pseudo–null point can be seen in adduction with latent or manifest latent nystagmus, but the direction of the fast phase will change depending on which eye is fixating with the fast phase jerking toward the fixating eye. The patterns of the slow phase velocities of each are distinctive: Increasing velocity is associated with infantile nystagmus and decreasing velocity is associated with latent nystagmus. Infantile nystagmus amplitudes or frequencies are seldom influenced by which eye is covered; however, the amplitudes of latent nystagmus or manifest latent nystagmus often change as the right versus the left eye fixates. The pattern of the right or left eye's fixation causing larger amplitude latent nystagmus is variable among patients but usually is consistent in the same patient, but may change with patching for amblyopia (H. J., Simonz personal communication, 1990).

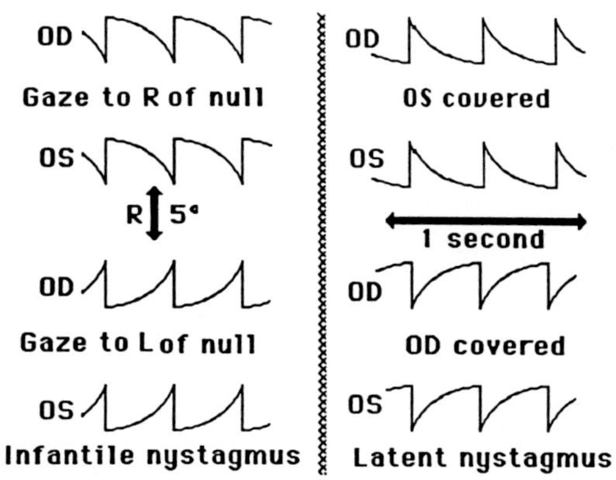

Figure 6 The diagrams contrast the increasing velocity of the slow phase of infantile nystagmus on the left to the decreasing velocity of the slow phase of latent (and manifest latent) nystagmus on the right.

B. Visual Acuity

My experience with visual acuity associated with infantile nystagmus is as follows: If the patient has nystagmus with or without mild oculocutaneous albinism, we often find about 20/100 visual acuity by age 5 years. The improvement in vision continues so that by age 8 years the vision is 20/40 to 20/80. Thus any treatment alleged to improve vision must be compared with what would have developed naturally by age 8 years—a difficult task. Continued data collection on these children, better nystagmus classification, and improved eye movement recordings are necessary.

As the parents are counseled, mention should be made that as the child becomes an adult the trend continues for even better visual acuity with age unless some sight-robbing problem unrelated to their nystagmus develops.

Over the last 5 years, I have had the opportunity to see patients whom I had examined 15 years ago or more. Some had Kestenbaum surgery and others were followed without treatment. As these patients reach age 50 years and older, their vision continues to improve. One patient had a vision of 20/50 at age 40 and at age 65 has 20/25 vision. Other patients have reported similar improvements with age.

The goal of most young adults, particularly men, is to have 20/40 vision by age 16 so that they can acquire an unlimited driver's license. We have looked for clues toward the prediction of this vision. Although the following factors are by no means certain, they may be of some help. If the patient has any of the following signs, the chances are improved toward attaining 20/40 vision:

OKN in all directions
Nystagmus present at birth
Dual jerk nystagmus
Periodic alternating nystagmus
Long flat portions of eye movement recordings
Demonstrating good foveation

The signs that suggest eventual vision worse than 20/40 include:

Outline of lens seen through the iris; that is, pronounced albinism
Blood vessels crossing the macula, usually in albinism
No macular pigment and no foveal reflex
Flash visual evoked potential positive for albinism
Absence of OKN in all directions

The genes of albinism, astigmatism, and nystagmus seem to be clustered together, since the three conditions often are found in the same subject. The three entities should be considered as separate, for they may or may not be associated. Examples of most forms of albinism can be found without nystagmus;

however, I have never seen a complete albino without nystagmus. The development of the albino's nystagmus usually follows the course I have outlined for infantile nystagmus. The more severe forms of albinism may never develop the jerk form of nystagmus seen to evolve from the usual infantile nystagmus triangular and pendular waveforms.

A commonly missed treatment opportunity is the careful refraction and correction of the astigmatism. Often the child with nystagmus has large amounts of astigmatism. Failure to correct these large astigmatic errors will cause bilateral amblyopia. Early correction of the astigmatism occasionally gives surprisingly good results. No special considerations are present other than care to cycloplege the child completely to assure measurement and prescription of the full astigmatic error. The parents should be warned that the child may not appreciate the astigmatic correction for months or years. The opportunity for the development of good vision should be seized, for to pass it by may condemn the child to poor amblyopic vision.

II. CONGENITAL NYSTAGMUS

Four types of nystagmus are usually present at birth, and hence may be called congenital as contrasted to infantile nystagmus, which usually develops after about age 4 months. The congenital nystagmus includes dual jerk nystagmus, X-linked nystagmus, vertical nystagmus, and torsional nystagmus. Parents often hope and believe that the nystagmoid eye movements will become normal and thus often seek attention only after several months. These four types of nystagmus tend to be consistent in their waveform and amplitude if present at birth, although the fixation patterns gradually become more stable.

Dual jerk is the most common nystagmus present at birth (Fig. 7). Typically, this nystagmus is observed in the first few hours after birth and remains relatively constant. There is enough variability in this nystagmus that repeat eye movement recordings are sometimes necessary to be sure of the condition. Once established as a dual jerk nystagmus waveform, its presence can be used as a reassuring fact that the vision probably will be relatively good; that is, better than 20/50. We

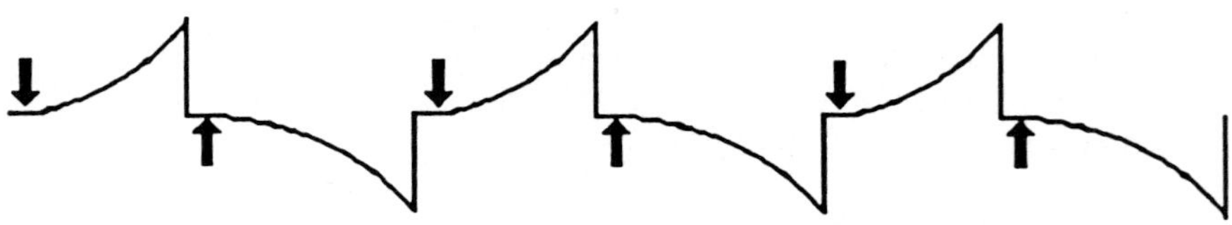

Figure 7 The diagram represents dual jerk nystagmus with both eyes having the same pattern. The arrows note the jerk returning the eyes to foveation and doing so in each direction.

have followed four such children and have seen no exceptions to this natural history. We have 10–12 such patients who have been seen initially as older children who evidence this good vision as well. As the child ages, the foveation increases until there are often long stretches of steady fixation. It is not uncommon for these patients with dual jerk nystagmus to have 20/20 vision and the nystagmus noted only incidentally in an eye examination. Since no known pathology has been reported to cause dual jerk nystagmus, reassurance can be given that this nystagmus is benign.

Torsional nystagmus typically is noted when the child is older and some other eye condition prompts a detailed eye examination. A child who has had recent strabismus surgery may have the first slit lamp examination postoperatively where the torsional nystagmus is noted for the first time. The torsional nystagmus is seen with the slit lamp magnification and consultation may be sought. If the child is thriving and no other form of nystagmus is seen, reassurance can be given. Since multiple sclerosis and vestibular disease can cause torsional nystagmus, some caution is appropriate. However, both vestibular disease and multiple sclerosis typically cause a nystagmus with oscillopsia, whereas the congential variety does not. The recording of torsional nystagmus can be done with a contact lens of the coil recording system. Such a recording requires a scleral coil contact lens that few children will tolerate. Television tape recordings are usually adequate to document the torsional nystagmus. The congenital torsional nystagmus is about 3 degrees and beats, usually concomitantly, at three to four cycles per second.

III. SPASMUS NUTANS

The hallmark of spasmus nutans is the asymmetry of the nystagmus in a child. Typically the onset is 6 months of age or older. Since the waveform, amplitude, and frequency are similar to the pendular stage of infantile nystagmus, an eye movement recording is often necessary to document the asymmetry. The asymmetry may be in phase, frequency, or direction. It is often intermittent particularly at its onset or at its resolution. At the onset of spasmus nutans or at its resolution, the amplitudes between the two eyes may be so different that it seems to be uniocular. Eye movement recordings usually show bilateral involvement. The presence of horizontal optokinetic nystagmus often helps establish the diagnosis of spasmus nutans, for OKN is seldom present in the horizontal plane in infantile nystagmus. If spasmus nutans is present, either an magnetic resonance imaging or a computed tomographic scan is appropriate to rule out central nervous system (CNS) lesions (3). We have termed spasmus nutans, in the presence of a CNS lesion, to be the spasmus nutans–like syndrome. We will continue to collect data in the hope of finding clinical signs and symptoms

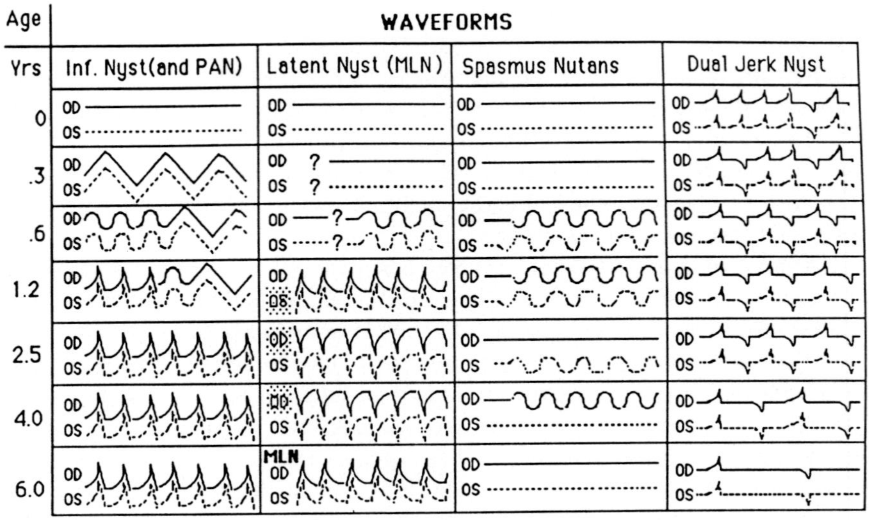

Figure 8 The waveforms are diagrammed as well as the changes in the nystagmus as the child ages.

that will distinguish the spasmus nutans, which is benign from the spasmus nutans–like syndrome, which has significant CNS pathology.

IV. MANIFEST LATENT NYSTAGMUS

The diagnosis of manifest latent nystagmus is important, for it is the one form of nystagmus that is treatable. Manifest latent nystagmus is distinguished by the decreasing velocity of the slow phase of the jerk nystagmus. The latent variety becomes manifest only when binocular vision is interrupted. When a strabismus or amblyopia is present, then the latent nystagmus becomes manifest. It is treated by the restoration of single binocular vision (4). Thus another reason for eye movement recordings is to distinguish the manifest latent nystagmus from infantile nystagmus.

V. NYSTAGMUS BLOCKAGE SYNDROME

Nystagmus blockage syndrome is important and often difficult to diagnose. The excessive convergence blocks the nystagmus so an esotropia, but no or little nystagmus, is seen. Careful extended recordings will show the presence of nystagmus. The diagnosis can be suspected when the patient has a recurrence of an esotropia as if no surgery were done. An unusual variant of the nystagmus blockage syndrome is at least one explanation for the horizontal dissociated deviation syndrome. In this entity, the amount of nystagmus blockage is dependent on the amount of nystagmus present, and which eye is fixating. If such a patient has nystagmus that has its amplitude and frequency dependent on which eye is fixating, the esotropia also will vary depending on which eye is fixating, and thus requiring increased convergence to block the increased nystagmus. Such a patient acts much like an anisometropic accommodative esotrope whose amount of esotropia is dependent on which of two dissimilar hyperopic eyes is fixating (5).

In summary, the typical development of nystagmus waveforms are outlined as well as some signs for final predictive estimates of the child's vision (Fig. 8). Eye movement recordings on most children may be productive when the nystagmus is noted and periodically thereafter in an effort to further characterize treatment measures and the natural histories of the nystagmus entities.

REFERENCES

1. Reinecke RD, Guo S, Goldstein HP. Waveform evolution in *infantile* nystagmus: an electro-oculo-graphic study of 35 cases. Binocular Vis 1988; 3:191–202.
2. Dell'Osso LF. Congenital, latent and manifest latent nystagmus—similarities, differences and relation to strabismus. Jpn J Ophthalmol 1985; 29:351–68.
3. Gottlob I, Zubcov A, Catalano RA, Reinecke RD, et al. Signs distinguishing spasmus nutans (with and without central nervous system lesions) from infantile nystagmus. Ophthalmology 1990; 97:1166–75.
4. Zubcov AA, Reinecke RD, Gottlob I, et al. Treatment of manifest latent nystagmus. Am J Ophthalmol 1990; 110:160–7.
5. Zubcov AA, Reinecke RD, Calhoun JH. Asymmetric horizontal tropias, DVD, and manifest latent nystagmus: an explanation of dissociated horizontal deviation. J Pediatr Ophthalmol Strabismus 1990; 27:59–64.

14

Management of Strabismus

Michael X. Repka
Johns Hopkins University School of Medicine, Baltimore, Maryland

Strabismus, or ocular misalignment, may be caused by a diverse array of neuro-ophthalmologic problems. These include thyroid eye disease affecting the extraocular muscles directly, ocular motor pareses affecting the cranial nerves, and demyelinating disease affecting internuclear ocular motor control within the brainstem. The causes of infantile and acquired comitant strabismus are not known. The intent of this chapter is to summarize the available treatment for a patient with strabismus of neuro-ophthalmological cause. These treatments may be both medical and surgical. The former are occlusion, prism correction, and spectacles. The latter are injection of botulinum neurotoxin A and strabismus surgery. The goal of any strabismus treatment is enhancement of ocular motility and enlargement of the field of binocular vision.

I. MEDICAL TREATMENT

Medical treatment is indicated for nearly every strabismus produced by a neuro-ophthalmological disorder. Many cases of ocular motor dysfunction will be temporary and resolve spontaneously or following neurosurgical intervention. Therefore, a definitive correction is not needed, but rather a temporary intervention is necessary. For most patients with comitant or incomitant strabismus, the initial treatment will be occlusion. This mainstay of therapy will eliminate double vision and allow the patient to function at a nearly normal level. Occlusion may be applied to either eye, although usually to the eye with poorer vision. There is no benefit proven to using the paretic or nonparetic eye. Alternate eye occlusion on a daily basis is not recommended, as the patient will have increased spatial difficulty because of the need to readapt constantly to the new ocular alignment. Occlusion may be achieved using a rectangular adhesive bandage, an eye patch available from a pharmacy (e.g., Opticlude, 3M, St. Paul, MN), or a black "pirate" patch available from many optical shops. Alternatively, a patient may gain adequate relief, while maintaining a degree of cosmesis, by applying a single layer of opaque tape to the back of their spectacles. A film of opaque nail polish may be applied to the back of glass spectacles to afford similar relief. A patient could also have their lenses frosted commercially. Special care must be taken when a child (<8 years of age) is being patched to ensure that the patient is not developing occlusion amblyopia. Alternation of the eye being occluded or reexaminations to measure visual acuity are needed at intervals of 1 week per year of age when prolonged occlusion is needed.

Occlusion during the period of initial rapid change in alignment is the most expedient approach. Patching may be continued for as long as the patient is symptomatic and some patients prefer this treatment for the rest of their lives. However, once a degree of stability of the size of the deviation is achieved, trying to regain binocularity in most instances is worthwhile. The initial approach is prism correction. Prisms are most useful for patients with small comitant deviations ($<15^{\Delta}$). Comitant deviations are of similar magnitude in all directions of gaze. As a prism provides only one size correction, prisms tend to be poorly tolerated by patients with large deviations or variability of their deviation in different positions of gaze (e.g., cranial nerve IV pareses) or when the size changes over the course of a day (e.g., myasthenia gravis). Prismatic effect can be produced by "ground-in" prism lenses, by lens decentration, or by the application of plastic Press-On (Optical Sciences Group, Petaluma, CA) Fresnel membrane prism.

Ground-in prism provides the best optical clarity, although there is some image distortion because of differential magnification from different parts of the lens and chromatic aberration. About seven prism diopters can typically be placed in each lens. Thus a total of 14 prism diopters of correction may be obtained. Prisms may be oriented vertically, horizontally, or at oblique angles to achieve the desired result. Practically it is best to experiment with both the size and the orientation of the prism in a trial frame before prescribing.

Prismatic correction may also be achieved by decentering a spectacle lens. If the visual axis of the patient's eye passes through a lens away from the optical center of that lens, there will be induced prism. For example, a patient wearing myopic correction who has the right lens decentered superiorly will experience base-down prism effect. The magnitude of the induced prism is proportional to the amount of decentration in centimeters and the power of the lens. With this method, most patients may obtain up to four prism diopters from each lens.

My preferred method of prism therapy for patients with neuro-ophthalmological disorders is the use of membrane prisms. These prisms are available in powers from 0.5^{Δ} to 30^{Δ}. They may be placed in any orientation and in any combination of power by placing one on each of the patient's lenses. Further, they may be rapidly and inexpensively interchanged. A patient could achieve a total effect of 60^{Δ} by wearing 30^{Δ} lenses oriented oppositely over each eye. These lenses are applied to the back of the spectacle lenses while immersed in warm water. The prisms are properly positioned on the back surface of the spectacle lenses, which are removed from the water and carefully dried. The prism may be removed, cleaned with contact lens cleaner, and changed if necessary. It is most convenient to select a power and orientation by trial and error from a set of stock lenses. A set of trial frame mounted Fresnel lenses is available from the manufacturer.

A second advantage of membrane prisms is that a different amount of correction may be employed at distance than at near. For example, a patient with a sixth cranial nerve paresis has a deviation greater at distance than at near. Therefore a larger power Fresnel lens is used on the top of the spectacle, and a lower power on the bottom. Membrane prisms do have the disadvantage of blurring vision. This is particularly significant for prisms of 15^{Δ} or more. Some patients will need to wear a separate pair of glasses to drive.

For many patients, prismatic correction will be satisfactory for many years. For others, prism correction serves only as a bridge between the onset of double vision and further treatment with surgery, botulinum toxin, or occlusion after stabilization of deviation.

II. BOTULINUM TOXIN

More than 20 years ago, the treatment of strabismus using botulinum toxin was reported by Scott (1). Since then the results of multiple pilot projects have been reported that suggest a number of applications for botulinum toxin (2–9).

There are seven distinct botulinum toxins. Botulinum toxin type A is currently approved by the U.S. Food and Drug Administration as a therapeutic agent for the treatment of strabismus. This toxin binds to presynaptic cholinergic nerve terminals, which are then taken up into the axon, where the toxin inhibits the release of acetylcholine. There is a loss of junctional acetylcholine receptors and secondary muscular atrophy. Shortly following administration of the toxin, new axonal terminals sprout and make new sypnaptic contacts on the muscle fibers and restore neuromuscular transmission. Theoretically, the drug works because new length-tension relationships are created by the period of paralysis in normal strabismic muscle. For paretic muscles, injection of antagonist muscles prevents contraction. Clinical resistance does not develop following repeated administrations of botulinum neurotoxin A in the doses used for the treatment of strabismus. Such resistance has been noted when much larger amounts of drug are used in the treatment of dystonias.

The dosage of botulinum neurotoxin A (Botox, Oculinum, Oculinum, Inc., Allergan Pharmaceuticals, Irvine, CA) necessary for strabismus treatment is based on the size of the deviation and the patient's weight. Currently, 2.5–10.0 U of botulinum neurotoxin A are recommended for a single rectus muscle. A treatment involves administration of three drops of proparaciane 0.5% at 1- min intervals as well as one to two drops of 2.5% phenylephrine hydrochloride. The latter drug blanches the conjunctiva and may reduce the likelihood of subconjunctival hemorrhage. The patient may be seated or in the prone position. Botulinum is injected directly into the orbital portion of the muscle using a mono-polar Teflon-coated needle (Allergan, Inc., Berkeley, CA) attached to an electromyographic (EMG) detector (Allergan, Inc., Berkeley, CA). The patient is asked to keep the eye straight ahead while the needle penetrates the conjunctiva. In some cases, it may be necessary to assist by fixating the globe with a forceps. Once the needle is 5–10 mm into the muscle, the patient is asked to look in the field of gaze of the muscle being injected. An enhancement of the basal EMG response is heard confirming localization of the needle in the muscle. The drug is then injected. The injection requires sedation for children and other patients who are unable to tolerate the injection with just topical anesthesia. Ketamine hydrochloride is preferred as a sedative, as it does not attenuate the EMG response and thereby facilitates the injection. No serious systemic complications have been reported. The ocular complications include ptosis (<5%), vertical strabismus after injection of a horizontal muscle (<5%), subconjunctival hemorrhage (10%), and retrobulbar hemorrhage (<1%). Rare cases of ocular penetration and perforation have been reported.

Essentially every eye movement condition has been treated with botulinum neurotoxin A. Most have been horizontal deviations. The successful treatment with vertical strabismus has been limited, because the superior rectus cannot be injected without inducing an upper eyelid ptosis. Injection of the inferior rectus for thyroid occular myopathy has been only occasionally successful. The oblique muscles have only been rarely injected. The treatment of infantile onset strabismus has had a variable response (2,3,9). Magoon reported an 85% success rate at 2 years of follow-up (2). Magoon's results, however, were not duplicated in a study by Biglan and colleagues (9), in which only 33% of children were satisfactorily aligned at similar duration follow-up. However, Scott and coworkers have recently reported on improved success rate of 65% (3). The relative efficacy of this drug compared with strabismus surgery for infantile strabismus remains to be proven in a randomized clinical trial.

The treatment of comitant exotropic deviations has been unsatisfactory. Less than 50% of patients are successfully treated and often the patient's ocular alignment returns to the same or nearly the same size deviation as they had prior to the injection (3,9,10).

Despite the difficulties in treating comitant strabismus, botulinum toxin has had more success for the treatment of patients with incomitant strabismus, particularly following acquired third or sixth nerve pareses (3,4,9). Once the third or sixth nerve paresis has been evaluated with appropriate neuroimaging and there is no evidence of recovery 4–6 weeks after onset, the patient is a candidate for injection. The botulinum injection is designed to prevent contracture of the unopposed antagonist muscle allowing more complete restoration of function should there be spontaneous restoration of function. For the patients who do not recover, the toxin may also serve as an adjunct to surgery by keeping the antagonist at normal length until strabismus surgery is performed. The toxin is not effective in my experience for patients who do not show substantial return of function. Studies of botulinum to date for paretic incomitant strabismus have been uncontrolled. In general, patients with binocular fusion and small angles of deviation have the greatest likelihood of achieving ocular alignment with botulinum neurotoxin A alone.

The toxin has a well-documented use in the surgical management of sixth nerve pareses. When there is complete loss of abduction ability, it has become conventional to perform a transposition of the entire inferior rectus and superior rectus tendons. At the same time, an adjustable medial rectus recession has been utilized. Thus three rectus muscles are disinserted increasing the chance of anterior segment ischemia. In a variation using botulinum and surgery, the horizontal transposition of the vertical rectus muscles is performed, but rather than recess the medial rectus muscle, 5–10 U of botulinum neurotoxin A is injected into this muscle. The injection occurs either 2 days prior to surgery or on the day of surgery (5,6). These investigators have reported achieving larger single binocular fields than in patients undergoing the transposition with medical rectus recession. The rationale for this procedure having a lessened risk of anterior segment ischemia is not absolute. Keech and colleagues have reported a case of anterior segment ischemia using this technique (11).

Botulinum toxin has also been used for patients who are over corrected following traditional strabismus surgery. Biglan and colleagues found that seven of eight patients treated in this fashion were satisfactorily aligned at 6-month follow-up (9). I have had a similar positive experience in two patients with consecutive esotropia with this treatment.

Botulinum toxin has also been used for the management of unremitting nystagmus with oscillopsia (8). The treatment is transient with return of symptoms after about 3 months.

III. STRABISMUS SURGERY

The mainstay of strabismus therapy for neuro-ophthalmological disorders continues to be surgical. The surgical techniques are identical to those used for comitant strabismus (e.g., infantile esotropia). Several additional techniques are available for patients with certain neuro-ophthalmological disorders. In this section, the surgical management of strabismus secondary to thyroid eye disease, myasthenia gravis, chronic progressive external ophthalmoplegia, internuclear ophthalmoplegia, and ocular motor neuropathies are reviewed.

A. Thyroid Eye Disease

Occlusion and prism therapy are used to treat the diplopia until the deviations have been stable for at least 6 months and the patient has not had radioablative therapy of the thyroid or orbital radiation therapy for at least 6 months.

The surgical management of the strabismus secondary to thyroid eye disease has the primary goal of releasing restriction to eye movement and consequent diplopia caused by inelastic extraocular muscles. Thyroid eye disease predominantly affects the inferior rectus muscle limiting upgaze and the medial rectus muscle limiting abduction. Strabismus surgery is delayed until at least 6 months after the patient's acute symptoms of congestive orbitopathy have resolved and the patient has concluded radiation therapy or orbital decompression surgery.

The appropriate medial or inferior rectus muscle is dissected free of all attachments to Tenon's capsule for at least 20 mm and placed on an adjustable suture. Special care must be taken not to pull hard enough to rupture the muscle. Surgery is usually performed under local anesthesia. It is common to recess the inferior rectus muscle 7 mm to gain appropriate elevation of the eye (12). During the suture adjustment, the surgeon attempts to maintain single vision in primary position as well as in the reading position. One should not sacrifice single vision in the reading position to gain perfect elevation. In my experience, it is common for a patient successfully to undergo inferior rectus recession of one eye and then develop a symptomatic contralateral restriction in the fellow eye that was not obvious prior to surgical correction. A second surgery will be needed.

B. Myasthenia Gravis and Progressive External Ophthalmoplegia

Initial therapy consists of occlusion and prism therapy. If these measures are unsatisfactory, then surgical correction is needed.

The surgical management of the strabismus induced by myasthenia gravis and chronic progressive external ophthalmoplegia (CPEO) is controversial. Some authorities feel these patients should not undergo surgery, as the effect of surgery will be transient. Nonetheless, strabismus surgery with adjustable sutures is able to restore binocular vision for these patients. Often a reasonable 25- to 30-degree field of single vision can be achieved. There is the ancillary benefit of improved appearance and self-esteem. The most common deviation is an exotropia. Bilateral lateral rectus recessions tend to be ineffective, so recess-resect operations are performed utilizing a large resection of one or both medial rectus muscles.

C. Internuclear Ophthalmoplegia

Patients with internuclear ophthalmoplegia (INO) may benefit from an initial trial of prism over the involved eye. With the help of a compensating head posture, many patients will achieve single vision. However, the exotropia secondary to intranuclear ophthalmoplegia infrequently may be treated surgically. Unilateral INO responds well to a recession of the ipsilateral lateral rectus muscle and resection of the involved medial rectus muscle often with both muscles on adjustable sutures. For bilateral INOs, I prefer to perform surgery on one eye, assess the effect, and if the patient is undercorrected, schedule a second operation on the fellow eye.

D. Ocular Motor Neuropathy

Trochlear nerve (cranial nerve IV) pareses are by far the most common abnormality and often the easiest to repair. Prior to surgical repair, a trial of prism may be beneficial. I have found that deviations of less than 8^{Δ} respond well to prism correction, but the patient needs to wear glasses constantly. Prior to surgical correction, the clinician should attempt to determine whether or not there is bilateral involvement (13,14). Bilateral involvement occurs frequently after trauma or on a congenital paresis, but one side may be masked. A clue to binocular involvement is the presence of a large V-pattern when there is an exotropia in up gaze and an esotropia in down gaze and no horizontal deviation in primary position. Other clues to bilateral involvement are a large angle of subjective excyclotorsion (>10 degrees) and bilateral objective torsion (seen with the indirect ophthalmoscope). Another feature to search for is a reversal of the hyperdeviation when the patient looks up and to the side of the presumed solely affected eye. For example, a patient with a large right hypertropia in left gaze who has a 2 prism diopter left hypertropia up and to the left likely has bilateral involvement. Appropriate counseling of the patient about the need for bilateral surgery is necessary when this diagnosis is considered. The surgical management of the hypertropia associated with the trochlear nerve paresis depends on the size of the deviation (15,16). Several general tenets are useful. If the deviation is largest in up gaze because of secondary inferior oblique overaction, a weakening operation of the inferior oblique muscle is preferred. A recession of the ipsilateral superior rectus muscle might also be considered. If the deviation is largest in down gaze, a recession of the contralateral inferior rectus muscle on an adjustable suture should be performed. Other surgeons have utilized a superior oblique tendon tuck (17). I have found the inferior rectus operation to be reliable and more easily fine tuned during the adjustment phase. For patients with large deviations in primary position (>15 prism diopters), a combination of both of these procedures is necessary. If the patient has little measurable heterotropia but continues to be bothered by diplopia or the inability to see clearly, consideration of torsional diplopia is necessary. This can be diagnosed readily using double Maddox rods. A white Maddox rod is placed before one eye and a red Maddox rod before the other eye. The patient is then asked to align the line images. When the images are more than 10–15 degrees divergent, torsional diplopia will result. A Harada-Ito procedure would be necessary to cure the torsional diplopia without producing a hypodeviation. This procedure involves advancement of the most anterior portion of the superior rectus tendon. The reader is advised to consult a text on strabismus for further information (17).

Abducens nerve pareses (cranial nerve VI) require a varied therapeutic approach. For the first 6 months, occlusion or prism may be tried. Prism should be effective for patients with primary deviation of 10^{Δ} or less. For fusing patients with small angles ($<20^{\Delta}$), botulinum should be considered. For large deviations, surgery will be necessary. If a patient has regained 15 or more degrees of abduction with a positive force generation test (the pull of the lateral rectus muscle is felt on attempted abduction), a maximal recession of the ipsilateral medial rectus muscle and resection of the ipsilateral lateral rectus muscle usually with adjustable sutures is necessary to align the patient. If the patient has poor to absent abduction, then a transposition procedure is necessary. A complete transposition of the superior rectus muscle tendon and inferior rectus muscle tendon to positions just above and below the lateral rectus muscle is preferred, although tendon-muscle–splitting operations have also been utilized. Simultaneously, a large adjustable recession of the medial rectus muscle is performed or botulinum neurotoxin A (10 U) is injected into the medial rectus muscle (6,7). In several studies of the use of botulinum toxin, the drug has been at least as good as recession in the management of abducens pareses.

Oculomotor nerve palsies (nerve III) are extremely difficult to treat medically or surgically. For a patient with a complete deficit, it is difficult to restore any significant field of binocular single vision. The surgical goal is to place the eye into primary position of gaze. However, the eye will move poorly and not yield any significant field of binocular vision. After surgery aligns the eye, the diplopic image can be minimized by blurring the image in this eye with a change in the power of the spectacle lenses. If the patient has an incomplete paresis, surgical treatment is more successful but must be individualized. Procedures usually involve weakening of the superior oblique.

If the patient develops aberrant regeneration of the oculomotor nerve, correction of misalignment is difficult. In some cases with aberrant regeneration of the lid, the third nerve ptosis may be treated by performing a recession of the contralateral lateral rectus muscle and resection of the contralateral medial rectus muscle. The patient will need to increase abduction of the contralateral eye and thus increase innervational flow intended for the ipsilateral medial rectus muscle. Because of the aberrancy, some flow will also go to the levator muscle thereby improving the ptosis.

REFERENCES

1. Scott AB, Rosenbaum A, Collens CC. Pharmacologic weakening of extra ocular muscles. Investigative Ophthalmology 1973; 12:924–7.
2. Magoon EH. Chemodenervation of strabismic children. A 2- to 5-year follow-up study compared with shorter follow-up. Ophthalmology 1989; 96:931–4.
3. Scott AB, Magoon EH, McNeer KW, Stager DR. Botulinum treatment of childhood strabismus. Ophthalmology 1990; 97:1434–8.
4. Wagner R, Frohman LP. Long-term results: botulinum for sixth nerve palsy. J Pediatr Ophthalmol Strabismus 1989; 26:106–8.
5. Scott A, Kraft SP. Botulinum toxin injection in the management of lateral rectus paresis. Ophthalmology 1985; 96:676–83.
6. Fitzsimmons R, Lee F, Elston J. The role of botulinum toxin in the sixth nerve paresis. Eye 1989; 3:391–400.
7. Rosenbaum AL, Kushner BJ, Kirchen D. Vertical rectus muscle transposition and botulinum toxin (Oculinum®) to medial rectus for abducens palsy. Arch Ophthalmol 1989; 107:820–3.
8. Helveston EM, Pogrebniak AE. Treatment of acquired nystagmus with botulinum A toxin. Am J Ophthalmol 1988; 106:584–6.
9. Biglan AW, Burnstine RA, Rogers GL, Saunders RA. Management of strabismus with botulinum A toxin. Opthalmology 1989; 96:935.
10. Magoon E. Long-term efficacy of botulinum treatment for adult horizontal strabismus. Ophthalmology 1990; 97 (Sept Suppl):107.
11. Keech RV, Morris RJ, Ruben JB, Scott WE. Anterior segment ischemia following vertical muscle transposition and botulinum toxin injection. Arch Ophthalmol 1990; 108:1733 (letter).
12. Scott WE, Thalacker JA. Diagnosis and treatment of thyroid myopathy. Ophthalmology 1981; 88:493–8.
13. von Noorden GK, Murray E, Wong Sy. Superior oblique paralysis. A review of 270 cases. Arch Ophthalmol 1986; 104:1771–6.
14. Kushner BJ: The diagnosis and treatment of bilateral masked superior oblique palsy. Am J Ophthalmol 1988; 105:186–94.
15. Scott WE, Kraft SP. Classification and surgical treatment of superior oblique palsies. Unilateral superior oblique palsies. Transactions of the New Orleans Academy of Ophthalmology. New York: Raven Press, 1986:5.
16. Scott WE, Kraft SP. Classification and surgical treatment of superior oblique palsies. II. Bilateral superior oblique palsies. Transactions of the New Orleans Academy of Ophthalmology. New York: Raven Press, 1986:265.
17. Del Monte MA, Wright KW: Superior oblique strengthening procedures. In: Wright KW, ed. Color atlas of ophthalmic surgery. Strabismus. Philadelphia: Lippincott, 1991:145–72.

15

Visual Symptoms of Otolith Dysfunction

G. M. Halmagyi
Royal Prince Alfred Hospital, Sydney, New South Wales, Australia

Ian S. Curthoys
University of Sydney, Sydney, New South Wales, Australia

Otolith dysfunction is relevant to the practicing neuro-ophthalmologist because there is close correspondence between the visual and vestibular perception of posture and movement. Consequently patients with central or peripheral vestibular disorders involving the otoliths can present primarily with visual problems. The aim of this chapter is to describe these problems, their clinical features, and possible mechanism. To understand human otolith dysfunction, it is first necessary to understand certain critical aspects of normal otolith function. For more details of this subject, see the original articles by Fernandez and Goldberg (1–2) and the review by Goldberg and Fernandez (3).

I. OTOLITH STRUCTURE AND FUNCTION

The balance organs in the inner ear—the vestibular sensory regions—are the gyros of the human body and unnoticed they function continuously in an almost perfect fashion providing the brain with information about head position and head movement. Until the balance organs fail, no one really appreciates their significance for daily life, but anyone who has experienced an attack of vertigo can attest to their importance. These biological gyros detect forces: the forces imposed by gravity and the forces generated when we move. They are constructed in such a way that different regions of the inner ear can detect rotational and linear forces in almost every possible direction. Until recently, it was assumed that the information about angular and linear forces was treated quite separately by the nervous system, but it is now clear that the brain synthesizes the information from these separate force detectors to provide a global integrated summary of where we are and how we are moving. That realization is of great clinical importance because it implies that disease affecting only one isolated region of the inner ear may have consequences for the overall integration of all of the vestibular sensory input. In this section, we deal only with those structures that respond to linear forces, such as the force of gravity or the "straight line" acceleration experienced while accelerating at traffic lights; that is, the otoliths.

A. Structure

The basic element of all vestibular transducers is the receptor hair cell that is remarkably similar in both the angular and the linear force sensing systems. The semicircular canals and the otoliths detect these two different forces because of the way the structures surrounding hair cells are affected by the stimulating force and not because of any differences in the intrinsic properties of the hair cells themselves. Each receptor cell has numerous fine hairlike cilia projecting from the cell body into a gelatinous mass called the otolithic membrane (Fig. 1d). The longest cilium is called the kinocilium. It is located at one side of the receptor cell, and it has a specialized cross-sectional structure. The remaining cilia are of uniform cross-sectional structure and are called the stereocilia. They are arranged in a series of increasing height as they approach the kinocilium. Forces cause the otolithic membrane to slide so that the cilia of the receptor hair cells are bent. The following outlines these processes.

Each labyrinth consists of endolymph-filled tubes and sacs containing receptor structures. The two specialized sacs are the utricular sac and the saccular sac. Contained within each of these sacs is a plate of specialized receptor hair cells and connective tissue, the *macula*. Each macula takes its name from the sac in which it is located, so that in each inner ear there is a utricular macula and a saccular macula. The terms *utricle* and *saccule* are often used to refer to the utricular and saccular maculae, although strictly speaking *utricle* and *saccule* refer to the membranous sacs that contain the maculae.

Both utricular and saccular maculae have similar gross features (Fig. 1e). Overlying the macula is a gelatinous *otolithic membrane* (Fig. 2). Embedded on the outer (free) surface of this membrane are dense crystals of calcium carbonate, *otoconia*. On the inner surface of this membrane, the cilia of the hair cells project into the membrane. The density of the otolithic membrane itself is similar to that of the surrounding endolymph—1.0 g/cm^3, but the density of the otoconia is almost three times greater—2.7 g/cm^3. These two receptor structures are together called the *otoliths*, because their construction is similar and because both detect forces according to the same physical principle; namely, an imposed linear force

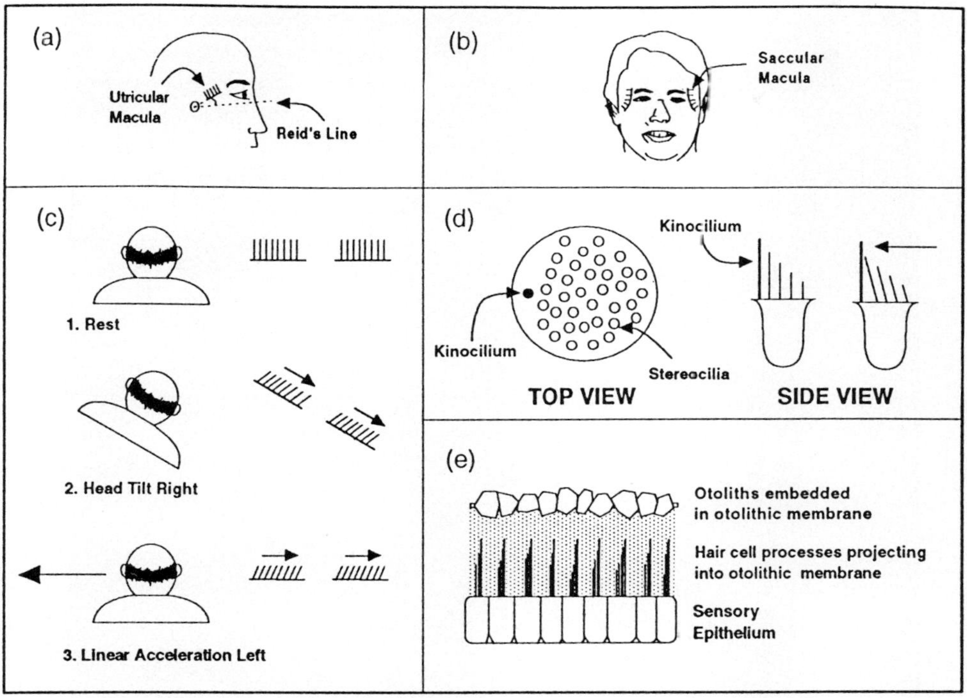

Figure 1 The structure and function of the otolithic system. (a,b) Schematics showing the approximate orientation of the utricular and saccular maculae in the head. Reid's line is a standard reference line joining the center of the external ear and the lower edge of the bony orbit. (c) Three cartoons show how different linear force stimuli affect the utricular receptor hair cells. The upper diagram (1) shows the back view of a person at rest with the cilia upright. Head tilts cause the cilia to be deflected (2) and similarly a linear acceleration (arrow) causes a deflection of the cilia (3). (d) Schematic diagram of a top view down on single receptor hair cell to show the polarization pattern of a single receptor cell. The kinocilium is located at one extreme of the upper surface of the cell. If the stereocilia are bent toward the kinocilium, as shown at the right, the receptor cell is facilitated. (e) Schematic illustration of the organization of a macula surface. The crystals of calcium carbonate (the otoliths) are embedded in one side of the gelatinous otolithic membrane and the tips of the cilia project into the other side of this membrane. Forces cause the membrane to slide so that the cilia are bent thus stimulating the receptor cells.

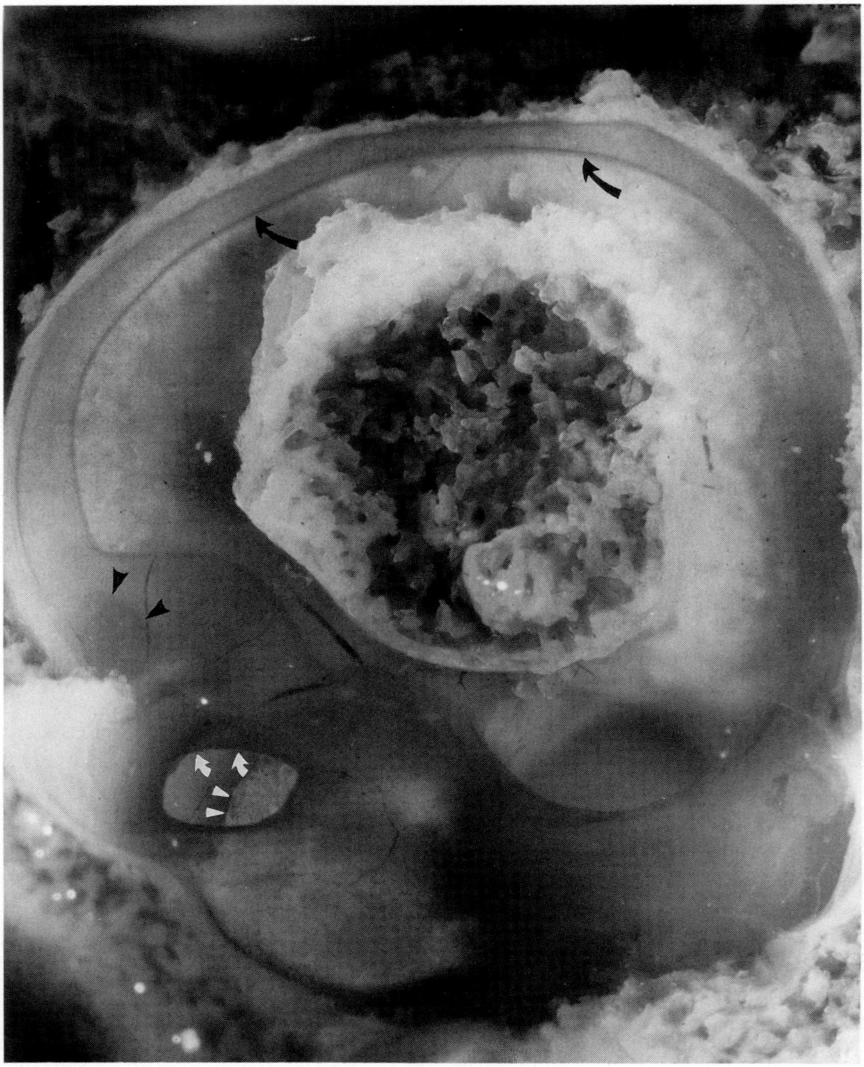

Figure 2 The human utricle. Dissection of the membranous labyrinth from a full-term human fetus showing the horizontal semicircular canal duct (curved black arrows) ampulla (black arrowheads) and the utricle. The point of view is from directly above the duct looking perpendicular to the plane of the horizontal canal. The utricular macula can be seen through the membranous wall of the labyrinth. The otoconial membrane (white arrowheads) is visible through the defect where the crus of the anterior semicircular canal was removed (curved white arrows).

displaces the relatively dense otoliths embedded in the otolithic membrane. The otolithic membrane then tends to *slide* across the surface of the macula displacing the cilia of the receptor hair cells that project into the otolithic membrane and thus producing a change in hair cell resting membrane potential (Fig. 1c). The displacements of the otolithic membrane generated in this way by natural head movements in a 1-*g* environment are in fact minute; on the order of 1 μm.

The utricular and saccular maculae are almost perpendicular to one another. With the head erect, the utricular macula is tilted by about 30 degrees (open anterior) with respect to the horizontal plane of the head (Fig. 1a and b), whereas the saccular macula is almost vertical. These different orientations mean that the receptors on each macula will respond maximally to forces in different directions. The surface area of the human utricular macula is only about 4.2 mm^2 and of the human saccular macula is only about 2.2 mm^2. But within this small space there is a large array of receptor hair cells: about 33,000 in the utricular macula and about 19,000 in the saccular macula. As in other sensory systems, there is considerable convergence of receptors to primary afferent fibers, and in the case of the otoliths this convergence is of the order of 6:1, so that only about 6000 afferents leave the utricle. The situation is similar in the saccule. There are about half as many saccular receptor hair cells on the saccular macula, which is about half the area of the utricular macula, and the number of afferent fibers is reduced correspondingly; only 4000 saccular primary afferents supply these 18,000 receptors, with an average ratio of about five receptors to each afferent fiber.

B. Normal Function

Intracellular recordings from single isolated otolithic receptor hair cells subjected to controlled forces in precisely defined directions have shown that each receptor hair cell is "polarized": It responds most strongly to forces in one particular direction and as the direction of the force deviates from that optimal direction, so the response of the receptor declines. This optimum direction is referred to as the cell's *polarization vector*. This physiological polarization corresponds to a morphological polarization in that receptor cells respond optimally when the imposed force shears the stereocilia toward the kinocilium (Fig. 1d). Receptor hair cells are arranged in a regular fashion across each macula, so that the direction of the kinocilium of each cell shifts in direction by only a small amount relative to its neighbors with the result that there is a highly ordered arrangement of polarization vectors across each macula.

Primary afferent neurons synapse on a number of adjacent receptor hair cells, so that some of the precision of tuning of the individual receptors is lost: Afferent fibers respond to forces over a greater range of directions than do the individual receptors. Each afferent fiber exhibits a preference for forces in a particular direction presumably reflecting the preferred orientation of the receptor hair cells on which the fiber synapses. For afferent fibers, just as for receptors, as the force direction deviates from the optimal direction, the fiber's firing frequency declines. Utricular afferents in general show a preference for forces directed across the plane of the macula; in other words, for laterally directed forces and similarly saccular afferents show a preference for forces directed vertically across the plane of the macula.

1. Primary Otolithic Afferents

Recordings from primary otolithic afferent neurons in the vestibular nerve of experimental animals show a number of important characteristics.

1. Primary otolithic afferents have a resting discharge rate. They fire at about 50 spikes/s even when there is no imposed force stimulus.
2. Primary otolithic afferents have a *functional polarization vector*. This means that linear accelerations oriented in one particular direction will most effectively activate the afferent neuron. As the direction of the imposed force deviates from this optimum direction so the response of the afferent neuron declines. If the stimulus is directed exactly opposite to the preferred direction, then the firing of the cell will be maximally suppressed.
3. Primary otolithic afferents show a marked asymmetry in bidirectional sensitivity. This characteristic results in a larger *increase* in firing rate for forces in the excitatory direction than *decrease* in firing rate for the same magnitude of force in the opposite disfacilitatory direction.
4. The spatial distribution of the directional preferences of all otolithic afferents is not uniform. In the squirrel monkey, there is a directional preponderance, so that more otolith afferents prefer ipsilaterally directed forces than contralaterally directed forces. There is 3:1 preponderance of ipsilateral force preferring utricular afferents, whereas there is about a 1:1 distribution of up-and-down force preferring saccular afferents.
5. At rest some otolithic afferents have a regular interspike interval, whereas others show an irregular pattern of firing. The dynamic response characteristics of these two groups of neurons are quite different. Regular neurons show little adaptation to maintained forces, whereas the irregular neurons show a transient mode of responding: They fire vigorously during the change in the stimulus but adapt rapidly for a maintained stimulus. This means that even at the level of the afferent neurons leaving the macula, functional specialization has already taken place in that different aspects of the force stimulus are being signaled by these different parallel pathways.

2. Projections

Primary otolithic afferent neurons project to secondary vestibular neurons mainly in the lateral, medial, and descending vestibular nuclei. In some regions, these otolithic projections show considerable overlap with the projections of horizontal semicircular canal afferents. The predominant response of lateral vestibular nucleus neurons is an increase in firing rate in response to ipsilateral tilts. Just as horizontal semicircular canal neurons in the medial vestibular nucleus are interconnected to the contralateral medial vestibular nucleus via commissural fibers that play a major role in the neural operation of the system, so otolith-responsive neurons also are interconnected to similar neurons in the opposite vestibular nucleus. However, the interconnections in the otolithic system are indirect and the functional mode of the bilateral interconnections is predominantly excitatory rather than inhibitory as is the case of the horizontal semicircular canal system. Some cells in each vestibular nucleus can be activated both by semicircular canal and by otolithic stimulation. These convergent neurons integrate linear and angular acceleration input and so help maintain posture and equilibrium. The pathways from the otolithic regions of the vestibular nuclei to the ocular motor nuclei are poorly understood. Trochlear motoneurons can be disynaptically activated by electrical stimulation of the utricular nerve and increasing attention is being paid to two midbrain regions close to the oculomotor nuclei—the interstitial nucleus of Cajal (4) and the rostral interstitial nucleus of the medial longitudinal fasciculus (5), which generate torsional and vertical eye movement responses to vertical canal and otolithic stimulation. In particular, it seems that the interstitial nucleus of Cajal has a major role in integrating input for coordinated eye and head responses to the linear forces detected by the otoliths. The neural substrate for the compensatory postural movements required by a linear acceleration are mediated by otolith-spinal projections—the lateral vestibulospinal tract arising in the lateral vestibular nucleus and the medial vestibulospinal tract arising in the medial vestibular nucleus.

C. Function of Otolithic Input

Suzuki et al. (6) showed that high-frequency electrical stimulation of the utricular nerve in the cat causes a distinct pattern of eye movement: a torsion of both eyes so that the upper poles of the eyes roll away from the side being stimulated. Complementing that result are studies that have shown that unilateral section of the vestibular nerve causes a torsion of both eyes toward the operated side (7). In natural movements, the otoliths are activated and generate compensatory eye and postural responses. For example, tilting the head toward one shoulder causes the gravity vector to activate particular regions of the utricular and saccular maculae and as a consequence the eyeball *torts* (or *rolls*) around the visual axis in a compensatory direction. At the same time, there is a complex pattern of activation of neck and trunk muscles acting to oppose this challenge to the equilibrium of the head. The degree of this countertorsion or ocular *counterrolling* is only about 10% of the head tilt, but it does depend on otolith function, since subjects without otoliths do not show such counterrolling (8).

II. OCULAR TILT REACTION

A. Definition

The ocular tilt reaction is a head-eye postural synkinesis consisting of three distinct components: head tilt, skew deviation, and binocular torsion, all toward the same side (Fig. 3). For instance, a leftward ocular tilt reaction comprises a leftward head tilt, a left skew deviation (i.e., a left hypotropia), and leftward eye torsion (i.e., excyclotorsion of the left eye and incyclotorsion of the right eye).

The finding of an ocular tilt reaction indicates an otolithic lesion, peripheral or central. Partial and complete, tonic and phasic ocular tilt reactions have been described following lesions and stimulations of the central and peripheral vestibular system in humans and in animals. The ocular tilt reaction is a compensatory postural reflex *righting reflex* arising from stimulation of the otoliths. Clinical and experimental evidence suggests that the ocular tilt reaction depends on a crossed graviceptive pathway that arises from excitation of the dependent utricle and then projects via the ipsilateral vestibular nucleus to the

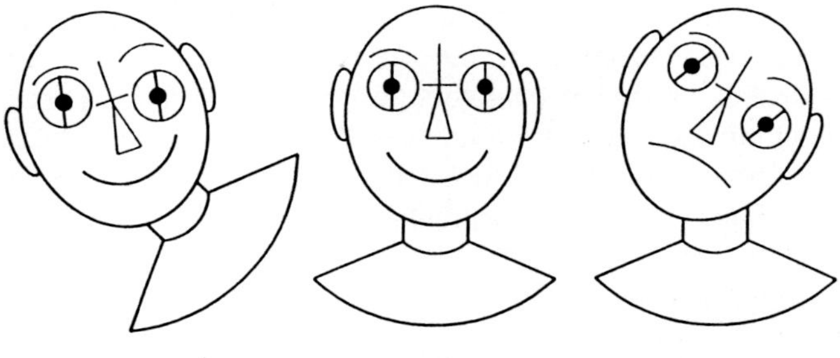

Figure 3 Control of eye-head posture and the ocular tilt reaction. Head-eye posture in a normal spatially vertical subject (center); in a normal subject tilted to the right (left); and in a patient with a leftward ocular tilt reaction (right). The left panel shows the normal compensatory leftward ocular tilt reaction in response to rightward tilt stimulation. The right panel shows a pathological tonic leftward ocular tilt reaction that could be due to a destructive lesion of the left utricle, or the left utricular nerve, or the left vestibular nucleus or the right mesodiencephalon. The normal subject's response to rightward tilt stimulation is leftward ocular tilt reaction comprising leftward head tilt, leftward eye torsion (i.e., counterrolling) and a left skew deviation (left hypotropia). Note that alone, and even together, the head tilt and eye torsion is normally incompletely compensatory. (From Ref. 10).

contralateral interstitial nucleus of Cajal and then to ocular and spinal motoneurons.

B. Clinical Features

1. Symptoms

Generally, the only symptom of an ocular tilt reaction is vertical diplopia due to skew deviation (9). The head tilt is always asymptomatic and the binocular torsion is usually asymptomatic. If the degree of ocular torsion is much larger in one eye than in the other, as it is in some patients with vestibular nucleus lesions, then there can also be an additional torsional element in the diplopia. Patients with partial ocular tilt reactions, such as some of those with acute peripheral vestibular lesions, are usually completely asymptomatic from a neuro-ophthalmic point of view (7). These patients have no skew deviation and little difference in the degree of torsion in the two eyes.

There are two surprising aspects to these observations. The first is that patients may be unaware of surprisingly large degrees of binocular torsion; as much as 40 degrees (10) so long as they are in a normal visual environment and so long as the degree of torsion is not too different in the two eyes. Presumably some of these patients will experience a visual tilt illusion (see Sec. II.H), but in fact most of them do not. If, on the other hand, patients with ocular tilt reaction are tested in a visually impoverished environment, for example, viewing a dimly lit light bar in an otherwise totally dark room, they will see a spatially vertical light bar as being tilted opposite to the direction of eye torsion, and when asked to align the light bar with the spatial vertical (called the *subjective visual spatial vertical*), they will in fact align it close to the rotated vertical meridian of the viewing eye.

The second aspect is that patients may be unaware of surprisingly large degrees of torsional disparity. With the eyes dissociated, it is common to be able to show up to 8 degrees of torsional disparity in patients with peripheral vestibular lesions and even more in patients with vestibular nucleus lesions (11). Perhaps it is not so surprising when one considers the amount of torsional disparity patients with superior oblique muscle palsies will ignore (12).

2. Signs

Head Tilt. A lateral head tilt is usually present early in an ocular tilt reaction but may disappear before the skew deviation and ocular torsion do so that it may no longer be present at the time a patient with an ocular tilt reaction presents with vertical diplopia. With peripheral vestibular lesions, the tilt may be only slight (10–20 degrees), and with interstitial nucleus lesions, it is usually larger (30–40 degrees).

Skew Deviation. A manifest primary position vertical strabismus is usually present early in the course of an ocular tilt reaction. The strabismus can be comitant or incomitant. If it is incomitant, it can increase on adduction or abduction, or on elevation or depression of the hypotropic eye, and it can mimic many different individual vertical muscle palsies. The head tilt test is usually negative, but if it is positive, it is on tilting the head toward the hypertropic eye (13) (Fig. 4). Nonetheless, the hypotropic eye is always ipsilateral to the spontaneous head tilt and is always the excyclotropic eye.

Ocular Torsion. Binocular torsion is the sine qua non of the ocular tilt reaction. Although the degree of torsion can be unequal in the two eyes, it is always in the same direction in the two eyes and is always toward the side of the hypotropic eye and of the head tilt. (The direction of torsion is given as the side of the patient to which the 12 o'clock point of the eye rotates.) In patients with acute unilateral peripheral vestibular lesions, the magnitude of the ocular torsion varies between 5 and 25 degrees (7). The degree of torsion is generally

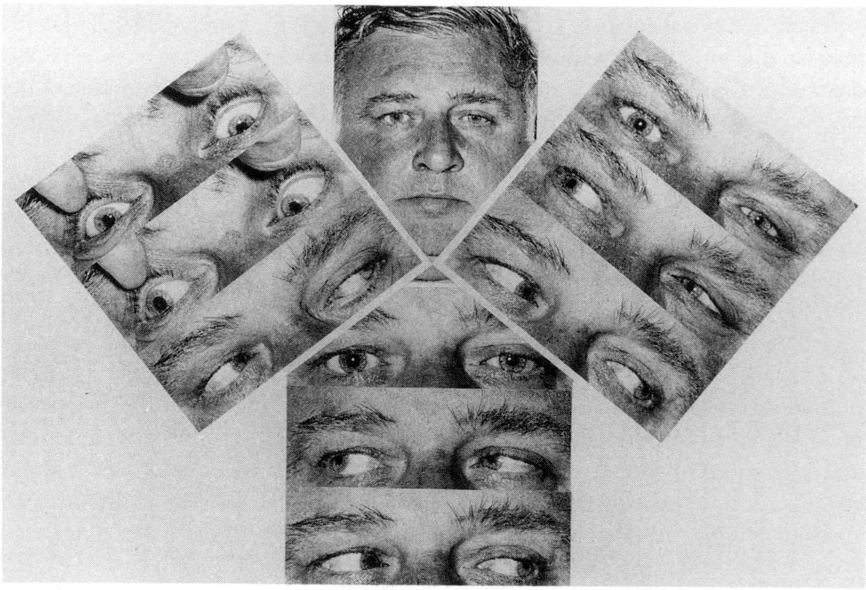

Figure 4 Skew deviation with a positive head tilt test due to acute left vestibular nucleus lesion. The patient had 2 days previously sustained a left lateral medullary infarction—note the left Horner's syndrome. He was orthotropic in all gaze positions while upright (bottom middle figures). During rightward head tilt (left figures), he developed vertical diplopia due to a skew deviation with 12 degrees of left hypotropia in the primary position increasing to 24 degrees in rightward gaze and decreasing to 2 degrees in leftward gaze. During leftward head tilt (right figures), the patient remained orthotropic.

the same in the two eyes but there can be up to 8 degrees of difference with larger torsion either in the extorted ipsilesional eye or the intorted contralesional eye. In patients with acute vestibular nucleus lesions, the degree of torsion is similar to that in patients with acute peripheral vestibular lesions except that the degree of torsion is usually different in the two eyes and is usually larger in the ipsilesional eye (11). In patients with acute interstitial nucleus lesions, the degree of torsion can be surprisingly large (up to 45 degrees) and is generally the same in the two eyes (10).

Ocular torsion is easy to miss unless carefully sought with specific methods. Detecting and measuring ocular torsion falls right into the scope of the neuro-ophthalmologist. There are several different methods and techniques of measuring ocular torsion. Each measures a different aspect of ocular torsion and is subject to different limitations and pitfalls. The three methods of measuring ocular torsion are described below.

Method 1: Ocular fundus photography. To demonstrate ocular torsion objectively, it is necessary to estimate the angle between the horizontal axis of the eye and the horizontal axis of the head. The most accurate way to do this is to take fundus photographs (Fig. 5). Then by constructing on the photograph a line between the fovea and the anatomical center of the optic disc, it is possible to define a horizontal ocular meridian or axis. The angle between this axis and the horizontal border of the photographic film (which is taken to be the same as the horizontal axis of the head) represents the *ocular tilt angle*. There are two potential pitfalls with this method. The first is the problem of defining the point on the optic disc that lies on the horizontal axis. Considering the anatomical center of the optic disc to be on the horizontal axis, the horizontal axis is normally extorted; that is, each eye is excyclotropic. Bixemann and von Noorden (14) found the mean ocular tilt angle to be 7.25 $\pm$ 2.57 (1 SD) of excyclotropia in each eye, whereas Dieterich and Brandt (9) found it to be 5.7 $\pm$ 2.9 degrees for the left eye and 4.9 $\pm$ 2.9 degrees for the right eye. (See Notes Added in Proof (p. 223), No. 2.) The second potential pitfall is technical and concerns possible misalignments in the position of the head with respect to measuring apparatus, namely, the camera and the film. If the vertical axis of the head is not exactly at 90 degrees to direction of the film transport, that is, if the head is slightly tilted or the camera is slightly rotated, errors of measurement could occur. Our own experience, however, is that with care but without special precautions, this source of error is small: it is possible to reproduce fundus photographs with an accuracy 1 degree.

Method 2: Plotting the location of the blind spot. Demonstrating that the blind spot has rotated is in cooperative patients a quick and easy way of detecting ocular torsion. In theory, this method should give similar results to fundus photography, but at this stage there are no data available on the sensitivity or reproducibility of the measurements (15).

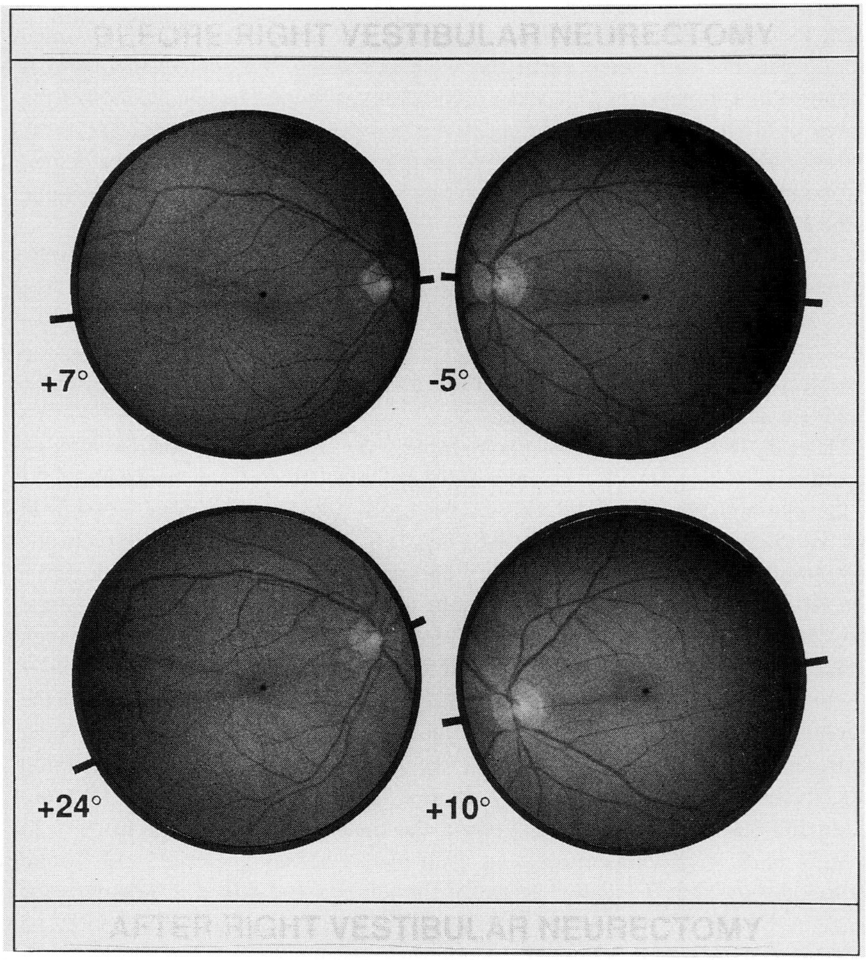

Figure 5 Rightward ocular torsion after right vestibular neurectomy. Fundus photographs of the left and right eye taken in a patient just before (top row) and 1 week after (bottom row) right vestibular neurectomy. Following vestibular neurectomy, both eyes developed tonic rightward eye torsion. The right eye developed 17 degrees of excyclotropia, whereas the left eye developed 15 degrees of incyclotropia. Note that before operation both eyes were excyclotropic by an amount that is within the normal range (11,12).

Method 3: Setting the subjective visual spatial vertical. Even in an otherwise dark room, normal subjects can accurately align a visible line to within ±1 degree of the spatial vertical. This method depends on a correspondence, presumably acquired, between the visual and the vestibular perception of the spatial vertical. Consider a patient sitting upright in a dark room. He or she has no visuospatial cues to verticality such as walls, doors, etc. Viewing with one eye at a time, the patient is then asked to set a visible line to the perceived spatial vertical. Setting of the subjective visual spatial vertical will not only be determined by the otolithic perception of spatial vertical but also by the torsional alignment of the eye with respect to the line. If the patient's eyes are tilted, the bar will be set closer to the anatomical vertical of the eye than to the true spatial vertical. It is possible to measure the subjective visual spatial vertical using several different techniques: a rotatable light bar (16,7), a Maddox rod (17), a rotating dome (11), or a *cadran* (18). The method using alternating Maddox rods is the easiest. The aim of the test is for the patient to align the Maddox rod with each eye in turn to his or her perceived spatial vertical. It is *not* the aim to align the vertical of one eye with that of the other—that is, simply measuring torsional disparity and not absolute torsional position. There are two pitfalls with using Maddox rods. The first is that if the test room is not perfectly dark, the patient will have visual cues to verticality such as a doorframe, a table, almost anything, and will align the Maddox rod with these. The second is that if the patient's head is tilted even slightly, then almost all the head tilt angle (minus the 10% or so of counterrolling) will be added to the measured ocular tilt angle producing an erroneous result. To use Maddox rods to measure the ocular tilt angle, it is essential to have the head perfectly vertical (17).

Following acute unilateral peripheral vestibular and vestibular nucleus lesions there is invariably a deviation of the subjective visual spatial horizontal or vertical (7). (For the purpose of indicating the ocular tilt angle, there seems to be no important differences between measures of the subjective visual vertical and the subjective visual horizontal.) The deviation is invariably toward the side of the lesion; that is, in the same direction as the ocular torsion. The degree of deviation ranges from 2 to 20 degrees. Although there is a significant correlation between the degree of rotation of the subjective visual spatial vertical and the degree of ocular torsion in each eye of each patient, there can be large discrepancies (Fig. 6). For example, in a patient with a peripheral vestibular lesion and say a 10 deviation of the visual spatial vertical, the actual ocular tilt angle could vary from 5 to 15 degrees.

There could be several reasons for such discrepancies. There could be visual sensory adaptation for the tonic ocular torsion. Although this could explain those cases where the subjective visual spatial vertical was less than the ocular tilt angle, it would not explain those cases where the subjective visual spatial vertical

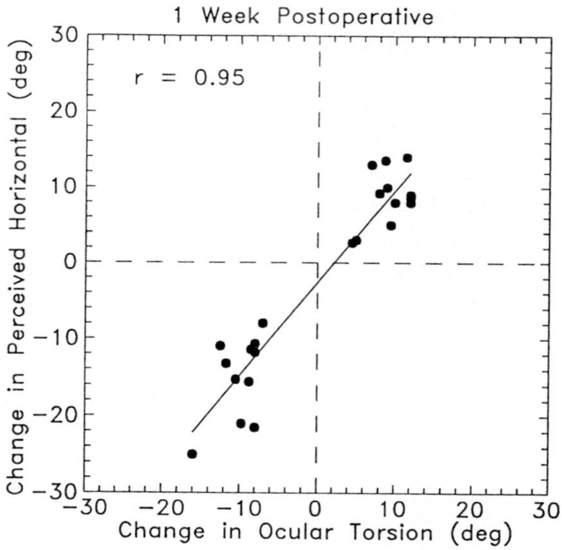

Figure 6 Subjective visual spatial horizontal as a function of ocular torsion. The relationship between the change in the degree of ocular torsion and the corresponding change in the subjective visual spatial horizontal 1 week after unilateral vestibular neurectomy in 23 patients. The average value of the torsion was calculated for each patient and plotted as a function of the patient's average change in the subjective visual spatial horizontal. The correlation (r = 0.95) is statistically significant. There is no significant difference in this case between the visual horizontal and vertical. (From Ref. 7.)

is greater than the ocular tilt angle. Second, the setting of the subjective visual spatial vertical not only reflects the ocular tilt angle but also the otolithic perception of the body vertical—that is, the subjective somatosensory spatial vertical. This is illustrated by the observation that during asymmetrical otolithic stimulation by centrifugation, normal subjects can accurately align a light bar with the true spatial vertical despite the profound deviation of the subjective somatosensory vertical, with a small degree of ocular counterrolling notwithstanding. Following a unilateral vestibular lesion there will also be asymmetrical otolithic activation and there can be a deviation of the subjective somatosensory spatial vertical resulting in lateropulsion. If a patient with a unilateral vestibular lesion sets the subjective visual spatial vertical to conform with his or her deviated perception of the somatosensory vertical, then the setting could exceed the degree of ocular torsion.

C. Differential Diagnosis

1. Fourth Nerve Palsy

The main differential diagnosis of ocular tilt reaction is a unilateral (or bilateral) superior oblique palsy. The similarity can be impressive, especially if in a patient with an ocular tilt reaction the skew deviation increases on gaze to the hypertropic eye, and on head tilt toward the hypertropic eye. However, the most telling difference between an acute unilateral superior oblique palsy and an ocular tilt reaction is that whereas in an *ocular tilt reaction there is incyclotropia of the hypertropic eye* and excyclotropia of the hypotropic eye, with *an acute superior oblique palsy there is excyclotropia of the hypertropic eye* and no cyclotropia of the hypotropic eye (9). (See Notes Added in Proof (p. 223), No. 1.)

2. Skew Deviation

A vertical disparity—that is, a skew deviation—can occur with lesions throughout the brainstem and cerebellum. The question arises as to whether all these skew deviations are in fact due to an ocular tilt reaction. Unfortunately, there is as yet no reliable data on ocular tilt angle in patients with skew deviation due to various brainstem lesions. However, recent data from Brandt and Dieterich (11) show that significant deviations of the subjective visual spatial vertical commonly occur in patients with brainstem and thalamic lesions (19,20). Athough many of these patients do not have a skew deviation, it does raise the possibility that a partial ocular tilt reaction is much more common than formerly assumed in patients with brainstem and thalamic lesions.

Other causes of vertical strabismus such as myasthenia, dissociated vertical deviation, and orbital lesions need to be considered in the differential diagnosis but will not be discussed here.

D. Tonic Versus Phasic Ocular Tilt Reactions

An ocular tilt reaction can assume two different temporal profiles. It can either be continuously present for days to weeks, in which case it is called "tonic," or it can be brief and recurring lasting each time from seconds to minutes, in which case it is called "paroxysmal." It is generally assumed that whereas a tonic ocular tilt reaction is due to a prolonged unilateral decrease in the activity of the graviceptive pathways, a paroxysmal ocular tilt reaction is due to a temporary unilateral increase in the activity of the graviceptive pathways. Since a lesion at any particular level of the graviceptive otolithic system can cause either a tonic or a paroxysmal ocular tilt reaction, lesions that produce a tonic ocular tilt reaction have been called "destructive," whereas lesions that produce a paroxysmal ocular tilt reaction have been called "irritative." The clearest example of lesions in one location causing a tonic ocular tilt reaction in one direction or a paroxysmal ocular tilt reaction in the opposite direction occurs with unilateral mesodiencephalic lesions involving the interstitial nucleus or its connections. This subject is discussed below.

E. Localization of the Ocular Tilt Reaction

Lesions both destructive and "irritative" of the graviceptive otolithic pathways from the otoliths in the labyrinth to the interstitial nucleus in the midbrain can all produce an ocular tilt reaction (Fig. 7).

1. Destructive Unilateral Peripheral Vestibular Lesions

The tonic (i.e., persistent) ipsiversive ocular tilt reaction that invariably follows acute unilateral vestibular deafferentation was first documented in different species by Magnus and his coworkers (21). There have been subsequent reports of this phenomenon in the scientific (22), clinical (23), and veterinary literature (Fig. 8) (24,25). Our own data show that a partial tonic ipsiversive ocular tilt reaction invariably develops in patients with acute destructive lesions of a functioning labyrinth (7). The partial ocular tilt reaction consists of excyclotropia (i.e., extorsion) of the ipsilateral eye and incyclotropia (i.e., intorsion) of the contralateral eye. The magnitude of the ocular torsion is usually the same in the two eyes but can vary from 5 to 25 degrees depending on preexisting vestibular function and on how long after the lesion was made the measurements are taken. Only some patients develop a complete tonic ocular tilt reaction with ipsiversive head tilt and ipsilateral hypotropia as well as ipsiversive ocular torsion. The tonic ocular tilt reaction that occurs after unilateral vestibular deafferentation invariably and largely resolves in much the same way as does the horizontal nystagmus. The development and resolution of the ocular tilt reaction after unilateral vestibular deafferentation could be an index of vestibular compensation (26).

2. Unilateral "Irritative" Peripheral Vestibular Lesion

In some patients with a hypermobile stapes, footplate acoustic stimulation of the labyrinth, presumably the utricle, can produce a paroxysmal contraversive ocular tilt reaction. This has been called the *otolithic Tullio* phenomenon (27,28). In the cat, a phasic (i.e., paroxysmal) contraversive ocular tilt reaction is produced by electrical stimulation of the utricular nerve (6).

3. Unilateral Destructive Vestibular Nucleus Lesion

A unilateral vestibular nucleus lesions produces a tonic ipsiversive ocular tilt reaction. In patients with lateral medullary infarcts (Wallenberg's syndrome), there is invariably an ipsiversive ocular tilt reaction (11). The ocular tilt reaction may be partial with just excyclotorsion of the ipsilateral eye or it may be complete with binocular ipsiversive torsion of 20 degrees or even more, ipsiversive head tilt, and ipsiversive skew deviation. Generally, the ipsiversive torsion is different in the two eyes. The excyclotropia of the ipsilesional eye is greater than the

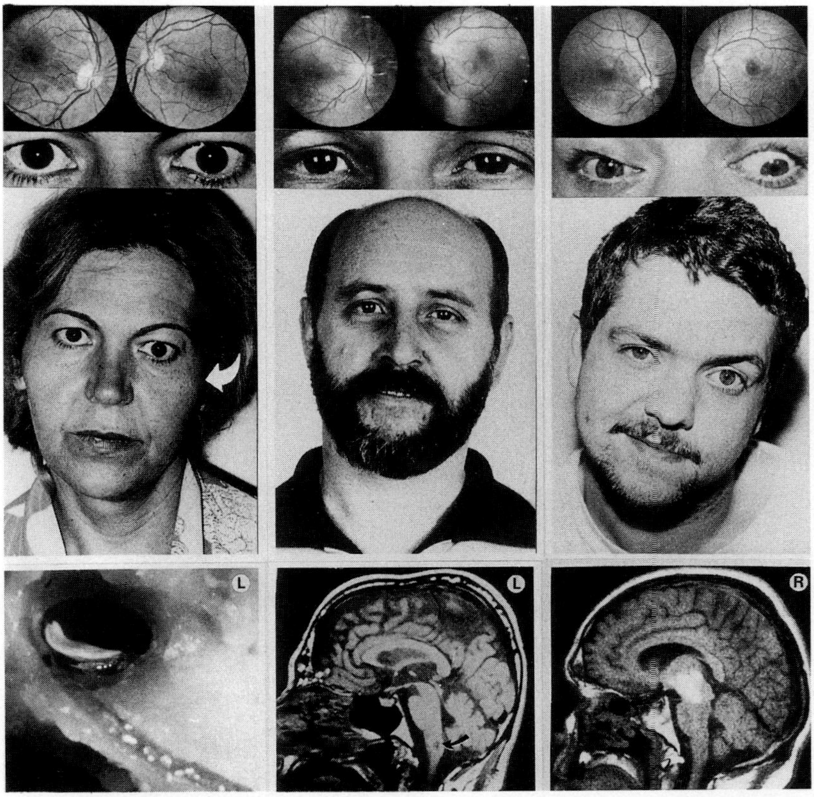

Figure 7 **Tonic leftward ocular tilt reaction; possible sites of lesion. Left column: Tonic leftward ocular tilt reaction in a patient 1 week after left vestibular lesion involving the utricle. There is 25 degrees of tonic leftward ocular torsion. There also is a left skew deviation with 10 degrees of left hypotropia in the primary position, and about 20 degrees of leftward head tilt. (From Ref. 23.) Bottom figure is a dissection of a guinea pig's left utricle showing the anterior curvature of the otolithic membrane. Center column: Tonic leftward ocular tilt reaction due to a left vestibular nucleus lesion. There is tonic leftward torsion of the eyes with 28 degrees of left excyclotropia and 7 degrees of right incyclotropia. There is also a left skew deviation with 6 degrees of left hypotropia in the primary position, and about 15 degrees of leftward head tilt. The bottom figure shows a T_1-weighted magnetic resonance image (MRI) of a left lateral medullary infarct involving the vestibular nucleus. (Courtesy of Professor T. Brandt.) Right column: Tonic leftward ocular tilt reaction due to a right mesodiencephalic hemorrhage from a thalamic arteriovenous malformation. There is tonic leftward ocular torsion with 26 degrees of left excyclotropia and 16 degrees of right incyclotropia. There is also a left skew deviation with 25 degrees of left hypotropia in the primary position and 30 degrees of leftward head tilt. The bottom figure is a T_1-weighted MRI of the lesion in the right thalamus. (From Ref. 10.)**

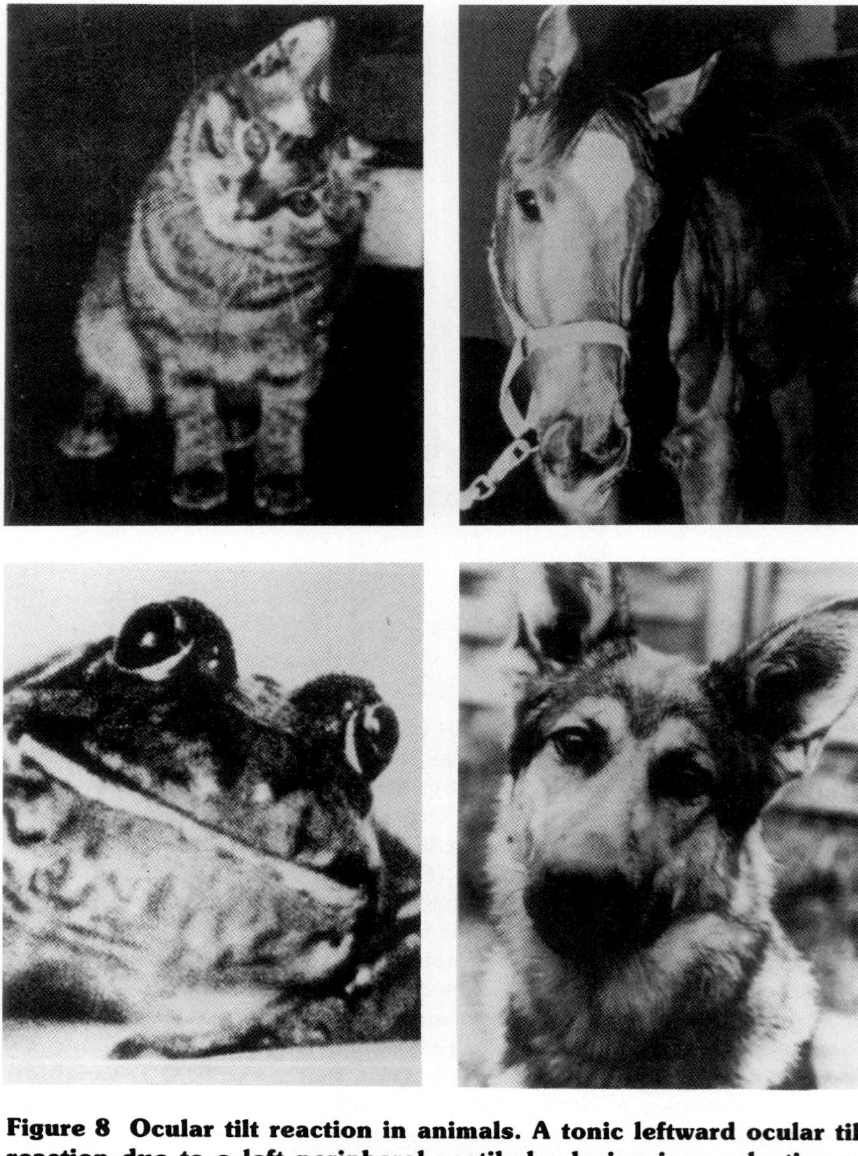

Figure 8 Ocular tilt reaction in animals. A tonic leftward ocular tilt reaction due to a left peripheral vestibular lesion in a selection of vertebrates. In the cat and the frog, the lesion was experimental, whereas in the horse and the dog, it was spontaneous (24,25). Although the head tilt is obvious, the ocular torsion is only discernible in animal pupils that are not circular. (Top right figure from Ref. 25.)

incyclotropia of the contralateral eye. Unilateral vestibular nucleus lesions also produce an ipsiversive tonic ocular tilt reaction in the monkey (29).

4. Unilateral Irritative Vestibular Nucleus Lesion

Slavin and LoPinto (30) reported the unique case of a patient with vascular compression left medulla, and presumably the left vestibular nucleus, who had what appeared to be a paroxysmal rightward ocular tilt reaction associated with a left visual tilt illusion. The case is unique in that there are no other reports of a contraversive ocular tilt reaction with a unilateral medullary lesion and no other cases with a visual tilt illusion in whom an ocular tilt reaction has been found—probably because it has not been sought.

5. Unilateral Destructive Interstitial Nucleus Lesion

Clinical (10) and experimental (31,32,4) unilateral lesions in the region of the interstitial nucleus of Cajal (INC) produce a tonic contraversive ocular tilt reaction. Lesions near the INC in the zona incerta or medial thalamus (33) as well as lesions restricted to the INC also can produce a tonic contraversive ocular tilt reaction. (See Notes Added in Proof (p. 223), No. 3.) A subsequent acute unilateral peripheral vestibular lesion ipsilateral to the INC lesion will abolish the tonic ocular tilt reaction produced by the INC lesion (22). (See Notes Added in Proof (p. 223), No. 4.)

6. Unilateral "Irritative" Interstitial Nucleus Lesion

Electrical stimulation in the region of the INC produces a phasic ipsiversive ocular tilt reaction in cats (4,34) and in humans (35). Although stimulation of the INC alone will produce a phasic ipsiversive ocular tilt reaction, stimulation of other regions (36), including zona incerta (37) and medial thalamus (33), can also produce the same ipsiversive ocular tilt reaction. In some patients, unilateral lesions in the region of the INC produce a paroxysmal ipsiversive ocular tilt reaction rather than a tonic contraversive ocular tilt reaction (38) (Figs. 9 and 10). This is possibly due to intermittent disinhibition of the normal ocular tilt reaction pathways passing through the INC rather than due to persistent disfacilitation as occurs with the tonic ocular tilt reaction.

F. Mechanism and Significance of the Ocular Tilt Reaction

The ocular tilt reaction is a compensatory postural reflex, a righting reflex, of otolithic origin (21). In frontal-eyed animals such as humans, it may only have a vestigial role (39,40). It is normally elicited by changes in the direction and magnitude of the linear acceleration vector acting on the head; that is, by angle of head tilt in the coronal plane with respect to the gravitational vertical. Its three components, head tilt, eye torsion, and skew deviation, are all in the compensatory direction (see Fig. 3). The head tilt component is most prominent

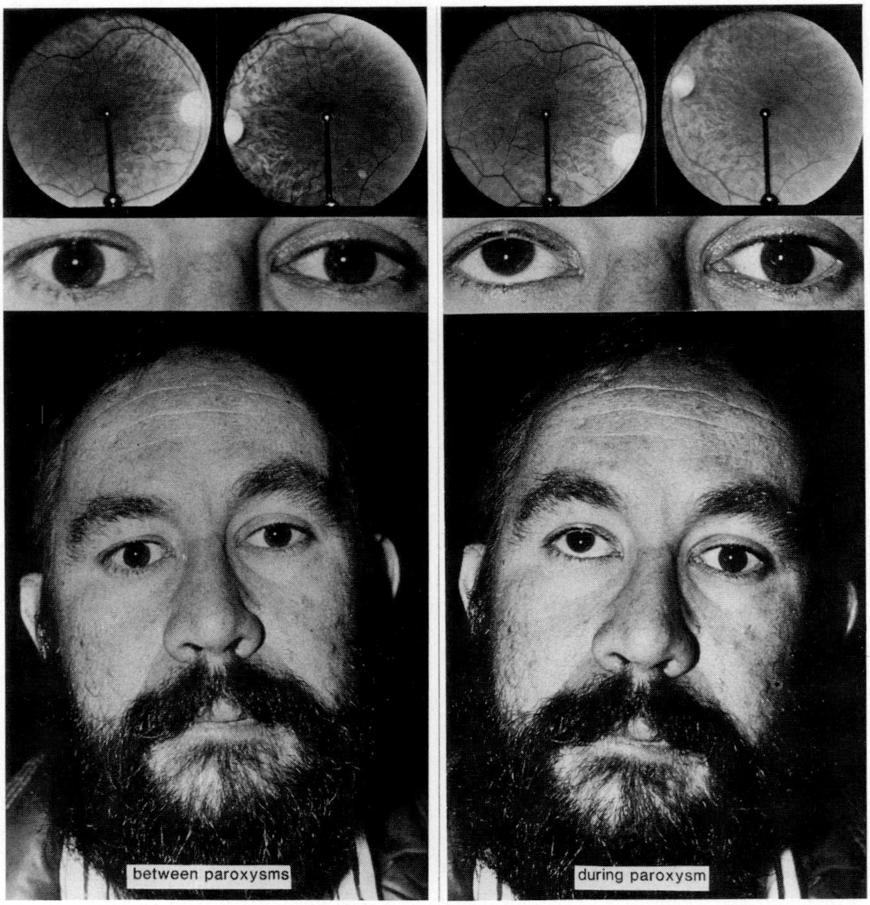

Figure 9 Paroxysmal ipsiversive ocular tilt reaction with mesodiencephalic lesion. A patient with a left mesodiencephalic lesion who has for the last 10 years experienced several times a day paroxysms of a leftward ocular tilt reaction with 25 degrees of leftward ocular torsion in each eye, a left skew deviation with 30 degrees of left hypotropia in the primary position, and about 25 degrees of leftward head tilt. Between paroxysms he was orthotropic but had about 10 degrees of rightward head tilt and about 4 degrees of rightward ocular torsion, representing a slight tonic contraversive ocular tilt reaction. (From Ref. 38.)

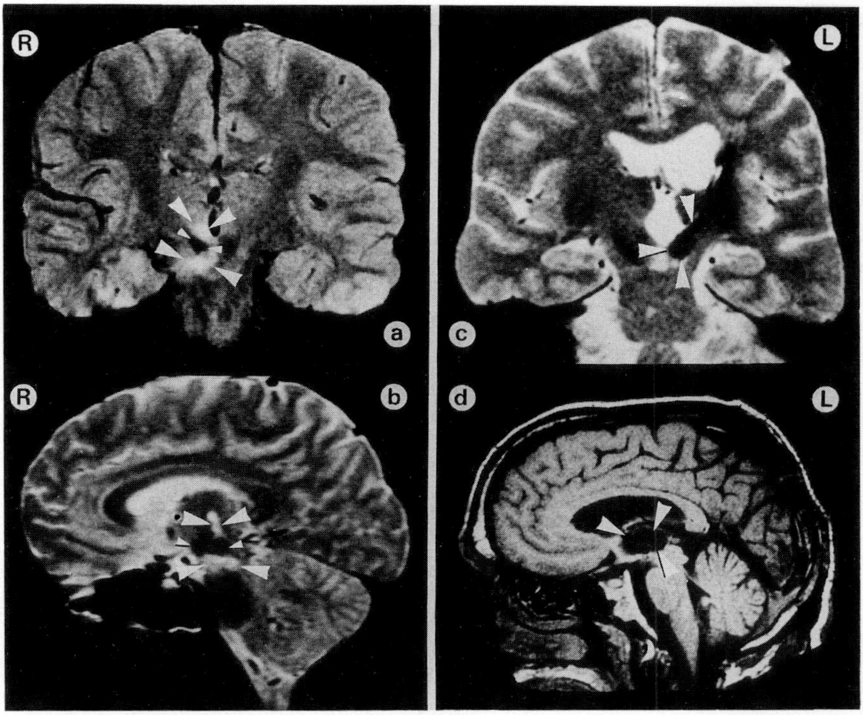

Figure 10 The mesodiencephalic lesions that produce a tonic contraversive or a paroxysmal ipsiversive ocular tilt reaction. Left column: Proton-density, coronal (a), and right parasaggital (b) MR images from a patient with a tonic leftward (i.e., contraversive) ocular tilt reaction due to right paramedian mesodiencephalic infarction. The upper large arrows indicate a lesion in the medial thalamus, whereas the lower large arrows indicate another lesion in the midbrain. The small arrows indicate the red nucleus, which is intact between these two lesions. The upper lesion is responsible for the leftward ocular tilt reaction, whereas the lower lesion causes a fascicular third nerve palsy. Right column: T_2-weighted coronal (c) and T1-weighted left parasaggital (d) MR images from the patient shown in Fig. 9 who had a paroxysmal leftward (i.e., ipsiversive) ocular tilt reaction due to a previous left mesodiencephalic abscess. The three white arrows indicate a cystic lesion in the medial thalamus and subthalamus extending rostrally through the internal capsule into the striatum. (The hemosiderin in the lesion is the result of a previous stereotactic needle aspiration.) The common area of involvement in all these lesions is the medial thalamus, subthalamus, and the midbrain including the interstitial nucleus of Cajal. (From Ref. 10.) This figure shows that a unilateral mesodiencephalic lesion can cause either a paroxysmal ipsiversive or a tonic contraversive ocular tilt reaction depending perhaps on whether rostral inputs to, or caudal outputs from, the interstitial nucleus of Cajal are involved.

in animals with little or no eye movements such as certain birds (41). For example, a chicken or an owl will keep its head gravitationally vertical during large tilt displacements of the trunk. The skew component is most prominent in animals that have mobile, laterally placed eyes but have no head movements in roll, such as fish. Tilting a fish about its long axis produces a compensatory skew deviation with hypotropia of the uppermost eye (42,43). In response to tilting in the coronal plane, the eye torsion component is most prominent in frontal-eyed animals, since in lateral-eyed animals tilting in the sagittal plane rather than in the coronal plane is the adequate stimulus for compensatory eye torsion. However, even in frontal-eyed animals, the eye torsion component, that is, the ocular counterrolling, is incompletely compensatory; 6–7 degrees at most in response to a 90-degree head tilt (8). Furthermore, in a frontal-eyed animal, any compensatory head tilt reduces the need for compensatory eye torsion. In the limiting case if the head tilt were fully compensatory, no eye torsion would be required.

A spontaneous or abnormal ocular tilt reaction, that is, an ocular tilt reaction appearing in a spatially vertical subject, is due to an imbalance in spontaneous neural activity arising in peripheral or central graviceptive, otolithic neurons (see Fig. 3). A tonic ocular tilt reaction in this case would be due to a persistent lesion-induced decrease in resting neural activity, whereas a phasic or paroxysmal ocular tilt reaction would be due to a transient lesion-induced increase in neural activity. In this way, the mechanism of the ocular tilt reaction is similar to the mechanism of the spontaneous nystagmus that occurs after unilateral vestibular deafferentation and reflect decreased resting activity in secondary vestibular neurons in the ipsilesional vestibular nucleus due to loss of input from primary vestibular neurons.

1. Anatomical Substrate of the Ocular Tilt Reaction

The clinical and experimental evidence indicates that the labyrinth, vestibular nucleus, and interstital nucleus of Cajal are all involved in the ocular tilt reaction. However, it is not obvious what pathways connect these three structures and mediate the ocular tilt reaction. The pathways from the labyrinth to the vestibular nucleus that have the capacity to mediate the ocular tilt reaction are well known: Primary vestibular neurons from the utricle project to secondary vestibular neurons in the lateral vestibular nucleus (44). In contrast, there is uncertainty about the location of the graviceptive pathway between the lateral vestibular nucleus and the contralateral INC. Although contralateral projections from the medial vestibular nucleus to the oculomotor, trochlear, and interstitial nuclei have been identified (45), there is no evidence that these pathways transmit otolith information and furthermore there is little data so far on the tilt sensitivity of INC neurons themselves (4). Although the details of graviceptive connections between the vestibular nucleus and the INC require further experimental evidence, from the clinical evidence presented here there can be little doubt that there is a pathway between the vestibular nucleus and the contralateral interstitial nucleus and that it decussates either in the pons or the caudal midbrain.

G. Ocular Tilt Reaction and Vestibular Compensation

One of the most remarkable aspects of the ocular tilt reaction, particularly the ocular tilt reaction produced by unilateral destructive peripheral vestibular lesions, is that the ocular tilt reaction invariably resolves, albeit not completely. Acute total unilateral deafferentation or destruction of an intact labyrinth—unilateral vestibular deafferentation—invariably causes a profound and stereotyped disturbance of perception posture and movement in species as diverse as amphibians, birds, rodents, and primates, including humans. The disturbances attributable to the unilateral loss of horizontal semicircular canal function are well known and include horizontal nystagmus and a deficit of horizontal vestibulo-ocular reflexes (46). In contrast, the disturbances due to unilateral loss of otolith function are not so well known.

Recent data from humans indicate that unilateral loss of otolith function causes disturbances in the control of head-eye posture and perception of gravitoinertial force, all in the coronal plane (47). Perhaps the most intriguing aspect of unilateral vestibular deafferentation is that although the unilateral vestibular deafferentation is permanent—the ipsilesional vestibular nucleus will never again receive input from the lesioned labyrinth—many of the disturbances that follow unilateral vestibular deafferentation are temporary. For example, in humans there is little overt evidence of any vestibular disturbance 1 month after unilateral vestibular deafferentation. The process of recovery from the consequences of unilateral vestibular deafferentation is termed vestibular compensation.

Following unilateral vestibular deafferentation there is invariably tonic conjugate ipsiversive ocular torsion. One week after unilateral vestibular deafferentation, there is up to 15 degrees of ocular torsion, and the magnitude of the ocular torsion is closely correlated ($r = 0.95$) with the magnitude of the tilting of the visual horizontal (7) (see Fig. 6). In the subsequent month, both the torsion and the tilting of the subjective visual spatial vertical gradually resolve, so that 1 month after unilateral vestibular deafferentation both the ocular torsion and the tilting of the visual horizontal are only half the 1-week value. A slight but statistically significant ocular torsion (4–5 degrees) appeared to be a permanent legacy of unilateral vestibular deafferentation. The ocular torsion and tilting of the subjective visual spatial vertical that occur after unilateral vestibular nucleus lesions resolve in a similar fashion.

H. Visual Tilt Illusion

Some patients with acute unilateral vestibular nucleus lesions temporarily see the visual world tilted sideways or even upside down. The symptom occurs in patients with lateral medullary infarcts (Wallenberg's syndrome) (48–50) and can last from a few minutes to a few hours and up to a day or 2 after the stroke. During that period, it can be continuous or intermittent—occurring for a minute or so and then is gone. There may or may not be other symptoms or signs of spatial disorientation such as vertigo, nystagmus, ocular tilt reaction, and lateropulsion.

There is no general agreement on the direction of the visual tilt illusion: the patients reported from Sweden saw the world as tilted away from the side of the vestibular nucleus lesion (46); Ropper's patients (49), cases 1 and 2, and Slavin and LoPinto's (30) patient saw the world tilted toward the side of the lesion. Because of this uncertainty, it is difficult to postulate a mechanism for the visual tilt illusion. Perhaps the simplest explanation is that it represents the sensory consequence of ipsiversive ocular torsion. A patient with a leftward ocular tilt reaction following a left vestibular nucleus lesion could develop a rightward tilt illusion. This explanation is, however, difficult to reconcile with the observation that most patients with the ocular tilt reaction, some with very large degrees of ocular torsion, do not complain of a tilt illusion. Furthermore, it appears that it is possible to have a visual tilt illusion with a lesion restricted to the vestibulocerebellum (50).

ACKNOWLEDGMENTS

This work was supported by the National Health and Medical Research Council of Australia and by the RPAH Neurology Department Trustees.

REFERENCES

1. Fernandez C, Goldberg J. Physiology of peripheral neurons innervating the otolith organs of the squirrel monkey. I. Response to static tilts and to long-duration centrifugal force. J Neurophysiol 1976; 39:970– .
2. Fernandez C, Goldberg J. Physiology of peripheral neurons innervating the otolith organs of the squirrel monkey. II. Directional selectivity and force-response relations. J Neurophysiol 1976; 39:985– .
3. Goldberg JM, Fernandez C. The vestibular system. In: Handbook of physiology. The nervous system III. Washington, D.C.: American Physiologic Society, 1982:977–1022.
4. Fukushima K. The interstitial nucleus of Cajal and its role in the control of movements of the head and eyes. Prog Neurobiol 1987; 29:107–92.
5. Vilis T, Hepp K, Schwartz U, Henn V. On the generation of vertical and torsional rapid eye movements in the monkey. Exp Brain Res 1989; 77:1–11.

6. Suzuki JI, Tokumasu K, Goto K: Eye movements from single utricular nerve stimulation in the cat. Acta Otolaryngol 1969; 68:350–62.
7. Curthoys IS, Dai MJ, Halmagyi GM. Human ocular torsion before and after unilateral vestibular neurectomy. Exp Brain Res 1991; 85:218–25.
8. Diamond SG, Markham CH. Ocular counterrolling as an indicator of vestibular otolith function. Neurology 1983; 33:1460–69.
9. Dieterich M, Brandt Th. Ocular torsion and perceived vertical in oculomotor, trochlear and abducens nerve palsies. Brain 1993; 116:1095–1104.
10. Halmagyi GM, Brandt T, Dieterich M, Curthoys IS, Stark RJ, Hoyt WF. Tonic contraversive ocular tilt reaction due to unilateral meso-diencephalic lesion. Neurology 1990; 40:1503–9.
11. Dieterich M, Brandt T. Wallenberg's syndrome: lateropulsion, cyclorotation, and subjective visual vertical in thirty-six patients. Ann Neurol 1992; 31:399–408.
12. Ruttum M, von Noorden GK. Adaptation to tilting of the visual environment in cyclotropia. Am J Ophthalmol 1983; 96:229–37.
13. Silferskiold BP. Skew deviation in Wallenberg's syndrome. Acta Neurol Scand 1965; 41:269–82.
14. Bixemann WW, von Noorden GK. Apparent foveal displacement in normal subjects and in cyclotropia. Ophthalmology 1983; 89:58–62.
15. Locke JC: Heterotopia of the blind spot in ocular vertical muscle imbalance. Am J Opthalmol 1968; 65:362–74.
16. Friedmann G. The judgement of the visual vertical and horizontal with peripheral and central vestibular lesions. Brain 1970; 93:313– .
17. Safran AB, Mermoud A: Frame with spirit level for evaluating visual tilt. J Clin Neuro Ophthalmol 1991; 11:74–5.
18. Safran AB, Hausler R, Issoua D, Stepanian E, Chiari M, Vibert D, Roth A. Strabisme induits par des lesions vestibulaires peripheriques. Klin Mbl Augenheilk 1992; 200:418–20.
19. Dieterich M, Brandt Th. Ocular torsion and tilt of subjective visual vertical are sensitive brainstem signs. Ann Neurol 1993; 33:292–94
20. Dieterich M, Brandt T. Thalamic infarctions: differential effects on vestibular function in the null plane (35 patients). Neurology 1993; 43:1732–40.
21. Magnus R. Korperstellung. Berlin: Julius Springer 1924:289–469. (English translation by Rosnoff WR, van Harreveld A. Body posture. New Delhi: Amerind Publishing Company, 1988.)
22. Toczek S, Hyde JE. Effect of vestibular nerve section on torsion and evoked rotatory movements. Exp Neurol 1963; 8:143–54.
23. Halmagyi GM, Gresty MA, Gibson WPR. Ocular tilt reaction with peripheral vestibular lesion. Ann Neurol 1979; 6:80–3.
24. Schunk KL, Averill DR. Peripheral vestibular syndrome in the dog: a review of 83 cases. J Am Vet Med Assoc 1983; 182:1354–7.
25. Watrous BJ. Head tilt in horses. Vet Clin North Am: Equine practice. 1987; 3:353–70.
26. Flohr H, Bienhold H, Abeln W, Macskovics I. Concepts of vestibular compensation. In: Flohr H, Precht W, eds. Lesion-induced neuronal plasticity in sensorimotor systems. Berlin: Springer-Verlag, 1981:153–72.

27. Deecke L, Mengner T, Plester D. Tullio phenomenon with torsion of the eyes and subjective tilt of the visual surround. Ann NY Acad Sci 1981; 374:650–5.
28. Dieterich M, Brandt T, Fries W. Otolith function in man. Results from a case of otolith Tullio phenomenon. Brain 1989; 112:1377–92.
29. Uemura T, Cohen B. The effect of vestibular nuclei lesions on vestibulo-ocular reflexes and posture in monkeys. Acta Otolaryngol 1973; 315(Suppl.):1–71.
30. Slavin ML, LoPinto RJ. Isolated environmental tilt associated with lateral medullary compression by dolichoectasia of the vertebral artery. J Clin Neuro Ophthalmol 1987; 7:29–33.
31. Hess WR. Charakter der im Zwishenhirn ausgelosten Bewengungseffekte. (The nature of the movements elicited by electrical stimulation of the diencephalon.) Pflugers Arch Ges Physiol 1941; 244:767–86. (English translation in selected works of Hess WR, Akert K, eds. Biological order and brain organization. Berlin: Springer-Verlag, 1981:223–42.)
32. Anderson JH. Ocular torsion in the cat after lesions of the interstitial nucleus of Cajal. Ann NY Acad Sci 1981; 374:865–71.
33. Jung R, Hassler R. The extrapyramidal system. In: Field J, Magoun HW, Hall VE, eds. Handbook of physiology. Neurophysiology, Vol. II. Washington, D.C.: American Physiological Society, 1960:863–927.
34. Hassler R. Supranuclear structures regulating binocular eye and head movements. Bibl Ophthalmol 1972; 82:207–19.
35. Lueck CJ, Hamlyn P, Crawford TJ, Levy IS, Brindley GS, Watkins S, Kennard C. A case of ocular tilt reaction and torsional nystagmus due to direct stimulation of the midbrain in man. Brain 1991; 114:2069–79.
36. Westheimer G, Blair SM. The ocular tilt reaction—a brainstem oculomotor routine. Invest Ophthalmol 1975; 14:883–839.
37. Hyde JE, Toczek S. Functional relation of interstitial nucleus to rotatory eye movements evoked from zona incerta stimulation. J Neurophysiol 1962; 25:455–66.
38. Hedges TR, Hoyt WF. Ocular tilt reaction due to an upper brainstem lesion: paroxysmal skew deviation, torsion and oscillation of the eyes with head tilt. Ann Neurol 1982; 11:537–40.
39. Simpson JI, Graf W. Eye muscle geometry and compensatory eye movements in lateral-eyed and in frontal-eyed animals. Ann NY Acad Sci 1981; 374:20–30.
40. Roberts TDM. The neurophysiology of postural mechanisms, 2d ed. London: Butterworths, 1978:247–58.
41. Steinbach MJ, Money KE. Eye movements of the owl. Vision Res 1973; 13:889–91.
42. Monnier M. The functions of the nervous system. Amsterdam: Elsevier, 1970:277–99.
43. Spiegel EA, Sommer I. Neurology of the eye, ear, nose and throat. New York: Grune & Stratton, 1944:82–95.
44. Precht W. Neuronal operations in the vestibular system. Berlin: Springer-Verlag 1978:76–8.
45. Precht W. Neuronal operations in the vestibular system. Berlin: Springer-Verlag, 1978:170–8.
46. Smith PF, Curthoys IS. Mechanisms of recovery following unilateral labyrinthectomy: a review. Brain Res Rev 1989; 14:155–80.

47. Dai MJ, Curthoys IS, Halmagyi GM. Perception of linear acceleration before and after unilateral vestibular neurectomy. Exp Brain Res 1989; 77:315–28.
48. Hornsten G. Wallenberg's syndrome: Part I. General symptomatology with special reference to the visual disturbances and imbalance. Acta Neurol Scand 1974; 50:434–46.
49. Ropper AH. Illusion of tilting of the visual environment. J Clin Neuro Ophthalmol 1983; 3:147–51.
50. Charles N, Froment C, Rode G, Vighetto A, Turjman F, Trillet M, Aimard G. Vertigo and upside down vision due to an infarct in the territory of the medial branch of the posterior inferior cerebellar artery causes by dissection of a vertebral artery, J Neurol Neurosurg Psychiatry 1992; 55:188–9.
51. Lopez L, Ochoa S, Lacman M, Mesropian H, Granillo R. Acute transient upside-down inversion of vision with brainstem-cerebellar infarction. (Neuro-ophthalmology, in press).
52. Halmagyi GM, An ST, Dehaene I, Curthoys IS, Todd MJ. Jerk waveform seesaw nystagmus due to unilateral mesodiencephalic lesion. Brain 1994; 117:789–804.
53. Fukushima K, Ohashi T, Fukushima J, Kase M. Ocular torsion produced by unilateral chemical inactivation of the interstitial nucleus of Cajal in chronically labyrinthectomized cats. Neurosci Res 1992: 13:301–305.

NOTES ADDED IN PROOF

1. Furthermore, with an acute superior oblique palsy the patient will set the monocular, subjective, visual vertical (but not the binocular) in extension with either the paretic or nonparetic eye. With chronic superior oblique palsies, the findings are more complex (9).

2. Thus normal subjects can have up to 12 degrees excyclotropia of each eye, making measurement of excyclotropia difficult. On the other hand, it means that more than 2° incyclotropia could be considered pathological.

3. Lesions of the INC, sparing the rostral interstitial nucleus of the medial longitudinal fasciculus produce a jerk-waveform seesaw nystagmus as well as an ocular tilt reaction (52).

4. A unilateral INC lesion after bilateral labyrinthectomy will still produce a tonic ipsiversive ocular tilt reaction (53).

16

Management of Acquired Nystagmus and Oscillopsia

R. John Leigh
Case Western Reserve University and Veterans Affairs Medical Center, Cleveland, Ohio

I. PATHOGENESIS OF NYSTAGMUS AND ITS VISUAL CONSEQUENCES

A. Pathogenesis of Nystagmus

Although many therapies for nystagmus and its visual consequences remain empirical, a few do have a logical basis. Furthermore, it seems likely that better understanding of the cause of nystagmus may bring more treatments to light. In thinking about the pathogenesis of nystagmus, recall that it is usually the *slow phase* that reflects the underlying abnormality (see Ref. 1 for a review). Thus, disorders of those mechanisms that normally function to hold gaze steady may cause the eyes to drift in a slow phase of nystagmus. With the head still and the eyes close to primary position, the visual fixation system is of primary importance for holding gaze steady. When the eyes are turned to an eccentric position in the orbits, a gaze-holding mechanism (the neural integrator) permits steady fixation. During head rotations, vestibular, optokinetic, and pursuit eye movements work together to keep the eyes pointed at a stationary object. Often the characteristics of the slow-phase drift indicate the ocular motor subsystem that is at fault. Reliable measurements of the nystagmus waveform are always advisable before treatment is started, since they often help identify the nature of the oscillation (see below). For example, imbalance of vestibular drives causes constant velocity drifts (Fig. 1a). If the gaze-holding mechanism is deficient, the eyes cannot be

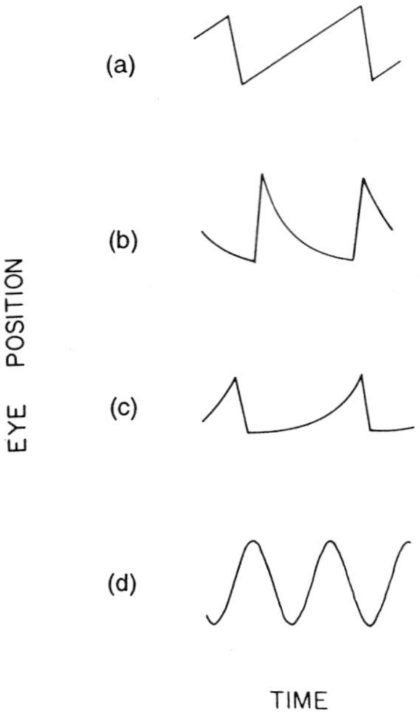

Figure 1 Four common slow-phase waveforms of nystagmus. (a) Constant velocity drift of the eyes. This occurs in nystagmus caused by peripheral or central vestibular disease and also with lesions of the cerebral hemisphere. The added quick-phases give a "saw-tooth" appearance. (b) Drift of the eyes back from an eccentric orbital position toward the midline (gaze-evoked nystagmus). The drift shows a negative exponential time course with decreasing velocity. This waveform reflects an unsustained eye position signal caused by an impaired neural integrator. (c) Drift of the eyes away from the primary position with a positive exponential time course (increasing velocity). This waveform suggests an unstable neural integrator and is encountered in the horizontal plane in congenital nystagmus and in the vertical plane in cerebellar disease. (d) Pendular nystagmus, which is encountered as a type of congenital nystagmus and with acquired disease. (From Ref. 1.)

held steadily in an eccentric orbital position, and they drift back to the midline with a decreasing velocity waveform (gaze-evoked nystagmus [Fig. 1b]). Because the gaze-holding mechanism in part depends on the vestibular nuclei, nystagmus due to brainstem lesions often shows characteristics of both vestibular imbalance and disturbed gaze holding. Such nystagmus may be present in primary position but its slow phase changes when the eyes are deviated (Alexander's law). Instability in the gaze-holding mechanism may lead to a slow-phase drift that increases in velocity (Fig. 1c).

Disorders of the visual fixation, smooth pursuit, and optokinetic systems may influence nystagmus in two ways. First, long-term deprivation of vision (e.g., optic nerve disease) may lead to jerk nystagmus with slow phases that are variably linear and decrease or increase in velocity (Fig. 1a–c). Pendular nystagmus (Fig. 1d) may also result and, especially in the vertical plane, irregular drifting movements of the eyes—"ocular motor noise"—may be superimposed. Second, nystagmus due to vestibular imbalance or disturbance of the gaze-holding mechanism will be more evident if visual fixation is abnormal; vestibular and gaze-evoked nystagmus are damped if the visual fixation mechanism is intact. An important corollary is that sometimes the slow phase has velocity or frequency components that are above the range within which the fixation and pursuit systems can cope; if treatment measures are able to damp the nystagmus to the point that fixation mechanisms can once again exert their effects, nystagmus may be completely suppressed.

It should be noted that saccadic abnormalities may also disrupt steady gaze; these disorders are frequently mistaken for nystagmus (unless records of the movements are made), but their pathogenesis and treatment are different. In addition, superior oblique myokymia, an unexplained condition of adults, may cause recurring episodes of monocular oscillopsia or diplopia accompanied by tremulous sensations in the affected eye (1). It is best seen with the ophthalmoscope or slit lamp when the patient is symptomatic.

B. Pathogenesis of the Visual Consequences of Nystagmus

Acquired nystagmus commonly causes impaired vision and oscillopsia—illusory movement of the environment. These symptoms, which are due to drift of images of stationary objects on the retina, interfere with reading and watching television, and the oscillopsia may be distressing to the patient. The relationship between retinal image velocity and visual acuity is a direct one: Image motion in excess of about 4 degrees/s impairs vision. On the other hand, the relationship between retinal image velocity and the development of oscillopsia is less consistent and varies among subjects. For example, individuals with congenital nystagmus, who often have images moving across the retina with speeds exceeding 100 degrees/s, seldom complain of oscillopsia. With acquired nystagmus, the magnitude of oscillopsia is usually less than the magnitude of nystagmus. For example, in patients with downbeat nystagmus, oscillopsia is on average about one third of the amplitude of the nystagmus. This latter finding implies that the brain compensates for the excessive retinal image motion by using an extraretinal signal, such as efference copy, to maintain visual constancy. Nonetheless, we have shown experimentally in patients with nystagmus that if retinal image drift can be reduced below about 5 degrees, oscillopsia is usually abolished and vision is improved (2).

It should be noted that apart from nystagmus oscillopsia can also be caused by an inappropriate (hypoactive or hyperactive) vestibulo-ocular reflex and due to weakness of an extraocular muscle. In these cases, oscillopsia is induced by head movements. However, when oscillopsia is caused by ocular oscillation such as nystagmus, it occurs even when the head is still. Rarely, oscillopsia is the complaint in patients who do not have excessive retinal image motion (i.e., have no nystagmus) but rather seem to have a disorder of those central mechanisms that normally ensure a sense of visual constancy.

II. EVALUATION OF THE PATIENT WITH ACQUIRED NYSTAGMUS

Before starting a patient on medication or other treatment for their nystagmus, it behooves the physician to look carefully for an underlying cause. Sometimes this may be obvious (e.g., multiple sclerosis), but it is worthwhile looking carefully for any remedial underlying condition such as the Arnold-Chiari malformation. A systematic eye movement examination should be carried out, noting the magnitude of the nystagmus in the nine cardinal gaze angles, and any other abnormality of ocular motility (e.g., internuclear ophthalmoplegia). Note that nystagmus causing oscillopsia is not always obvious on gross examination. A sensitive and convenient way to detect instability of gaze is to view the retina with an ophthalmoscope.

Measurement of the nystagmus, if possible, is worthwhile. First, it identifies the type of nystagmus and, in particular, is invaluable in identifying congenital nystagmus (see Chap. 17). It also helps differentiate nystagmus from saccadic intrusions. Finally, it provides an objective record of the nystagmus before treatment is started so that its efficacy can be measured. The average amplitude of the nystagmus, slow-phase velocity, and frequency should be measured with the eye close to primary position and in the other cardinal gaze angles. Properties of each class of eye movement and the effects of convergence and removal of fixation (darkness or Fresnel goggles) on the nystagmus should also be recorded. A video record, although not capable of measuring nystagmus waveforms, is essential.

In addition, a systematic evaluation of visual function is warranted prior to starting treatment. Measurement of visual acuity at far and near, ophthalmoscopy, testing of visual fields, color vision, and pupillary responses should all be performed. Finally, an attempt to record the oscillopsia (if present) should be made. One method is to ask the patient to fixate a small light in a dark room and to indicate the direction of the perceived movement of the stationary light; the patient can be asked to draw the trajectory of the oscillopsia.

III. TREATMENT OF NYSTAGMUS

A. Drug Treatments

Of the various drugs reported to suppress nystagmus, only a few reliably improve symptoms. *Baclofen* is usually effective in treating acquired periodic alternating nystagmus (PAN). Acquired PAN is a spontaneous horizontal nystagmus present in primary gaze that reverses its direction approximately every 2 min (1). Because the period of oscillation is 4 min, the disorder is often missed unless the examiner observes the nystagmus for several minutes. As the nystagmus finishes one half cycle (e.g., of right-beating nystagmus), a brief transition period occurs during which there may be downbeating or upbeating nystagmus or square wave jerks before the next half cycle (e.g., of left-beating nystagmus) starts. Acquired PAN has been reported in association with a variety of conditions, many of which involve the cerebellum. Experimental ablation of the nodulus and uvula of the cerebellum in monkeys causes PAN when they are put into darkness; baclofen abolishes this nystagmus. Thus, the gamma-aminobutyric acid (GABA) agonist baclofen is able to abolish PAN due to experimental or clinical lesions of the nodulus and uvula. Although baclofen has been tried in a variety of other forms of nystagmus, its effect is unreliable.

A second drug that often has an effect on nystagmus in the rare syndrome of familial periodic ataxia with nystagmus is *acetazolamide* (1). Other reports of drug treatments of nystagmus mainly concern success in one or two individuals. *Clonazepam* has received a controlled (but not blinded) evaluation and been reported to be useful in the treatment of downbeat nystagmus (3). *Isoniazid* has been reported to suppress acquired nystagmus in some patients (4). We conducted a randomized, double-blind crossover trial of two *anticholinergic agents*, trihexyphenidyl (Artane) and tridihexethyl chloride (Pathilon—a quaternary anticholinergic that does not cross the blood-brain barrier) in patients with acquired nystagmus (5). We measured visual acuity and nystagmus prior to and at the end of 1 month on each medication. Of the 10 patients admitted to the study, only 5 completed trials of both drugs because of intolerance of medication or intercurrent illness. Of six patients who completed the trial of trihexyphenidyl, only one showed an improvement. Of six patients who completed a trial of tridihexethyl chloride, four showed improvement. An example is shown in Figure 2. Although the response of nystagmus to tridihexethyl chloride was an unexpected and interesting result, no patient wished to continue with this medication at the end of the study because of the anticholinergic side effects. We concluded that, first, trihexyphenidyl is not a reliable treatment for acquired

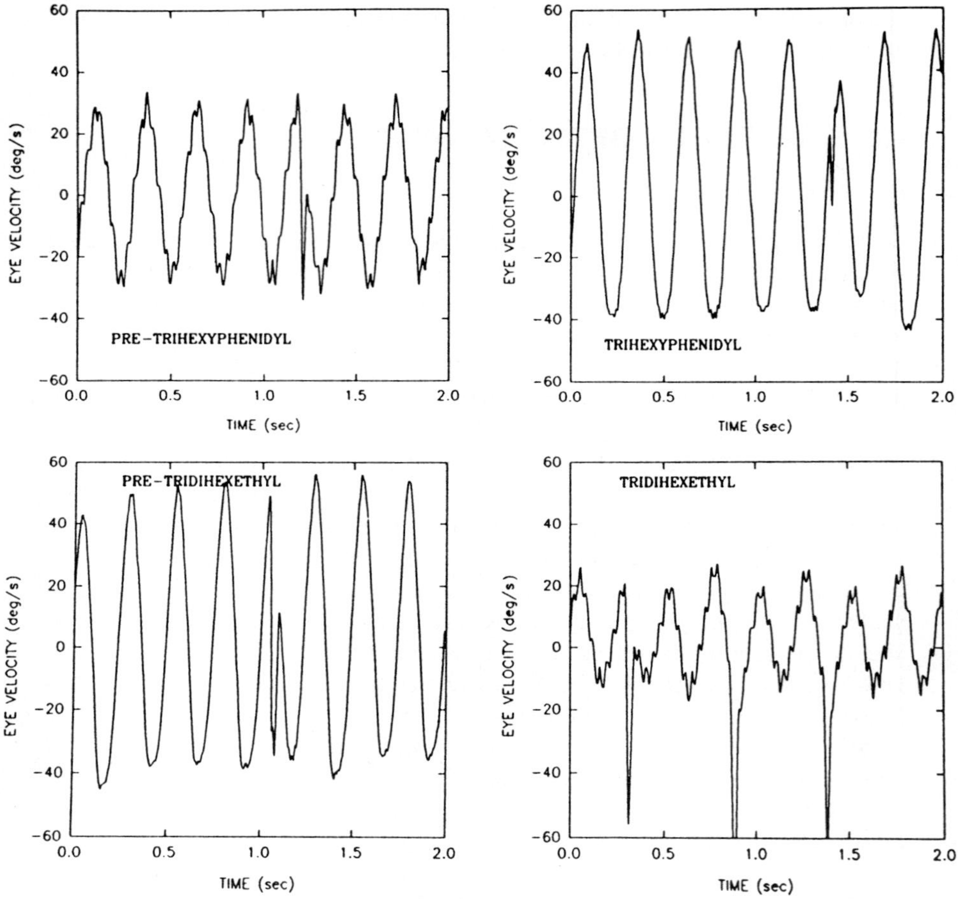

Figure 2 **Comparison of horizontal position of the left eye of a patient with acquired pendular nystagmus due to multiple sclerosis prior to treatment with trihexyphenidyl (top left); at the end of 1 month of treatment with trihexyphenidyl, maximum dose 20 mg/day (top right); prior to treatment with tridihexethyl chloride (bottom left); and at the end of 1 month treatment with tridihexethyl, maximum dose 100 mg/day (bottom right). Note that the nystagmus was mildly increased by trihexyphenidyl but reduced by tridihexethyl chloride. Upward deviations indicate eye rotations to the right. See text for details. (From Ref. 5.)**

nystagmus, although occasional patients may benefit; second, anticholinergic agents may suppress nystagmus by peripheral rather than central mechanisms (since tridihexethyl chloride probably does not cross the blood-brain barrier in appreciable quantities); third, the side effects of anticholinergic agents limit their effectiveness in the treatment of nystagmus. These reservations may not apply to all anticholinergic agents, however (8).

Certain drugs may influence the frequency of saccadic intrusions of the "square wave" type. *Benzodiazepines* and *barbiturates* have been reported to suppress macro–square wave jerks and *amphetamines* to suppress square wave jerks. *Clonazepam*, *propranolol*, and *thiamine* have been reported to diminish ocular flutter (saccadic oscillations without an intersaccadic interval) in individual patients (1). Superior oblique myokymia in some patients may be effectively treated with *carbamazepine*, *baclofen*, or *propranolol*.

B. Optical Treatments

A number of optical devices have been suggested for treatment of nystagmus. Patients whose nystagmus suppresses with convergence may benefit by wearing base-out prisms (6). Although convergence-suppression is common in congenital nystagmus, certain patients with a variety of acquired ocular oscillations may show the same phenomenon. Similarly, acquired nystagmus may be less prominent in one gaze angle (e.g., up gaze for some cases of downbeat nystagmus); in these individuals, prisms that turn the eyes toward the gaze direction of least nystagmus may be useful.

Another approach has been the development of an optical system to stabilize images on the retina (2,7). This system consists of a high-plus spectacle lens worn in combination with a high-minus contact lens (Fig. 3). Theoretically, stabilization could be achieved if the power of the spectacle lens focused the primary image close to the center of rotation of the eye. A contact lens would then be required to extend back the focus onto the retina. Since the contact lens moves with the eye, it does not negate the effect of retinal image stabilization produced by the spectacle lens. With such a system it is possible to achieve up to about 90% stabilization of images on the retina. One disadvantage of this system is that it disables the vestibulo-ocular reflex and voluntary eye movements.

We have attempted to treat 10 patients with acquired nystagmus with the optical stabilization device. In practice, only two patients were able to persevere with it for more than a few months, and none has used it for more than a year. One reason is that the hard contact lens is not well tolerated. Recently, however, we have been able to develop a gas-permeable contact lens made of Fluoroperm 90 material of powers up to –58 diopters that is more comfortable for patients to wear (9).

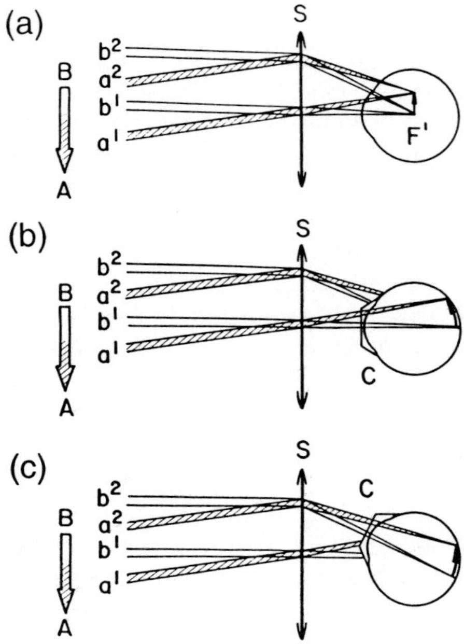

Figure 3 An optical method for stabilizing images of stationary objects upon the retina. (a) When viewing a distant object, AB, a convergent spectacle lens, S, will focus rays of light (b^1, b^2) from a point of interest B, on its focal point F^1, which is close to the center of rotation of the globe. Thus, if the eyeball were to rotate, light rays from point B would remain focused at the same point as in the eye. (b) A strongly divergent contact lens, C, extends back the focus from the center of the globe to the retina. (c) Since the contact lens moves with the eye, it does not negate the effect of retinal image stabilization produced by the spectacle lens, and rays of light from point B remain focused on the foveal region of the retina. (From Ref. 2.)

C. Invasive Procedures

Surgical operations such as the Kestenbaum procedure, which effectively treat certain patients with congenital nystagmus (see Chap. 17) are of uncertain value in the treatment of acquired forms of nystagmus. Neurosurgery does have a clear role in the therapy of the Arnold-Chiari syndrome; suboccipital decompression is reported to improve downbeat nystagmus and to prevent progression of other neurological deficits.

Attempts to stop the eyes moving, either by detaching the extraocular muscles or by injecting them with botulinum toxin, are invasive measures that may help in some cases but suffer from a number of limitations (10).

Table 1 Etiology of Oscillopsia

Oscillopsia due to ocular oscillations	
	Acquired nystagmus (especially pendular, upbeat, downbeat, see-saw, dissociated, periodic alternating nystagmus)
	Saccadic oscillations (ocular flutter, microsaccadic flutter and opsoclonus, psychogenic flutter/voluntary nystagmus)
	Superior oblique myokymia (monocular oscillopsia)
	Congenital nystagmus (uncommon under natural illumination)
Oscillopsia with head movements: Abnormal vestibulo-ocular reflex	
	Peripheral vestibular hypofunction
	Central vestibular dysfunction
Central oscillopsia	
	With cerebral disorders: seizures, occipital lobe infarction

IV. CONCLUSIONS

At present, there are few forms of acquired nystagmus for which there is reliable, effective treatment. The prognosis is generally better if an underlying condition that can be treated, such as the Arnold-Chiari malformation, is present. A number of drugs have been reported to help individual patients. There is a great need

Table 2 Treatments for Nystagmus and Its Visual Consequences

Drugs	
	Baclofen
	Acetazolamide
	Clonazepam
	Isoniazid
	Trihexyphenidyl
	Valproic acid
	Carbamazepine
	Barbiturates
	Alcohol
Optical Devices	
	Base-out prisms
	Other prism arrangements
	Spectacle lens-contact lens combination (for retinal image stabilization)
Invasive Procedures	
	Operative treatment of Arnold-Chiari malformation
	Botulinum toxin

for double-blind trials of such drugs before they can be recommended for more general use. The role of botulinum toxin in the treatment of acquired nystagmus requires systematic and careful evaluation before it can be recommended as a therapy.

ACKNOWLEDGMENTS

Supported by USPHS grant EY06717, the Department of Veterans Affairs, and the Evenor Armington Fund.

REFERENCES

1. Leigh RJ, Zee DS. *The neurology of eye movements*. 2d ed. Philadelphia: Davis, 1991.
2. Leigh RJ, Rushton DN, Thurston SE, Hertle RW, Yaniglos SY. Effects of retinal image stabilization on acquired nystagmus due to neurological disease. Neurology 1988; 38:122–7.
3. Currie JN, Matsuo V. The use of clonazepam in the treatment of nystagmus-induced oscillopsia. Ophthalmology 1986; 93:924–32.
4. Traccis S, Rosati G, Monaco MF, Aiello I, Agnetti V. Successful treatment of acquired pendular elliptical nystagmus in multiple sclerosis with isoniazid and base-out prisms. Neurology 1990; 40:492–4.
5. Leigh RJ, Burnstine TH, Ruff RL, Kasmer RJ. The effect of anticholinergic agents upon acquired nystagmus: a double-blind study of trihexyphenidyl and tridihexethyl chloride. Neurology 1991; 41:1737–1740.
6. Lavin PJM, Traccis S, Dell'Osso LF, Abel LA, Ellenberger C Jr. Downbeat nystagmus with a pseudocycloid waveform: improvement with base-out prisms. Ann Neurol 1983; 13:621–4.
7. Rushton D, Cox N. A new optical treatment for oscillopsia. J Neurol Neurosurg Psychiatry 1987; 50:411–5.
8. Barton JJS, Huaman AG, Sharpe JA. Muscarinic antagonists in the treatment of acquired pendular and downbeat nystagmus: a double-blind, randomized trial of three intravenous drugs. Ann Neurol 1994;35:319–325.
9. Yaniglos SS, Leigh RJ. Refinement of an optical device that stabilizes vision in patients with nystagmus. Optom Vis Sci 1992; 69:447–450.
10. Leigh RJ, Tomsak RL, Grant NP, Remler BF, Yaniglos SS, Lystad L, Dell'Osso LF. Effectiveness of botulinum toxin administered to abolish acquired nystagmus. Ann Neurol 1992; 32:633–642.

17

Management of Congenital Nystagmus

L. F. Dell'Osso
Case Western Reserve University, Cleveland, Ohio

Congenital nystagmus (CN), as the term is used herein, is a specific type of nystagmus that usually presents in early infancy; there are other types of nystagmus of infancy that are *not* CN. The word *congenital* means "with birth," and although CN may be present at birth, it may also become manifest later in infancy, childhood, or even adulthood. Thus, this term should not be taken literally but rather as a description of a congenital predisposition toward a specific ocular motor instability that may be manifest at birth, in early infancy, or occasionally later in life. It is pointless to attempt to change the name of this motor sign to one that merely shifts the time of onset (such as "infantile" nystagmus), since this is a variable with a wide range in individuals. If the name is to be changed at all, and I am not advocating that it should be, the chosen name should reflect the waveform(s) that are intimately related to the underlying mechanism(s) rather than some arbitrary time of onset; the latter only serves to exclude those with the *same* disorder but different timing. To paraphrase Marshall M. Parks (discussing "congenital" versus "infantile" esotropia), "To adopt another term in place of the widely used congenital *nystagmus*, just because the *nystagmus* cannot be proven to be present at birth may not be in the best interest of *nystagmography*" (italics added to indicate changed words). The most important factor in the management of CN is not its name but its accurate diagnosis and differentiation from other benign types of nystagmus of infancy and from symptomatic acquired types.

I. DEFINITION AND DIFFERENTIAL DIAGNOSIS

CN is a motor eye sign and is defined as follows: either a pendular or jerk nystagmus resulting from a slow eye movement instability producing periodic motion of the eyes away from an intended visual target and back to the target (*not* across the target). The pendular waveforms look sinusoidal but they are usually distorted by both flattening and presence of small foveating saccades on the peaks corresponding to where the foveation occurs. The jerk waveforms are caused by an instability that leads to an acceleration of the eyes away from the intended gaze angle or target and requires a saccade ("braking" saccade) in the opposite direction to stop that runaway. This saccade might return the eyes back to the target ("foveating" saccade) or initiate a slow eye movement back to the target for refoveation. The direction of nystagmus is defined by the direction of that saccade despite the fact that it is the slow eye movement that causes the nystagmus. CN is usually horizontal but occasionally may have vertical components in some patients; torsional components are not uncommon.

Also common are associated sensory defects (Table 1) that may accompany CN of all waveforms. One cannot equate pendular CN with a sensory defect or jerk CN with a motor defect; *all* CN waveforms are due to a primary motor defect. We have determined that the etiology and the mechanisms of these nystagmus waveforms are independent of accompanying sensory defects and therefore, although there is an association between many sensory defects and the presence of CN, it is not a causal relationship. The sensory defect is neither the primary cause of the nystagmus nor is the nystagmus the primary cause of the defect. Sensory defects appear to be secondary factors provoking the manifestation of CN in individuals in whom there is already a primary predisposition for the latter. Thus, although sensory defects are not the primary cause of CN, they appear to be the precipitating factors in the manifestation of CN in many patients. The observation, that *any* of several different sensory abnormalities can result in the developing motor system becoming unstable, leads to the following possibilities: (1) a small percentage of individuals are born with a motor system

Table 1 Sensory Defects Associated with Nystagmus

Achromatopsia
Albinism
Aniridia
Congenital stationary night blindness
Disorders of the media
Optic atrophy (developmental/hereditary)
Optic nerve disease (aplasia/dysplasia/hypoplasia/atrophy/colobomas)

that is precariously close to oscillation, or (2) nature has evolved the ocular motor system in such a way that the horizontal system is close to instability in many individuals. The reason for the latter hypothesis may lie in our need for rapid horizontal eye motion to survive. Whatever the underlying reason, the motor system seems to require early visual input to assure its stability and any sensory defect interfering with vision might result in the instability we call CN. In those individuals actually born with CN, the system may have developed with such a strong instability (due to hereditary or spontaneous genetic factors) that even the presence of adequate visual input after birth is not enough to stabilize it.

When there is a sensory defect, it rather than the nystagmus may be the limiting factor for acuity, and even halting eye motion using forceps may not result in an acuity improvement in some patients; in others, acuity can be improved by damping the CN. One must perform the necessary diagnostic tests (e.g., the electroretinogram [ERG]) to assess correctly the functional integrity within the visual system and diagnose any sensory abnormalities present, but that diagnosis is *not* sufficient to describe the motor defect causing the nystagmus. The latter requires motility recordings for absolute diagnosis. If a patient with nystagmus has a visual acuity uncorrectable to better than 20/60, one should look carefully for afferent defects. Sensory defects may be more prominent in pediatric patient populations than in adult populations where there is a higher incidence of idiopathic CN. It is possible that there are two different genes with variable probabilities of the one causing the slow eye movement instability CN and the other causing the afferent defect. The presence of either of these genes might be related to the presence of the other by some third probability. Another possibility is that there is one gene with different probabilities for an afferent defect and CN; a patient may have both or one or the other. The diagnosis and treatment of sensory abnormalities will not be covered in this chapter that concentrates on the proper management of CN and other forms of infantile nystagmus.

In addition to CN, other types of nystagmus (and saccadic oscillations) may also occur at or shortly after birth and should not be confused with, or lumped with, CN. They are different from CN in waveform (mechanism) and clinical characteristics. Some of these other benign types of infantile nystagmus are: latent/manifest latent nystagmus (LMLN), spasmus nutans, and the nystagmus blockage syndrome (NBS). The physician need not be concerned with whether the nystagmus appeared at birth or in the first few weeks after birth. More important is (1) determining whether this is a benign nystagmus or one that is indicative of disease, and (2) if the nystagmus is benign, determining whether it is CN, LMLN, spasmus nutans, or NBS. Those types of nystagmus that have been determined to be symptomatic types are downbeat nystagmus (due to structural brain stem abnormalities), epileptic nystagmus, uniocular nystagmus (due to optic nerve glioma), vestibular nystagmus (due to any number of vestibular problems), and "nystagmus" of the blind; the latter is not truly a nystagmus but rather wandering eye movements. Table 2 lists both benign and symptomatic forms of nystagmus of infancy. Another instance when it is important to distinguish between CN or a benign or symptomatic nystagmus is when an adult is first seen after trauma or for some unrelated condition and a correct history is unavailable. Under these conditions, it may be unclear whether the nystagmus was present before the trauma or especially if it occurred following the trauma.

Manifest latent nystagmus (MLN) is present with both eyes open but only one being used for fixation. There is always a tropia, and vision from the tropic eye is suppressed in the cortex. The slow phase is a decreasing-velocity exponential, and the corrective fast phase is always in the direction of the eye that is fixating; that is, the straight eye. MLN is the same nystagmus as the rare, latent nystagmus that only appears with occlusion of one eye. In MLN, the subject "occludes" one eye by cortically suppressing it while fixating with the other eye. Thus, the term *latent/manifest latent nystagmus* refers to this type of nystagmus that is present in most patients with both eyes open while one is fixating but, in some patients, may only be present when one eye is occluded.

Spasmus nutans may appear at or after birth. It is pendular and usually, but not necessarily, ceases by the age of 3 years. It also is usually monocular or disconjugate and is commonly accompanied by a head oscillation. Reports of "spasmus nutans" accompanying neurological disease have not included recordings to document that the nystagmus was that of spasmus nutans.

The nystagmus blockage syndrome is the source of some misunderstanding. NBS waveforms are those of CN when the patient is looking in the distance and the eyes are straight. When there is a purposive esotropia (this is *not* a strabismus that occurs transiently but one that the patient willfully imposes because he or she has found that acuity is better under that condition) the waveform can either become a damped CN waveform (one type of NBS) or a small-amplitude MLN (another type of NBS). Thus, there are two types of blockage syndrome. NBS

Table 2 Types of Nystagmus of Infancy

Benign	Symptomatic
Congenital (CN)	Downbeat (structural brain stem abnormalities)
Latent/manifest latent (LMLN)	Epileptic
Spasmus nutans	Uniocular (optic nerve glioma)
Nystagmus blockage syndrome (NBS)	Vestibular
	"Nystagmus" of the blind[a]

[a]Wandering eye movements, *not* true nystagmus

is often misdiagnosed in patients with LMLN and alternating fixation who place their fixating eye in adduction.

Unfortunately, for the diagnostician, there exist individuals with both CN and LMLN (it is not usual, but some patients have a combination of CN and LMLN); one or the other might be dominant and result in complex waveforms and variations of nystagmus type with gaze angle. These become very difficult to diagnose and the best approach is first to learn to diagnose accurately the more straightforward types.

II. DIAGNOSTIC CRITERIA

Unambiguous, diagnostic characteristics exist for each of the benign types of nystagmus of infancy. Simple eye movement recordings differentiate these types and simultaneously provide the data necessary for effective therapeutic intervention.

A. Waveform

The waveforms recorded from infants with CN where the nystagmus was noted at birth are the same as those seen in infants where they were noted to appear later. Since the waveforms are the same, the mechanism in both instances is the same; there is only one CN, independent of time of onset. With the aid of recorded eye movements, the diagnostic criteria for CN are definitive. Any of the 12 waveforms (Table 3) that have been identified in CN are pathognomonic of CN except pure pendular; that could be an acquired nystagmus. Usually the pendular nystagmus of CN is distorted so the patient can foveate, whereas in acquired nystagmus it is not. In acquired nystagmus, the slow phases can be linear, of increasing velocity, of decreasing velocity, or pendular. CN slow phases can be pendular, increasing velocity, or some may look linear. Within the pendular or jerk major types of CN, we identified three different forms of pendular and eight jerk, four unidirectional and four bidirectional. One waveform, dual jerk, is a superimposition of pendular on a jerk waveform with increasing velocity slow phases; illustrations and examples are available in the literature. In a group of patients with CN, 87% had more than one waveform; they had any number of the 12 waveforms. A small percentage of patients (13%) exhibited only one waveform.

One specific group of patients who usually have CN are those with albinism. Here, as with CN, what was once a "clinical" diagnosis can now be made definitively by a simple diagnostic test based on the visual evoked potential (VEP). If performed properly using the paradigm developed by Apkarian, the VEP is virtually 100% free of both false positives and false negatives. This paradigm uses full-field, monocular pattern (checkerboard) onset/offset stimuli

Table 3 Nystagmus Waveforms

Congenital	Latent
Pendular	
Pendular	
Asymmetric pendular	
Pendular with right/left foveating saccades	
Unidirectional jerk	
Jerk right/left	Jerk right/left
Jerk right/left with extended foveation	
Right/left pseudocycloid	
Pseudo jerk right/left	
Bidirectional jerk	
Pseudopendular	
Pseudopendular with right/left foveating saccades	
Triangular	
Bidirectional jerk right/left	
Dual	
Dual jerk right/left	Dual jerk right/left latent

rather than pattern reversal stimuli; the latter contain motion artifacts and should *not* be used in individuals with CN or any other nystagmus. For children below the age of about 3 years, reliable results are obtained with a luminance flash paradigm. Appropriate VEP testing demonstrates the unequivocal dissociation between the misrouted fibers found in albinos and their CN, since no individuals with hereditary or idiopathic CN had misrouting. Thus, the hypothesis that misrouting can cause CN lacks scientific foundation.

The diagnostic criterion for LMLN also is the waveform (see Table 3); recordings reveal a decreasing velocity exponential slow phase. All patients (100%) with latent (LN) or manifest latent nystagmus (MLN) have strabismus. I include in the definition of strabismus the latent strabismus (phoria) resulting when you cover an eye. Thus, there is pure LN, where the eyes are straight with both eyes open and when you cover one eye, it will develop an esophoria or exophoria followed by LN. The LN waveform has decreasing velocity slow phases. Pure latent nystagmus (i.e., no nystagmus with both eyes open) is very rare. If you occlude the left eye and the right eye is fixating, jerk-right LN with decreasing velocity slow phases results and vice versa. Latent nystagmus implies strabismus but the reverse is not true.

The diagnostic criteria for spasmus nutans have also been defined. We can now diagnose spasmus nutans immediately by recording; it is no longer necessary to wait 3 or 4 years before making the diagnosis based on its possible disappearance. The waveform is a dissociated pendular nystagmus and this dissociation may be so great that the nystagmus is uniocular. The diagnostic key is the variable phase difference between the oscillations in both eyes; unlike CN and LMLN that are conjugate. The spasmus nutans waveform can vary anywhere from pure conjugacy to pure disconjugacy; 0- to 180-degree phase shift. It varies during the recording, usually from minute to minute.

The nystagmus blockage syndrome criteria, as indicated above, are twofold: In one type, CN changes to damped CN, so acuity is better (i.e., why the patients induce the esotropia); in the other type, the CN becomes LMLN and even though that is usually a waveform unsuitable for good acuity (because there are no long foveation periods), it is of low amplitude and acuity increases. Obviously to accomplish this patients must have a variable strabismus. If one is binocular, one cannot turn one eye in without diplopia resulting. These patients turn one eye in and they do not experience diplopia (they suppress that eye); they have a variable, purposive strabismus. When they are looking in the distance they are orthotropic; they become esotropic by design and then they either exhibit one (CN) or the other (MLN) low-amplitude waveform along with better acuity.

There is a very small group of patients who present a diagnostic nightmare—CN and LMLN together. Some of them have mostly CN (CN/LMLN) and their waveforms are any of the CN waveforms (i.e., pendular or increasing velocity slow phases) and one other waveform called "dual jerk latent" (see Table 3). The latter is a waveform where pendular is superimposed on a decreasing velocity slow phase jerk waveform. They do not have pure latent waveforms (i.e., decreasing velocity slow phases) so therefore CN is predominant. The other group has LMLN/CN, and their waveforms are latent and dual jerk latent. There are some patients who have equally CN and LMLN. At various times they exhibit the CN waveform, latent waveform, or the dual jerk waveform. A linear slow phase is not diagnostic of either CN or LMLN. If the slow phase is accelerating, it is a congenital dual jerk. If the slow phase is decelerating and a pendular waveform is superimposed, it is a dual jerk latent. One has to determine carefully what is happening to the axis of the pendular slow phase (is it decelerating or accelerating?) to categorize properly the nystagmus. This small but difficult group of patients must be recorded for accurate diagnosis.

Summarizing, there is a large category of pure CN, a significant category of pure LMLN, and a small category that is a mixture of the two; all are easily diagnosed with the aid of recordings. There are 12 CN waveforms, one latent waveform and one mixed waveform (dual jerk latent). If a patient walks into your office with wiggling eyes and you wish to guess what they have before you record them, your best guess would be CN. A large percentage (80%) will be CN and 15% LMLN with only a small percentage being mixtures. If you look at just patients with CN, 94% will be pure CN and only 6% a mixture. If you just look at patients with LMLN, three quarters of them will just have LMLN, but there is a significant number of patients who will have mixtures. Thus, more patients with predominantly LMLN will also have some CN than patients with predominantly CN have LMLN.

III. CLINICAL CHARACTERISTICS

A. Congenital Nystagmus

In addition to the quantifiable and diagnostic characteristics of CN available through eye movement recordings, there are clinical signs one can look for in the office. In CN, one should look for a null angle; an indication of this is the presence of a head turn. A teenager or an adult may not show a head turn because of societal pressures. They have learned to keep their heads straight at the expense of vision because it is not "appropriate" to walk around with their head turned, but a child will have a head turn. A positive family history and negative neurological examination are indicative of CN.

If patients hold reading material close, one should suspect that converging the eyes will damp the nystagmus. They may have a latent component; this can be checked by the cover test. If the nystagmus direction reverses, one still does not know whether it is LMLN or CN with a latent component (they *are* different). Such patients may also have head nodding that is not compensatory.

The CN magnitude damps at a specific gaze angle if there is a null. The definition of a null (a true null) is that the nystagmus must get larger on either side. This is in contrast to LMLN where monotonic variation with gaze angle (Alexander's law) causes patients to keep their eyes deviated to one side where the nystagmus is low. This is not a true null, because there is no increase on both sides. In CN, the position of the null is a function of the angle of gaze and also a function of the velocity of the eyes. The null angle during fixation does not usually equal the null angle during pursuit, optokinetic nystagmus, or head movement (where the vestibulo-ocular reflex is stimulated). Usually, the null is shifted in the direction opposite to the eye movement. During pursuit to the left, the null moves to the right of the static null; and during pursuit to the right, the null moves to the left. In the CN population, 48% have both convergence and gaze angle nulls, 29% only convergence nulls, 9% only gaze angle nulls, and there are 14% with no nulls.

Children with CN automatically adopt a head turn to see better. They do not have to wait to be told about the null, they know where it is because things appear clearer when they turn their head. One may think of the null as a region of ocular motor equilibrium. The brainstem (left and right) generates forces pulling the eyes both ways and there is a position of equilibrium of forces, not necessarily in primary position, where the nystagmus is minimal. When viewing targets at the null angle, acuity should increase; when there is a severe afferent defect, the acuity may not increase measurably.

Sometimes the patient will tilt the head and sometimes turn the head (vertically or horizontally) and tilt it. Perhaps the oblique muscles are involved; this has not really been studied well. It represents innervation of muscles other than the horizontal muscles that are somehow helping to reach equilibrium in what are basically horizontal oscillations. Most CN is horizontal with little or no vertical components. Few patients have significant vertical components, and many may have small torsional, components. Again, acuity increases with vertical or torsional head positions, especially if there are no afferent defects.

The CN might reverse direction on covering an eye, because (similar to when the person pursues) the null moves, and therefore you may see a direction reversal of the CN if gaze went from one side of the null to the other. MLN mimics latent nystagmus exactly if it is bidirectional. When MLN is unidirectional and the patient fixates with one eye, there will be no nystagmus and the other eye will be esotropic, but when the patient fixates with the other eye and the formerly fixating eye is esotropic, he or she will have MLN. Although CN with a latent component looks like LN or MLN, it is not because the waveform remains CN; only the CN direction changes, because the null has moved with occlusion.

Many children with CN exhibit spontaneous head oscillations. When adults with CN concentrate on a visual task (real or imaginary), they may also have spontaneous head oscillations, but they usually learn to keep the head still because it is socially unacceptable to allow the head to shake. These head oscillations use existing pathways in the neck muscles. EMG in the neck muscles show that when normal individuals make saccades to the left, the innervation is seen in the left-turning neck muscles, and when they made them to the right, it is seen in the right-turning neck muscles. Normally, when we look left, we are going to turn the head left. The pathways exist and, if there is an instability causing the eyes to oscillate and one records from the neck muscles, the same waveform is seen. When the oscillation grows large enough, the head will start oscillating. This is not something willed by the patient to accomplish anything; it is a manifestation of an existing oscillation on existing pathways to the neck. It used to be thought that head oscillations were compensatory. The head was supposed to be moved equally and oppositely to the CN to stabilize the eye in space. If that were true, the VOR gain would have to be zero. A VOR is incompatible with a head movement that compensates for an eye movement. With no VOR the head would have to move in very complex ways opposite to the CN waveforms to achieve stability, which is clearly impossible. The head has too much mass to duplicate the waveforms of CN. When you understand the VOR, you know this compensatory hypothesis cannot work. For realistic compensation, one could suppress a normal VOR to near zero and only move the head equally and oppositely to any movements of the eye during the CN foveation periods.

This would achieve stability only during that part of the waveform and is a possible form of compensation useful only when the foveation periods do not result in stable eyes with the head still.

In patients with CN, the VOR is normal; it is not affected by CN. The head oscillations are merely an extension of the CN, and during the foveation periods, the eyes do not move and acuity is unaffected by head movements. The head oscillations in CN with a normal VOR are equivalent to those of a normal person moving the head and acuity does not change. In a few patients, if the VOR is suppressed and the head moves opposite to the eyes only during the foveation periods, these periods become motionless in space, because they were not so before the head was moving; here acuity can increase. Thus, if the CN waveform does not contain good foveation periods, the head might oscillate in a compensatory way so that during the foveation period, gaze remains stable in space (i.e., the eye movement recording is flat). If patients have good foveation periods, there is no reason to shake the head. Thus, if the foveation periods are flat, head motion cannot help the patient.

B. Strabismus

What is the relation of strabismus to nystagmus (to the CN or the LMLN)? The presence of LMLN means that there is strabismus. Of all patients with strabismus, 50% do not have any nystagmus. The other 50% do have nystagmus of some type; the question is, what type? Of that 50% of the total, 26.5% will have CN, only 17% will have LMLN, and 6% will be mixed. If one considers 100 patients who walk into the office with both nystagmus and strabismus and one has to guess (even though all patients with manifest latent nystagmus must have strabismus), the best guess is CN, because there are many more patients with CN than with LMLN. For 100 patients with both CN and LMLN, 43% had strabismus and 57% had no strabismus. So, the patient who has nystagmus probably does not have strabismus; more than half will not. If one considers just patients with CN (including those with some LMLN), almost three quarters do not have strabismus; thus, most patients with CN do not have strabismus. If one considers only those with pure CN, the great majority of patients do not have strabismus. We have recorded all 12 CN waveforms in patients with binocular alignment, so it is not necessary to have strabismus for any particular CN waveform. Of 43% of patients with strabismus in the first 100 mentioned above, more than half had CN even though most patients with CN do not have strabismus. Summarizing, for strabismus with nystagmus: 53%—CN, 35%—LMLN, and 12%—mixed.

C. Latent/Manifest Latent Nystagmus

Pure latent nystagmus is extremely rare. That is, when you record pure LN, you will find no nystagmus with eyes open at all gaze angles. There have been only a couple of cases proven by recordings to have pure LN. Many patients thought clinically to have pure LN actually have MLN. When one records them or examines them with an ophthalmoscope, the MLN is visible. More common is pure LN in primary position with MLN in lateral gaze; most common is MLN at all gaze angles.

The intensity of LMLN is greatest with gaze toward the direction of the fast phase (Alexander's law). Jerk-right nystagmus is greater in right than in left gaze and vice versa. These are not true nulls—one cannot show increased nystagmus because the patient is at the end of the excursion of the eye; this is an example of a monotonic relationship of gaze and amplitude. It would not be uncommon for a person who fixates with one eye to have MLN with that eye in adduction where Alexander's law will reduce the nystagmus. In CN, there is a null and increased amplitude (with increasing velocity exponentials) as gaze is directed away from the null in both directions, whereas in LMLN (right eye or left eye fixating), there is an Alexander's law relationship and decreasing velocity exponentials. Patients with LN usually place their fixating eye in adduction to minimize the nystagmus and thereby maximize acuity. Some might also place the fixating eye in abduction because of a perverted non–Alexander's law variation. As in CN, the head turn minimizes the nystagmus and maximizes acuity. A patient could place the eye in other than the minimum position of nystagmus if he or she had an "angle kappa" that required eccentric fixation. Better acuity results despite the fact that the nystagmus might be a little higher where the patient places the gaze. We have never recorded the LN waveform in patients with orthophoria; they all had latent strabismus (when you cover one eye, the other does not remain straight). MLN has never been recorded in patients with binocular alignment; all had manifest strabismus. Both eyes are open, but one eye must be turned in or out to have MLN. If patients can straighten their eyes, the MLN disappears; in the blockage syndrome, patients have CN. Therefore, LN and MLN imply strabismus. Of course, strabismus does not imply LMLN (50% have no nystagmus at all), but if an individual has LN, strabismus also is present. Even if it is not evident clinically (it may be a microstrabismus that can be recorded), it is there. Strabismus is a necessary, but not sufficient, condition for LMLN. It is either a latent strabismus, in those rare patients with pure LN, or a tropia for MLN. Thus, CN can occur with or without strabismus; all patients with MLN have strabismus.

D. Spasmus Nutans

In spasmus nutans, unlike CN, the head nodding is compensatory. The ocular oscillations are asymmetrical between the two eyes and, contrary to what is commonly believed, it does not always disappear. There have been 10- or 12-year-old patients who still had spasmus nutans. Many times spasmus nutans disappears to clinical observation (again, like MLN), but when recorded, a pendular dissociated nystagmus will be found. The head nodding in spasmus nutans is very curious. The VOR of these patients is normal, but by shaking the head willfully, the nystagmus is switched off and the eyes become stable in space because of a good VOR; their acuity increases. A patient may have convergence nystagmus, with one eye going left and the other eye going right at the same time (180 degrees out of phase) while the head is still. When the head starts shaking, the nystagmus stops; owing to a normal VOR, the eyes begin moving conjugately equally and oppositely to the head, so gaze remains constant. Thus, patients cancel the disconjugate pendular oscillation of spasmus nutans (present with a still head) and substitute a conjugate VOR when the head is moving and acuity increases.

E. Nystagmus Blockage Syndrome

Patients with NBS can willfully become esotropic at distance. This is something a person with CN cannot do unless they have the ability partially to suppress the eye they purposely make esotropic. If patients with CN with normal binocularity made an eye esotropic they would have diplopia—oscillating diplopia. Patients with NBS can turn one of their eyes in and suppress it; their nystagmus damps and they adopt a head turn to place their viewing eye in adduction. The CN is either reduced in amplitude or converted to a low-amplitude LMLN by this purposive esotropia; the greater the esotropia, the lower the nystagmus and, as the fixating eye moves from adduction to abduction, the nystagmus increases and esotropia decreases. These patients usually put the fixating eye in adduction.

IV. THERAPEUTIC OPTIONS

What are the therapeutic options for the various types of benign nystagmus of infancy? In CN, we have found that a strong fixation reflex maintains foveation despite slow acceleration off the target. This again is juxtaposed to the mistaken idea that CN is caused by poor fixation reflexes. We have found that fixation in CN is very accurate (<13 min of arc). In LMLN, the fixation reflexes seem to be ineffective, since the slow phase immediately takes the eyes away from the target as soon as a fast phase is completed. These patients seem to have no ability to use the fixation system to keep the eye on the target. One can increase the visual acuity of patients with CN (if they have no foveal defects) if there is a null angle or a convergence null and if there are good waveforms with long foveation periods. In such patients, prisms or surgery may be effective, but if a patient does not have these characteristics, these methods are not likely to be successful. One could still straighten the head, but these characteristics are necessary for an increase in acuity. If one can minimize the attempt to fixate, acuity will be maximized, because in CN, the greater the effort to see, the higher the level of nystagmus. Even in turning the head to find the null, the level of nystagmus of that null is higher than if the null is placed straight ahead surgically. That null is better because there is no effort involved. Visual acuity is proportional to how much time in each cycle the target is foveated. The longer the eyes remain on the target, the more visual detail is obtainable. The retinal slip during this time should be less than 4 degrees/s. Data from normal individuals show that when retinal slip stays below 4 degrees/s, acuity is the greatest. Also important is the stability of the foveation periods. The eyes must be in exactly the same position from cycle to cycle; the extent to which that is not so is called "jitter" in engineering terms. Jitter must be minimized otherwise, even with long foveation periods, one cycle might fall to the left of the target and the next to the right. All of these characteristics must be present for good acuity—long foveation periods with low retinal slip velocities that are repeatedly positioned accurately on target. The nystagmus foveation function (NFF = duration of foveation period/product of the standard deviations of the mean position and velocity of the foveation periods) is the best method for determining the conditions under which acuity will be maximum. It can be used to plan surgery, optical correction, or other therapy.

A. Optical Therapy

Prisms can be used to shift gaze and take advantage of nulls within 5 degrees of primary position. If there is a null to the left, base-right prisms will move the eyes leftward into the null. Accurate measurements of the gaze-angle and convergence nulls can be translated directly to prisms. To converge the eyes, use base-out prisms with added minus to compensate for the induced accommodation; to move the eyes laterally and converge them, use compound prisms. Prisms are not substitutes for head turns; they yield higher acuity than head turns, because there is less fixation attempt. Fresnel prisms are not good substitutes for properly ground optical plastic. It should be noted that many patients with CN have both convergence and gaze-angle nulls and the former usually result in greater CN damping. This is important to know when the gaze-angle null is large; here base-out prisms (with –1.0 spheres) can be used to converge the eyes and the resulting damping will preclude a head turn.

Feedback of the eye motion from the inside of the eyelids may also damp CN. This effect can be taken advantage of by inserting soft contact lenses in a patient with CN. Contact lenses with an anesthetic (to block afferent input) do not damp the CN. There is a simple office procedure that may indicate if contact lenses will damp a patient's CN. Take a cotton swab and just touch the eyelid to see if the nystagmus damps; do not press on the eyelid. It is a quick way to tell whether the soft lenses might work. Contact lenses should be beneficial to patients without a null. Even if the cotton swab does not produce damping (perhaps due to anxiety in the patient), it is easy to try contact lenses. Unfortunately, for many years contact lenses have not been prescribed for patients with nystagmus. Soft contact lenses at least are *not* contraindicated by CN and may be indicated as a good therapy.

B. Surgery

Large-angle nulls are best treated surgically. Kestenbaum and Anderson independently developed the recess and resect operation. This effectively rotates both eyes opposite to the null angle such that the same innervation that preoperatively put the eyes at the null postoperatively puts them in primary position and, therefore, the nystagmus is nulled.

If the patient not only has a null angle but also has strabismus and surgery is desired to minimize the nystagmus and straighten the eyes, the best approach is to operate on the good eye first, the fixating eye, not the strabismic eye. Any remaining tropia can be corrected after the initial operation. Sometimes the surgery performed on the fixating eye reduces or eliminates the tropia; sometimes it is made worse. Moving the tropic eye so it is straight will not affect the nystagmus. If the strabismic eye was esotropic and the null was in adduction of the fixating eye, the surgical rotation has to be abduction. That will result in less esotropia and is the most common case. Esotropia is more common than exotropia and the combination of esotropia and a null in adduction is more common than esotropia and a null in abduction. This causes in a good surgical result on the tropic eye without surgery of that eye.

One should never use head turn to assess the results of surgery. The young patient realizes the parents are spending a lot of money and hears the physician say that the surgery is going to make his or her head straight; one cannot trust the patient's postoperative head turn on the first visit after the surgery because that patient is going to keep the head straight. This scenario is probably the cause of the myth that the surgery was correct (no head turn) and 6 months later the head turn came back. The head turn cannot be used to assess the surgical result because it is under control of the child who is subject to all kinds of input; the patient may want to please the parents or the surgeon. It is best to measure the null by having the patient fixate at different gaze angles with the head fixed both before and after the operation, so that there is no input from the patient. This is preferably done by recordings before the surgery to document the null and after the surgery to see where the null shifted. Evaluated that way, whatever null is measured on day 1 after the operation will be measured 5 years later; it will not have moved because it was fixed by the surgery. The surgery itself, luckily for the surgeon, broadens the null (so even if the null was slightly miscalculated, the results will not be off by much) and lateral to the null the nystagmus is much less than before surgery. It appears to be a self-fulfilling prophecy that any surgical rotation of a patient with CN with a null produces a better result than not doing the surgery; furthermore, the null is broader because the CN has damped at all gaze angles. Therefore, surgery moves the null angle, increases the null area, and decreases off-null nystagmus and the new null is stationary. If surgery does not totally move the null to primary position and there is a new null a few degrees to one side, another surgery is not always necessary. Prisms could shift the visual world to the new null and fine-tune the surgery.

Another surgical approach is a bimedial recession. This is artificial divergence created by weakening both medial recti. It might be contraindicated if the patient has strabismus, since it depends on the ability to fuse to straighten the eyes. Perhaps in the blockage syndrome it would still work because this is a different kind of strabismus—a purposive strabismus. Weakening both medial recti creates an artificial divergence and the convergence innervation required to turn the eyes to primary position nulls the nystagmus. This, of course, is in a person who has a convergence null; this is the condition under which this operation would be successful. It should also be considered when there are both convergence and gaze-angle nulls, since the convergence null will probably yield the greatest CN damping. Bimedial recession may also help those with NBS; this has been suggested but published studies are lacking.

The Faden operation times four weakens all four horizontal muscles (developed by Cüppers). Double vision in lateral gaze may be a problem with this operation, but some say it does not matter because the patient is happy. Weakening the muscles reduces the effect of all innervation. Whether the nystagmus, or anything else, is going to be affected so that the nystagmus will damp in primary position (or in all positions) requires the muscles to have less efficiency. This operation is useful in patients without nulls.

A minority of patients with CN adopt a vertical or torsional head position to damp the nystagmus. They can be treated with either prisms or surgery on the vertical or torsional extraocular muscles. Those with both CN and LMLN may be helped by the methods discussed above if they exhibit primarily CN and by those methods discussed below if they exhibit primarily LMLN. The key to these cases is in the accurate diagnosis.

It is also possible to enhance surgically the acuity of some patients with LMLN. If a patient has LMLN and a constant head turn to take advantage of an Alexander's law reduction of the nystagmus, he or she is fixating with the adducted eye (the other being in a tropic position and suppressed). Under these conditions, one may operate on the fixating eye to move the low-amplitude LMLN from the eccentric gaze position to primary. That is, rotate the fixating eye to an abducted position so the innervation that previously placed it in adduction will result in a gaze straight ahead. If the strabismus accompanying the LMLN was esotropia (the most common case), the strabismic eye will assume a less tropic position after rotation of the fixating eye owing to the innervation required to straighten the latter; this procedure may correct the strabismus in addition to reducing the nystagmus in primary position. Any remaining strabismus can be corrected later by rotating the strabismic eye. If the strabismus is exotropia, this procedure will tend to worsen it, but a second operation on the strabismic eye can also correct this condition. If the patient with LMLN exhibits two head turns and alternately fixes with the adducted eye, this procedure should not be used. Here, a Faden operation may prove useful.

C. Other Therapies

Biofeedback has been shown to be useful in damping CN and it is claimed that with repeated training the effect can be used by the patient outside the laboratory without the biofeedback. This remains to be demonstrated under conditions of stress when higher acuity is needed for an important task.

Drugs are *not* beneficial in the treatment of CN. Despite reports of some CN damping with barbiturates or baclofen, the secondary effects of these drugs preclude their recommendation.

The injection of botulinum toxin into the extraocular muscles has also been reported to damp CN, but this procedure must be repeated every few months to remain effective.

Finally, we have discovered that stimulation of the ophthalmic division of the trigeminal nerve may damp CN. This response, when present, is robust and stimulus independent; touch, pressure, vibration, and subliminal electrical stimulation have all been found to damp CN. Making the transition from experimental to therapeutically useful methods of stimulation remains.

V. CONCLUSIONS

The importance of electrophysiological tests (ERG and VEP) to assess afferent visual system function at both the retinal and central levels is now accepted. Unfortunately for the patient with nystagmus, the use of accurate ocular motility recording for the dual roles of diagnosis and treatment is not widely used. Only in selected centers of ophthalmological or neuro-ophthalmological research are such motility recordings routinely made. Years ago, cardiologists realized that they could not rely solely on their ears accurately to diagnose complex disorders of cardiac function. Too many ophthalmologists are still attempting to use only their eyes for the same purpose; it simply cannot be done reliably for ocular motor disorders.

In this chapter, I have summarized the results of the past 20 years of ocular motor research relevant to the diagnosis and treatment of CN and other benign types of nystagmus of infancy. Analogous to the utility of ERG and VEP, definitive diagnostic motility criteria have been established for all types of nystagmus. The purely clinical signs of these types of nystagmus are often ambiguous and reliance on them without quantitative motility data will continue to cause diagnostic errors that may be compounded by the wrong choices for therapeutic intervention. In many cases, visual acuity can be improved, or binocularity restored, by the correct therapy applied in a timely manner. The patient's complete diagnosis must include the motility diagnosis in addition to the afferent system diagnosis, as must the therapeutic plan. This will require the addition of eye movement recordings in the clinical setting to augment the ERG and VEP.

ACKNOWLEDGMENT

This work was supported in part by the Department of Veterans Affairs.

The author wishes to thank Dr. P. Apkarian for discussion of the VEP and Dr. R. Tomsak for reviewing the manuscript.

SELECTED READINGS

1. Apkarian P, Shallo-Hoffmann J. VEP projections in congenital nystagmus, VEP asymmetry in albinism: a comparison study. Invest Ophthalmol Vis Sci 1991; 32:2653–2661.
2. Apkarian P, Spekeijse H. The use of the electroretinogram and visual evoked potentials in ophthalmogenetics. In: Desmedt JE, ed. Visual evoked potentials. Amsterdam: Elsevier, 1990:169–223.
3. Daroff RB, Dell'Osso LF. Periodic alternating nystagmus and the shifting null. Can J Otolaryngol 1974; 3:367–71.
4. Del'Osso LF. Congenital, latent and manifest latent nystagmus—similarities, differences and relation to strabismus. Jpn J Ophthalmol 1985; 29:351–68.
5. Dell'Osso LF. Evaluation of smooth pursuit in the presence of congenital nystagmus. Neuro Ophthalmology 1986; 6:383–406.
6. Del'Osso LF, Daroff RB. Congenital nystagmus waveforms and foveation strategy. Doc Ophthalmol 1975; 39:155–82.
7. Dell'Osso LF, Daroff RB. Abnormal head position and head motion associated with nystagmus. In: Keller EL, Zee DS, eds. Adaptive processes in visual and oculomotor systems. Elmsford: Pergamon Press, 1986: 473–8.
8. Dell'Osso LF, Ellenberger Jr C, Abel LA, Flynn JT. The nystagmus blockage syndrome: congenital nystagmus, manifest latent nystagmus or both? Invest Ophthalmol Vis Sci 1983; 24:1580–7.
9. Dell'Osso LF, Flynn JT. Congenital nystagmus surgery: a quantitative evaluation of the effects. Arch Ophthalmol 1979; 97:462–9.
10. Dell'Osso LF, Flynn JT, Daroff RB. Hereditary congenital nystagmus: An intrafamilial study. Arch Ophthalmol 1974; 92:366–74.

11. Dell'Osso LF, Leigh RJ, Daroff RB. Suppression of congenital nystagmus by cutaneous stimulation. Neuro Ophthalmology 1991; 11:173–175.
12. Dell'Osso LF, Schmidt D, Daroff RB. Latent, manifest latent and congenital nystagmus. Arch Ophthalmol 1979; 97:1877–85.
13. Del'Osso LF, Traccis S, Abel LA. Strabismus—A necessary condition for latent and manifest latent nystagmus. Neuro Ophthalmology 1983; 3:247–57.
14. Dell'Osso LF, Traccis S, Abel LA, Erzurum SI. Contact lenses and congenital nystagmus. Clin Vision Sci 1988; 3:229–32.
15. Dell'Osso LF, Van der Steen J, Collewijn H, Steinman RM. Foveation dynamics in congenital nystagmus. Invest Ophthalmol Vis Sci (ARVO Suppl.) 1988; 29:166.
16. Flynn JT, Dell'Osso LF. Surgery of congenital nystagmus. Trans Ophthalmol UK 1981; 101:431–3.
17. Gresty MA, Bronstein AM, Page NG, Rudge P. Congenital-type nystagmus emerging in later life. Neurology 1991; 41:653–6.
18. Weissman BM, Dell'Osso LF, Abel LA, Leigh RJ. Spasmus nutans: a quantitative prospective study. Arch Ophthalmol 1987; 105:525–8.

18

Neuro-Ophthalmic Implications of Vestibular Disorders

James A. Sharpe
University of Toronto and The Toronto Hospital, Toronto, Ontario, Canada

Vestibular disorders that arise from the labyrinths or their projections in the brainstem affect vision by altering the vestibulo-ocular reflex (VOR). The VOR serves vision by generating conjugate smooth eye movements that are equal in speed and opposite in direction to head movements. If the reflex is accurate, the eyes remain stationary with respect to the world, and images are stable on the retina. The accuracy of vestibular smooth eye movements determines visual acuity during head motion. As the eyes and head move in opposite directions, the ratio of eye velocity to head velocity, the VOR gain, must approximate unity. The phase of the VOR must be such that the eyes are 180 degrees out of phase with the head. This phase difference is called zero. Slippage of images on the retina over 2–3 degrees/s reduces visual acuity.

If the gain of the reflex is too much above or below its ideal value of 1.0, a retinal image remains off the fovea, although it may be transiently stable on the retina. If there is a phase lead of the eyes before the head or a phase lag of the eyes behind the head, the target image is never stationary on the retina. Saccades or nystagmus quick phases opposite to vestibular smooth eye movements are dispatched to bring the fovea toward a new target when the VOR takes them away from it. Abnormal phase or gain of the reflex causes visual blurring or oscillopsia during head motion. Imbalance of the VOR that persists when the head is still causes nystagmus, which is not discussed here; for extensive discussions of vestibular disorders, the reader is referred to other sources (1,2).

I. TESTS OF THE VOR

A. Caloric Testing

Caloric testing assesses the low-frequency response of the VOR. It is useful in detecting the side of unilateral peripheral labyrinthine damage, since one labyrinth at a time is tested. Patients with bilateral peripheral vestibular damage may have no response to caloric stimulation or low-frequency rotational testing, yet have normal rotational responses at high frequencies (above 1 Hz) (3). Cool water irrigation causes contralateral nystagmus, whereas warm caloric stimulation evokes ipsilateral nystagmus. Nystagmus is named according to the direction of the quick phase, but the caloric stimulation induces vestibular imbalance in the direction of the slow phase. The quick phases are compensatory saccades that bring the fovea toward a target.

Nystagmus is best recorded with the eyes open in darkness. Electro-oculography (EOG) is usually employed to measure the movements. The nystagmus is measured by its slow-phase velocities. A familiar mnemonic for caloric nystagmus direction is COWS—cold-opposite, warm-same—referring to the direction of the quick phase. Bithermal caloric testing (warm and cold water at 44° and 30°C) detect unilateral "canal paresis" or vestibular nerve damage. Central (brainstem) disease typically causes bidirectional impairment of caloric responses or leaves it intact. Ongoing "spontaneous nystagmus" causes the phenomenon of directional preponderance of the direction of warm and cold caloric responses from either ear toward the side of spontaneous nystagmus.

B. Rotatory Tests

Impulsive rotation of the patient while seated in a vestibular chair to a constant velocity can provide a measurement of the time constant of the VOR. Once the chair reaches constant velocity, the VOR begins to fade away. The time for the slow-phase velocity to decline to 37% of the maximal value is the time constant of the reflex. The time constant is decreased by vestibular lesions. Comparison of the slow-phase velocity during rightward and leftward constant velocity rotation can identify unilateral vestibular loss particularly only in the acute stages. After several weeks, the VOR rebalances so that asymmetry may not be detected during low acceleration stimulation. Impulsive, constant velocity rotation often fails to identify partial peripheral vestibular lesions.

Sinusoidal rotation at low frequencies (0.0125–0.25 Hz; 0.05 Hz is a routine screening frequency) identifies a phase lead of the eyes before the head after unilateral, bilateral peripheral, or central vestibular lesions. Phase lead does not have localizing value. Moreover, it is a nonspecific finding that can occur in normal subjects who are habituated to prolonged rotation. Symmetry of nystagmus slow phases between rightward and leftward rotation is often within the normal range even in patients with complete unilateral peripheral lesions, since compensation occurs at low frequencies.

The responses to low-frequency rotation are similar though to those obtained with caloric testing. A patient with bilateral peripheral vestibular disease may have loss of caloric responses but normal VOR function during high-frequency head motion. Patients may not experience any vertigo or oscillopsia when only the response to low-frequency components is lost. Inability of labyrinthine receptors to respond to low frequencies can be compensated for by visual (optokinetic and smooth pursuit) tracking systems that stabilize the eyes. In order to assess the VOR independently of visual following responses, it must be assessed in darkness or during very high-frequency motion (well over 1 Hz) where visual following reflexes become ineffective.

Only laboratories with high-torque motor chairs can deliver high-frequency stimuli, but similar information can be obtained by passive ballistic movements or by head shaking at the bedside.

C. Bedside Tests of VOR

1. Inspection of the Eyes

The function of both labyrinths together and their central projections can be tested in the clinic or at the bedside by having the patient shake the head from side to side while viewing a stationary target. At low rates of head motion (under 1 Hz), optokinetic and smooth pursuit movements add to the VOR. In order to assess the VOR without these visual influences, the patient is instructed to shake the head rapidly (about 2–3 Hz) through an excursion of about 20–40 degrees. If the VOR is normal, eye movements will appear smooth, without corrective saccades or nystagmus quick phases, and the patient perceives images to be stable. If the VOR is abnormal, the patient perceives movements of images in the direction of the nystagmus quick phases, which correct for abnormal vestibular smooth eye movements. If the VOR is hypoactive (eye movements too slow), nystagmus fast phases are directed opposite to head motion. The fixation target appears to move opposite to the direction of head movement. If the VOR is hyperactive (smooth eye movements too fast), nystagmus fast phases appear in the same direction as head motion (4). Eye movements are more readily seen if the patient wears Fresnel lenses, plus 20 diopter lenses worn in an illuminated goggle frame, which serve to magnify and illuminate the eyes; they also blur fixation impairing visual cancellation of nystagmus.

Head Shaking Nystagmus. Patients with unilateral peripheral vestibular lesions have nystagmus directed away from the affected side after vigorous head shaking. The patient is instructed to shake the head through 80 degrees of range at about 2 Hz for 20–30 s (5,6). Then when the head is stopped, the observer examines the patient's eyes under Fresnel lenses. It is preferable to record the eye movements in darkness, but Fresnel lenses enable the physician to examine the nystagmus in the clinic or at the bedside. Ophthalmologists may use their 20-D indirect ophthalmascope lens over one eye while occluding the other eye to look for nystagmus with the head still. Slow phases of head-shaking nystagmus (HSN) are initially directed toward the impaired ear. It is initially brisk and lasts less than 20 s, but high-resolution oculography reveals that it is often followed by a low-amplitude reversed HSN with slow phases away from the impaired ear (6). Central lesions, including stroke, spinocerebellar degeneration, and multiple sclerosis, also cause HSN (5). Central lesions may, however, damage the velocity storage mechanism by involving the nucleus prepositus hypoglossi and medial vestibular nucleus, precluding the appearance of HSN.

Excitation of a semicircular canal is a more effective stimulus than inhibition (Ewald's law). That is, stimulation of the left lateral semicircular canal by leftward head movement is a more potent vestibular stimulus than inhibition of input from the right lateral semicircular canal by leftward head movement. If a patient with only one remaining labyrinth (say the left side) is rotated to the left (exciting the left labyrinth), a better vestibular response is evoked than from rotation to the right (inhibiting the left labyrinth). Inability of inhibitory stimuli to decrease vestibular nerve firing rates to less than zero accounts for the greater efficacy of canal excitation than inhibition. Most fibers in one vestibular nerve can be driven to a firing rate of close to zero during rotation of the head in the opposite direction at only 180 degrees/s. At higher head velocity, the excitatory response from the normal left labyrinth during leftward heard rotation overwhelms the inhibitory response. As the head moves from side to side, the imbalanced response from the left side charges a velocity storage mechanism (7) in the vestibular and prepositus hypoglossi nuclei so that it stores a net predominance of slow phases directed toward the right. After the head and cupula come to rest, discharge of the velocity storage mechanism leads to leftward HSN, with quick phases beating away from the right-sided lesion.

2. *Visual Acuity During Head Shaking*

When a normal person shakes the head at 2–3 Hz while viewing a Snellen chart, visual acuity should remain the same as that recorded with the head immobile. If acuity falls by several lines, the VOR is overactive or underactive (i.e., its gain is above or below the ideal value of 1.0) or its phase is abnormal. In our clinics, we attribute a drop of 3 or more lines of Snellen acuity (e.g., 20/20 to 20/60) to an abnormal VOR. If the patient does not maintain adequate voluntary head motion, the examiner may move it for him or her. This passive testing has the advantage of eliminating preprogrammed smooth eye movements that can compensate partially for an impaired VOR when labyrinthine defective patients move the head actively (8), but some patients object to having the head moved rapidly in a sinusoidal pattern.

3. Ophthalmoscopic Assessment of the VOR

The VOR can also be assessed during ophthalmoscopy with the pupil dilated. The patient is instructed to shake the head from side to side through an excursion of about 20 degrees. The nonvisualized eye is covered. If the VOR functions normally, the optic disc is seen to remain still during head rotation. If the VOR is overactive or underactive, the disc oscillates. If its gain is too high, the optic disc is seen to move in the same direction as the head. If it is underactive, the disc appears to move opposite to the head (4). Care must be taken that the head does not shift from side to side, since translation of the head causes movement of the optic disc even when the VOR is normal.

During all bedside tests of the VOR, the patient should wear customary distance spectacles, since the gain (ratio of eye velocity to head velocity) is adapted to the power of corrective spectacles (9). For clear vision with spectacles, the brain must adapt VOR gain to their magnification power, which is approximated by the relation 40/40–D, where D is the lens power in diopters (D); thus a 6-D myopic patient would have a VOR gain of about 0.87, where- as a 6-D hyperopic patient would have a gain of 1.18 during high-frequency head shaking. If the patient did not wear his or her usual glasses, nystagmus would appear. Spectacles make ophthalmoscopic assessment of the reflex difficult.

4. Oculocephalic Maneuvers

Movement of the patient's head passively with the examiner's hands is termed the oculocephalic maneuver and the ocular response is often called the doll's eye reflex. In unconscious patients, oculocephalic maneuvers assess the VOR in the absence of visual following reflexes. Nystagmus quick phases are abolished in coma of any cause, so that eye movements appear smooth and excursion of the eyes may be full in range, even if the VOR gain is subnormal. Moreover, in alert patients full ocular excursion does not necessarily indicate that the VOR is normal. If the head is moved at low accelerations, intact smooth pursuit and optokinetic following reflexes may compensate for a defective VOR and elicit full excursion of the eyes despite a subnormal, even absent, VOR. Nonetheless, oculocephalic responses are useful in detecting the range of VOR excursion; if saccades and pursuit are paralyzed, the presence of active oculocephalic reflexes indicates at least partial sparing of the VOR and signifies that the ophthalmoplegia is caused by supranuclear damage to saccadic and pursuit pathways. In normal humans, cervico-ocular reflexes are rudimentary or absent, but in patients with bilateral loss of labyrinthine function there is an adaptive increase in their gain that compensates, in part, for loss of the VOR (8). In the rare comatose patient with bilateral labyrinthine damage, preserved responses to oculocephalic maneuvers do not specify sparing of the VOR.

5. Rapid Passive Head Movements to Test Peripheral Function

The examiner briskly moves the patient's head to one side while the patient fixates a distant object. Normally the eyes should stay on target and the examiner should see only a smooth compensatory eye movement in the orbit. Patients with unilateral vestibular loss make one or more saccades to bring the eyes on target when the head is moved toward the side of the impaired ear. Saccades in the same direction as the VOR signify an inability of vestibular smooth eye movements to match head velocity (10). Thus, a patient with right vestibular neurectomy will make visible leftward saccades during rightward head movements but no saccades during leftward head movements (11). Oppositely directed, compensatory, refixation saccades during rapid horizontal head rotations indicate a severe horizontal semicircular canal lesion on the side toward which the head is being rotated. The head must be moved at high velocity, because the VOR eventually becomes balanced for low-velocity head movements after unilateral peripheral vestibular damage.

6. Visual Cancellation of the VOR

During pursuit of an object with both the head and eyes, the VOR must be canceled. Otherwise, the VOR would move the eyes opposite to the head motion away from the object. During cancellation the head and eyes move simultaneously toward the target. VOR cancellation is tested clinically by rotating the patient to and fro en bloc while the patient fixates an object moving with him or her such as a finger of an outstretched arm. This is not a test of the VOR but rather of its interaction with vision. If cancellation is adequate, the eyes remain stationary in the orbit.

Patients with impaired visual cancellation of the VOR exhibit nystagmus during this test. Vestibular smooth eye movements take the eyes off their target and quick phases (saccades) bring them back to it. Oscillation must be performed at less than 1 Hz; at higher frequencies, VOR cancellation is defective in normal subjects. Impaired visual cancellation of the VOR typically corresponds clinically to defective smooth pursuit (12,13), but defective smooth pursuit and cancellation can be dissociated (14). Testing VOR cancellation has an advantage of over testing smooth pursuit in patients with gaze-evoked nystagmus, which confounds the visualization of saccadic pursuit, since normal cancellation keeps the eyes near the primary position in the orbit.

Two caveats should be borne in mind when assessing cancellation: If VOR gain is low, cancellation is readily achieved, even if smooth pursuit (or a distinct cancellation system) is impaired. Conversely, if VOR gain is abnormally high, cancellation can be impaired when smooth pursuit (or a cancellation system) is normal.

II. THE DORSAL AND VENTRAL PRETECTAL SYNDROMES AND THE VERTICAL VOR

Infarcts, hemorrhages, demyelination, or neoplasms in the pretectum dorsal to the aqueduct of Sylvius often paralyze upward saccades; retraction saccades elicited by attempted upward saccades and light near dissociation of the pupils are accompanying features. The eponym Parinaud's syndrome is not appropriate for this constellation of neuro-ophthalmic signs, since Parinaud neither described it nor recognized that dorsal pretectal damage was responsible for palsy of upward gaze (15,16). Pretectal lesions ventral to the aqueduct of Sylvius paralyze downward saccades or both upward and downward saccades; the pupils are usually of medium size and poorly reactive to both light and accommodation. I term these distinct ocular motor defects the dorsal and ventral pretectal syndromes.

In both the dorsal and ventral syndromes, the vertical VOR and smooth pursuit may appear to be spared. However, reduced gain, limited amplitude, and abnormal phase lead of the vertical VOR were measured in a patient with a unilateral ventral infarct involving the interstitial nucleus of Cajal and rostral interstitial nucleus of the medial longitudinal fasciculus and confirmed by neuropathological examination (17). The lesion spared the ocular motor nuclei indicating that *supranuclear* lesions of the rostral midbrain can impair the vertical VOR; this varies from the prevailing concept that supranuclear lesions spare the vertical VOR. This misconception results from the usual method of testing the vertical VOR at the bedside: the oculocephalic maneuver, in which the patient's head is passively flexed and extended while fixating on a target in a well-lit room. As noted above, the eye movements that result represent not only the vertical VOR but visual enhancement of this reflex by smooth pursuit and optokinetic smooth eye movements. Moreover, although the examiner may judge the amplitude of oculocephalic eye movements to be normal, the gain and phase of the vertical VOR cannot be measured at the bedside. Complete assessment of vertical VOR dysfunction requires oculographic recording and quantification of vertical VOR eye movements performed in darkness.

Quantitative study of the vertical VOR, and its control by vision in a series of patients with focal lesions that caused dorsal or ventral pretectal syndromes (18) also refuted the clinical aphorism that supranuclear palsies of vertical gaze spare the vertical VOR. We (18) recorded reduced vertical VOR gain and abnormal phase lead, although many patients had full ranges of smooth eye movements to passive oculocephalic maneuvers tested in the clinic. Cervico-ocular reflexes and preprogrammed smooth eye movements may have contributed to the VOR that we measured during active head motion. Moreover, measurement of visual enhancement of the reflex, which simulates oculocephalic (doll's eye) maneuvers in the clinic, revealed subnormal enhancement of the reflex by a visual target despite a normal range of excursion. Normality of the vertical VOR and its visual enhancement cannot be assured by gross integrity of oculocephalic reflexes.

III. THE VERTICAL VOR IN INTERNUCLEAR OPHTHALMOPLEGIA

Bilateral lesions of the medial longitudinal fasciculi cause bilateral internuclear ophthalmoplegia (INO), which consists of binocular paresis of adduction and gaze-evoked nystagmus of the eye in abduction. INO is associated with impairment of the vertical VOR and smooth pursuit and vertical gaze-evoked nystagmus (19,20). We recorded reduced gain of upward and downward smooth vestibular movements and abnormal phase lag at frequencies up to 2 Hz in a group of patients with unilateral or bilateral INO (20). VOR gain increases when patients view a stationary target but remains below the ideal gain of unity, which indicates defective visual enhancement of the reflex. Despite a subnormal vertical VOR patients with INO are unable adequately to cancel this reflex when they pursue a target with combined head and eye motion (20). Impairment of the vertical VOR and its cancellation in patients witn INO provides evidence that vertical VOR, vertical eye position, and VOR cancellation signals in humans are transmitted from the vestibular nuclei to the third nerve and fourth nerve nuclei, at least in part, in the MLF.

IV. VESTIBULO–OCULAR HYPERREFLEXIA

Brainstem tegmental lesions typically abolish the VOR or reduce its gain (Table 1). The converse, high VOR gain, is a manifestation of cerebellar system disease (13,21) that has been attributed to loss of inhibition of the vestibular nuclei by the vestibulocerebellum (flocculonodular lobe). Flocculectomy increases the gain to 1.17 in the monkey (22) and in humans with cerebellar degeneration the highest horizontal VOR gain recorded is 3.0 (23) (normal $\leq$1.0). In one reported patient, physostigmine, an acetylcholinesterase inhibitor, reduced the gain and improved visual acuity during head shaking (23). Reversible chemical lesions of the olivocerebellar climbing fiber pathway made with lidocaine cause a reversible increase of VOR gain in cats (24), which suggests that involvement of this pathway is responsible for vestibulo-ocular hyperreflexia in humans with cerebellar system disease. A third possible mechanism of gain elevation is adaptation of the reflex to impaired smooth

Table 1 Vestibulo-Ocular Reflex Gain Changes

Low gain	High gain
Bilateral labyrinthine damage	Floccular lesions
Brainstem tegmental lesions	Olivocerebellar lesions
Severe metabolic coma	Adaptation to impaired pursuit
Drugs	
amytriptiline	
phenytoin (Dilantin)	
sedatives	

pursuit; smooth pursuit movements enhance VOR gain during head motion at low frequency, and when they are impaired by cerebellar disease, the VOR, which is remarkably plastic (10), may undergo adaptive enhancement to compensate for poor smooth pursuit (13).

V. POSITIONAL VERTIGO AND NYSTAGMUS: STATIC AND PAROXYSMAL

Paroxysmal positional vertigo is the most common cause of vertigo (25). It is typically a benign disorder that may be explained by cupulolithiasis in the posterior semicircular canal. However, paroxysmal vertigo and nystagmus may also be evoked in patients with central lesions (26) by rapid changes in head position, such as reaching for an object on a shelf or rolling over in bed, and demonstrated in the clinic by quickly placing the head in the supine or hanging position. In contrast to the benign paroxysmal positional nystagmus (BPPN) of peripheral origin, central paroxysmal positional nystagmus (CPPN) typically begins immediately, does not fatigue after the head-hanging maneuver is repeated several times, and lasts longer than 30 s (Table 2). Nonetheless, central lesions involving the caudal brainstem or vestibulocerebellum, such as ependymoma,

Table 2 Central Versus Peripheral Paroxysmal Positional Nystagmus

Type	Direction	Latency(s)	Fatigue	Brainstem Signs	Duration(s)
Peripheral	Torsional-upbeat, dysconjugate	4–10 s	Typical	Absent	<30 s
Central	Horizontal or vertical conjugate	<4 s	Uncommon	Usual	>30 s

can cause paroxysmal positional nystagmus with features of the peripheral "benign" type (26). Patients with apparent BPPN should have neurological examinations and careful follow-up to exclude CPPN. I advocate cranial computed tomograph (CT) or magnetic resonance imaging (MRI) only for patients who have atypical features (Table 2) that suggest CPPN. A caveat is a rare type of horizontal canal BPPN which is purely horizontal, occurs without latency, and lasts more than 30 s (27); it may be mistaken for CPPN.

Central positional vertigo is characterized by little dizziness and prominent nystagmus in contrast to benign paroxysmal positional vertigo. Either direction-fixed or direction-changing positional nystagmus usually arises from labyrinthine disease, although both can also be manifestations of central disease. *Paroxysmal positional nystagmus* that lasts less than 30 s or so after assuming a head-hanging position should be distinguished from *static positional nystagmus*, which persists as long as the head position is maintained (Table 3). Static positional nystagmus more often results from central (brainstem) disease than the paroxysmal type, but both static and paroxysmal positional nystagmus are usually caused by labyrinthine disorders. Peripheral static positional nystagmus is probably caused by damage to otolithic receptors, and central static positional nystagmus likely arises from disruption of their projections within the brainstem and cerebellum, since the otolithic organs are sensitive to changes in head position with respect to gravity. Primary position upbeat or downbeat nystagmus, both signs of central disease, may appear only upon assuming the supine position, or they may reverse directions between erect and supine postures (28).

Static and paroxysmal positional nystagmus are tested in the recumbent position with the head hanging to the right and then to the left. Static and paroxysmal nystagmus of central origin is often evoked with the head supine in the midposition, but BPPN typically requires the head to be accelerated into a head-hanging posture with the affected ear undermost so as to maximally stimulate a posterior semicircular canal. The nystagmus of BPPN has its slow phase directed in the plane of action of the offending posterior canal; the right posterior canal excites the ocular muscles that act in its plane, the left inferior

Table 3 Central Versus Peripheral Static Positional Nystagmus

Type	Direction	Effect of fixation	Brainstem signs
Peripheral	Torsional, upbeat dysconjugate	Suppression	Absent
Central	Upbeat or down-beat conjugate	None	Usually present

rectus, and the right superior oblique causing extorting jerk nystagmus in the right eye and upbeating nystagmus in the left eye. CPPN, on the other hand, is typically conjugate and often downward toward the lower eyelids (see Table 2).

Nystagmus is inspected with the eyes open and preferably under Fresnel lenses. Accompanying vertigo, if severe, often prompts the patient to close the eyes and prior instructions must be given to keep the eyes open and maintain a steady viewing direction. Fixation inhibits or stops BPPN but has little effect on CPPN, since central lesions that affect otolithic or posterior semicircular canal projections also damage brainstem and cerebellar circuits that mediate smooth pursuit and cancellation of the VOR. Patients with cupulolithiasis may experience terrible positional vertigo but not exhibit nystagmus when examined without Fresnel lenses.

Management of central positional vertigo is addressed at treating the brainstem or cerebellar lesions that cause it. There is no rationale for positional exercises or maneuvers that are sometimes employed in BPPN (29). Antivertiginous drugs such as meclizine or phenergan can be used to suppress pervasive dizziness that occurs in particular head positions.

ACKNOWLEDGMENT

This work was supported by Medical Research Council of Canada grant MT5404.

REFERENCES

1. Sharpe JA, Barber HO. The Vestibulo-Ocular Reflex and Vertigo. New York: Raven Press, 1993.
2. Baloh RW, Honrubia V. Clinical neurophysiology of the vestibular system. Philadelphia: Davis, 1990.
3. Baloh RW, Honrubia V, Yee RD, Hess K. Changes in the human vestibulo-ocular reflex after loss of peripheral sensitivity. Ann Neurol 16:222–8, 1984.
4. Zee DS. Ophthalmoscopy in evaluation of vestibular disorders. Ann Neurol 3:373, 1978.
5. Kamei T, Kornhuber H. Spontaneous and head-shaking nystagmus in normals and in patients with central lesions. Can J Otolaryngol 3:372–80, 1974.
6. Hain TC, Fetter M, Zee DS. Head-shaking nystagmus in patients with unilateral peripheral vestibular lesions. Am J Otolaryngol 8:36–47, 1987.
7. Demer JL. Hypothetical mechanism of head-shaking nystagmus (HSN) in man: asymmetrical velocity storage. Soc Neurosci. 11:1038, 1985 (abstract).
8. Kasai T, Zee DS. Eye-head coordination in labyrinthine-defective human beings. Brain Res 144:123–41, 1978.
9. Cannon SC, Leigh RJ, Zee DS, Abel LA. The effect of rotational magnification of corrected spectacles on the quantitative evaluation of the VOR. Acta Otolaryngol 100:81–8, 1985.

10. Gauthier GM, Robinson DA. Adaptation of the human vestibulo-ocular reflex to magnifying lenses. Brain Res 92:331–5, 1975.
11. Halmagyi M, Curtoys IS. A clinical sign of canal paresis. Arch Neurol 45:737–9, 1988.
12. Zee DS, Suppression of the vestibulo-ocular reflex. Ann Neurol 1:217, 1977.
13. Sharpe JA, Goldberg HJ, Lo AW, Herishanu YO. Visual-vestibular interaction in multiple sclerosis. Neurology 1981; 31:427–33.
14. Peterson BW, Leigh RJ. Modulation and cancellation of the vestibulo-ocular reflex: physiological and clinical considerations. In: Barber HO, Sharpe JA, eds. Vestibular disorders. Chicago: Year Book, 1988:24–34.
15. Parinaud H. Paralysie des mouvements associes des yeux. Arch Neurol 1883; 5:145–172.
16. Parinaud H. Paralysis of the movement of convergence of the eyes. Brain 1886; 9:330–41.
17. Ranalli PJ, Sharpe JA, Fletcher WA. Palsy of upward and downward saccadic, pursuit and vestibular movements with a unilateral midbrain lesion: patho-physiological correlations. Neurology 1988; 38:114–22.
18. Sharpe JA, Ranalli PJ. Vertical vestibulo-ocular reflex control after supranuclear midbrain damage. Acta Otolaryngol 1991; 481(Suppl.):194–8.
19. Evinger LC, Fuchs AF, Baker R. Bilateral lesions of the medial longitudinal fasciculus in monkeys: effects on the horizontal and vertical components of voluntary and vestibular induced eye movements. Exp Brain Res 1977; 28:1–20.
20. Ranalli PJ, Sharpe JA. Vertical vestibulo-ocular reflex, smooth pursuit and eye-head tracking dysfunction in internuclear ophthalmoplegia. Brain 1988; 111:1277–95.
21. Baloh RW, Jenkins HA, Honrubia V, Yee RD, Lau CJY. Visual-vestibular interaction and cerebellar atrophy. Neurology 1979; 29:116–9.
22. Zee DS, Yamazaki A, Butler PH, Gucer G. Effects of ablation of flocculus and paraflocculus on eye movements in primates. J Neurophysiol 1981; 446:878–99.
23. Thurston SE, Leigh RJ, Abel LA, Dell'Osso LF. Hyperactive vestibulo-ocular reflex in cerebellar degeneration: pathogenesis and treatment. Neurology 1987; 37:53–57.
24. Demer JL, Robinson DA. Effects of reversible lesions and stimulation on olivocerebellar system on vestibulo-ocular reflex plasticity. J Neurophysiol 1982; 47:1084–1107.
25. Baloh RW, Honrubia V, Jacobson K. Benign positional vertigo. Clinical and oculographic features in 240 cases. Neurology 1987; 37:371.
26. Watson P, Barber HO, Deck J, Terbrugge K. Positional vertigo and nystagmus of central origin. Can J Neurol Sci 1981; 8:133–7.
27. Baloh RW, Jacobson K, Honrubia V. Horizontal semicircular canal variant of benign positional vertigo. Neurology 1993; 43:2542–2549.
28. Hirose G, Kawada J, Tsukada K, Yoshioka A, Sharpe JA. Upbeat nystagmus: clinicopathological and pathophysiological considerations. J Neurol Sci 1991; 105:159–167.
29. Herdman SJ, Tusa RJ, Zee DS, Proctor LR, Mattox BE. Single treatment approaches to benign paroxysmal vertigo. Arch Otolaryngol Head Neck Surg 1993; 119:450–454.

19

Management of Ocular Myasthenia Gravis

Daniel B. Drachman
Johns Hopkins University School of Medicine, Baltimore, Maryland

Myasthenia gravis (MG) is an autoimmune disorder of neuromuscular junctions characterized by weakness and fatigability of skeletal muscles. The extraocular muscles and elevators of the eyelids are often affected early producing symptoms of diplopia and/or ptosis. The term *ocular myasthenia gravis* (OMG) is used when the clinical manifestations of MG are limited to these muscles. It is useful to consider *ocular* MG, as distinct from generalized MG, for several reasons: (1) The ophthalmologist is commonly the physician consulted first when MG presents with ocular symptoms. (2) Certain conditions that may mimic ocular features of OMG require special diagnostic testing. (3) Both the treatment and the prognosis of OMG differ in some respects from those of MG with generalized manifestations. However, despite the restricted localization of its *clinical* features, OMG is a *systemic* disease: The pathogenesis of OMG involves a *systemic* autoimmune reaction. Associated *systemic* factors may influence the manifestations of OMG. Finally, OMG may require treatment with *systemically* active agents.

I. PATHOGENESIS

Rational treatment of OMG requires an understanding of its pathogenesis. The basic abnormality in MG is a reduction of available acetylcholine receptors (AChRs) at neuromuscular junctions. This results in impairment of neuromuscular transmission clinically manifested by weakness and muscular fatigue. Autoimmune mechanisms mediated by antibodies to AChR play a key role in this process. The autoantibodies act to decrease the number of available AChRs by three distinct mechanisms that have been well described. Anti-AChR antibodies are detectable in the serum of approximately 90% of patients with generalized MG but only about 50% of patients with OMG. The reason for this difference is not clear, but it has been suggested that the autoantibodies in OMG may selectively bind to determinants on extraocular muscle AChR, and bind less well to limb muscle AChR, which is used in the standard radioimmunoassay. Although antibodies to AChR are clearly implicated in the pathogenesis of MG, their absolute serum concentration does not correlate with the clinical severity of the disease. However, in a given patient, treatment-induced reduction of AChR antibody levels usually parallels clinical improvement.

II. CLINICAL FEATURES AND DIAGNOSIS OF OMG

The diagnosis of OMG may be difficult in some cases, even for experienced clinicians. There are no pathognomonic features on physical examination, and diagnostic testing may give inconclusive results. Nevertheless, it is of great importance to establish the diagnosis of OMG unequivocally and to exclude other possible conditions that may mimic it. Perhaps the most common error encountered in consultation is the failure of the physician to establish the diagnosis of OMG unequivocally, or to exclude other related conditions, before beginning treatment. The diagnosis of myasthenia usually commits the patient to medical and/or surgical therapy that entails significant risks. On the other hand, a missed diagnosis of another condition simulating OMG may result in delayed treatment, with serious medical (and occasionally legal) consequences. Therefore, before initiating treatment of OMG, it is essential (1) to establish the diagnosis as definitively as possible; (2) to exclude conditions that may imitate, or occur in addition to, OMG; and (3) to search for associated conditions that may exacerbate OMG or influence the choice of treatment.

The cardinal features of MG are weakness and fatigability of muscles. Weakness increases after repeated use ("fatigue") and improves following rest or sleep. The course of MG is often variable, with exacerbations and remissions, particularly during the first few years after onset of the disease. Remissions are rarely complete or permanent. Unrelated infections or systemic disorders can lead to increased weakness.

The distribution of muscle weakness has a characteristic pattern. The cranial muscles, particularly the elevators of the lids and the extraocular muscles, are often involved early, giving rise to initial symptoms of diplopia and ptosis.

Table 1 Diagnosis of Ocular Myasthenia Gravis

History
- Ptosis, diplopia
- ?Weakness in other cranial or limb muscles
- Fluctuation and fatigue: worse with repeated activity, improved by rest
- Effects of previous treatments

Physical Examination
- Ptosis on forward gaze; on sustained upward gaze
- Diplopia—distribution and extent of EOM limitation
- ?Cranial and generalized muscle involvement
- Absence of other neurological signs.

Laboratory Testing
- AChR antibody radioimmunoassay: ~50% positive in OMG
  - Definite diagnosis if positive. Negative result does not exclude OMG
- Anti-ChE: Edrophonium (Tensilon) 2 mg + 8 mg i.v.
  - Pyridostigmine (Mestinon) 60 mg orally
    - Highly probable diagnosis if unequivocally positive. Beware equivocal response.
- Repetitive nerve stimulation (face, proximal muscles):
  - Decrement of >15% at 3 Hz—highly probable
- Single fiber EMG: jitter or blocking with normal fiber density: confirmatory, but not specific

However, in approximately 85% of patients, the weakness eventually becomes generalized and affects the bulbar, limb, and trunk muscles as well.

The diagnosis of OMG is suspected on the basis of weakness of the lids and extraocular muscles, particularly when it is variable. The weakness often involves multiple ocular muscles that are innervated by different cranial nerves. The diagnosis should always be confirmed definitively before treatment is undertaken.

A. Anticholinesterase Test

Drugs that inhibit the enzyme acetylcholinesterase (AChE) allow acetylcholine (ACh) to interact repeatedly with the limited number of AChRs producing improvement in the strength of myasthenic muscles. Edrophonium (Tensilon) is used most commonly for testing, because of the rapid onset (30 s) and short duration (about 5 min) of its effect. It is essential that an objective endpoint be used to assess the effect of edrophonium. The examiner should focus on one or more unequivocally weak muscle groups and evaluate them objectively. For example, the pattern of extraocular muscle or lid weakness should be defined prior to the test dose. An initial dose of 2 mg of edrophonium is given intravenously. If definite improvement occurs, the test is considered positive and

Table 2 Exclusion of Conditions That Mimic OMG

Parasellar or orbital neoplasm or aneurysm: MRI or CT of head and orbits
Thyroid ophthalmopathy: Thyroid functions; thyroid stimulating immunoglobulin
Progressive external ophthalmoplegia, oculopharyngeal syndrome: Muscle biopsy: "ragged red" fibers; "red-rimmed vacuoles"; mitochondrial abnormalities

terminated. If there is no change, the patient is given an additional 8 mg intravenously. The dose is administered in two parts, because some patients react to edrophonium with unpleasant side effects such as nausea, diarrhea, salivation, and rarely syncope. Atropine (0.6 mg) should be available for intravenous administration if these symptoms become troublesome. False-positive tests occur occasionally in patients with other neurological disorders and in placebo reactors. False-negative or equivocal tests may also occur in OMG. In some cases, it is helpful to use a longer acting drug such as pyridistigmine (60 mg orally), since this permits more time for detailed evaluation of muscle function. In virtually all instances, it is desirable to carry out further testing to establish the diagnosis of MG definitively.

B. Electrodiagnostic Testing

Repetitive nerve stimulation may provide further diagnostic evidence of MG. Anti-ChE medication should be stopped at least 6 h prior to testing. Weak muscles or proximal muscle groups most often give positive results. Therefore, in OMG we frequently stimulate the facial nerve or the nerves to the deltoid or biceps muscles. Supramaximal stimuli are delivered at a rate of three or five per second, and action potentials are recorded from the muscles. In normal individuals, the amplitude of the evoked muscle action potential does not change at these rates of stimulation. In myasthenic patients, a decrease in the amplitude of the evoked responses of 15% or more is considered positive. As a further test, a single dose of edrophonium may be given to determine whether it abolishes or diminishes the decremental response.

C. Anti-AChR Antibody

Anti-AChR antibodies are detectable in the serum of approximately 90% of patients with generalized myasthenia but in only about 50% of patients with weakness confined to the ocular muscles. The finding of anti-AChR antibodies is virtually diagnostic of MG, but a negative test does not exclude the disease. The measured level of anti-AChR antibody does not correlate with the severity

Table 3 Disorders Associated with Myasthenia Gravis

History
Other autoimmune disorders: lupus erythematosus, rheumatoid arthritis, thyroiditis, skin disorders, family history of autoimmune disorder
Conditions that may exacerbate MG: hyper- or hypothyroidism, occult infection, medications (aminoglycoside antibiotics, penicillamine, antiarrhythmics)
Disorders that may interfere with therapy: tuberculosis, diabetes, ulcer disease, hypertension, asthma, osteoporosis
Laboratory Tests
LE preparations, antinuclear antibody, rheumatoid factor, antithyroid antibodies
Thyroid function tests
Pulmonary function tests
Tuberculin test
Chest radiograph
Fasting blood sugar
MRI or CT scan of mediastinum
Bone densitometry in older patients

of MG in different patients. However, in an individual patient, a treatment-induced fall in the antibody level often parallels clinical improvement.

D. Differential Diagnosis

Several other conditions that cause weakness of the cranial musculature must be considered in the differential diagnosis of MG, including drug-induced myasthenia, hyperthyroidism, botulism, intracranial mass lesions or aneurysms, and progressive external ophthalmoplegia. Treatment with *penicillamine* may result in true autoimmune MG, but the weakness is usually mild, and recovery occurs within weeks or months after discontinuing its use. Other drugs such as *aminoglycoside antibiotics* in very large doses or *procaine amide* can cause neuromuscular weakness in normal individuals or exacerbation of weakness in myasthenic patients. Hyperthyroidism, or Graves' disease, can cause disturbances of extraocular motility. It is readily diagnosed or excluded by tests of thyroid function (including measurement of thyroid-stimulating immunoglobulin) that are routinely carried out in patients with suspected MG. Diplopia that mimics the symptoms of OMG may occasionally be due to *intracranial mass lesions* that compress nerves to the extraocular muscles (e.g., sphenoid ridge meningioma or cavernous sinus aneurysm). Magnetic resonance imaging (MRI) or computed tomographic (CT) scans of the head and orbits usually reveal the lesions. *Progressive external ophthalmoplegia* is a relatively uncommon condition resulting in weakness of the extraocular muscles, which may be accompanied by weakness of the proximal muscles of the limbs, and a variety of other systemic features that are beyond the scope of this discussion. Most patients with this condition have mitochondrial abnormalities seen on muscle biopsy.

E. Search for Associated Conditions

Myasthenic patients have an increased incidence of several associated disorders. *Thymic abnormalities* occur in approximately 75% of patients. Of these, 65% are due to thymic hyperplasia, whereas the remaining 10% are neoplastic (thymoma). Thymic enlargement is best detected by MRI or CT scanning of the anterior mediastinum. Enlargement of the thymus in a patient over 40 years of age or progressive enlargement of the thymus on repeated scanning in any patient is highly suspicious of thymoma. *Hyperthroidism* occurs in 3–8% of patients with MG, and either hyper- or hypothyroidism may aggravate the myasthenic symptoms. Tests of thyroid function should therefore be obtained. Because of the *association with other autoimmune diseases*, blood tests for rheumatoid factor and antinuclear antibodies should be carried out in all patients. Chronic infection of any kind can exacerbate MG and should be carefully sought.

Because of the side effects of adrenal corticosteroids and other immunosuppressive agents used in the treatment of MG, a thorough medical examination should be made searching specifically for evidence of chronic or latent infection (such as tuberculosis or hepatitis), hypertension, diabetes, renal impairment, cataract, glaucoma, and osteoporosis.

III. TREATMENT

A. Anticholinesterase Agents

Anticholinesterase (Anti-ChE) agents continue to be used first for treatment of most patients with OMG. They prolong the action of ACh released at neuromuscular junctions and thereby enhance neuromuscular transmission. There is no substantial difference in efficacy among the available anti-ChE agents; pyridostigmine bromide (Mestinon) is most widely used in the United States. Its action begins within 15–30 min and lasts for 3–4 h, but there are individual variations in the duration of response. The initial dosage is usually 60 mg (one tablet) every 4–6 h during the day. The dosage may be increased empirically, but the maximum useful dosage rarely exceeds 120 mg every 3 h. Although anti-ChE medication benefits many patients, the improvement is often incomplete. Therefore, anti-ChE mediation alone usually does not correct diplopia. The effectiveness of anti-ChE drugs is generally most impressive when treatment is begun, but later becomes less helpful in most patients. A majority of patients therefore require further therapeutic measures as described below.

The most common side effect of anti-ChE treatment is diarrhea, which can be controlled with diphenoxylate hydrochloride with atropine (Lomotil) or Imodium taken once or twice a day. Excessive amounts of anti-ChE medication may rarely cause increased weakness that is reversible after decreasing or discontinuing treatment. Anti-ChE treatment should be used with care in patients with asthma, since it may increase bronchospasm.

Ephedrine is sometimes helpful as an adjunct to anti-ChE medication and is thought to enhance ACh secretion from cholinergic terminals. The usual dose is 25 mg two or three times a day. If it causes agitation or insomnia, the dose may be reduced or the evening dose omitted entirely.

B. Thymectomy

As noted above, over 75% of patients with MG have thymic abnormalities. "Hyperplasia" is present in 65% of patients, with microscopic evidence of germinal centers (which are not normally present) or in some cases gross enlargement. The remaining 10% of patients have thymic tumors. The thymus may be removed surgically in myasthenic patients either (1) to prevent further spread of a thymoma or (2) for its beneficial effect on myasthenic weakness.

Surgery is indicated if a thymoma is found, since the tumor may spread locally and become invasive, although it rarely metastasizes. MRI or CT scanning of the mediastinum is used for the detection of thymomas, although the scan cannot distinguish between a tumor mass and thymic enlargement. However, an anterior mediastinal mass in a myasthenic patient over age 40 years or progressive enlargement of the thymic shadow on repeated scans in a patient of any age is strongly suggestive of a neoplasm and should lead to surgery. The tumor and the remaining thymus gland should be removed as completely as possible. If the thymoma cannot be completely removed, or if it is invasive, nonferromagnetic marker clips should be placed at the tumor site during surgery and postoperative irradiation should be directed toward this area.

Surgical thymectomy as a treatment for *generalized* MG has gained increasing acceptance and is now recommended by most authorities. However, the place of thymectomy in the treatment of OMG is still uncertain. In theory, thymectomy should be as useful in OMG as it is in generalized MG, since the pathogenetic mechanisms are the same. The former objection that the risks of thymectomy outweigh the benefits in a disease as mild as OMG no longer applies, since modern advances in management have greatly reduced the risks of surgical thymectomy. In one series of 18 patients with OMG, more than 75% improved with thymectomy and 3 of 18 patients achieved "complete" remission. For these reasons, it is likely that the present criteria for thymectomy may eventually be liberalized to include patients with symptoms limited to the extraocular muscles. However, the present practice of most experts is to recommend thymectomy only if the myasthenic weakness becomes generalized. If thymectomy is elected, it should be performed in an institution where there is extensive experience with the surgical technique as well as pre- and postoperative management of myasthenic patients. Under these circumstances, the mortality rate for the procedure is essentially that of anesthesia. The surgical approach should remove as much of the thymus as possible. A sternal-splitting incision allows exploration of the anterior mediastinum and the adjacent space extending into the neck, with removal of all thymic tissue and related fat. The results of thymectomy in generalized myasthenia indicate that remission occurs in approximately 35% of patients, with lesser degrees of improvement in another 50%. The benefits of thymectomy are usually experienced after a delay of months to years after surgery. In the meantime, other therapeutic measures as described below should be used.

C. Immunosuppressive Treatment

Immunosuppressive treatment should be considered for any patient whose symptoms are not satisfactorily controlled by anti-ChE medications. The definition of "satisfactory control" usually depends on the patient; for many individuals, mild ptosis or diplopia may interfere with their ability to function effectively.

1. Corticosteroids

Adrenal corticosteroids are the immunosuppressive agents used most widely for the treatment of MG. They produce improvement in the great majority of patients with all degrees of muscular weakness. Diplopia, which often fails to respond to anti-ChE medication, can usually be corrected by steroid treatment.

Relative contraindications to steroid therapy include hypertension, ulcer disease, diabetes, chronic infection, osteoporosis, and obesity, although these problems can usually be minimized by appropriate medical measures. Long-term treatment with steroids requires continued medical attention by an experienced physician. Patients who are unable or unwilling to be followed medically should *never* be treated for long periods with steroids.

Before beginning steroid treatment, the anti-ChE medication should be adjusted optimally. Patients with OMG may be treated on an outpatient basis. Since high doses of steroids during the early stages of treatment may exacerbate weakness, we use a gradually increasing dosage schedule. Prednisone is begun at a dosage of 15–20 mg per day and is increased by about 5 mg every second or third day until the patient achieves a satisfactory clinical response or reaches the level of 50 mg per day. The rate of increase should be guided by the patient's response and may be rapid in OMG. About 90% of myasthenic patients improve with steroid treatment. The clinical effect usually begins within 2–6 weeks, although it may take 6 months to a year or more to reach maximum benefit. Side effects of steroids can be minimized by the use of alternate-day treatment.

Accordingly, when the patient has shown definite improvement (usually 2–3 months after beginning treatment), the dosage is gradually shifted toward an alternate-day schedule. The amount given on the "on" day is increased by 5 mg, whereas that on the "off" day is decreased by the same amount until an alternate day regimen is established. In some patients, a small dose of prednisone must be used on the "off" day to prevent fluctuations in symptoms.

Steroid treatment must be continued indefinitely in nearly all patients, although the dose can usually be reduced over time. The goal is to establish the *minimum dosage* required by each patient, not to eliminate all medication. This usually ranges from 10–100 mg every other day and must be established by trial and error for the individual patient. Tapering steroids is a slow process, since the consequences of lowering the dose too much may not be apparent for several months. A common error in the treatment of myasthenic patients is to lower the dose of prednisone too rapidly or to too low a level.

Adverse side effects of prednisone occur in some patients, including cataracts, elevation of intraocular pressure, osteoporosis, aseptic necrosis of bone, reduced resistance to infection, ulcer disease, hypertension, exacerbation of diabetes, increased appetite and obesity, and salt and fluid retention. Consistent follow-up for all of these potential problems is the responsibility of the physician and the patient. Patients should be encouraged to notify their physicians at the first sign of infection or unexplained symptoms of any kind. Steroid-treated patients should be followed at intervals with routine measurements of blood pressure, blood sugar, serum electrolytes, and periodic chest radiographs as well as ophthalmological evaluation for cataract and glaucoma. To minimize the risks of osteoporosis, especially in older patients, I recommend moderate exercise and treatment with vitamin D (50,000 units twice a week) and calcium (1 g per day, in the form of calcium lactate, calcium gluconate, or the proprietary preparation, Tums).

2. *Azathioprine*

Azathioprine (Imuran) is effective in many patients, although its beneficial effects may take 6 months or more to appear. It is useful (1) in patients for whom corticosteroids are contraindicated, (2) in patients whose response to corticosteroids is insufficient, (3) as an adjunct to permit the reduction of steroid dosage, and (4) in patients who develop adverse side effects from the use of steroids.

The usual dose of azathioprine is 2–3 mg/kg per day or 125–300 mg for adult patients. In obese patients, the dose depends on total body weight (not lean body mass). About 10% of individuals develop an acute idiosyncratic reaction consisting of a flulike syndrome of fever and myalgia, which precludes the use of azathioprine. To identify these patients, a test dose of 50 mg per day should be given for the first week. If this is well tolerated, the dose is gradually raised while complete blood counts and liver function tests are followed. In patients who are not receiving steroids concomitantly, the dose of azathioprine can be increased until the white blood count (WBC) falls to approximately 3000/mm^3. The total WBC cannot be used in patients receiving prednisone because of leukocytosis induced by steroids, but a lymphocyte count below 1000/mm^3 is a useful indication of appropriate dosage in this situation. A rise in the mean corpuscular volume (MCV) of red blood cells above 100 is also indicative of a positive effect of azathioprine.

Side effects of azathioprine include abnormalities in hepatic function and leukopenia. If the transaminase level rises above two to three times the normal range, the dose of azathioprine should be reduced. Nausea or anorexia occur occasionally but can usually be controlled by administering azathioprine with meals. Pancreatitis occurs rarely and can be detected early by a rise in serum amylase levels. The prolonged use of immunosuppressive agents in patients who have had organ transplants may predispose to the development of malignancies, but this has not been reported in myasthenic patients treated for many years with azathioprine.

3. *Cyclosporine A*

Cyclosporine A (CsA) has recently been used alone or in conjunction with prednisone in the treatment of MG. It acts more promptly than azathioprine and has a different spectrum of side effects. CsA is usually begun at a dose of 4–5 mg/kg and is taken in two divided doses (morning and evening). It is supplied as capsules containing 25 or 100 mg. Adjustment of the dosage is based on periodic measurement of the serum "trough level" of CsA, which is measured in the morning before taking the drug. The therapeutic serum level depends on the method of assay, and standards for the clinical laboratory should be consulted for recommended values. Renal toxicity is the most important adverse side effect, and the dose of CsA should be reduced if the serum BUN and creatinine levels rise. Other side effects include hypertension, headache, hirsutism, and nausea. As with all immunosuppressive drugs, the dosage of CsA should be tapered very gradually once satisfactory clinical response has been attained. The present high cost of CsA limits its availability for some patients.

IV. PROGNOSIS AND MAINTENANCE OF PATIENTS WITH OMG

As noted above, many patients whose symptoms of myasthenia begin in the extraocular muscles later develop generalized MG. Therefore, all patients should be followed closely for the development of generalized weakness. If weakness remains confined to the extraocular muscles for 3 years or more, the likelihood of developing generalized MG is relatively small, although it is not completely excluded. Because of this possibility, as well as the risks of adverse side effects of the treatments, patients with OMG should be followed at regular intervals.

V. ADDITIONAL CAUTIONS

If surgery is necessary for an intercurrent problem, certain precautions should be taken. Curarelike drugs should never be used in myasthenic patients, because they may increase weakness. If the patient has been receiving prednisone prior to surgery, daily treatment with parenteral steroids (hydrocortisone or methyl prednisolone) or oral prednisone is used for 2–6 days following surgery in a dose equivalent to the "on" day dose of oral prednisone. Other drugs that should be used with caution in patients with MG include aminoglycoside antibiotics, procaine amide, quinine, quinidine, and β-adrenergic blocking agents.

SELECTED READING

1. Drachman DB. Myasthenia gravis. N Engl J Med 1994; in press.
2. Vincent A, Newsom-Davis J. α-Bungarotoxin and anti-acetylcholine receptor antibody binding to the human acetylcholine receptor. Adv Cytopharmacol 1979; 3:269–78.
3. Schumm FH, Weitholter H, Fateh-Moghadam A, Dichgans J. Thymectomy in myasthenia with pure ocular symptoms. J Neurol Neurosurg Psychiatry 1985; 48:332–7.
4. Penn AS, Richman DP, Ruff RL, Lennon VA, eds. Myasthenia gravis and related disorders. Experimental and Clinical Aspects. Ann NY Acad Sci 1993; 681:1–622.
5. Moorthy G, Behrens MM, Drachman DB, Kirkham TH, Knox DL, Miller NR, Slamovitz TL, Zinreich SJ. Ocular pseudomyasthenia or ocular myasthenia "plus": a warning to clinicians. Neurology 1989; 39:1150–4.
6. Seybold ME. The office tensilon test for ocular myasthenia gravis. Arch Neurol 1986; 43:842–3.

20

Diagnostic Workup and Management of Fourth Nerve Palsies

Edward G. Buckley
Duke University Medical Center, Durham, North Carolina

The fourth cranial nerve innervates the superior oblique muscle that lies along the nasal aspect of the superior orbit in close proximity to the ethmoid bone. It originates above the annulus of Zinn, travels anteriorly, and becomes tendinous as it passes through a trochlea located at the junction between the frontal and nasal bones near the superior orbital rim. The tendon then runs posteriorly traveling underneath the superior rectus muscle and attaching to the globe beginning approximately 8–9 mm from the limbus and fanning posteriorly for approximately 13–15 mm. Because of this unique anatomical arrangement, the superior oblique muscle acts as a depressor when the eye is in the adducted position. Its secondary actions are abduction and incyclotorsion. Injuries to the fourth cranial nerve often result in vertical, horizontal, and torsional diplopia.

I. NEUROANATOMY

The fourth cranial nerve is unique in that it is the only nerve to exit dorsally from the brainstem. The nucleus is at the level of the inferior colliculus just inferior to the third nerve nuclear complex. The nerve exists posteriorly in the anterior medullary velum located near the fourth ventricle. Both fourth nerves cross to the opposite side in this structure. The nerve continues around the brainstem and travels anteriorly in the subarachnoid space piercing the dura to enter the cavernous sinus. There it is attached to the lateral wall just below the oculomotor nerve and above the ophthalmic division of the trigeminal nerve. It enters the orbit through the superior orbital fissure outside of the muscle cone. The superior oblique muscle, therefore, is contralaterally innervated, since the right fourth nerve nucleus supplies innervation to the left superior oblique muscle. This trip from brainstem to target organ is the longest of any cranial nerve making it extremely susceptible to injury, especially from head trauma.

II. DIAGNOSIS

The clinical hallmark of a fourth nerve palsy is vertical diplopia. The diplopia is worse on lateral gaze away from the involved superior oblique muscle and is often associated with incyclodiplopia. The patient may manifest a head tilt to the side opposite of the involved fourth nerve in order to eliminate diplopia. The clinical diagnosis of a fourth nerve palsy is difficult because the palsy is rarely complete and, when testing ocular rotations, the superior oblique muscle may appear to be fairly normal in its function (Fig. 1). The "three-step test" was developed to help correctly make the diagnosis in cases of an isolated vertical muscle palsy and is very useful in confirming the suspicion of fourth nerve injury. The characteristics of a fourth nerve palsy using the three-step test are (Fig. 2):

Step 1: A vertical hypertropia on the side of the fourth nerve palsy (a right hypertropia with a right superior oblique palsy).

Step 2: The vertical deviation gets worse on gaze opposite the involved eye (i.e., vertical deviation of a right superior oblique palsy gets worse on left gaze).

Step 3: The vertical deviation gets worse when tilting the head toward the involved fourth nerve palsy (i.e., a right superior oblique palsy is a right hypertropia which gets worse on head tilt to the right).

A fourth step can be included to help confirm the diagnosis. Since the superior oblique muscle acts as a depressor, the hyperdeviation should become greater on down gaze as opposed to up gaze (see Fig. 2).

Although a fourth nerve palsy is the most common cause of a vertical deviation from a neurological cause, there are many local ocular and orbital etiologies. Table 2 lists the neurological and ocular causes of vertical double vision in order of frequency. In making the diagnosis of a fourth nerve palsy, one must consider these other possibilities.

III. DIAGNOSTIC WORKUP

A fourth nerve palsy can occur isolated or in conjunction with other neurological signs or symptoms. If there are other cranial nerves involved or additional neurological abnormalities, then the workup is directed toward the entities that

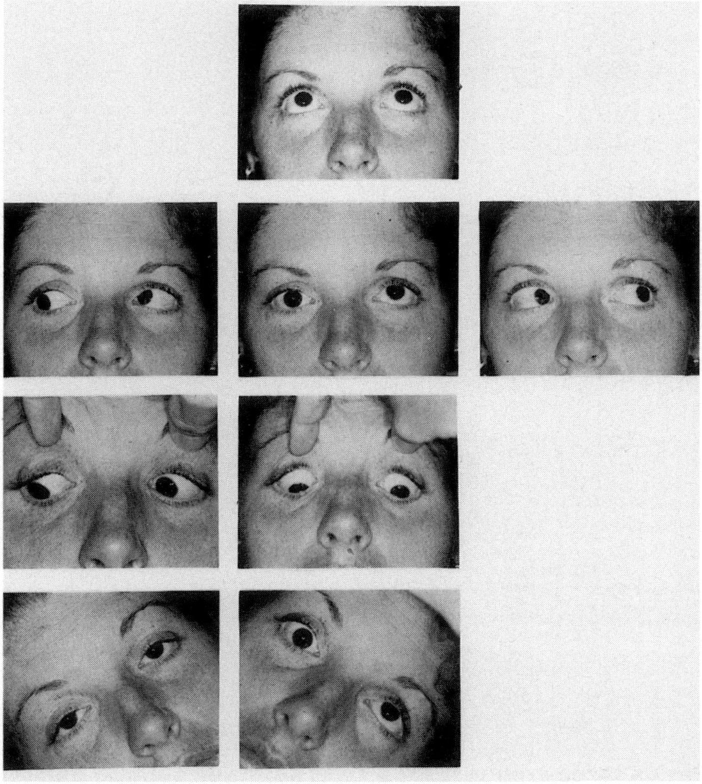

Figure 1 The patient with a right fourth nerve palsy. *Note:* Right hypertropia in the primary position that is worse on left gaze. The Bielschowsky head tilt test shows a right hypertropia worse on head tilt to the right (bottom photos). Hypertropia also is worse on down gaze as opposed to up gaze.

result in those combinations of findings. The evaluation becomes more difficult when the fourth nerve palsy is isolated. As shown in Table 1 there is a long list of possible causes but, fortunately, most of these are quite rare.

By far the most common cause of an isolated fourth nerve palsy is *trauma*. Because of the long intracranial course, the nerve is susceptible to injury at a variety of locations. One of the more common locations is the anterior medullary velum that often results in a bilateral fourth nerve palsy (see Fig. 2). Bilateral fourth nerve palsies can be difficult to recognize because the usual clinical signs of vertical diplopia and head tilt are absent. In this situation, the patient often uses a chin tuck with a gaze up position to eliminate diplopia. Suspicion of a

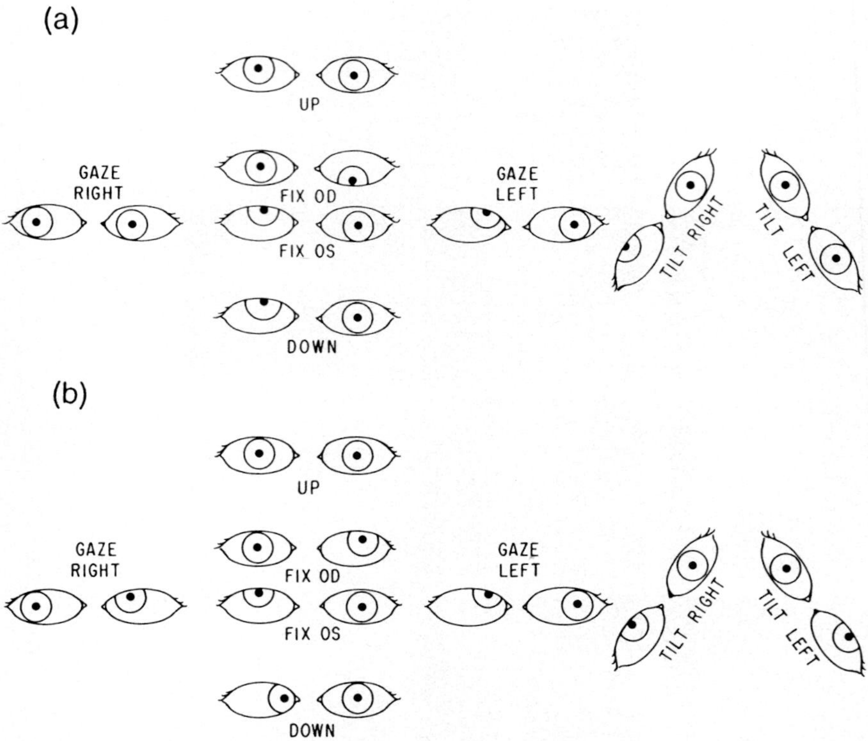

Figure 2 (a) Park's three-step test for a right superior oblique palsy. A right hypertropia is present in the primary position that is worse on left gaze and right head tilt. (b) Clinical findings of a bilateral superior oblique palsy. These are a "V"-pattern esotropia with a left hypertropia on right gaze and a right hypertropia on left gaze. The Bielschowsky head tilt test shows a right hypertropia on right head tilt with a left hypertropia on left head tilt.

bilateral fourth nerve palsy should be raised in any post–head trauma patient complaining of horizontal diplopia on down gaze combined with significant cyclodiplopia. The magnitude of the head trauma need not be severe, and often trivial trauma can result in injury to the fourth nerve. Cranial nerve palsies associated with minor head trauma often harbor undiagnosed intracranial tumors. If this is suspected, a computed tomographic (CT) or magnetic resonance imaging (MRI) scan should be performed to rule out an intracranial mass. If the fourth nerve palsy is isolated and there is a clear history of head trauma of a significant nature, then no further workup is necessary.

Table 1 Etiology of Isolated Trochlear Palsy

Trauma
congenital
Vascular disorders
diabetes
hypertension
aneurysms
arteriovenous malformations
migraine
Inflammatory disorders
acute meningitis
tuberculous meningitis
sarcoidosis
syphilis
encephalomyelitis
Guillain-Barré syndrome
herpes zoster ophthalmocus
botulism
diphtheria
Collagen vascular diseases
systemic lupus
polymyalgia rheumatica
temporal arteritis
Toxic substances
lead poisoning
quinoline posioning
vitamin deficiency
alcohol
Neoplasms
glioma
meningioma
pituitary tumors
schwannoma
pinealoma
metastatic
Neuromuscular disorders
myasthenia gravis

Table 2 Causes of Vertical Diplopia

Ocular	Neurological
Thyroid ophthalmopathy	Superior oblique palsy
Blow-out fracture	Skew deviation
Brown's syndrome	Myasthenia gravis
Progressive external ophthalmoplegia	Inferior oblique palsy
Orbital myositis	Double elevator palsy
Orbital pseudotumor	
Orbital tumor	
Previous orbital surgery	
Previous eye surgery	

Congenital fourth nerve palsies account for the second largest group of patients presenting with symptomatic vertical double vision. The etiology of these is unclear and probably secondary to birth trauma. These patients usually do not present until the third or fourth decades. Examination of old photographs will often reveal a head tilt present as a child or young adolescent, and they will have a history of increasing difficulties over many years. On examination, patients with congenital fourth nerve palsies will usually demonstrate extremely large vertical fusional amplitudes. Using the cross cover technique to measure motility deviations, the size of the vertical deviation will continue to increase with prolonged cross cover and sometimes end up double or triple the original measurement. Another useful clue is a grossly positive Bielschowsky head tilt test with a large vertical deviation seen when tilting the head to the side of the fourth nerve palsy. This is usually several magnitudes greater than that seen with acquired fourth nerve palsies.

Microvascular disease accounts for the bulk of the remaining causes of fourth nerve palsy and for the most part occurs in older individuals in the seventh and eighth decades who present suddenly with vertical double vision. These are usually small vertical deviations and the patients are very symptomatic because they lack vertical fusional amplitudes. As with other causes of neurological microvascular disease, the workup is somewhat limited and involves a search for hypertension, diabetes, and vascular inflammatory disorders such as temporal arteritis and collagen vascular disorders. A list of possible etiologies is shown in Table 1.

In a small percentage of patients, a fourth nerve palsy can be a sign of significant intracranial disease. However, in such cases, other cranial nerves are almost always involved. In a recent review, an isolated fourth nerve palsy was the first sign of metastatic disease in only one case. The most common primary brain tumor involving the fourth nerve is a glioma of the cerebellum or midbrain. Only 14 patients had fourth nerve involvement in a large series of over 300 patients with third, fourth, and sixth nerve palsies from intracranial neoplasms. Therefore, an isolated fourth nerve palsy does not require neuroradiological diagnostic procedures unless there are other additional signs of central nervous system abnormalities.

In summary, the workup of a fourth nerve palsy includes very thorough ophthalmological and neurological evaluations. If the palsy is thought to be "isolated," then no other evaluation is necessary expect for identifying treatable causes of microvascular disease in the appropriate age group. Nonisolated or atypical fourth nerve palsies require more extensive neurological and neuroradiological evaluations.

IV. TREATMENT

Treatment of fourth nerve palsies depends on a variety of factors, including the duration of the palsy, the size of the vertical deviation, field of gaze with the greatest vertical deviation, and the presence of cyclotorsion. In the case of an acute onset, either traumatic or microvascular, no intervention should be entertained until at least 4–6 months of documented stability of the deviation. During this period of time, three treatment modalities are available: patching, prisms, or botulinum toxin injections.

V. PATCHING

In deviations of unknown etiology, or ones that need to be followed closely, simply patching the involved eye temporarily will relieve the double vision. If the patient wears glasses, fogging the image by placing an opaque tape on the glass is usually sufficient. This allows the patient to retain peripheral vision while eliminating diplopia. Although effective, a patch placed on the face does not allow the patient to continue to use side vision, which is very useful in navigating through the environment. In the older patient, the *involved* eye should be occluded to avoid the instability that occurs when a patient is forced to use an eye that has a paralytic muscle. Such problems as, for example, pastpointing can occur, and there are no deleterious effects from patching one eye continuously in this patient population. In the young child, however, amblyopia can develop, and in this situation *alternate* patching or such regimens as 2:1 or 3:1 may be necessary to avoid amblyopia of the paralytic eye until the situation stabilizes. The goal in a young child is to eliminate suppression, muscle contracture, and the development of amblyopia while the palsy is stabilizing.

VI. PRISMS

Prisms can be helpful in small vertical deviations of less than 10 prism diopters when only mild variations exist in different fields of gaze. Such patients routinely will have 5–6 prism diopters of a vertical deviation in the primary position with only 7–8 on lateral gaze and can obtain temporary relief from a Fresnel prism placed in front of the paralytic or poorer seeing eye. Since most of these patients will improve with time, the need for prism therapy is usually temporary. If a permanent small-angle vertical strabismus remains, prism ground into the glasses will eliminate the double vision circumventing the need for surgical intervention. The amount of prism selected should be the smallest amount that enables the patient to gain the largest area of singular binocular vision. Having the patient wear a trial prism in the office will often help determine the exact power necessary. In some of older patients, there will be both a vertical and small horizontal deviation. The prism can be tilted either base in or base out in order to gain both a horizontal and vertical vector. Fresnel prisms should not be placed on both eyes, as they cause a significant decrease in visual function and will not be tolerated by the patient. Occasionally the patient will see single straight ahead and have diplopia only on down gaze. Fresnel prisms can also be used on the lower half of the glasses to take care of such situations. With the judicious use of prism therapy, many patients can be controlled symptomatically until the deviation improves or requires more definitive intervention.

VII. BOTULINUM TOXIN

Botulinum toxin injections have a role in the treatment of both acute and chronic fourth nerve palsies. The two muscles that are most easily treated with this technique are the ipsilateral antagonist inferior oblique muscle and the contralateral yoke inferior rectus muscle. Injection of botulinum toxin into the inferior oblique muscle may eliminate the vertical deviation to a point where the patient can regain fusion. The duration of the toxin lasts approximately 8–12 weeks, which is about the same rate at which the fourth nerve tends to regain its function. The patient remains relatively comfortable with the diplopia kept to a minimum. The second muscle that is amendable to this type of treatment is the contralateral inferior rectus. This is especially helpful if the patient's symptoms are worse on down gaze. By injecting botulinum toxin into the inferior rectus of the other eye, the patient's diplopia in down gaze can often be reduced or totally eliminated. Again, the toxin tends to wear off as the palsied superior oblique muscle function improves resulting in a permanent correction of the double vision.

In patients with a chronic fourth nerve palsy, botulinum toxin can be used as an alternative to surgery. In this situation, injection into the inferior rectus muscle is usually more effective than the inferior oblique. The patients selected for botulinum toxin injection into the interior rectus muscles are those with small vertical deviations in the primary position (less than 10 prism diopters) that gets worse on down gaze. Because of the variable response of botulinum toxin injections, these patients must be willing to experience instability of ocular motility for up to 3 or 4 months postinjection and be willing to receive more than one injection in order to get adequate relief.

VIII. SURGICAL TREATMENT

After the vertical deviation has remained stable for 4–6 months, surgical intervention can be contemplated. Depending on the size, type, location, and magnitude of the deviation, there are many options available (Fig. 3). If the diplopia is mainly vertical in nature with very little torsion, then either an ipsilateral inferior oblique weakening procedure or a contralateral inferior rectus weakening procedure can be utilized. If there is marked superior oblique weakness and significant cyclotorsion, a superior oblique strengthening procedure will be necessary. If the diplopia is mainly torsional, superior oblique surgery such as a Harato-Ito procedure may be necessary. Ultimately combinations of all three procedures may be required.

Inferior oblique weakening procedures for superior oblique palsies involve either an inferior oblique myectomy or an inferior oblique recession. Both procedures are extremely safe in that they rarely overcorrect the deviation, will always provide some improvement in the patient's symptomatology, are equally

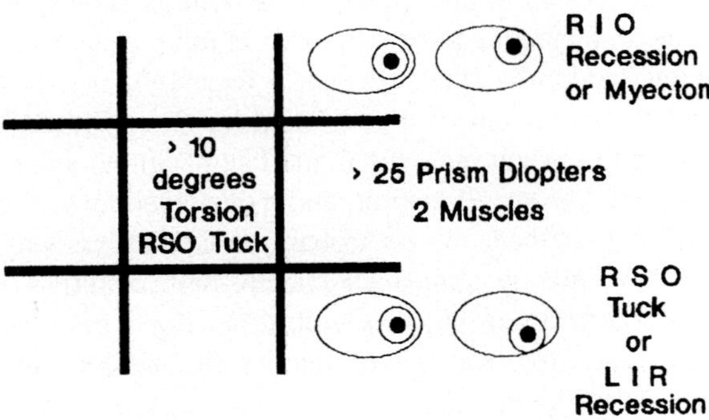

Figure 3 The surgical approach of a right fourth nerve palsy. A right inferior oblique recession or myectomy for a right hypertropia worse on up and left gaze. A right superior oblique tuck or left inferior rectus recession for a right hypertropia worse on down gaze. If the lateral deviation is greater than 25 prism diopters, both a right inferior oblique recession or myectomy and a left superior oblique tuck or inferior rectus recession needs to be performed. If greater than 10 degrees cyclotorsion, a right superior oblique tuck is needed.

effective in reducing a vertical deviation in the primary position by approximately 10 prism diopters, and can eliminate as much as 20–25 prism diopters in lateral horizontal gaze. Neither procedure will eliminate significant excyclotorsion. In reviewing my own experience and those of others, there is no advantage of one procedure over the other. Graded weakening of the inferior oblique appears to be of little value and the maximum surgery should be performed. Almost all patients will show a residual vertical deviation on lateral gaze indicating less than 100% effectiveness of these procedures.

An alternative to inferior oblique weakening procedures is a contralateral inferior rectus recession. This is useful in eliminating a small vertical deviation in the primary position that is worse in lateral and down gaze. The advantage of an inferior rectus recession is that it can be done with the adjustable suture technique that allows immediate postoperative manipulation in order to maximize a good result. Care must be taken not to overrecess the inferior rectus muscle as, unlike inferior oblique surgery, it can result in an overcorrection. I tend to reserve an inferior rectus recession for a small primary vertical deviation (<8 prism diopters), especially if it increases on down and lateral gaze.

If there is significant weakness of the superior oblique muscle combined with a torsional component or a very large vertical deviation on lateral gaze, a superior oblique tucking procedure is very effective. Superior oblique tucks are not widely used, as they are more complicated than inferior oblique weakening procedures and run the risk of overcorrection. A common postoperative complication from a superior oblique tuck is an iatrogenic Brown's syndrome from overtucking the tendon. There are no clear guidelines as to how much of the tendon should be tucked, but most surgeons agree that creating a small limitation in up gaze is the goal. After the superior oblique tendon has been tucked, a forced duction test can be done to assess ultimately how much of a restriction has been created. This technique involves grasping the eye at the medial and lateral limbal areas, retropulsing the globe, rotating the eye into adduction, and then elevation. If the eye cannot be elevated past the midline, the tendon is probably tucked excessively and needs to be adjusted. Postoperatively almost all patients will experience diplopia in up and lateral gaze that tends to improve with time. For a bilateral superior oblique palsy, it is very effective in eliminating the torsion and esodeviation on down gaze.

Individuals who have little or no vertical diplopia but cannot fuse because of excessive excylotropia will require a Harato-Ito procedure. The anterior portion of the superior oblique tendon controls mainly torsional movements of the eye, whereas the posterior portion involves depression and abduction. In such cases, the anterior portion of the tendon is split and advanced from underneath the superior rectus muscle to the superior border of the lateral rectus muscle of the involved eye. This procedure can also be done using the adjustable suture technique with good results.

IX. CONCLUSIONS

Diagnosis of fourth nerve palsies should be suspected in any patient who complains of vertical diplopia. By far the most common cause of a fourth nerve palsy is trauma (or congenital), which accounts for over 70% of the cases. The remainder of isolated fourth nerve palsies are generally not a sign of significant intracranial abnormality and are usually associated with microvascular disease. The workup is directed toward detecting treatable causes such as diabetes, hypertension, and collagen vascular disorders. The majority of acquired fourth nerve palsies will clear relatively quickly and symptoms are usually gone by 3 or 4 months. In those patients whose symptoms remain, treatment modalities can vary from prisms to botulinum toxin injections and, ultimately, surgery. Fortunately, the results of these therapeutic interventions are quite rewarding and the majority of patients can expect to get significant relief.

SELECTED READINGS

1. Carpenter MD, Sutin J, eds. Human neuroanatomy. 8th ed. Baltimore: Williams & Wilkins, 1983.
2. Ellis FD, Helveston EM. Superior oblique palsy: diagnosis and classification. In: strabismus surgery. Boston: Little, Brown, 1976:127–135.
3. Scott WE. Differential diagnosis of vertical muscle palsies. In: Helveston EM, et al., eds. New Orleans Symposium. St. Louis: Mosby, 1978:118–34.
4. Rucker CW. The causes of paralysis of the third, fourth and sixth cranial nerves. Am J Ophthalmol 1966; 61:1293–8.
5. Rush JA, Young BR. Paralysis of cranial nerves III, IV, and VI: cause and prognosis in 1000 cases. Arch Ophthalmol 1981; 99:76–9.
6. Jampolsky A. Management of vertical strabismus. In: Crawford JS, Flynn JT, Haik BG, et al., eds. Pediatric ophthalmology and strabismus: Transactions of the New Orleans Academy of Ophthalmology. New York: Raven Press, 1986:141–71.
7. Kraft SP, Scott WE. Masked bilateral superior oblique palsy, clinical features and diagnosis. J Pediatr Ophthalmol 1986; 23:264.

III

CAVERNOUS SINUS/ORBIT

21

Cavernous Sinus/Orbital Apex Syndrome

Lanning B. Kline
University of Alabama School of Medicine, Birmingham, Alabama

I. NOMENCLATURE

Cavernous sinus syndrome consists of a combination of ipsilateral neurological deficits, including oculomotor (III), trochlear (IV), and abducens (VI) nerve palsies, involvement of the ophthalmic (V^I) and occasionally maxillary (V^{II}) divisions of the trigeminal nerve, and oculosympathetic paralysis (Horner's syndrome). This syndrome has been given a variety of names, including superior orbital fissure syndrome, parasellar syndrome, and sphenocavernous syndrome. The term *orbital apex syndrome* is applied when there is optic nerve involvement in addition to cavernous sinus findings. Proptosis is often present, since the pathological process also involves orbital structures.

II. CLINICAL FEATURES

Because multiple cranial nerves are affected in cavernous sinus and orbital apex syndromes, patients present with a variety of clinical findings. Generally, not all cranial nerves are equally affected, and thus incomplete syndromes are the rule. The clinical features may be divided into five categories: (1) eyelid and pupil abnormalities, (2) extraocular muscle palsy, (3) orbital signs, (4) optic neuropathy, and (5) pain.

A. Eyelid and Pupil Abnormalities

Involvement of these structures is due to sympathetic or parasympathetic denervation. Oculosympathetic paralysis causes 2–3 mm of ptosis, 1–2 mm of "upside down" ptosis, and ipsilateral miosis. Cavernous sinus disease causes interruption of the third-order neuron of the oculosympathetic pathway. These fibers originate in the superior cervical ganglion and course alongside the extracranial and intracranial portions of the internal carotid artery forming the carotid plexus. Within the cavernous sinus, the sympathetic fibers join the ophthalmic division of the trigeminal nerve prior to entering the orbit. Involvement of the third-order neuron may be confirmed by topical hydroxyamphetamine hydrobromide (Paredrine) drops.

Oculomotor nerve dysfunction within the cavernous sinus may also lead to eyelid and pupillary abnormalities. Ptosis may be partial or complete. It may, at times, only be associated with superior rectus weakness; thus causing a "superior division third nerve palsy." This is due to the bifurcation of the ocular motor nerve into the superior and interior divisions either within the cavernous sinus or the superior orbital fissure.

Pupillary changes from parasympathetic involvement in cavernous sinus disease are usually minimal. This may be due to slow progression of most cavernous sinus processes, aberrant reinnervation of the iris sphincter, simultaneous occurrence of ipsilateral Horner's syndrome, or "sparing" of the inferior division of the oculomotor nerve. In cases of combined sympathetic and parasympathetic paralysis, the pupil is midposition and sluggishly reactive to both light and near stimuli.

Aberrant regeneration of the oculomotor nerve is thought to result from "miswiring" of the oculomotor fibers to the pupillary sphincter, extraocular muscles, and eyelid. Signs of misdirection are seen during recovery of an oculomotor nerve palsy, usually weeks to months after onset. Frequent causes include trauma or compression either from tumor or aneurysm. Occasionally, primary aberrant regeneration may occur in which insidious development of oculomotor nerve palsy is seen with accompanying signs of misdirection. Primary aberrant regeneration has only been reported with intracavernous lesions: meningioma, aneurysm, neurinoma.

B. Extraocular Muscle Palsy

Cavernous sinus disease is the most likely cause of simultaneous deficits in two or more ipsilateral ocular motor cranial nerves. Careful clinical testing is essential in evaluating such patients, with examination for sensory involvement along the ophthalmic and maxillary nerves. Early in the evolution of cavernous sinus/orbital apex disease, an ocular motor cranial nerve palsy may be isolated. The decision to pursue extensive evaluation must be based on clinical judgement. For example, if a patient with vasculopathic risk factors (e.g., hypertension, diabetes mellitus) presents with an isolated sixth nerve paresis, medical evaluation and careful follow-up appears warranted. If other signs of parasellar cranial nerve dysfunction appear, then thorough evaluation of the cavernous sinus is indicated.

C. Orbital Signs

Signs of orbital disease are unusual in cavernous sinus syndromes. The major exception is vascular causes, particularly fistulas of the cavernous sinus. Clinical findings include proptosis, at times pulsatile, chemosis, venous engorgement of the lids and neighboring face, arterialization of episcleral vessels, and retinal vascular changes, including venous engorgement and retinal hemorrhages. Carotid-cavernous fistula is characterized by obvious orbital changes and an audible bruit. Low-flow dural cavernous fistula may present in a more subtle fashion and requires a high index of suspicion for correct diagnosis. If orbital congestion is significant, ocular motility disorders may result from passive congestion of the extraocular muscles. In addition, elevated intraocular pressure may occur with development of secondary glaucoma.

Ophthalmological signs of cavernous sinus thrombosis include proptosis, orbital congestion, chemosis, ptosis, ophthalmoplegia, and corneal hypesthesia. At times the eyelids may develop a purplish hue due to venous congestion. Bilateral changes also suggest cavernous sinus thrombosis, indicating spread of infection to the contralateral side through connecting venous channels. This condition represents a potentially life-threatening disorder that necessitates prompt recognition and aggressive treatment.

D. Optic Neuropathy

Visual loss is not usually considered in a discussion of cavernous sinus syndrome, since the optic nerve and chiasm are located outside of the cavernous sinus. Nevertheless, these structures lie in close proximity. Disease processes of the superior orbital fissure may extend into the orbital apex and damage the optic nerve, or expanding lesions within the cavernous sinus may compress the intracranial optic nerve or chiasm.

Signs of optic nerve involvement include reduced visual acuity, defective color vision, and an afferent pupillary defect. Visual field abnormalities include central and nerve fiber bundle defects. Early in the clinical course, compressive optic neuropathy is characterized by a normal disc, with the eventual appearance of disc pallor within weeks to months. Impairment of orbital venous drainage, as in cavernous sinus fistula or thrombosis, may lead to optic disc edema and dilation and tortuosity of retinal vessels with associated retinal hemorrhages. The occurrence of central retinal artery occlusion with cavernous sinus syndrome is highly suggestive of an orbital vasculitis, and mucormycosis should be included in the differential diagnosis.

E. Pain

Retro-orbital pain may be the first indication of cavernous sinus disease. Characterizing the pain, as well as looking carefully for other signs and symptoms, may facilitate arriving at the correct diagnosis for the patient's painful ophthalmoplegia.

Pain is a typical finding of pituitary apoplexy, which may produce a cavernous sinus syndrome often accompanied by visual failure. The syndrome is composed of the triad of acute, severe bitemporal headaches, partial or complete ophthalmoplegia, and meningismus due to subarachnoid hemorrhage. Pain also is the hallmark of the Tolosa-Hunt syndrome, nonspecific granulomatous inflammation affecting the cavernous sinus. This pain usually begins subacutely, is constant and boring, and is well localized behind the affected eye. Intracavernous internal carotid artery aneurysm usually expands slowly and is associated with unilateral ophthalmoplegia and retro-orbital pain that is severe and throbbing. More insidious pain, which has a gnawing or burning quality, develops when the trigeminal nerve is invaded by a malignant process such as nasopharyngeal carcinoma. The pain frequently radiates to the forehead (ophthalmic nerve) or cheek (maxillary nerve).

Although periorbital pain is not always associated with cavernous sinus disease, its presence along with other cranial nerve abnormalities should alert the clinician to possible disease in the parasellar region.

III. ETIOLOGY

The causes of cavernous sinus/orbital apex syndrome are listed in Table 1. Certain facts in the patient's history may aid in narrowing the potential causes, such as a history of craniocerebral trauma, or a history of systemic disease, possibly malignant, infectious, or a connective tissue disorder. Physical examination may demonstrate signs of orbital congestion, suggestive of a vascular cause (fistula), whereas a skin eruption along the distribution of the ophthalmic nerve would support the diagnosis of herpes zoster. Patients who are diabetic or immunosuppressed or patients with cavernous sinus syndrome accompanied by blindness should be aggressively evaluated for mucormycosis.

IV. DIAGNOSTIC STUDIES

Table 2 summarizes the diagnostic studies of particular value in evaluating cavernous sinus/orbital apex syndrome. Current neuroimaging studies of mag-

Table 1 Causes of Cavernous Sinus/Orbital Apex Syndrome

Trauma
Vascular
intracavernous carotid artery aneurysm
posterior cerebral artery aneurysm
carotid-cavernous fistula
carotid-cavernous thrombosis
Neoplasm
primary intracranial tumor
pituitary adenoma
meningioma
craniopharyngioma
sarcoma
neurofibroma
gasserian ganglion neuroma
epidermoid
primary cranial tumor
chordoma
chondroma
giant-cell tumor
local metastases
nasopharyngeal tumor
cylindroma
adamantinoma
squamous cell carcinoma
distant metastases
lymphoma
multiple myeloma
carcinomatous metastases
Inflammation
bacterial: sinusitis; mucocele; periostitis
viral: herpes zoster
fungal: mucormycosis
spirochetal: treponema pallidum
mycobacterial: mycobacterium tuberculosis
unknown cause: sarcoidosis, Wegener's granulomatosis, eosinophilic granuloma, Tolosa-Hunt syndrome

Table 2 Diagnostic Evaluation of Cavernous Sinus/Orbital Apex Syndrome

Hematologic tests
complete blood count
erythrocyte sedimentation rate
serum chemistry
fluorescent treponemal antibody test
antinuclear antibody
lupus erythematosus cell preparation
serum protein electrophoresis
human immunodeficiency virus
Cerebrospinal fluid
opening pressure
cell count and differential
protein
glucose
culture: bacterial, fungal, mycobacterial
serology
cytology
Neuroradiological studies
magnetic resonance imaging
computed tomography
magnetic resonance angiography
cerebral angiography
Nasopharynx
examination
biopsy

netic resonance imaging (MR) and computed tomography (CT) have revolutionized evaluation of cavernous sinus disease. These studies currently allow direct visualization of the orbital apex and parasellar region. MR is the initial study that should be done on all patients suspected of cavernous sinus/orbital apex disease. Multiple projections (axial, coronal, and sagittal), thin tomographic slices, and contrast (gadolinium) enhancement are essential in evaluation of this area. MR will provide valuable information regarding the soft tissue structures, vascular anatomy, and paranasal sinuses. MR angiography provides a noninvasive method to detect cavernous sinus fistulas and aneurysms. If bone detail is required, the patient should undergo cranial CT scanning.

After obtaining neuroimaging studies, further patient evaluation may be required. Additional tests are summarized in Table 2. Hematological studies are helpful in detecting infectious, inflammatory, and neoplastic disease metastatic to the cavernous sinus. Careful examination of the peripheral blood smear is required when looking for leukemia or lymphoma. Cerebrospinal fluid testing may also provide valuable data regarding potential infectious or neoplastic causes of cavernous sinus syndrome. Multiple cytological studies may be required to detect carcinomatous or lymphomatous invasion of the central nervous system. Prior to the advent of current neuroimaging techniques, nasopharyngeal carcinoma often proved to be an elusive diagnosis. This neoplasm extends through basal foramina of the skull producing painful ophthalmoplegia. With the availability of detailed examination of subcranial soft tissue with MR or CT, the need for "blind" biopsy of the nasopharynx now seems to be rare.

Imitators of cavernous sinus/orbital apex disorders are summarized in Table 3. Each may produce some combination of ophthalmoplegia, visual loss, and pain. As with almost any eye movement disorder, myasthenia must be kept in the differential diagnosis. Ocular dysthyroidism and orbital disease should produce typical findings with neuroimaging studies. Diseases of the paranasal sinuses with spread into the orbit, particularly mucormycosis, must be vigilantly looked for, since they represent a potentially life-threatening disease. On occasion, diabetic ophthalmoplegia may present with simultaneous paralysis of multiple, ipsilateral ocular motor nerves. Often painful, this condition is not responsive to steroid therapy. Although giant cell arteritis is a well recognized cause of sudden visual loss, it may also produce painful ophthalmoplegia. This form of arteritis leads to ischemic necrosis of the extraocular muscles. Migrainous ophthalmoplegia is a rare and poorly understood form of complicated migraine. It typically occurs in a child or young adult affecting any of the ocular motor cranial nerves and may be recurrent. Posterior fossa aneurysms may cause either

Table 3 Conditions Simulating Disease of the Cavernous Sinus/Orbital Apex

Myasthenia gravis
Ocular dysthyroidism
Orbital disease
inflammation
infection
neoplasm
trauma
Diabetic ophthalmoplegia
Giant cell arteritis
Migrainous ophthalmoplegia
Posterior fossa aneurysm
Botulism
Fisher's syndrome

acute painful ophthalmoplegia (posterior communicating artery) or a subacute or more chronic ophthalmoplegia (basilar artery aneurysm). Botulism may produce ptosis, ophthalmoplegia, and poorly reactive pupils in a systemically ill patient with nausea and vomiting associated with facial, pharyngeal, and generalized proximal muscle weakness. Fisher's syndrome is a variant of Guillain-Barré syndrome characterized by the triad of ataxia, areflexia, and ophthalmoplegia. Involvement of pupils and accommodation may also occur.

V. TREATMENT

Treatment of patients with cavernous sinus/orbital apex disease must be done on a case by case basis depending on the specific etiology. In general, a "team approach" is required, including a variety of specialties: internal medicine, infectious disease, neurology, neurosurgery, radiation therapy, oncology, otolaryngology. One potentially life-threatening condition requiring emergent therapy is mucormycosis. Aggressive debridement of the involved paranasal sinuses should be coupled with systemic and at times local therapy with amphotericin B. Consultations with oncology and radiation therapy will provide valuable help in treating neoplastic causes of cavernous sinus/orbital apex disease. In general, metastatic malignancy to the parasellar area has a very poor prognosis, with mean survival less than 1 year. Interventional neuroradiology has revolutionized the therapy for fistulas and aneurysms of the cavernous sinus. An arterial or venous approach with embolization provides direct therapy for both low- and high-flow fistulas and results in a permanent cure.

The ophthalmologist is in a unique position to direct both diagnostic evaluation and therapeutic techniques in diseases of the cavernous sinus and orbital apex. In addition, ophthalmological follow-up will be essential in monitoring the patient's clinical response to treatment.

SELECTED READINGS

1. Bosley TM, Schatz NJ. Clinical diagnosis of cavernous sinus syndromes. Neurol Clin 1983; 1:929–53.
2. Harris FS, Rhoton AL. Anatomy of the cavernous sinus. A microsurgical study. J Neurosurg 1976; 45:169–80.
3. Kline LB: The Tolosa-Hunt syndrome. Surv Ophthalmol 1982; 27:79–95.

22

Fine-Needle Aspiration Biopsy of the Orbit

Dennis C. Matzkin and Thomas L. Slamovits
Albert Einstein College of Medicine and Montefiore Medical Center, Bronx, New York

Fine-needle aspiration biopsy (FNAB) is an accepted office procedure for cytological diagnosis in various anatomical sites, including breast, thyroid, lung, and prostate. In the mid 1970s, the application to orbital masses was popularized in Europe (1,2), and subsequently a large series consisting of 50 cases of orbital fine-needle aspiration biopsies (OFNAB) was reported by Kennerdell et al. in the United States in 1980 (3). This series was expanded on with a report of 156 cases in 1985 (4). Although recognizing the limitations of a cytological rather than histological diagnosis, we believe that in the appropriate clinical setting, in particular when neoplastic disease is suspected, orbital fine-needle aspiration biopsy is an appropriate and useful diagnostic technique.

I. ADVANTAGES

The specific advantage of OFNAB is that it is relatively safe and frequently avoids unnecessary surgery. The diagnostic yield of OFNAB in experienced hands is high—in the order of 80% when the clinical and radiological features of the orbital lesion is considered (4–6). It is generally a well-tolerated procedure with no need for local anesthesia or sedation. It has a relatively low level of invasion and low morbidity. It is cost effective and saves operating room–related expenses. The procedure is quick and the cytological interpretation is generally available in a short period of time. This speed of diagnosis can relieve patient anxiety, aid the clinician in convincing the patient of the necessity of immediate treatment or hospitalization, and streamline patient management. OFNAB has no adverse effects on the natural behavior of the tumor. Should it fail to provide a diagnosis, open orbital biopsy can then be embarked on to provide a tissue diagnosis. FNAB does not prevent a surgical biopsy because the needle tract does not change the characteristics of the tumor or the orbital anatomy.

II. DISADVANTAGES/LIMITATIONS

False-negative results will occur if the needle tip is not within the substance of the lesion. Misleading information may be obtained if the inflammatory component adjacent to the tumor is aspirated. Fibrous lesions cannot be readily sampled because of the scanty cellularity. In 156 cases of OFNAB in the Kennerdell series (4), 28 (18%) specimens were inadequate for interpretation and 3 gave incorrect results. Two nonspecific inflammations were identified as malignancies, and one malignancy (adenocarcinoma) was identified as nonspecific inflammation.

OFNAB provides a cytological and not a histological diagnosis. The distinction between benign and malignant lymphoid lesions is often extremely difficult to make on FNAB. The cytological report will rarely commit to a diagnosis of "benign lymphoid hyperplasia" or "lymphoma," and a question of malignancy will often still remain. Under such circumstance, an open biopsy is indicated in order to make a histological diagnosis and will also enable B- and T-cell populations to be determined.

Lacrimal gland lesions are often difficult to interpret cytologically. OFNAB in this site should be avoided unless the clinical picture and radiological appearance are almost diagnostic of a particular lesion (e.g., carcinoma) and confirmation is desired. If on clinical grounds a benign mixed tumor of the lacrimal gland is suspected, an excisional biopsy is the accepted method of treatment. In such cases, there is no need for prior histological or cytological confirmation of the diagnosis.

III. INDICATIONS

OFNAB is indicated in patients with an accessible orbital mass suspected of being metastatic, especially large unresectable lesions. It is a valuable technique in patients who are not good surgical candidates, especially where the risk for general anesthesia is high.

The objective of performing OFNAB is to establish the presence of a malignant process, and if the specific diagnosis cannot be made, to narrow down the differential. At times histological sections can be obtained via cell blocks, which may allow a more definitive diagnosis.

The greatest yield for positive diagnosis in OFNAB is in suspected cases of cancer. In the series by Kennerdell et al. (4), the most frequently diagnosed lesions were metastatic malignant orbital neoplasms, most of which were undifferentiated neoplasms or adenocarcinomas. Lymphoid lesions are readily diagnosed on OFNAB, but although the distinction between benign and malignant lymphoid lesions can be difficult to assess from a cytological specimen, the exclusion of another variety of neoplasm is useful. For lymphoid lesions, the demonstration of immunoglobulin light chains can help establish the diagnosis of a B-cell neoplasm. T-cell lymphomas can show loss of certain types of antigens, but these findings are not per se indicative of lymphoma (7,8). With the use of special immunoperoxidase staining, more accurate cytological identification is now possible in certain clinical situations. For metastatic neoplasm, "marker" studies can, in a few specific instances, establish the type of tumor; for example, prostatic specific antigen is present in prostatic carcinoma, neuronal specific enolase in neuroblastoma, and desmin in primary orbital rhabdomyosarcoma. Consultation with the cytopathologist with regard to the differential diagnosis based on the clinical impression may help direct the cytologist toward staining for a specific immunohistochemical marker. Despite advancement in the field of immunohistochemistry, most metastatic tumors cannot be classified by markers as to site of origin with certainty.

OFNAB is particularly rewarding and may be indicated under the following circumstances:

1. Metastatic lesions to the orbit and orbital lesions in which treatment is not expected to be surgical excision.
2. Recurrence of a previously treated orbital tumor. OFNAB can readily confirm the nature of the mass, especially if previous histological sections are available for comparison.
3. Small posterior apical lesions that are difficult to biopsy and associated with a greater incidence of hemorrhage. A successful biopsy in such an instance will avoid difficult surgery and most likely reduce morbidity.
4. Small intraconal masses that also are difficult to localize and hazardous to biopsy. Successful OFNAB has been described using computed tomographic (CT) scan to localize optic nerve meningiomas, astrocytoma, and optic nerve leukemic infiltrate (9). Similarly, orbital ultrasound has been used, but the probe is often found to be an impediment while simultaneously trying to localize an orbital mass with a needle.
5. Cavernous sinus lesions with spread into the orbital apex are amenable to OFNAB and has been used successfully to diagnose metastatic breast carcinoma (10), adenocarcinoma, and lymphoid lesions. Successful diag-

nosis of sino-orbital aspergillosis has been reported with CT-guided transorbital FNAB of the anterior cavernous sinus (11).
6. Where the distinction between nonspecific orbital inflammation (orbital pseudotumor) and orbital cellulitis is unclear.

IV. RELATIVE CONTRAINDICATIONS

1. Orbital lesions that are easily accessible surgically and that are likely to be biopsied or excised safely; that is, an anteriorly located lesion.
2. Lesions that are likely to be treated by total surgical excision; for example, neuroimaging suggests that the lesion is a cavernous hemangioma or schwannoma (neurilemoma).
3. Lesions in which cytology alone is likely to be nondiagnostic (e.g., cavernous hemangioma) or in which cytologic diagnosis may be inadequate (e.g., tumors requiring histological pattern such as lymphoid lesions).
4. Highly vascular lesions (suspected arteriovenous malformation).
5. Patients on anticoagulants.
6. Patients unlikely to cooperate in the office. Such patients might include the disabled, the elderly, or children, although good results (87% positive diagnostic yield) were reported in 15 children aged 1–15 years (6).

V. CASE HISTORIES (1–7)

Clinical examples best illustrate the potential usefulness of OFNAB.

Case 1

A 67-year-old man without any past medical history of malignancy presented with proptosis. CT scan showed a lytic lesion involving the lateral orbital wall with a surrounding soft tissue component extending into the posterior orbit (Fig. 1). OFNAB revealed sheets of plasma cells that narrowed the differential diagnosis to plasmacytoma versus multiple myeloma; a systemic workup confirmed the latter.

Case 2

A 55-year-old woman with a prior history of breast carcinoma presented with proptosis. CT scan revealed a hyperostotic lesion of the lateral orbital wall with extension into the posterior orbit (Fig. 2A). Neuroradiological differentiation between meningioma and metastatic carcinoma was not possible. OFNAB revealed numerous meningoendothelial whorl cells and absence of any malignant cells (Fig. 2B), and a diagnosis of meningioma was confidently made.

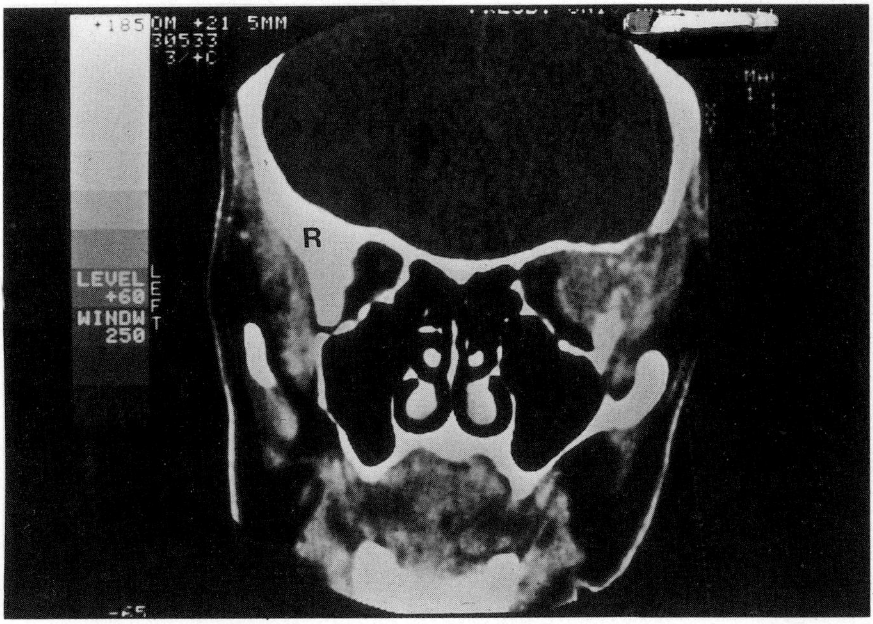

Figure 1 Coronal CT scan of a 67-year-old man demonstrating a lytic lesion involving the lateral wall of the left orbit. OFNAB revealed sheets of plasma cells compatible with the diagnosis of multiple myeloma.

Case 3

A 64-year old woman with a similar history and CT scan (Fig. 3) to case 2 yielded malignant cells on OFNAB suggestive of metastatic breast carcinoma. This led to a completely different treatment plan than the preceding case. In both cases 2 and 3, open biopsy of the orbit was avoided.

Case 4

An 81-year-old woman had undergone complete surgical excision of an adenoid cystic carcinoma of the lacrimal gland. Several years later she developed breast carcinoma. Subsequently she developed a superotemporal orbital mass with bony involvement (Fig. 4). Clinically, differentiation between metastatic breast carcinoma or recurrent lacrimal tumor could not be made. OFNAB revealed that she had recurrent lacrimal gland carcinoma and not metastatic breast carcinoma. The cytology of the OFNAB was compared with the histology of the original

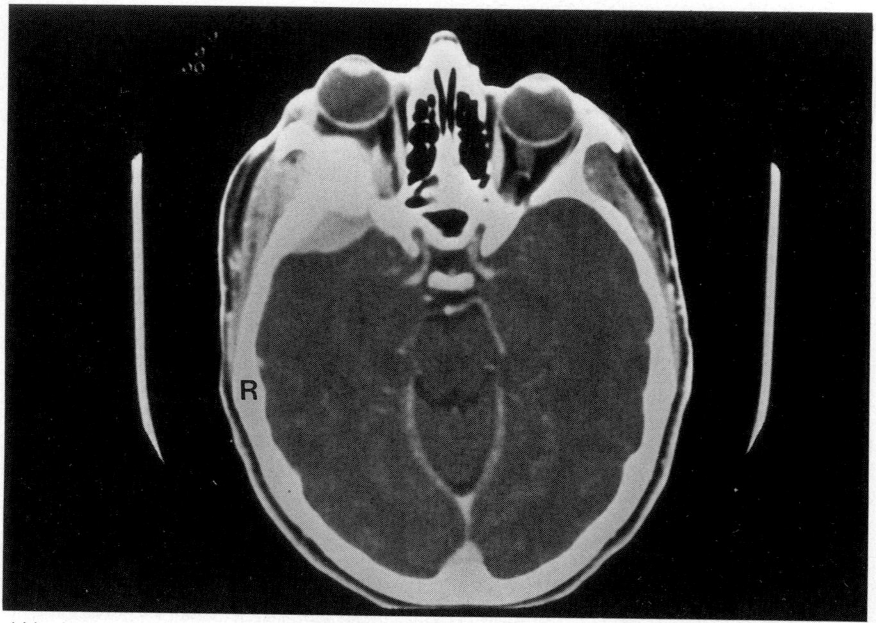

(A)

Figure 2 (A) Axial CT scan of a 55-year-old woman with a prior history of breast carcinoma demonstrates a lesion involving the right orbit adjacent to the lateral rectus muscle with hyperostosis of the lateral orbital wall. (B) Light microscopy from the OFNAB specimen demonstrates meningoendothelial whorl cells and absence of malignant cells compatible with the diagnosis of meningioma.

malignant lacrimal gland specimen and to that of the breast tumor and allowed a confident diagnosis of lacrimal gland tumor recurrence.

Case 5

An 80-year-old woman presented with the acute onset of a painful orbital apex syndrome unassociated with trauma or any underlying systemic disease. The clinical impression was that of either orbital cellulitis or pseudotumor. There was no evidence of either an external source of infection or sinus disease, and blood cultures were negative. CT scan failed to demonstrate an orbital mass or bony abnormalities, and the paranasal sinuses were clear. OFNAB revealed polymorphonuclear neutrophils with no lymphocytes or plasma cells. Gram-positive cocci in clusters were identified and subsequent cultures yielded *Staphylococcus aureus*. This rapid diagnosis of orbital cellulitis secondary to a presumed endogenous septicemia allowed prompt institution of medical treatment.

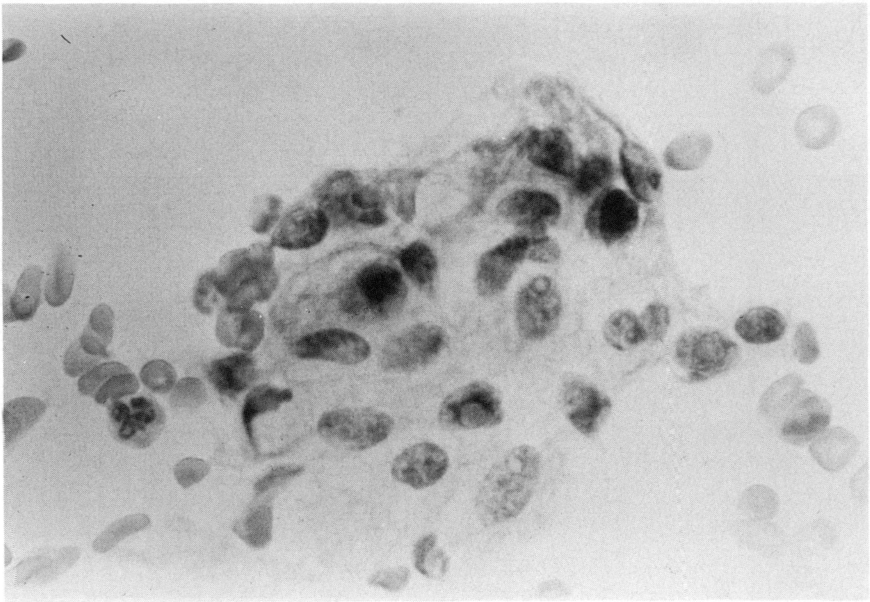

(B)

Case 6 (12)

A 3.5-year-old girl being treated for acute lymphoblastic leukemia was noted to have a right orbital mass on CT scan (Fig. 5A). The patient's elevated blood pressure raised the suspicion of neuroblastoma. OFNAB demonstrated rosettelike arrangements of cells with fibrillar cytoplasmic processors suggesting neuroblastoma (Fig. 5B). The tumor cells were antineuronal-specific enolase positive but common acute lymphoblastic leukemia antigen negative, which was consistent with neuroblastoma and not acute lymphoblastic leukemia. Further workup revealed a right suprarenal mass, as well as positive urinary catecholamines, vanillylmandelic acid, homovanillic acid, and metanephrines. Based on the OFNAB, the original diagnosis of acute lymphatic leukemia was revised in favor of neuroblastoma.

Case 7

A 74-year-old previously healthy man presented with diplopia and proptosis. CT scan showed hyperostotic lesions involving both orbits (Fig. 6A). OFNAB of the left orbit revealed malignant cells (Fig. 6B), which were acid phosphotase positive, establishing the diagnosis of metastatic prostatic carcinoma. Further workup confirmed the primary tumor as prostatic cancer.

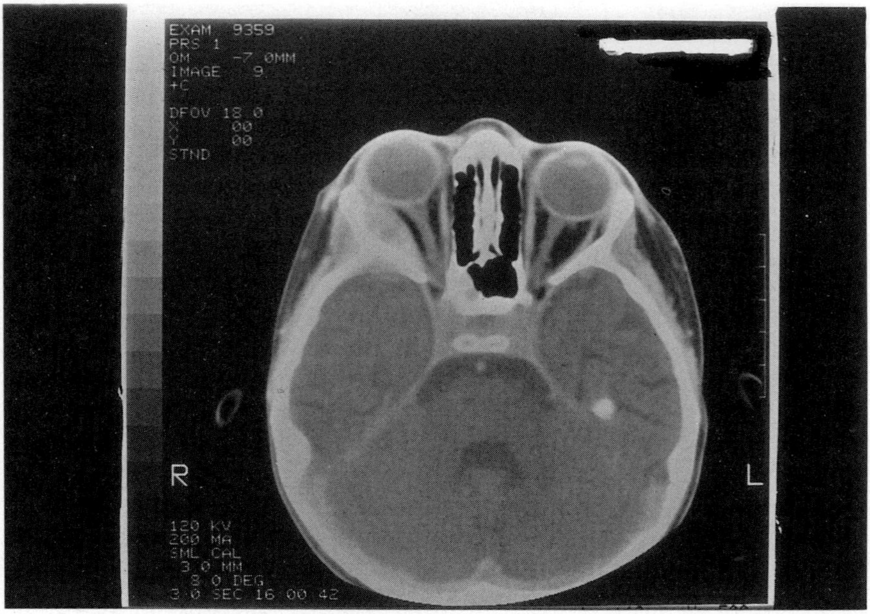

Figure 3 Axial CT scan of a 64-year-old woman with a history of breast carcinoma demonstrates a right orbital lesion with a soft tissue density surrounding an area of moderate hyperostosis of the adjacent orbital wall. OFNAB yielded malignant cells consistent with the diagnosis of metastatic breast carcinoma.

Case 8

A 10-year-old girl with proptosis underwent surgical biopsy for a CT-demonstrated anterosuperior orbital mass (Fig. 7). The tumor was very mucinous in content and easily crushed on attempted removal. At the time of surgery, a simultaneous OFNAB was obtained. The OFNAB revealed malignant cells suggesting rhabdomyosarcoma or neuroblastoma. Special stains with desmin led to the diagnosis of rhabdomysarcoma. Subsequent EM studies confirmed the diagnosis.

VI. SPECIFIC REQUIREMENTS

1. Complete familiarity and surgical experience pertaining to the anatomy of the orbit
2. Comfort with the clinical and radiological differential diagnosis

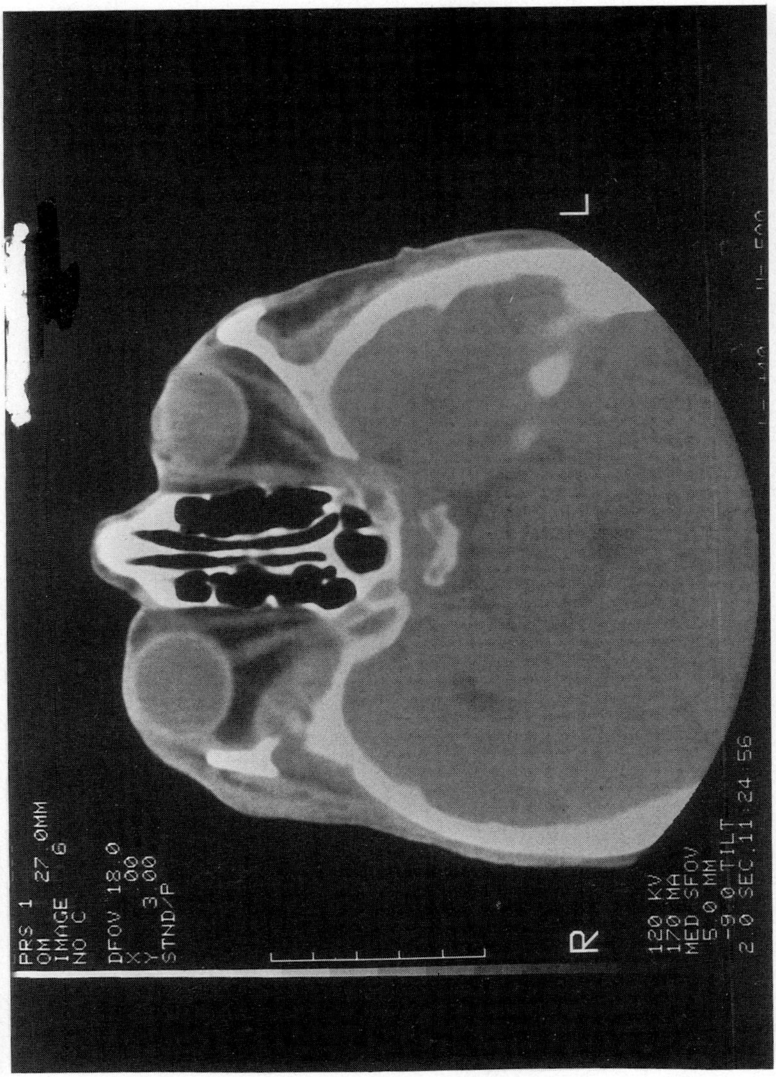

Figure 4 **CT scan of an 81-year-old woman with a history of adenoid cystic carcinoma of the lacrimal gland and subsequent breast carcinoma several years later. The axial view demonstrates a soft tissue mass in the lateral orbit with adjacent hyperostosis and extension of the mass into the temporal fossa through a defect in the orbital wall. OFNAB of the right orbit enabled a diagnosis of malignant lacrimal gland tumor to be made and ruled out metastatic breast carcinoma.**

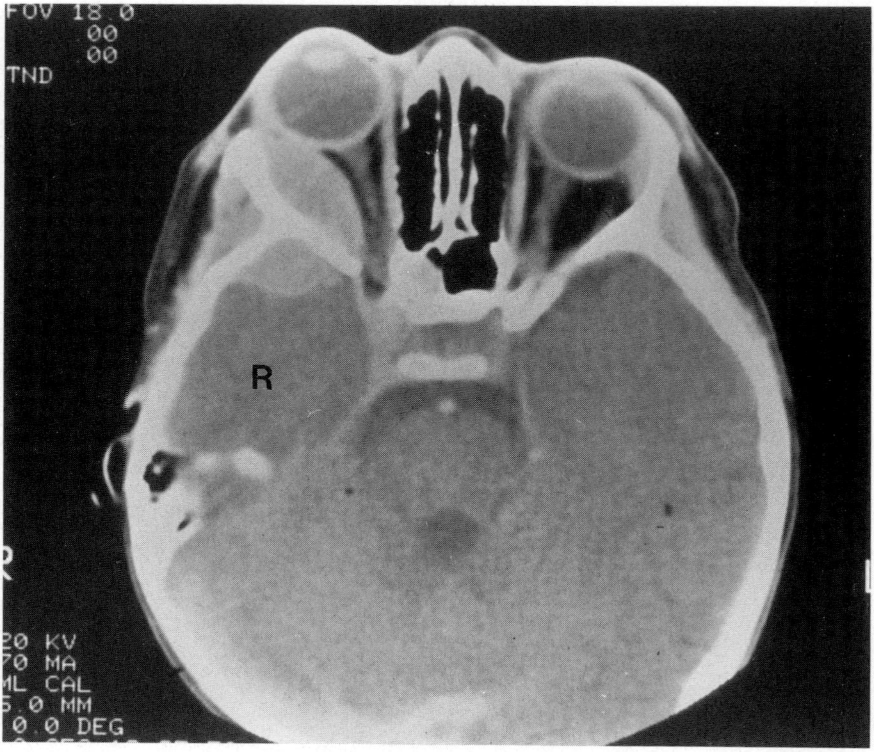

(A)

Figure 5 (A) Axial CT scan of a 3.5-year-old girl treated for lymphoblastic leukemia demonstrates a right orbital mass involving the lateral orbital wall and sphenoid wing. (B) Light microscopy from the OFNAB specimen of the above patient shows malignant small tumor cells in clusters with rosette formation characteristic of neuroblastoma. Special stains with antineuronal-specific enolase confirmed the diagnosis, and the original diagnosis of lymphoblastic leukemia was revised.

3. A team consisting of the following:
   a. Orbitologist (neuro-ophthalmologist, oculoplastic surgeon/orbital surgeon)
   b. Cytopathologist and technical support staff
   c. Neuroradiologist and state of the art neuroradiological facility
4. Familiarity in technique of OFNAB
5. Understanding the limitations of the procedure
6. Familiarity of the complications of the procedure and management thereof

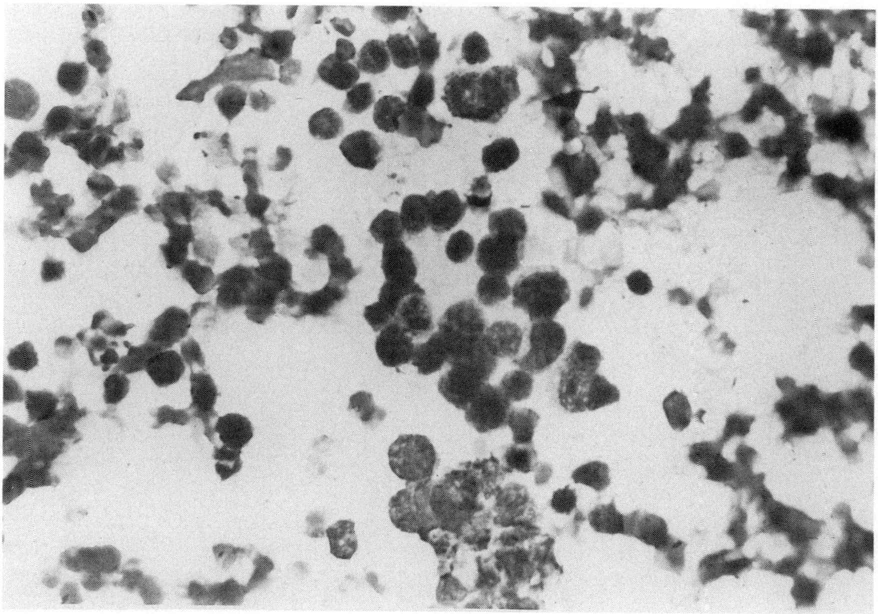

(B)

VII. TECHNIQUE

The procedure is performed in the office and no monitoring is usually required. Orbital CT or MRI scans are reviewed. A cytology laboratory technician with appropriate slides and fixatives are at hand. The patient is positioned comfortably in an examination chair with the head firmly positioned against the head-rest. Periorbital local anesthetic is avoided, as this causes orbital swelling and distortion and necessitates an extra needle penetration.

A 3.75-cm (1.5-inch) 25-gauge needle for adults or a 2.5-cm (1-inch) needle for shallow orbits and children is loaded into a 20-ml syringe that is attached in turn to a pistol-grip handle (Aspir-gun pistol grip, Everset Co., Linden, NJ). This allows a one-handed technique of aspiration while the other hand is free to stabilize the globe and localize the mass if palpable. Extraconal tumors are often large and their location within the orbit is not difficult to locate with the needle. For smaller tumors and those within the intraconal space, localization using B-scan ultrasound (13) or CT scan (14) has been found useful by some clinicians. Some surgeons prefer to place the needle into the tumor mass prior to attachment to the pistol-grip syringe for greater sensitivity and accuracy.

The needle is introduced into the orbital mass without local anesthesia and without pressure on the plunger or within the syringe. When the tip of the needle is felt to be in representative tissue, the surgeon aspirates by applying pressure

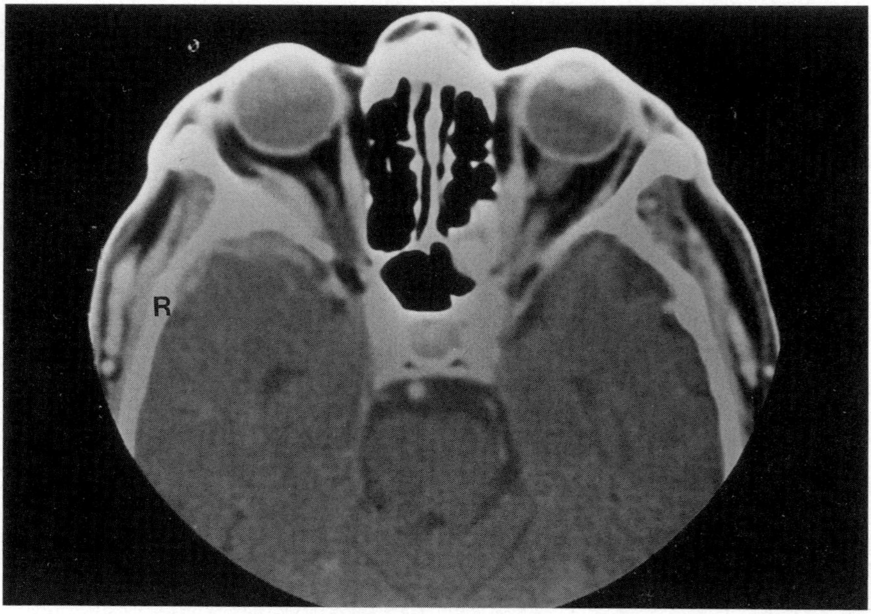

(A)

Figure 6 (A) CT scan of a previously healthy 74-year-old man who presented with double vision. The axial view demonstrates a medially displaced right lateral rectus with adjacent hyperostosis, as well as hyperostosis of the left orbital apex and medial wall. (B) Light microscopy from the OFNAB specimen of the left orbit of the above patient demonstrates malignant cells that were acid phosphotase positive consistent with the diagnosis of prostatic cancer. Further work-up confirmed this diagnosis.

to the trigger of the syringe. Simultaneously, the physician moves the needle back and forth within the tumor, minimally angled in different planes in an attempt to shear representative cells from the mass. During this to-and-fro motion, a vacuum is maintained within the syringe. Aspiration pressure is released before the needle is removed from the mass.

Preparation of the biopsy specimen requires skill and experience and should be done by a technician with the necessary skills. The needle is removed from the syringe. Air is drawn into the syringe, the needle repositioned into the same air-filled syringe, and the contents, with the specimen in the hub of the needle, squirted onto a glass slide. For "routine" studies the specimen is immediately spread with a second slide, fixed in 95% alcohol, and stained according to the Papanicolaou technique. Aspirate for special stains or lymphocyte studies may

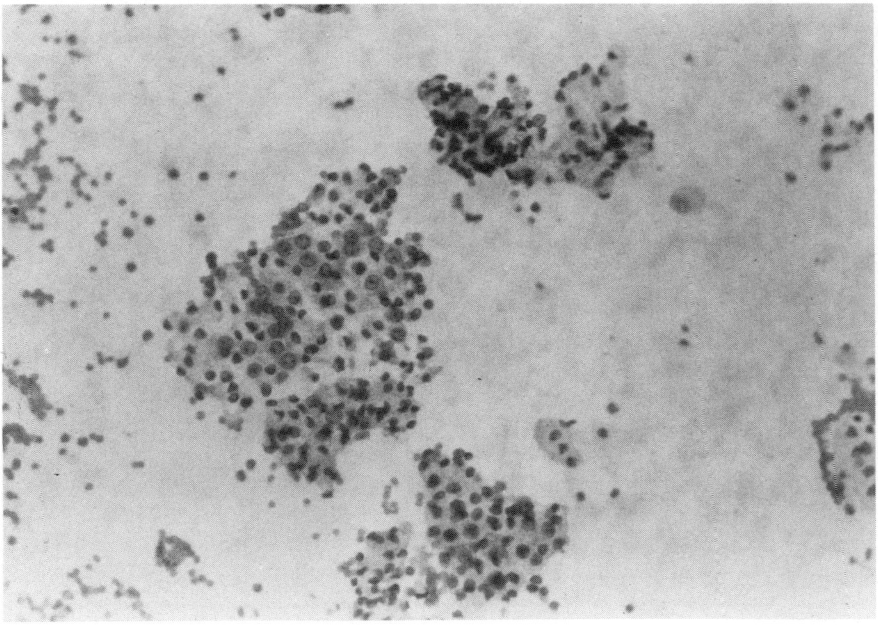

(B)

require other preparation. Any material remaining in the aspirate needle is removed and fixed for at least 20 min with 4% formaldehyde and then submitted as a cell block. The material is embedded in paraffin so that hematoxylin-eosin histological sections can be prepared.

Special stains can be planned for in advance based on preoperative suspicion. Examples of useful immunohistochemical stains include acid phosphotase, neuronal enolase, and desmin. Gram and Giemsa stains are used to identify bacteria and fungi in selected cases.

VIII. RISK FACTORS

1. Noncompliant patients such as children and elderly individuals who are unable to cooperate with instructions or requests to be relatively still.
2. Patients with bleeding tendencies are at risk for severe retrobulbar hemorrhage.
3. High myopes with posterior staphylomas are at risk for posterior globe perforation, especially if an intraconal mass is targeted.
4. Tumor Location:
   a. Lesions at the orbital apex are at risk for vital structure damage in particular the optic nerve, orbital arteries, and nerves. A long needle,

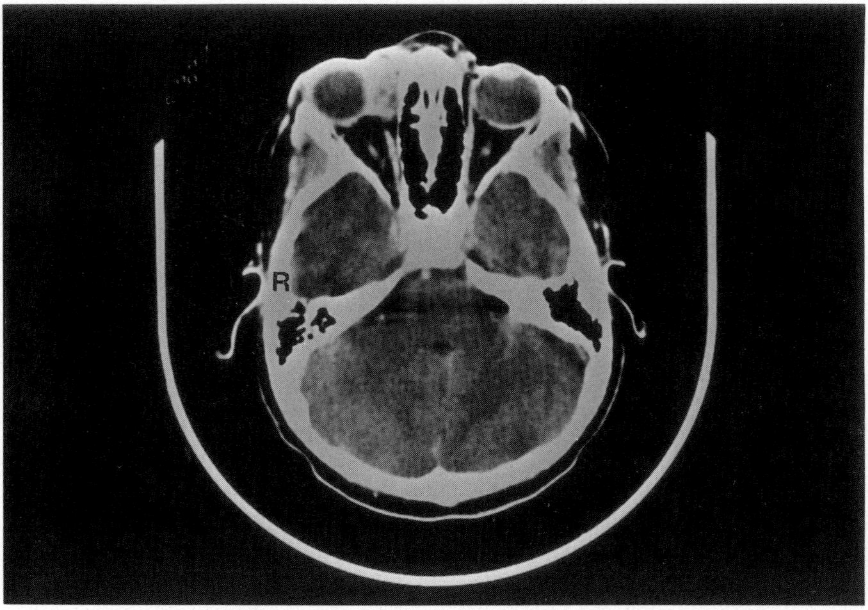

Figure 7 Axial CT scan of a 10-year-old girl with rapidly progressive proptosis demonstrates an anteromedially located solid mass with a cystic component. OFNAB performed at the time of a surgical biopsy, revealed malignant cells compatible with the diagnosis of rhabdomyosarcoma.

>4 cm (1.75 in) should not be used, since they can traverse the superior orbital fissure into the cavernous sinus with potential for serious sequelae.

b. Anterior located tumors of the muscle cone are at greater risk for globe penetration, especially if a superior approach is used. The superior orbital rim might limit the appropriate angulation necessary to biopsy such a lesion.

IX. COMPLICATIONS

Complications of FNAB are usually not serious, are reversible, and generally do not require intervention. Mild discomfort and a small retrobulbar hemorrhage account for the large majority of the complications. Severe complications are rare. In an uncontrolled survey by Lui involving 138 FNAB performed by 98 ophthalmologists, only 10 complications were reported (15). Diffuse retrobulbar hemorrhage occurred in seven patients, one patient had a ptosis, one a motility disturbance, and one a permanent scar. In the same report, a second group of 14 patients (from an unknown pool of patients) were seen in consultation because of complications arising from OFNAB. The complications in this group of patients included three orbital hemorrhages, one resulting in no light perception, two perforated globes, two motility defects, one ptosis, and three cases of blindness. Three cases of death occurred in this group. The deaths were presumed to have been due to an entirely inappropriate technique using needles longer than 5 cm (2 in.) that penetrated into the cavernous sinus though the superior orbital fissure causing meningitis and brain abscess. Although the serious complications such as death reported in this survey are of extreme concern, as pointed out by Kennerdell in the discussion following the paper, specific case details in the survey were lacking. Indeed, if the guidelines of experienced exponents of OFNAB are adhered to, complications should be minimal.

Retrobulbar hemorrhage is an expected complication (incidence approximately 10%) but should not lead to permanent sequelae.

Ocular perforation is a real risk, particularly to those unfamiliar with approaching the posterior orbit from all four quadrants. In the Kennerdell series of 156 patients (4), only two perforations occurred; both while the surgeon was trying to approach a deep orbital tumor from directly above the globe.

Seeding of tumor along the needle tract with the use of a fine needle is a complication that appears more of theoretical than of practical concern. The experience of investigators performing FNAB in a variety of other organs, including lung, prostate gland, salivary gland, and breast, suggests that the incidence of tract seeding is very small, with only isolated cases being reported (16). After experiencing one case of needle-tract seeding following FNAB of the liver, Glaser et al. (17) found 11 published reports of needle-tract seeding. It is felt that implantation metastases from needles with diameters over 1 mm might be more frequent (18), possibly because tumor cells and stroma are dragged into the channel and can support tumor proliferation (19). It is therefore recommended that a thin 0.6- to 0.9-mm needle diameter be used to minimize the risk of tract seeding.

X. CONCLUSIONS

Orbital fine needle aspiration biopsy is an effective, low cost, diagnostic tool. It can expedite patient care by avoiding invasive open biopsy and the morbidity associated with surgery and anesthesia. OFNAB is not intended for the occasional orbitologist. For it to be fully and accurately utilized, the clinician must understand not only the strengths and weaknesses of the procedure, but also the technical difficulties involved in obtaining diagnostic material. Patient selection and tumor characteristics will result in an accurate diagnostic yield in approximately 80% of patients. It is specifically recommended in cases of suspected metastatic malignancies, for recurrences of tumor and more rarely for primary orbital carcinoma and orbital. If OFNAB should fail to be diagnostic, further surgical exploration can be performed without undue disadvantage.

ACKNOWLEDGMENT

This work was supported in part by an unrestricted grant to the Department of Ophthalmology, Montefiore Medical Center/Albert Einstein College of Medicine, Bronx, NY, from Research to Prevent Blindness, Inc.

REFERENCES

1. Schyberg E. Fine needle biopsy of orbital tumors. Acta Ophthalmol (Copenh) 1975; 125 (Suppl.):11.
2. Westman-Naeser S, Naeser P. Tunors of the orbit diagnosed by fine needle biopsy. Acta Ophthalol 1978; 56:969–76.
3. Kennerdell JS, Dekker A, Johnson BL. Orbital fine needle aspiration biopsy: the results of its use in 50 patients. Neuro Ophthalmology 1980; 1:117–21.
4. Kennerdell JS, Slamovits TL, Decker A, Johnson BL. Orbital fine-needle aspiration biopsy. Am J Ophthalmol 1985; 99:547–51.
5. Tijl JWM, Koorneef L. Fine needle aspiration biopsy in orbital tumors. Br J Ophthalmol 1991; 75:491–2.
6. Arora R, Betharia SM. Fine needle aspiration of pediatric orbital tumors. Orbit 1988; 7:115–20.
7. Surhland MJ, Wieczorek R: Fine needle aspiration biopsy in the diagnosis of lymphoma. Cancer Invest 1991; 9:61–8.
8. Robey SS, Cafferty LL, Beschorner WE et al. Acta Cytol 1987; 31:453–9.
9. Czerniak B, Woyke S, Daniel B, et al. Diagnosis of orbital tumors by aspiration biopsy guided by computerized tomogaphy. Cancer 1984; 54:2385–9.
10. Slamovits TL, Cahill KV, Sibony PA, Dekker A, Johnson BL. Orbital fine needle aspiration biopsy on patients with cavernous sinus syndrome. J Neurosurg 1983; 59:1037–42.
11. Rowed DW, Kasel EE, Lewis AJ. Transorbital intracavernous needle biopsy in painful ophthalmoplegia. J Neurosurg 1985; 62:776–80.
12. Slamovits TL, Rosen CE, Suhrland MJ. Neuroblastoma presenting as acute lymphoblastic leukemia but correctly diagnosed after orbital fine-needle aspiration biopsy. J Clin Neuro Ophthalmol 1991; 11:158–61.
13. Spoor TC, Kennerdell JS, Dekker A, et al. Orbital fine needle aspiration biopsy with B-scan guidance. Am J Ophthalmol 1980; 89:274–7.
14. Kennerdell JS, Dubois PJ, Dekker A, Johnson BL. CT-guided fine needle aspiration biopsy of orbital optic nerve tumors. Ophthalmology 1980; 87:491–6.
15. Lui D. Complications of fine needle aspiration biopsy of the orbit. Ophthalmology 1985; 92:1768–71.
16. Medina E, Segato T, Piermarocchi S, Boccato P. Fine needle aspiration biopsy in ophthalmology. Surv Ophthalmol 1985; 29:410–22.

17. Glaser KS, Weger AR, Schmid KW, Bodner E. Is fine-needle aspiration of tumors harmless? Lancet 1989; 1:620.
18. Evans GHC, Harries SA, Hobbs KEF. Safety of and necessity for needle biopsy of liver tumors. Lancet 1987; 1:620.
19. Ryd W, Hagmar B, Eriksson O. Local tumor cell seeding by fine-needle aspiration biopsy. APMIS 1983; 9:17–21.

23

Cavernous Sinus Arteriovenous Fistula

Karl C. Golnik
The Storm Eye Institute and the Medical University of South Carolina, Charleston, South Carolina

Cavernous sinus arteriovenous fistulas (CSAVFs) may be separated into two types: direct and dural. A direct CSAVF is a communication between the intracavernous internal carotid artery and the cavernous sinus. Dural CSAVFs are communications between the cavernous sinus and the extradural branches of the internal carotid artery (meningohypophyseal trunk, inferior cavernous sinus artery), external carotid artery (middle meningeal artery, ascending pharyngeal artery), or both. Direct CSAVFs usually occur when a tear is traumatically or iatrogenically produced in the intracavernous internal carotid artery. However, a direct CSAVF may also arise spontaneously after rupture of an intracavernous carotid aneurysm or in association with systemic diseases that affect blood vessel walls, such as arteriosclerosis, fibromuscular dysplasia, and the Ehlers-Danlos syndrome. Dural CSAVFs most often become symptomatic spontaneously, often in middle-aged hypertensive women, and it is in such patients that the correct diagnosis is most often delayed. The etiology of these dural fistulas is not known.

I. CLINICAL MANIFESTATIONS

Consequences of CSAVFs are usually caused by compression and ischemia related to increased venous pressure in and around the orbit. Increased venous pressure is related, in part, to the velocity of flow within the fistula. High-flow fistulas are usually, but not always, direct; low-flow fistulas are usually dural. Ophthalmic manifestations of CSAVFs develop because orbital venous pressure rises when direct arterial-venous communication allows equilibration of the arterial and venous pressures. Higher flow rates, typically present in direct CSAVFs, result in more severe signs and symptoms unless the fistula drains posteriorly through the inferior and superior petrosal sinuses. CSAVFs that drain posteriorly produce no orbital consequences but may cause ocular motor nerve palsies (1). Most CSAVFs drain anteriorly through the superior and inferior orbital veins producing symptoms and signs of orbital and ocular ischemia and congestion. Thus, the severity and type of manifestations may vary considerably and are dependent on a fistula's flow rate and the direction of its venous drainage. Contralateral and bilateral ocular manifestations are unusual but can occur if there is significant blood flow to the contralateral cavernous sinus through the intercavernous or basilar sinuses.

The ocular manifestations of anteriorly draining CSAVFs include increased intraocular pressure (IOP), arterialization of conjunctival blood vessels, and conjunctival injection and chemosis (Fig. 1). Proptosis may be mild but is almost invariably present. Ocular or facial bruit may be noticed by the patient or may only be detected by auscultation. Facial bruit is often present in patients with high-flow direct fistulas, but low-flow dural CSAVFs usually do not produce a bruit. Headache and facial pain are frequent complaints of patients with both types of fistulas. Ischemia and/or compression of the ocular motor nerves often results in ocular motility disturbances and double vision. Alternatively, diplopia can occur if venous congestion of the extraocular muscles restricts ocular motility. Trigeminal nerve dysfunction (ophthalmic and maxillary divisions), acute visual loss (caused by central retinal vein occlusion, anterior ischemic optic neuropathy, retinal and choroidal detachment, or vitreous hemorrhage), and glaucoma (acute angle closure or neovascular) occur infrequently.

II. DIAGNOSIS

The differential diagnosis of CSAVFs depends on the severity of clinical manifestations. The diagnosis is seldom in doubt when proptosis, ophthalmoplegia, and facial bruit develop after head injury. However, patients with the gradual onset of mild episcleral injection and subtle proptosis may be inappropriately treated for chronic conjunctivitis or episcleritis. Moderate orbital congestion and motility disturbances may be mistaken for dysthyroid orbitopathy, orbital pseudotumor, orbital cellulitis, cavernous sinus thrombosis or a medial sphenoid wing meningioma.

Current noninvasive diagnostic techniques used to diagnose CSAVFs require either a high degree of technical proficiency or are expensive enough to prohibit widespread acquisition and office use. Orbital ultrasonography has been used to

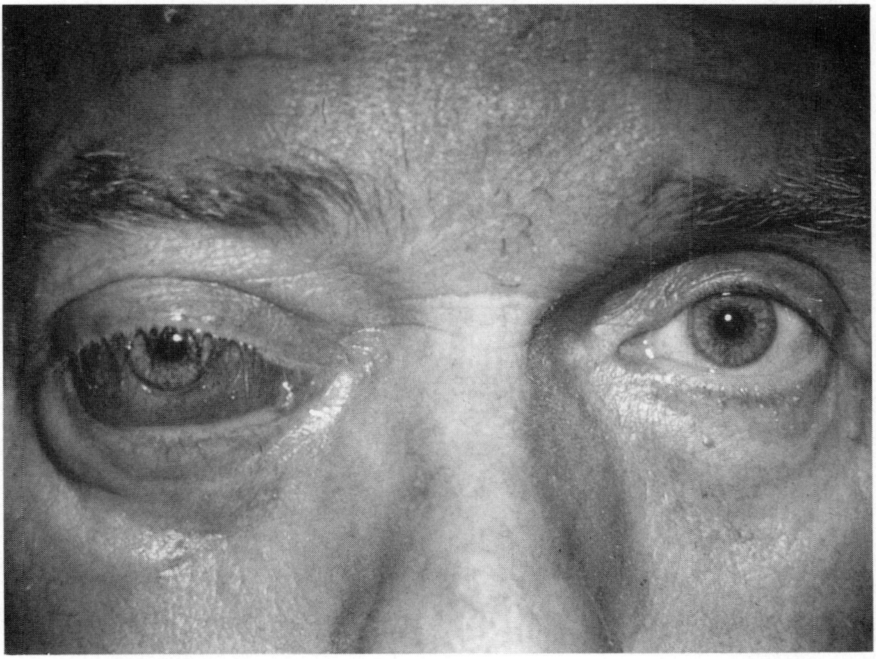

Figure 1 This 60-year-old man presented with a partial right oculomotor nerve palsy in addition to proptosis, chemosis, and conjunctival injection. Angiography demonstrated a right dural cavernous sinus fistula.

demonstrate dilation of the superior ophthalmic vein and congestion of the orbital tissues, particularly the extraocular muscles (2,3). Reversal of blood flow in the superior ophthalmic vein has been detected using Doppler techniques in combination with ultrasonography (4). Orbital color Doppler imaging has been used alone and in combination with Doppler flow measurements of the internal carotid arteries in the evaluation of patients with suspected CSAVFs (5). Orbital color Doppler imaging is able to identify retrograde blood flow in the superior ophthalmic vein ipsilateral to a CSAVF, but its advantage over established noncolor Doppler ultrasonography in the diagnosis of CSAVFs is unclear. Computed tomographic (CT) scanning and magnetic resonance (MR) imaging often show orbital congestion and an enlarged superior ophthalmic vein (Fig. 2). These techniques may also demonstrate a convexity of the lateral wall of the cavernous sinus or an abnormal flow void within the sinus (6). Unfortunately, these findings can result from other orbital and intracranial diseases and are not always present in patients with CSAVFs (7). MR imaging has demonstrated

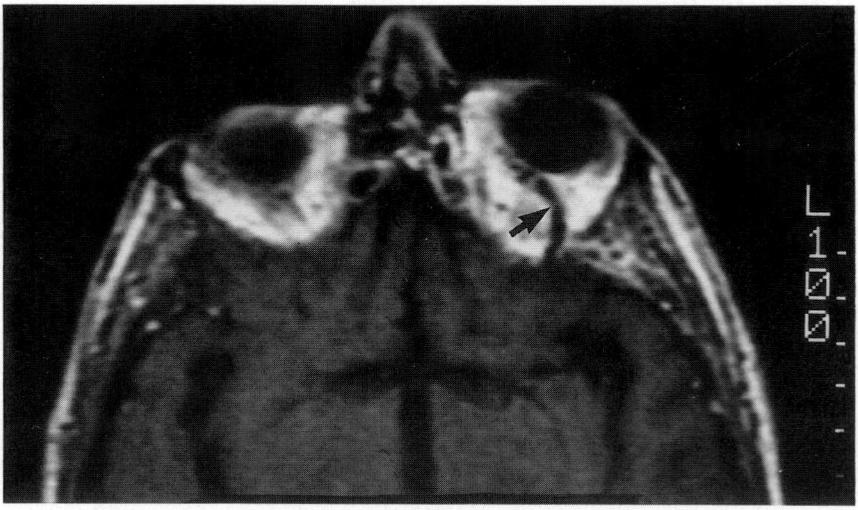

Figure 2 Magnetic resonance imaging of a patient with a left dural fistula showed an enlarged superior ophthalmic vein ipsilateral to the fistula (arrow).

decreased signal within the cavernous sinus (spin-echo technique) and dilation of the intercavernous sinus in patients with dural CSAVFs (8,9). A combination of two time-of-flight MR angiographic techniques, sequential two-dimensional slices and sequential acquisition of multiple thin volumes, may prove to be valuable in the diagnosis of CSAVFs and other intracranial vascular disease (10).

In 1930, Birch-Hirschfeld recognized that patients with CSAVFs had an increased ocular pulse (11). Subsequently, Boyes and Ralph reported two patients with CSAVFs in whom the Schiotz tonometer "described a to-and-fro arc of six to eight divisions on the scale . . .," whereas normal patients had movement of one to two divisions on the scale (12). More recently, several investigators have noted an increase in ocular pulse in patients with CSAVFs (13,14). The ocular pulse is synchronous with the cardiac cycle and has maximum and minimum values that correspond to the systolic and diastolic blood pressure. The ocular pulse amplitude (OPA) is defined as the difference between these maximum and minimum values and can be readily measured with a pneumotonometer. Golnik and Miller showed that the difference between the OPAs of an individual's eyes (▲OPA) is elevated in patients with CSAVFs (Fig. 3) (15). Furthermore, a ▲OPA greater than 1.6 mm Hg is 93% specific and 100% sensitive in identifying patients with CSAVFs. The increase in ▲OPA presumably occurs because the arterial pulse is transmitted directly to the ipsilateral orbital veins through the fistula; thus bypassing the normal blunting effect of the capillary bed. Orbital

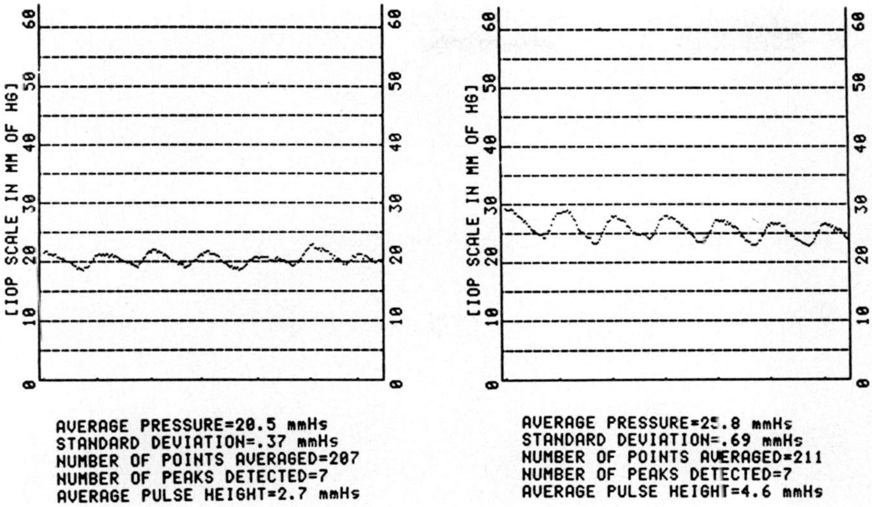

Figure 3 Pneumotonometry measurements of the patient in Figure 1 (right eye on the right). The difference between the maximum and minimum intraocular pressure is the "average pulse height" or ocular pulse amplitude (OPA). The difference between the OPAs in this individual's eyes (▲OPA) is 1.9 mm Hg (4.6–2.7 = 1.9). A ▲OPA greater than 1.6 mm Hg indicates the presence of a CSAVF.

and ocular conditions for which CSAVFs may be mistaken (e.g., conjunctivitis, thyroid orbitopathy) are not associated with a direct pulse transmission, and thus the ▲OPA is not increased.

Although these noninvasive techniques may be helpful, cerebral arteriography remains the "gold standard" for diagnosis of CSAVFs (Fig. 4). Selective arteriography of the internal *and* external carotid arteries on *both* sides must be performed completely to characterize the blood supply and drainage of the CSAVF. In this way, appropriate therapy can be determined and implemented. Although intravenous digital subtraction angiography has been used to evaluate CSAVFs, this technique does not provide the resolution necessary fully to characterize the hemodynamics of most CSAVFs. The risks and expense of conventional arteriography make careful patient selection essential.

III. NATURAL HISTORY

When untreated, direct CSAVFs usually produce progressive ocular difficulties and may cause potentially life-threatening events. Progressive, irreversible visual

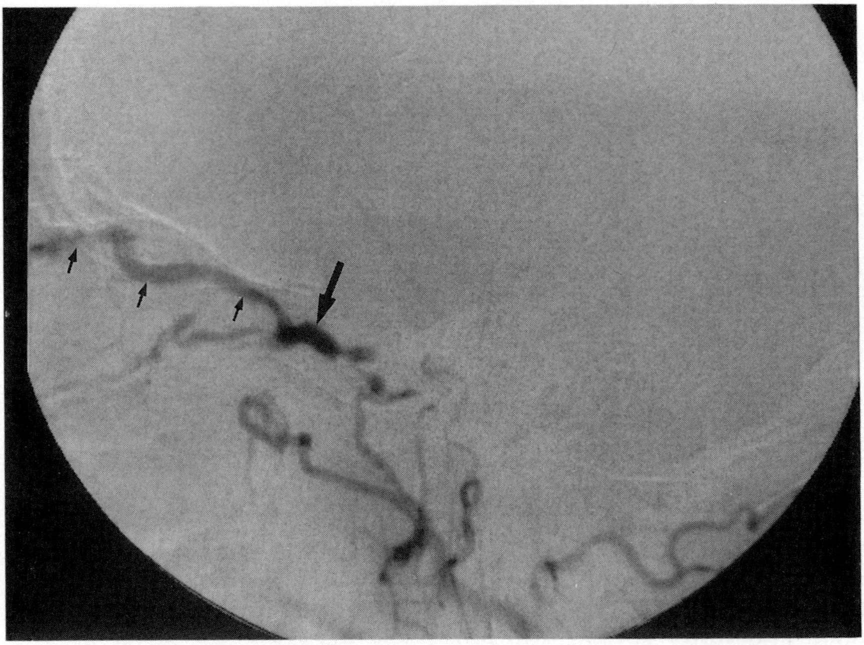

Figure 4 Selective right external carotid arteriography of the patient in Figure 1. There is early opacification of the cavernous sinus (large arrow) and dilatation of the superior ophthalmic vein (small arrows).

loss can occur from glaucoma or ischemic optic neuropathy. Intracerebral hematoma, subarachnoid hemorrhage, brainstem edema, and fatal epistaxis may occur (16,17). Halbach and associates reviewed 128 cases of direct CSAVF and found enlarged cortical veins, pseudoaneurysm, and cavernous sinus varix to be risk factors for intracranial hemorrhage (17). Although direct CSAVFs are not generally considered fatal, 5 of the 128 patients (3.9%) in this series died of hemorrhage associated with the fistula.

Dural CSAVFs generally have a more benign course. Occasionally, vision is lost from central retinal vein occlusion and rare patients with persistent fistulas have experienced intracranial hemorrhage (18,19). Dural CSAVFs resolve spontaneously or after angiography in at least 50% of patients. Symptoms can spontaneously resolve months to years after the initial diagnosis. Closure of the fistula is often heralded by transient worsening of symptoms apparently due to thrombosis of the superior ophthalmic vein and subsequent changes in orbital hemodynamics (20). MR imaging and MR angiography may show no cavernous sinus flow void and thrombosis of the superior ophthalmic vein (21). However,

petrosal sinus via a femoral vein approach (29). Occasionally, anatomical constraints prohibit this route and a more direct approach through the superior ophthalmic vein is necessary (30). Rarely, craniotomy and direct exposure of the cavernous sinus is necessary (31). Once entered, the cavernous sinus can be embolized with detachable balloons, metallic wire coils, or a variety of other agents. Rarely, dural CSAVFs are supplied only by ICA feeders. These fistulas are usually treated by transvenous embolization. Transvascular treatment modalities obliterate dural CSAVFs in 90–100% of patients. Radiation therapy has been used after unsuccessful CSAVF embolization (32). Favorable results have been reported, but it is difficult to interpret the results of this anecdotal report because dural CSAVFs frequently resolve without treatment.

Like patients with direct CSAVFs, patients with dural CSAVFs usually experience resolution of ocular symptoms days to months after successful treatment. However, dural fistulas can recanalize or recruit new arterial feeders. Measurement of the OPA can be helpful in determining the persistence or reopening of a dural CSAVF. Although the ▲OPA normalizes in patients who are successfully treated, a ▲OPA greater than 1.6 mm Hg indicates a patent fistula is present and further treatment may be necessary (15).

REFERENCES

1. Kosmorsky GS, Hanson MR, Tomsak RL. Carotid-cavernous fistulae presenting as painful ophthalmoplegia without external ocular signs. J Clin Neuro Ophthalmol 1988; 8:131–5.
2. Phelps CD, Thompson HS, Ossoinig KC. The diagnosis and prognosis of atypical carotid-cavernous fistula (red-eyed shunt syndrome) Am J Ophthalmol 1982; 93:423–36.
3. Spector RH. Echographic diagnosis of dural carotid-cavernous sinus fistulas. Am J Ophthalmol 1991; 111:77–83.
4. Rush JA, Blachshear WM, Grizzard WS. Doppler sonography in the diagnosis of a dural carotid cavernous fistula. J Clin Neuro Ophthalmol 1982; 2:39–42.
5. Flaharty PM, Lieb WE, Sergott RC, et al. Color doppler imaging: a new noninvasive technique to diagnose and monitor carotid cavernous sinus fistulas. Arch Ophthalmol 1991; 109:522–6.
6. Uchino A, Hasuo K, Matsumoto S, Masuda K. MRI of dural carotid-cavernous fistulas. Clin Imag 1992; 16:263–8.
7. Sergott RC, Glaser JS. Graves ophthalmopathy. A clinical and immunologic review. Surv Ophthalmol 1981; 26:1–21.
8. Hirabuki N, Miura T, Mitomo M, et al. MR imaging of dural arteriovenous malformations with ocular signs. Neuroradiology 1988; 30:390–4.
9. Elster AD, Chen MYM, Richardson DN, Yeatts PR. Dilated intercavernous sinuses: an MR sign of carotid-cavernous and carotid-dural fistulas. AJNR 1991; 12:641–5.

10. Lewin JS, Laub G. Intracranial MR angiography: a direct comparison of three time-of-flight techniques. AJNR 1991; 12:1133–9.
11. Birch-Hirschfeld A. Kurzes Handbuch der Ophthalmologie. Vol 1. Berlin: Julius Springer, 1930; 20–5.
12. Boyes TL, Ralph FT. Carotid-cavernous fistula. Am J Ophthalmol 1954; 37:262–6.
13. Knox DL. Ocular pressure studies in the diagnosis of carotid artery disease. Trans Am Ophthalmol Soc 1973; 71:459–87.
14. Gee W, Morrow RA, Stephens HW. Ocular pneumoplethysmography in carotid-cavernous sinus fistulas. J Neurosurg 1983; 59:40–5.
15. Golnik KC, Miller NR. The diagnosis of cavernous sinus arteriovenous fistula by ocular pulse amplitude. Ophthalmology 1992; 99:1146–52.
16. Teng MMH, Chang T, Pan DHC, et al. Brainstem edema: an unusual complication of carotid cavernous fistula. AJNR 1991; 12:139–42.
17. Halbach VV, Hieshima GB, Higashida RT, Reicher M. Carotid cavernous fistulae: Indications for urgent treatment. AJNR 1987; 8:627–33.
18. Pollack S, Miller NR. Central retinal vein occlusion complicating spontaneous carotid cavernous fistula. Arch Ophthalmol 1986; 104:331.
19. Harding AE, Kendall B, Leonard TJK, Johnson MH. Intracerebral hemorrhage complicating dural arteriovenous fistula: a report of two cases. J Neurol Neurosurg Psychiatry 1984; 47:905–11.
20. Sergott RC, Grossman RI, Savino PJ, et al. The syndrome of paradoxical worsening of dural cavernous sinus arteriovenous malformations. Ophthalmology 1987; 94:205–12.
21. Hirabuki N, Fugita N, Hashimoto T, et al. Follow-up MRI in dural arteriovenous malformations involving the cavernous sinus: emphasis on detection of venous thrombosis. Neuroradiology 1992; 34:423–7.
22. Debrun GM, Vinuela F, Fox AJ, et al. Indications for treatment and classification of 132 carotid-cavernous fistulas. Neurosurgery 1988; 22:285–9.
23. Vinuela F, Fox AJ, Debrun GM, Peerless SJ, Drake CG. Spontaneous carotid cavernous fistulas: clinical, radiological, and therapeutic considerations. J Neurosurg 1984; 60:976–84.
24. Barrow DL, Spector RH, Braun IF, et al. Classification and treatment of spontaneous carotid-cavernous sinus fistulas. J Neurosurg 1985; 62:248–56.
25. Grossman RI, Sergott RC, Goldberg HI, et al. Dural malformations with ophthalmic manifestations: results of particulate embolization in seven patients. AJNR 1985; 6:809–13.
26. Halbach VV, Higashida RT, Hieshima GB, et al. Dural fistulas involving the cavernous sinus: results of treatment in 30 patients. Radiology 1987; 163:437–45.
27. Kupersmith MJ, Berenstein A, Choi IS, et al. Management of nontraumatic vascular shunts involving the cavernous sinus. Ophthalmology 1988; 95:121–30.
28. Halbach VV, Higashida RT, Hieshima GB, Hardin CW. Embolization of branches arising from the cavernous portion of the internal carotid artery. AJNR 1988; 10:143–50.
29. Halbach VV, Higashida RT, Hieshima GB, et al. Transvenous embolization of dural fistulas involving the cavernous sinus. AJNR 1989; 10:377–83.

30. Monsein LH, Debrun DM, Miller NR, et al. Treatment of dural carotid-cavernous sinus fistulas via the superior ophthalmic vein approach. AJNR 1991; 12:435–9.
31. Debrun GM, Nauta HJ, Miller NR, et al. Combining the detachable balloon technique and surgery in imaging carotid cavernous fistulae. Surg Neurol 1989; 32:3–10.
32. Pierot L, Poisson M, Jason M, et al. Treatment of type D dural carotid-cavernous fistulas by embolization followed by irradiation. Neuroradiology 1992; 34:77–80.

24

Idiopathic Orbital Inflammation (Pseudotumor)

Phil A. Aitken
University of Vermont College of Medicine, Burlington, Vermont

Pseudotumor of the orbit presents a complex diagnostic and therapeutic dilemma to all physicians involved in the care of patients with orbital problems. It is important from the start to recognize that by the nature of the term *pseudotumor*, the diagnosis requires the exclusion of tumor as the source of adnexal signs and symptoms. One must be alert to not be lulled into a false sense of complacency that may lead to a less than efficient evaluation and treatment of an identifiable pathology requiring immediate attention.

Diagnostic advances, especially in the areas of imaging, including B-mode ultrasound, computed tomography (CT), and magnetic resonance imaging (MRI), have provided a quantum leap forward in the localization and identification of abnormalities in the orbit.

Idiopathic orbital inflammation was first described as "pseudotumor" of the orbit by Birch-Hirschfeld in 1930 (1). This term evolved to describe inflammatory swellings of the orbital contents that produced false clinical impression of an orbital tumor. These patients often presented with proptosis, ptosis, and motility disturbance. As the level of diagnostic sophistication and the knowledge of orbital diseases progressed, a number of patients could be separated as having a specific identifiable pathophysiology. Earlier studies undoubtedly included some noninflammatory cases. Jakobiec (2) points out that some investigators have categorized lymphoid tumors as lymphoid pseudotumor, which has further confused the natural history of each type of disease. He emphasizes that both benign and malignant lymphoid tumors should be distinguished from idiopathic orbital inflammations.

It is important that in dealing with a diagnosis of exclusion, one must recognize the place of the age of the patient in establishing a differential diagnosis. In children, conditions such as rhabdomyosarcoma and metastatic neuroblastoma are usually easily distinguishable. The difference between orbital pseudotumor and orbital cellulitis may not be so clear as to risk withholding antibiotic during the period of time of observation and investigation. At the same time, the need for tissue diagnosis and expedient therapeutic decisions following biopsy also may push us ahead in spite of the strong impression that the correct diagnosis is inflammatory pseudotumor of the orbit.

It seems that the more oriented toward ophthalmic pathology the investigator is, the more likely he or she is to be frustrated by the term *pseudotumor* and concerned about the possibility of a "pseudodiagnosis" (2–6). In spite of these concerns and considerations as well as the multiple "authors' denunciation of the term *pseudotumor*, it is embedded in the ophthalmology lexicon and will probably remain so until these disease processes are better understood" (3). Thus, our best efforts to obtain information and understanding of this condition with its multiple presentations and manifestations is mandatory if we are to decrease the incidence of pseudodiagnosis. Increasingly sophisticated methods of noninvasive as well as invasive investigation, including fine-needle aspiration biopsy, open biopsy, and surgical exploration, with appropriate pathology examinations will hopefully help us in our diagnosis and treatment of this condition.

I. CLINICAL MANIFESTATIONS

The presentation of the patient with orbital inflammatory disease of an idiopathic nature is most frequent in the 20–80 age group but may occur in children as well. The condition may present as an acute, subacute, or chronic condition, involve one or both orbits, and recur, as well as progress, from one side to the other. In addition, the condition may be diffuse or involve any segment or element of the orbit. There may be a myositis involving one or more of the extraocular muscles, dacryoadenitis, trochleitis, episcleritis, and perineuritis. Involvement may be concentrated anteriorly or apically, thus changing the spectrum of symptoms. The range of common symptoms and signs is outlined in Table 1.

II. DIFFERENTIAL DIAGNOSIS

The differential diagnosis of orbital pseudotumor is extensive, including essentially all orbital processes. Orbital pseudotumor is probably second only to Graves' disease as the etiology of proptosis. A second common process confused with orbital inflammatory disease, orbital cellulitis, may require parallel or simultaneous treatments until the correct diagnosis is made (Fig. 1A–C). This

Table 1 Symptoms and Signs of Target Hormone Deficiency

		Lacrimal	Myositis	Scleritis	Perineuritis	Diffuse	Apical
Symptoms	PAIN	+	++	++	±	+	+
	Diplopia	±	++	±	–	+	+
	Decreased vision	±	–	+	++	+	++
Signs	Proptosis	±	+	–	–	++	±
	Chemosis	±	±	+	–	+	–
	Injection	±	±	++	–	+	–
	Dystophia	++	±	–	–	–	–
	Lid swelling	++	±	±	–	+	–
CT	Involvement	Lacrimal gland	EOM enhancement insertion	Enhancement thickening sclera	Enlargement enhancement optic nerve	Stringy increase fat shadow	Apical mass with enhancement

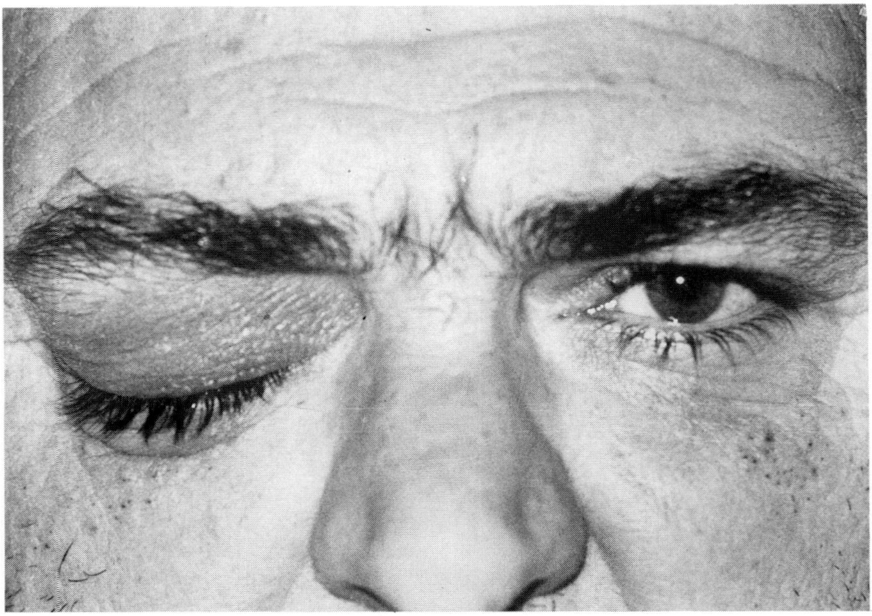

(A)

Figure 1 (A) A 42-year-old patient with acute onset of orbital pain, proptosis, ptosis, and ophthalmoplegia along with severe edema and chemosis. The patient failed to respond to an initial trial of intravenous antibiotics. He demonstrated a rapid resolution with the initiation of high dose corticosteroids. (B) Failure of attempted abduction as well as conjunctival chemosis of right eye. (C) Limited adduction of right eye. Patient had almost total reduction of pain in 24 h and return of full motility in 72 h of initiation of high dose corticosteroid therapy.

patient had received intravenous antibiotics for a presumed orbital cellulitis for about 5 days without response clinically. Imaging studies did not identify specific pathology and the decision was made to start the patient on high-dose systemic steroids. His response was dramatic and complete. The presence of ptosis is helpful in excluding Graves' orbitopathy, as most of these patients with lid retraction rather than ptosis.

As mentioned above, other lymphocytic conditions may also add to the confusion (Fig. 2A–E). This patient presented with recent onset of proptosis and diplopia with only modest pain. Although the patient had findings that might suggest Graves' disease or orbital pseudotumor, the contribution of imaging and subsequent lymph node biopsy led to the diagnosis of lymphoma. The lid position

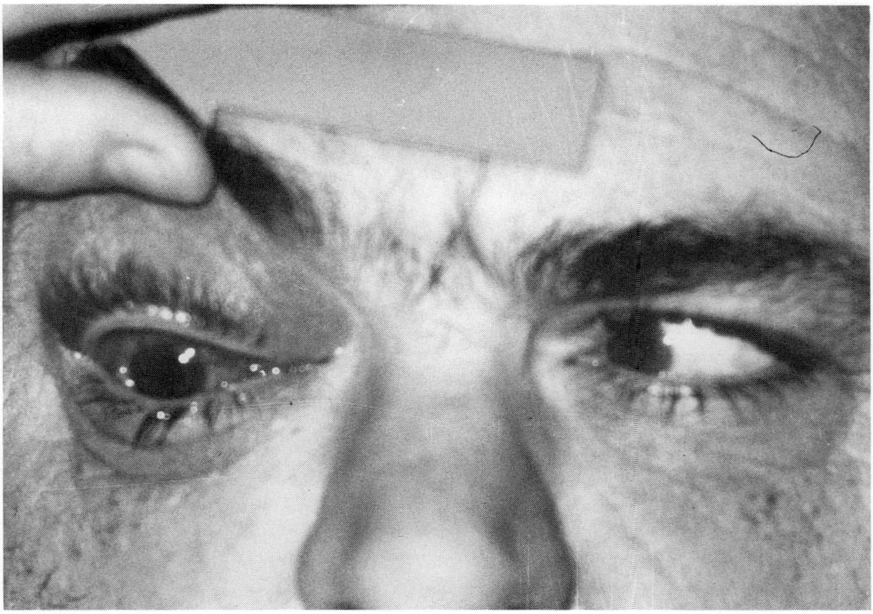

(B)

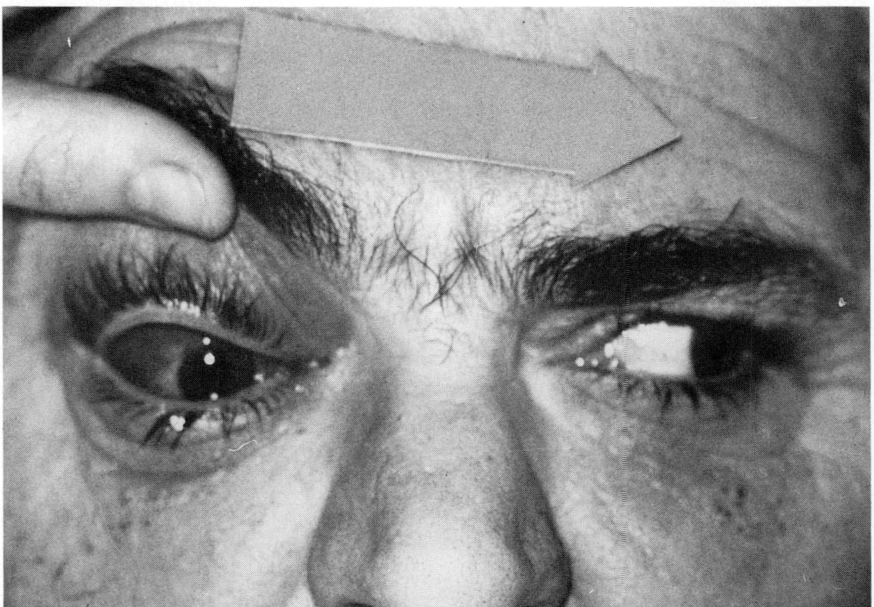

(C)

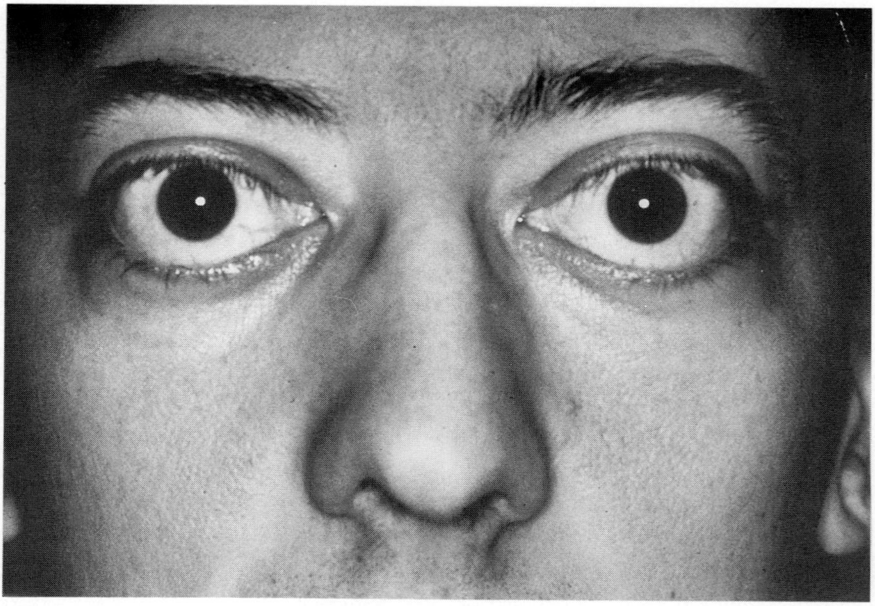

(A)

Figure 2 (A) A 32-year-old man with progressive exophthalmos and diplopia. There is no ptosis or injections. (B, C) The CT scan shows diffuse fluffy infiltrate of both orbits with molding around the globe. (D) CT of abdomen shows hepatosplenomegaly. (E) Lymph node biopsy diagnosed as non-Hodgkin lymphoma.

and the relatively modest pain were also important in pushing toward a correct diagnosis.

Muscle involvement in the patient with orbital inflammatory disease may be painful or painless occasionally affecting one but more commonly several muscles. There may be paresis or restriction of function. The patient with Graves' disease is likely to have more muscles involved and CT scan will show lack of involvement and enhancement of the tendinous insertion of the muscle into the sclera (Fig. 3A).

Evaluation of the patient should include axial and coronal CT views of the orbit, ultrasound where available, and thyroid evaluation (which will help as the clinical course becomes clearer). Attention should also be directed to the (paranasal) sinuses, especially if orbital cellulitis or a secondary neoplastic process is considered. Once the diagnosis by exclusion points toward orbital pseudotumor, the initiation of treatment with systemic corticosteroids will often result in a dramatic change in the patient's status. Although the majority of

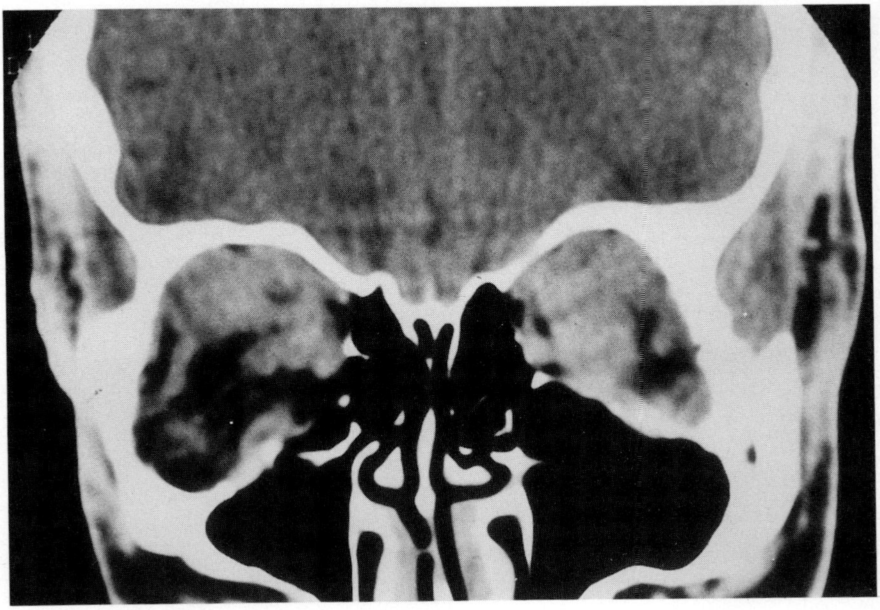

(B)

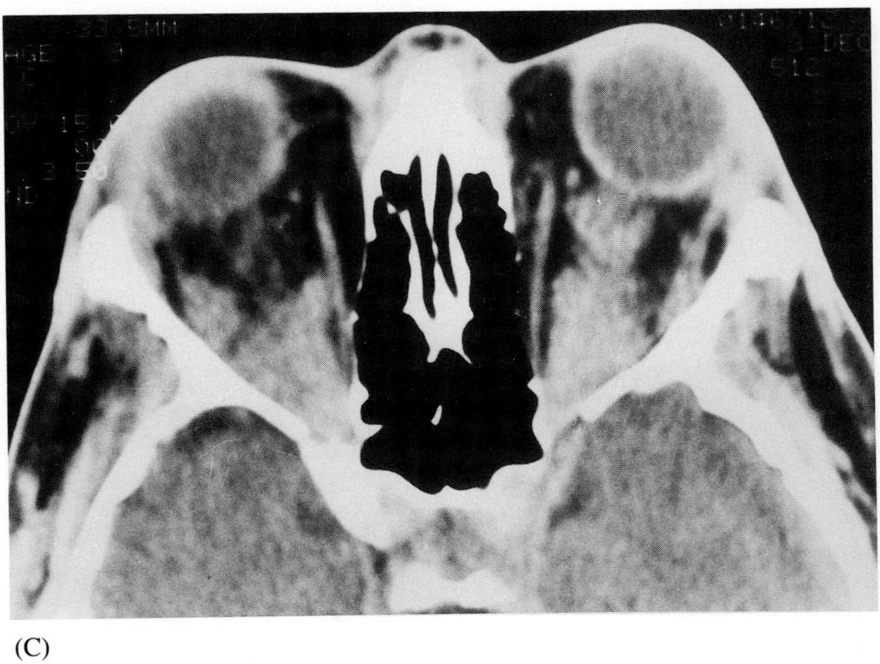

(C)

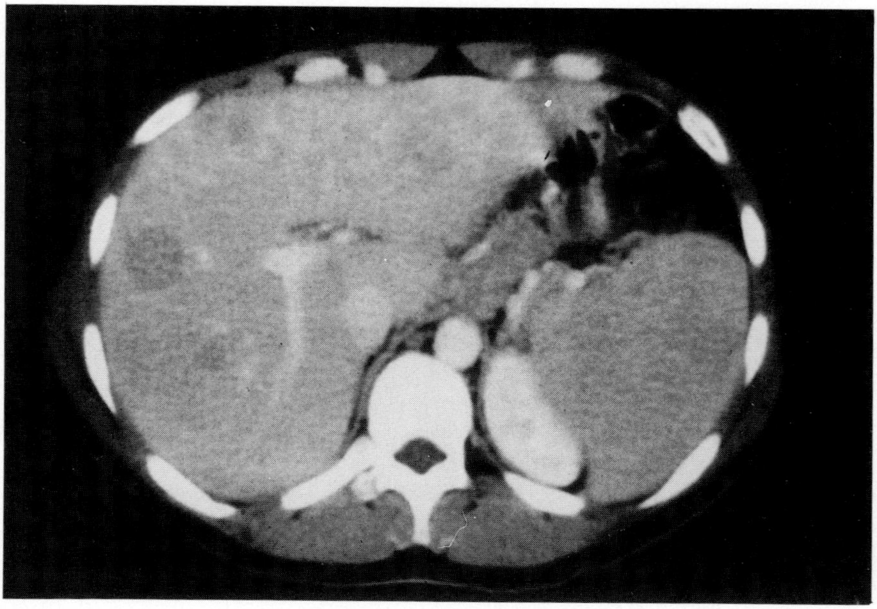

(D)

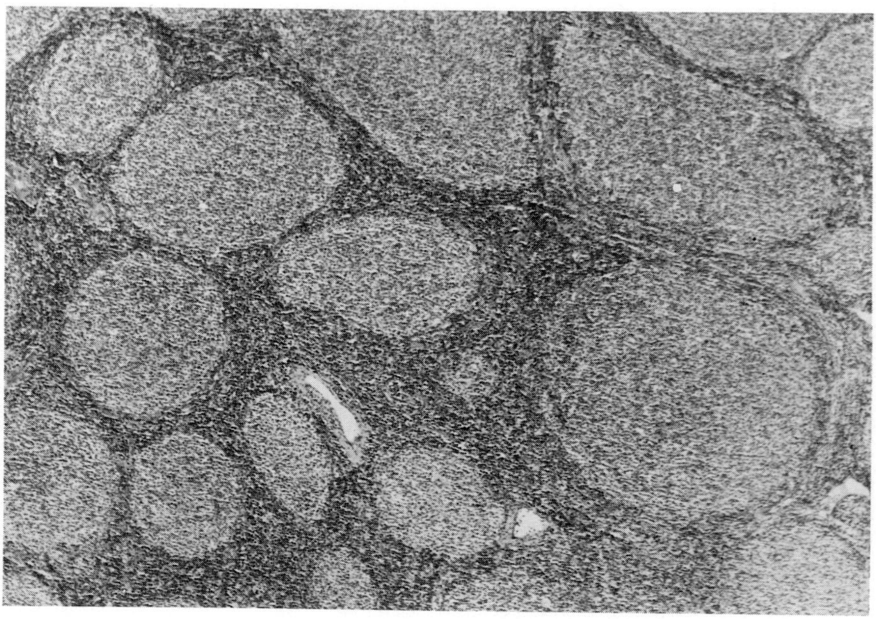

(E)

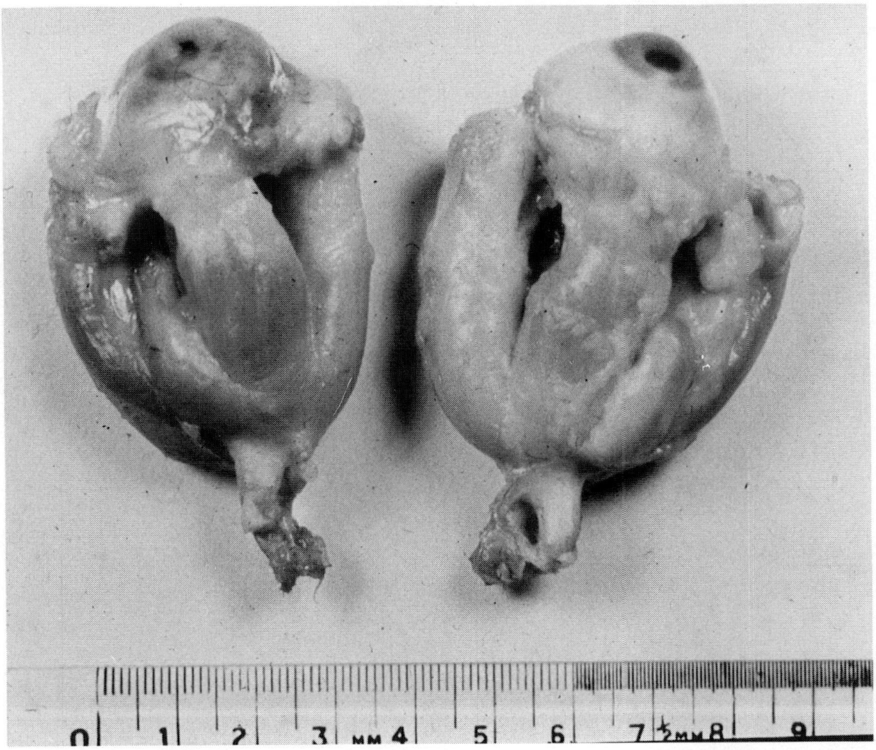

Figure 3 Autopsy specimen of patient with Graves' orbitopathy demonstrating diffuse enlargement of multiple extraocular muscles and relative sparing of the tendinous insertion to the globe (photograph courtesy of Michael Sanders).

patients with pseudotumor will respond promptly to steroids, those that do not may be on too low a dose for too short a period. Premature tapering of steroids not infrequently leads to symptomatic recurrence. One may find a threshold level of steroids that one has difficulty getting below. Very slow reduction or the addition of other therapeutic modalities may be important.

Primary or metastatic muscle disease is usually discovered on imaging study (Fig. 4A–C). These patients usually present with diplopia due to muscle dysfunction but may later develop pain and proptosis. This patient had a known primary tumor that only rarely metastasizes to extraocular muscle. Surgical biopsy demonstrated a myositis without evidence of metastatic disease. This patient stabilized and has remained asymptomatic for 4 years.

In addition to the extraocular muscles, other single structures such as the sheath of the optic nerve may be involved (Fig. 5A–C). In contrast, diffuse

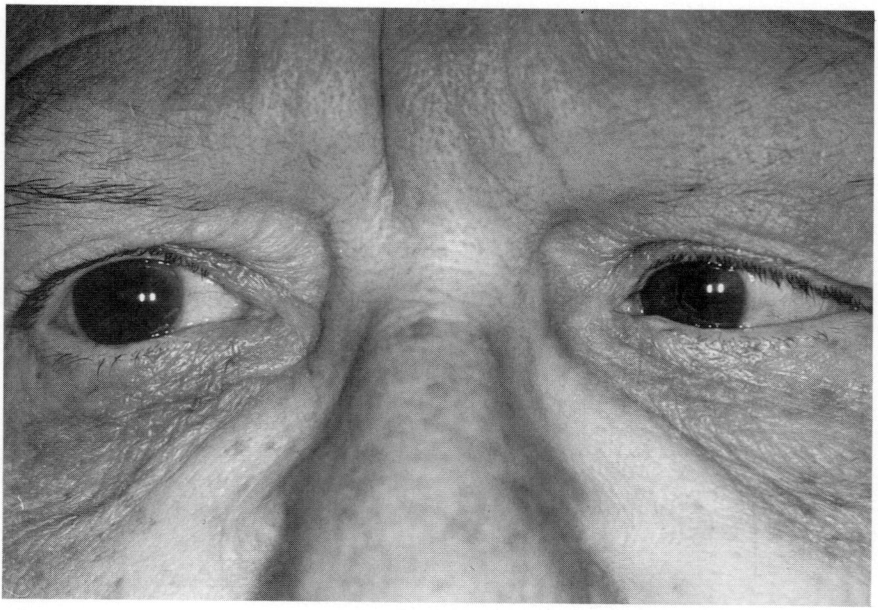

(A)

Figure 4 (A) A 62-year-old woman with recently diagnosed abdominal tumor and onset of fixed adduction of the left eye. The abdominal tumor was a epithelioid leiomyosarcoma. (B) CT scan shows selective enlargement of the left medial rectus. (Thyroid studies were negative.) (C) Surgical biopsy and recession carried out. The biopsy of the muscle demonstrated edema, decreased muscle fibers, and diffuse inflammation. No tumor was identified. The patient has remained asymptomatic for four years.

involvement may involve all of the tissues in the orbit to varying degrees. Figure 6A–B is representative of tissue obtained after a rather extensive orbitotomy on a patient with orbital pseudotumor. On presenting this information and the patient to Dr. David Cogan, he inquired, "why did you not just do a simple biopsy through the conjunctiva, the tissue would all show the same finding." The voice of experience again had something to say as we look for the etiology in these patients with a diffuse orbitopathy.

Discrete lesions may be present and surgical excisional biopsy is the most direct course to a diagnosis and well as a treatment (Fig. 7A–C). Findings of a lymphocytic response such as in this patient requires careful evaluation for possible systemic involvement. To this point, he has remained disease free, but the risk has been demonstrated (7). Local treatment may include steroids or

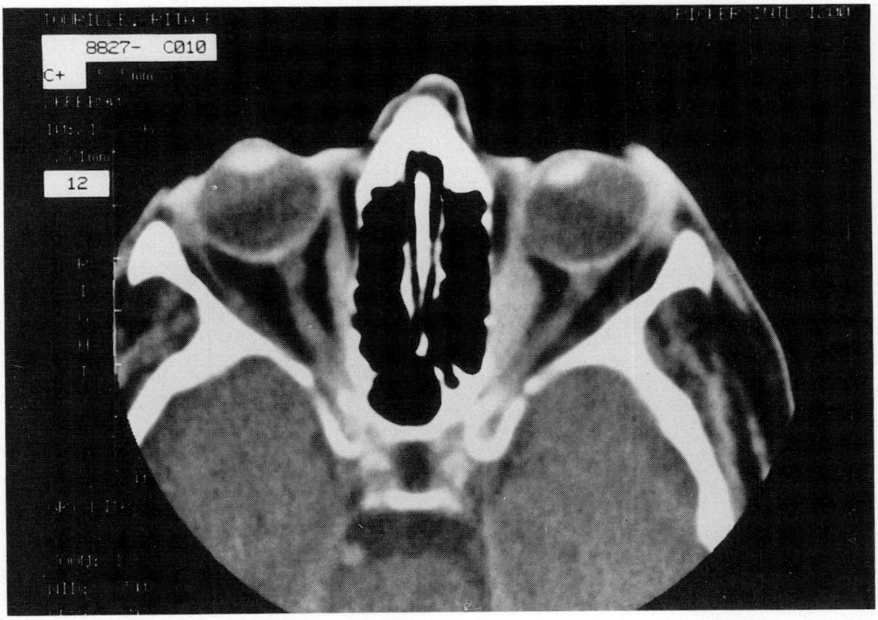

(B)

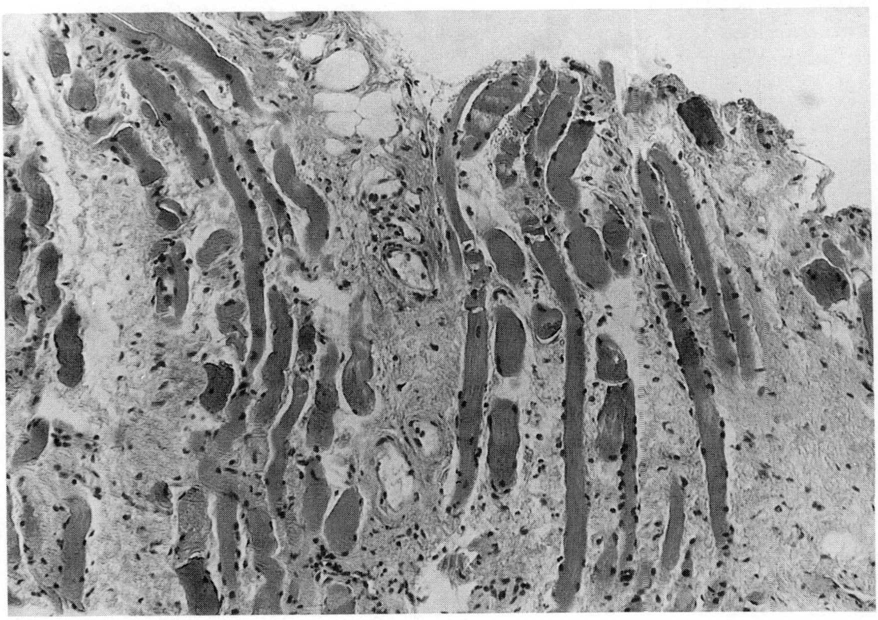

(C)

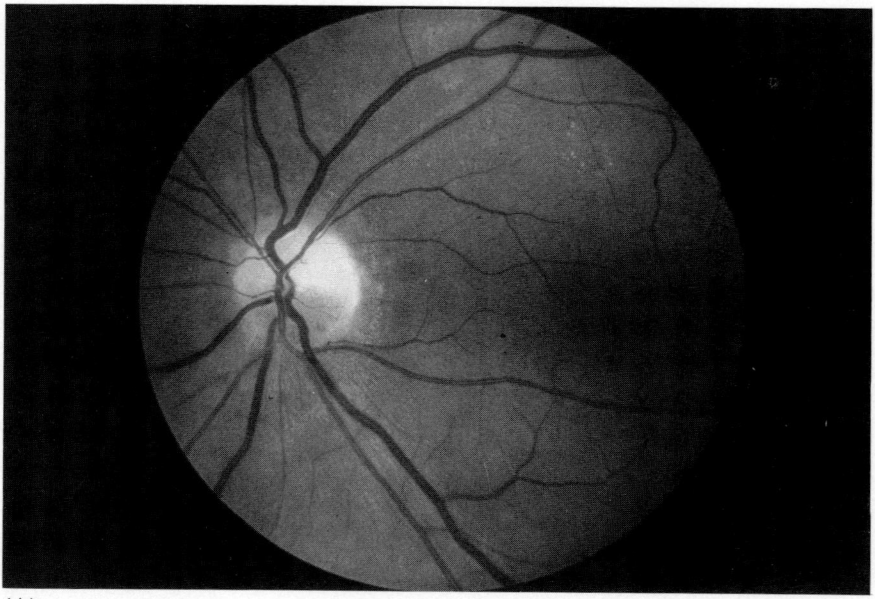

(A)

Figure 5 (A–C) A 49-year-old man with onset of orbital pain and superior altitudinal defect on the left side. CT scan demonstrated enhancement of the optic nerve on the left. This was felt to be an inflammatory pseudotumor confined to the optic nerve.

radiation. (If asymptomatic, benign lymphoid hyperplasia may simply be followed.)

One group of patients deserves special mention and consideration separate from the multiple presentations we have discussed. Figure 8A–H only partially tells the complete clinical story about patients with the sclerosing form of pseudotumor. In my experience, this condition has a relentless downward course in spite of extensive local and systemic therapy. Repeat biopsies have been carried out to rule out conditions such as Wegener's granulomatosis, and in spite of all efforts, the patient has ended with a blind painful eye eventually leading to exenteration for relief of pain. Evidence of involvement of the cavernous sinus and the tentorium has been present and there was subsequent involvement of the fellow eye with an equally malignant downhill course even with the most aggressive use of radiation, steroids, chemotherapy, and surgical decompression. This, fortunately uncommon form of orbital pseudotumor, has proven to be a particularly challenging problem when treating orbital inflammatory disease.

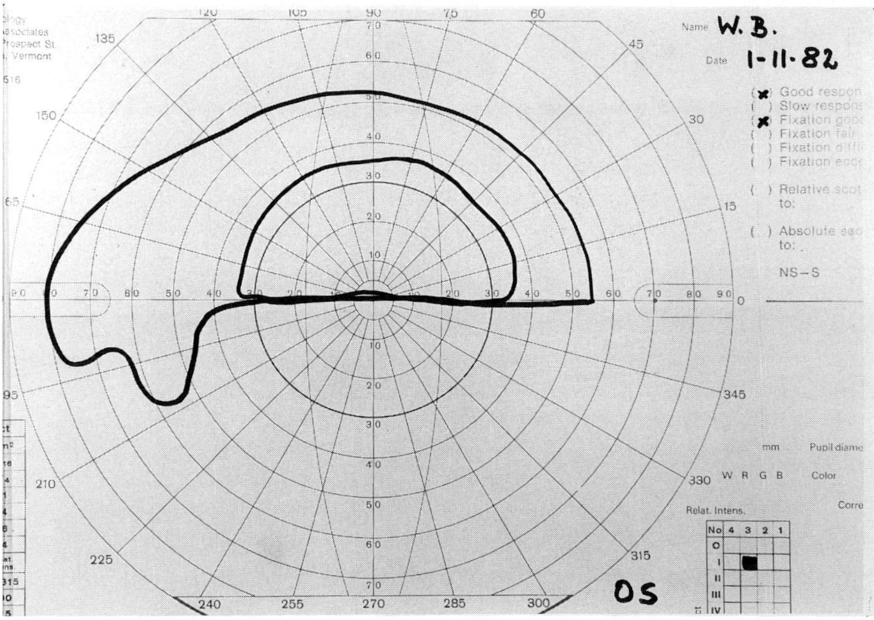
Name W. B.
Date 1-11-82
NS–S
OS
Relat. Intens.

(B)

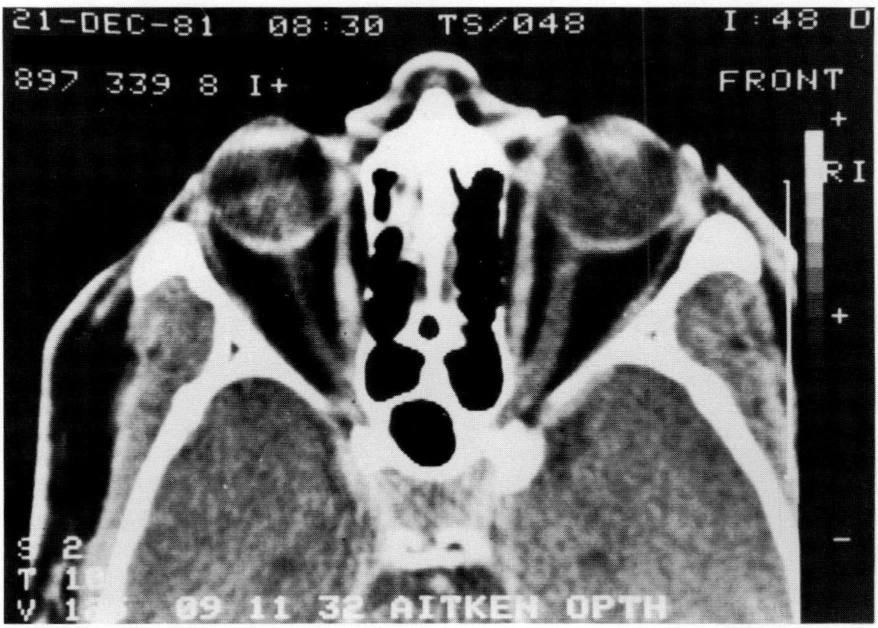
21-DEC-81 08:30 TS/048
I:48 D
897 339 8 I+
FRONT

(C)

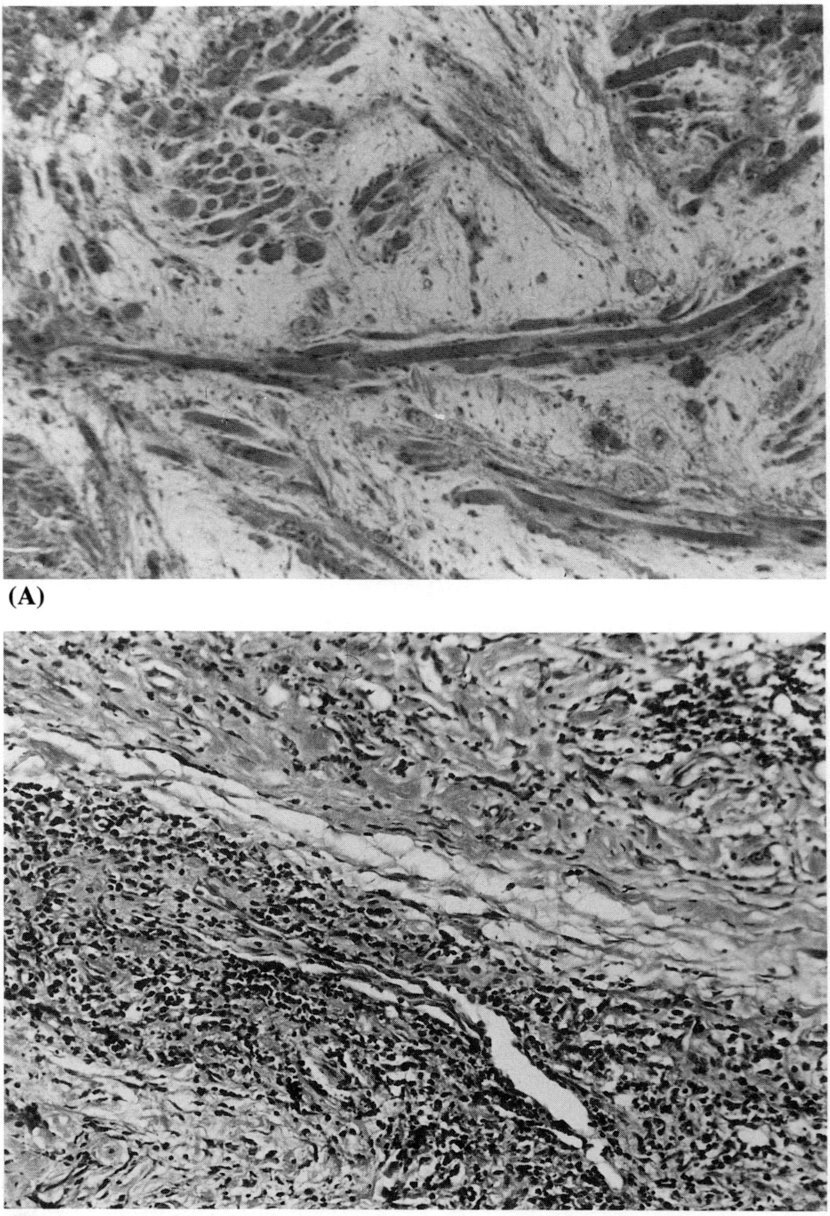

(A)

(B)

Figure 6 (A, B) Biopsy specimen from the orbit of a patient with inflammatory orbital pseudotumor demonstrating inflammatory cells and edema in muscle and fatty tissue of orbit.

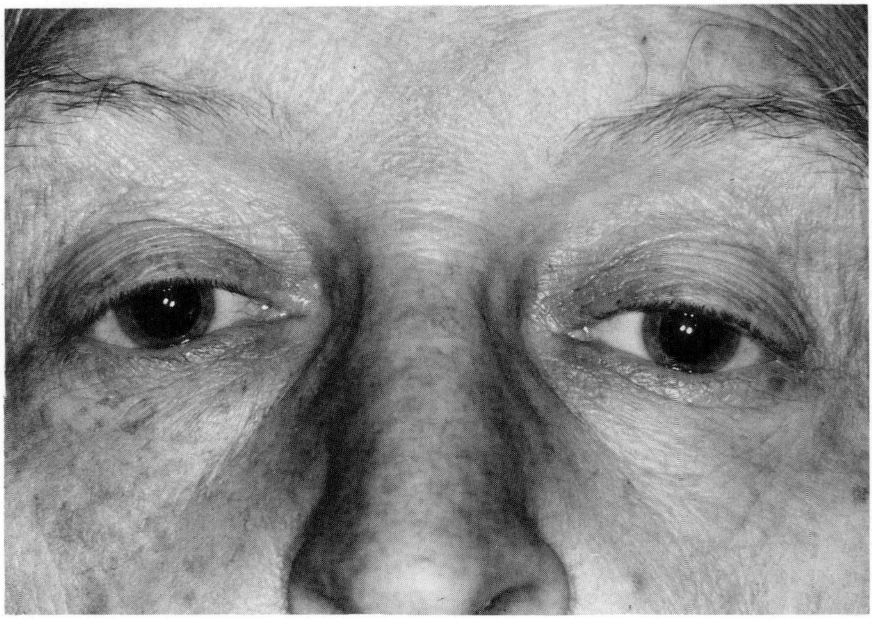

(A)

Figure 7 (A, B) A 60-year-old man with recent onset of pain in left orbit and mass that would prolapse with pressure on or below globe. This clinically and on CT scan was free of lacrimal gland. No mass visible on straight ahead gaze. Mass visible and easily palpated after gentle pressure on globe. (C) Surgical removal carried out with total removal of lesion with tissue clearly respecting anatomical tissue planes. Diffuse inflammatory tissue identified without evidence of lymphoma. Patient will be followed with anticipation.

III. TREATMENT

The treatment options in orbital inflammatory disease depend to a large part on the extent of the disease and the status at the time of intervention. Moderate- to high-dose corticosteroids are required to control an acute inflammatory response and reactivation may again require high doses to regain control. Steroid therapy must be tapered gradually over an extended period. Certainly the acute form of inflammation is much more sensitive to therapy with resolution with minimal fibrosis resulting. Jakobiec (2) suggests prednisone, 80–100 mg daily by mouth, with continuation at this level for 2–3 weeks to prevent relapse; then slow, steady tapering over an additional 3 weeks.

Recurrence with taper may require much slower reduction. When the patient

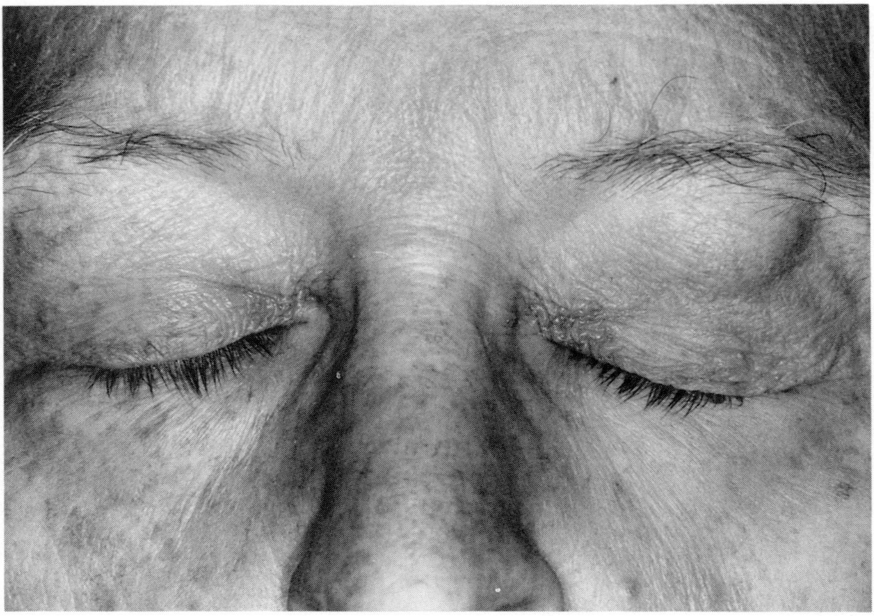

(B)

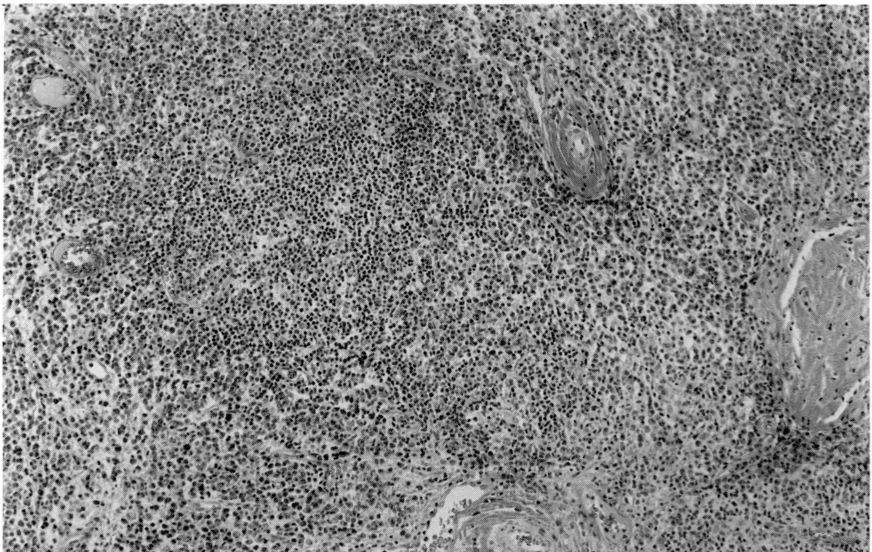

(C)

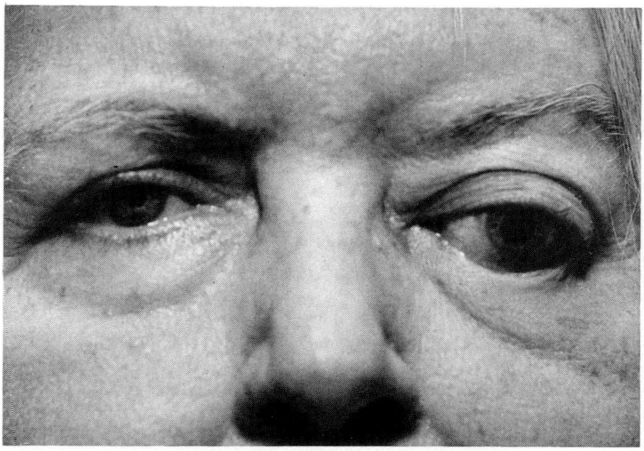

(A)

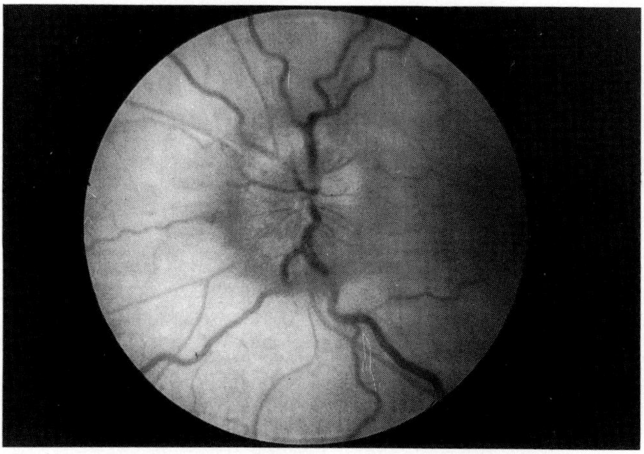

(B)

Figure 8 (A) A 42-year-old woman with sclerosing inflammatory pseudotumor initially of the left orbit. (B) Disc edema on left side with progressive loss of vision. (C) Early stage of involvement of left orbit. (D) Progression of involvement of left orbit with calcification in mass. Therapy has included multiple attempts with corticosteroids, radiation, chemotherapy, and surgical decompression without positive benefit. (E) Pathology subsequently demonstrated in cavernous sinus on CT scan. (F) CT of patient following orbital exenteration on left because of uncontrolled pain and total loss of vision. This CT now demonstrates a similar sclerosing pseudotumor in the right orbit. This has now progressed to involve the entire right orbit, and the patient is left with hand motion vision. (G, H) Pathology of sclerosing pseudotumor shows areas of inflammation in a sea of dense collagen. No evidence of a perivasculitis ruled out Wegener's granulomatosis.

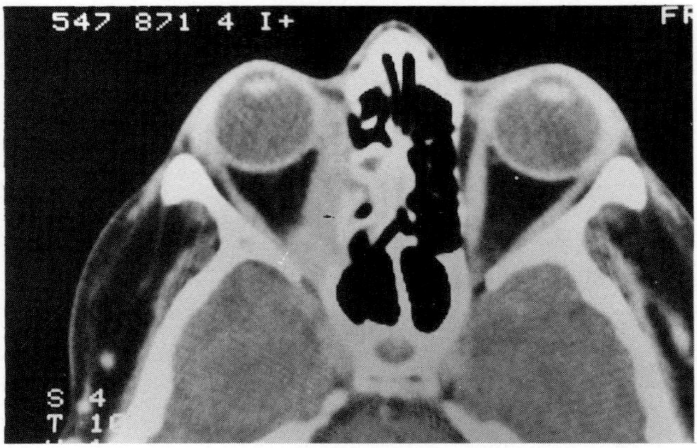

(C)

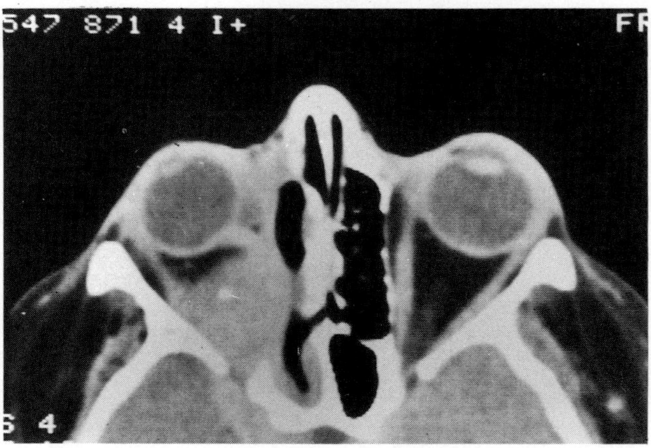

(D)

Figure 8 (*Continued*)

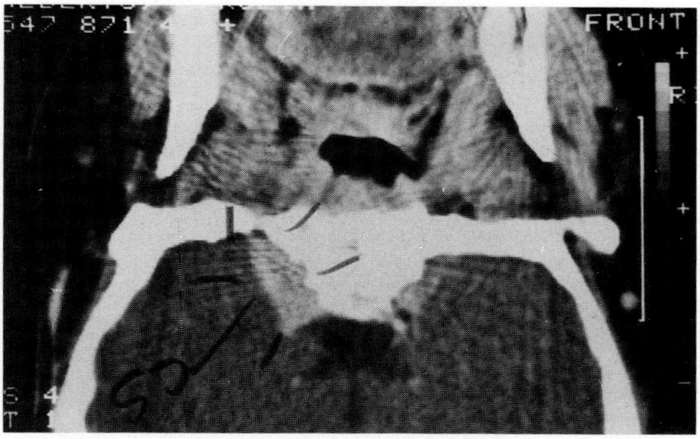

(E)

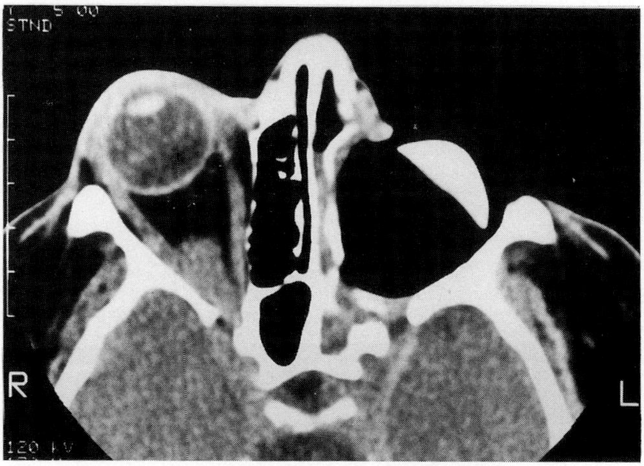

(F)

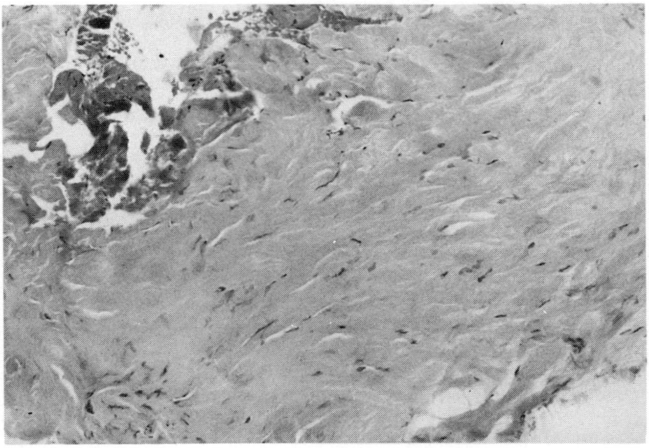

(G)

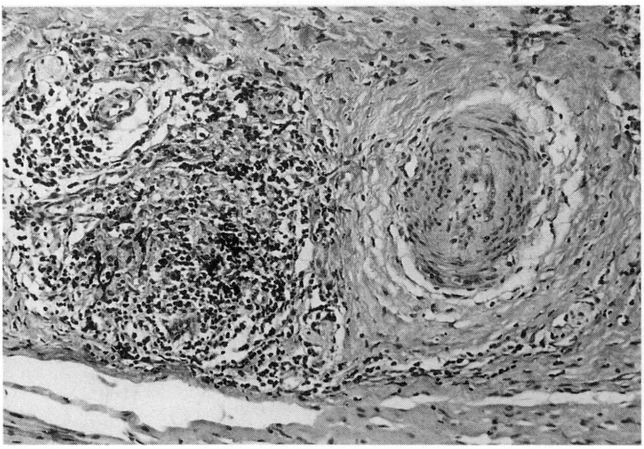

(H)

Figure 8 (***Continued***)

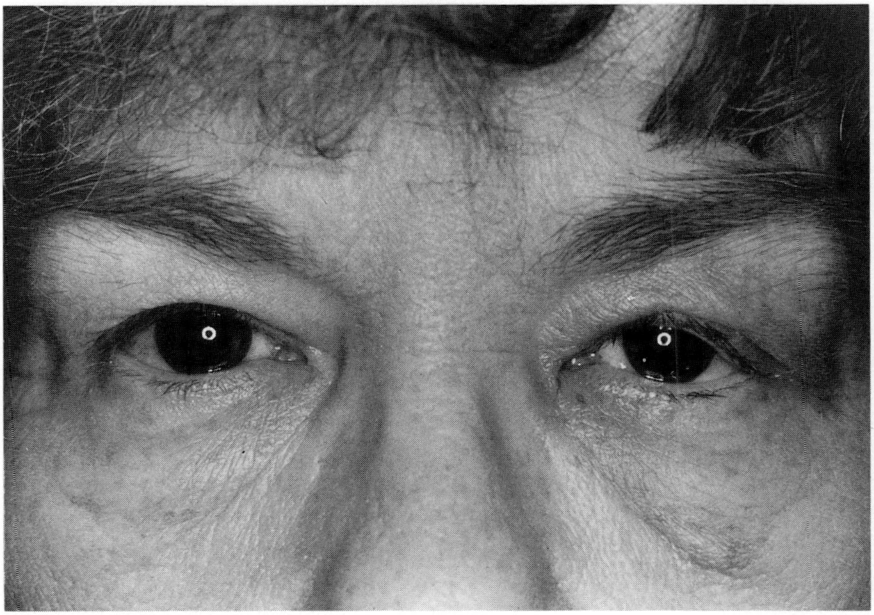

(A)

Figure 9 (A) Patient is a 50-year-old woman referred with left superolateral orbital mass. Slight superotemporal fullness noted. The patient had been explored in an outpatient setting with the thought that this was an unusual "chalazion." When it was observed to be larger and extend further, that procedure was discontinued. No biopsy was obtained. (B, C) CT scan shows left lacrimal fossa mass with slight flattening of the globe and larger lacrimal gland on left than right. (D, E) Left lateral orbitotomy was carried out. Lacrimal gland, both palpebral component and orbital component, were removed totally. The initial impression was that of inflammatory disease—lacrimal gland with marked acinar atrophy, chronic inflammation, and fibrosis. The tissue was reevaluated, and a diagnosis of lacrimal gland tumor made.

fails to respond to steroids, other pathophysiologies must be considered and a biopsy may be indicated. For patients who will not tolerate tapering of steroids or fail to improve on adequate steroid doses, radiation therapy and immunosuppressive agents may be effective. Radiation is usually delivered to the entire orbit shielding the anterior segment to a dose of 20 Gy in divided doses of 2 Gy (8). Attempts to treat with immunosuppressive therapy (e.g., cyclophosphamide) have met with some success in some patients with vasculitis. My personal experience with immunosuppressive therapy has been limited and not as rewarding as one might imagine.

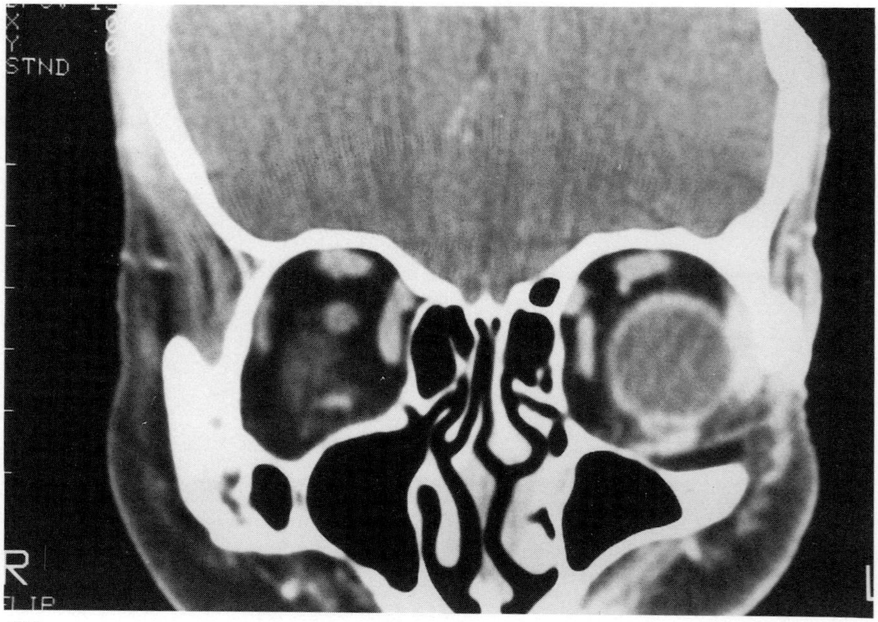

(B)

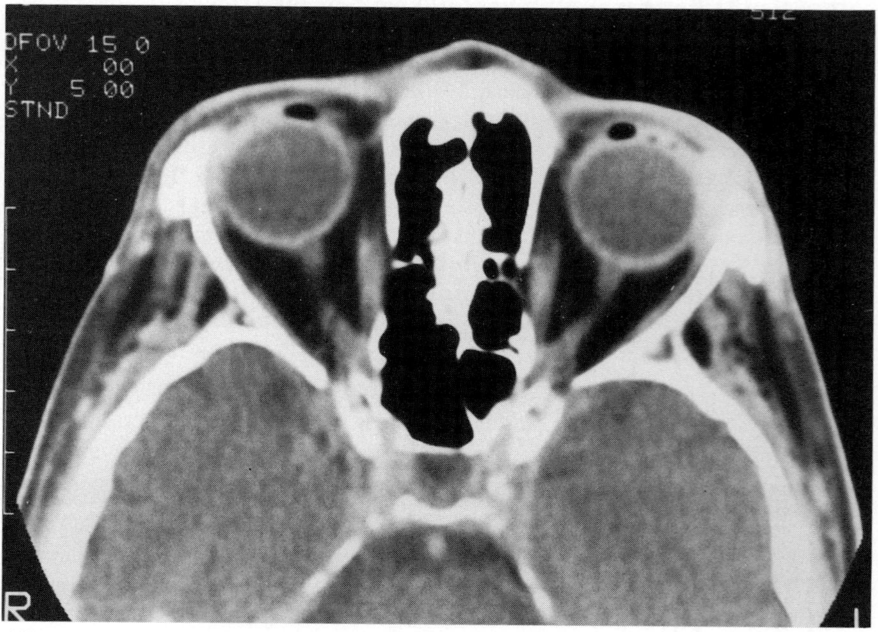

(C)

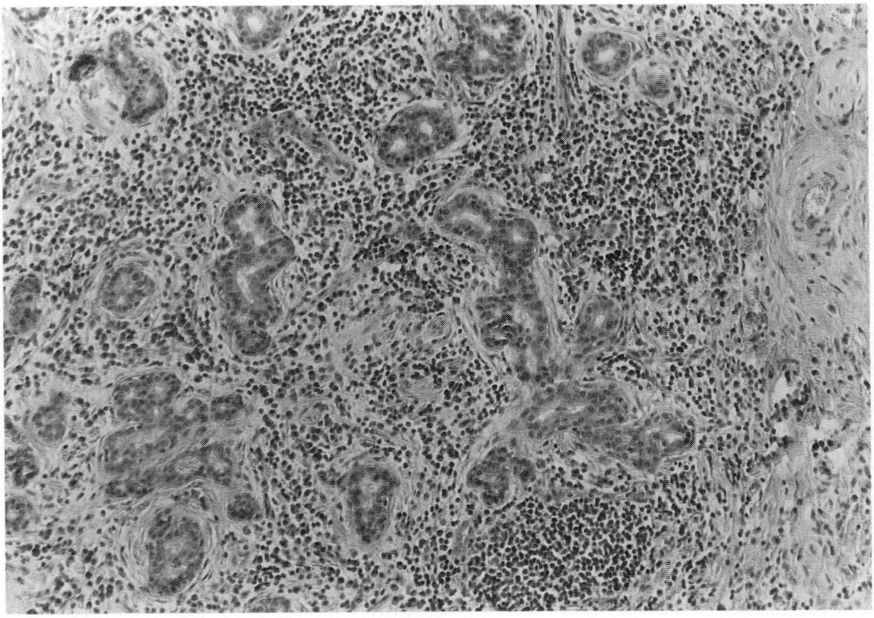

(D)

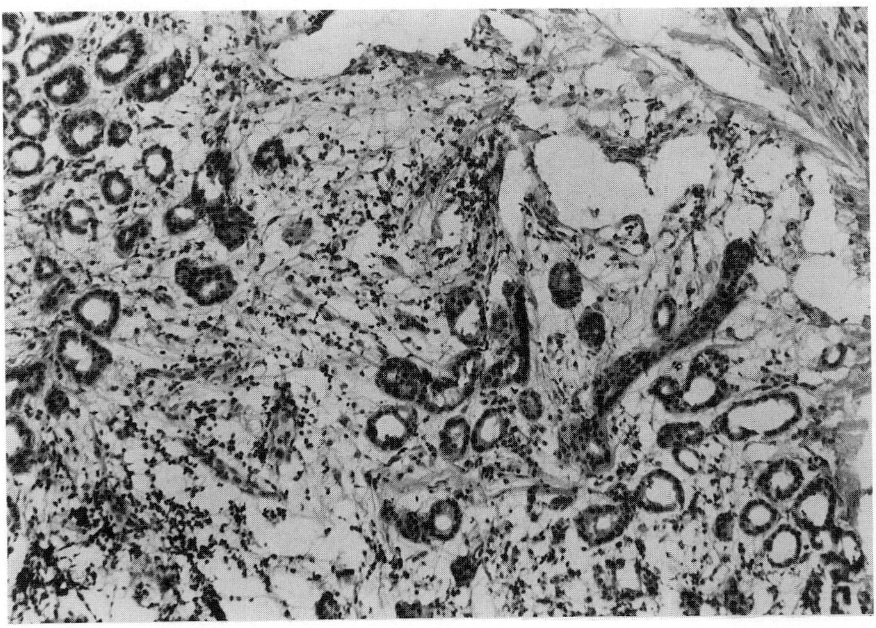

(E)

IV. CONCLUSIONS

This patient (Fig. 9A–E) was referred with lacrimal fossa mass that clinically appeared as a chalazion and was approached as such. At the time of surgery, it was noted that this extended well beyond the limits of the referring physician's initial expectations and he immediately abandoned the procedure. A CT scan was obtained which demonstrated an enlarged lacrimal gland on left side. It was elected to carry out an excisional biopsy and both the orbital and palpebral component of the lacrimal gland was removed via a left lateral orbitotomy. The tissue was submitted, and the initial impression was that of pseudotumor of the lacrimal gland. Subsequent reevaluation of the tissue and consultation regarding the tissue revealed this to be a lacrimal gland tumor. This patient's diagnosis went from originally a chalazion to inflammatory pseudotumor of the lacrimal gland to finally lacrimal gland tumor. A simple limited biopsy may well have been misleading, and lesions in the orbit need to be approached for thorough surgical evaluation and sampling.

With increasingly sophisticated diagnostic techniques, we hope to reduce the number of patients diagnosed as "idiopathic orbital inflammatory disease" by separating out specific pathophysiologies. Until that time, it is important that we continue to follow our patients with orbital pseudotumor involving any of the orbital tissues. The possibility of a misdiagnosis, reactivation, or transition to lymphoma needs to be considered. Even with the full armamentarium of chemotherapeutic agents, steroids, and radiation, we are not always successful in treating a condition that can range from trivial to one that can be severe and sight threatening, if not life threatening. With this spectrum of disease and with the multiple components of the orbit that may be involved, it will continue to be a challenge to those managing patients with orbital disease.

REFERENCES

1. Birch-Hirschfeld A. Die Krankheiten der Orbita. In: Graefe A, Saemisch T, eds. Handbuch der Gesamten Augenheilkunden. Vol 9, Part 1. Berlin: Julius Springer, 1930.
2. In: Spence WH, ed. Ophthalmic pathology. Vol 3. 3d ed. Philadelphia: Saunders, 1986: 2777–95.
3. Ophthalmology, Volume 100:1702-Number 11, Nov. '93. Orbital Pseudotumor, Devron H. Char MD, Miller Theodore, MD, pp 1702.
4. Rootman J. Orbital inflammation-evolving concepts. Perspectives in ophthalmic plastic surgery. American Society of Ophthalmic Plastic and Reconstructive Surgeons. Abstract from Featured Guest Lecture, 1993:72.
5. Char DH. Clinical ocular oncology. New York: Churchill Livingstone, 1989:349–66.
6. Rootman J. Diseases of the orbit. Philadelphia: Lippincott, 1988:165–79.

7. Alper MG, Bray M. Evolution of a primary lymphoma of the orbit. Br J Ophthalmol 1984; 68:225–60.
8. Orcutt JC, Garner A, Henk JM, Wright JE. Treatment of idiopathic inflammatory orbital pseudotumors by radiotherapy. Br J Ophthalmol 1983; 67:570–4.

SELECTED READINGS

In: Spaeth G, ed. Ophthalmic surgery: principles & practice. Philadelphia: Saunders, 1990:430–3.

McCord CD, Tanenbaum M, eds. Oculoplastic surgery. New York: Raven Press, 1987:238–240.

In: Hornblass A, ed. Oculoplastic, orbital, and reconstructive surgery. Vol. 2: Orbit and lacrimal system. Baltimore: Williams & Wilkins, 1990.

25

Diagnosis and Management in Thyroid-Related Orbitopathy

Gregory S. Kosmorsky
Cleveland Clinic Foundation, Cleveland, Ohio

I. DIAGNOSIS

A. History and Physical Signs

Thyroid-related orbitopathy (TRO) is a common disorder presenting to the ophthalmologist. The signs and symptoms may vary from mild to extreme. Initially patients may present with only nonspecific symptoms of pressure in and about the orbit, early morning periorbital swelling, and foreign body sensation. They may develop upper eyelid retraction and stare with or without lid lag. Proptosis is common and is caused mainly by enlargement of the extraocular muscles. The extraocular muscles become enlarged owing to in a predominantly perivascular lymphocytic and plasmocytic infiltration with subsequent endomysial fibrosis and deposition of glycosaminoglycans.

The Werner classification was an attempt to define TRO into predictable classes as follows:

Class 0: No signs or symptoms
Class 1: Only signs, no symptoms (signs limited to upper eyelid retraction and stare, with or without lid lag and proptosis)
Class 2: Soft-tissue involvement (symptoms and signs)
Class 3: Proptosis
Class 4: Extraocular muscle involvement

Class 5: Corneal involvement
Class 6: Sight loss (optic nerve involvement)

These classes may be recalled by the mnemonic "NOSPECS." However, any of these classes may precede the other and in fact, occur in combination quite frequently. The Werner classification is a useful tool to recall the signs and symptoms of TRO.

In class 0, patients have thyrotoxocosis but no signs of TRO. In classes 1 and 2, which do not separate distinctly on the basis of their clinical criteria, one may see lid retraction with the characteristic stare. Mild periorbital edema may occur in these stages. Unilateral proptosis may be misconstrued as a retrobulbar tumor by inexperienced observers. In fact, the most common cause of unilateral or bilateral proptosis is TRO. It is in these stages that lid retraction occurs in down gaze. Lid retraction certainly is not pathognomonic of Graves' ophthalmopathy and the differential diagnosis includes aberrant regeneration of the third nerve, Collier's sign secondary to midbrain disease, hyperkalemic periodic paralysis, chronic systemic steroid therapy, and unilateral ptosis with contralateral overaction of the levator palpebrae such as that seen in myasthenia gravis.

For many years it was thought that the retraction seen in TRO was due to the sympathetic overstimulation. However, studies have documented that this is not the case but rather that lid retraction is due to inflammation and cicatrization within the levator complex and Mueller's muscle.

A foreign body or gritty sensation may also be a part of these classes and is aggravated by infrequent blinking and proptosis. These symptoms are frequently exacerbated during sleep, which explains why many patients are worse in the morning.

In class 3, patients usually have at least 22 mm of proptosis. It is unusual for patients to have TRO-related proptosis and no other signs. A Hertel exophthalmometer is used to measure these patients and follow them. Asymmetrical proptosis of greater than 6 mm is very unusual in TRO and suggests a unilateral retrobulbar mass.

In class 4, the extraocular muscles become involved resulting in strabismus. This is usually first seen within the vertical plane, as the inferior rectus is the most commonly involved muscle. A very useful physical sign at this stage is the injection of the conjunctiva over the tendinous insertions of the recti muscles. It is very important to perform a forced duction test as TRO produces mechanical resistance to forced duction testing, whereas neurological disorders such as cranial nerve palsies or ocular myasthenia gravis do not cause mechanical restriction. A free forced duction is strong evidence against a diagnosis of TRO with manifest strabismus. A rise in intraocular pressure on up gaze is a useful clinical test and should be used routinely. Since the inferior rectus muscle is most typically involved, upward gaze produces compression of the globe by the thickened inferior rectus, thereby increasing intraocular pressure.

In class 5, the cornea is threatened by chronic exposure. Lid retraction and failure of up gaze on attempted lid closure (Bell's phenomenon) compound this problem. Corneal exposure in and of itself is annoying but not sight threatening. The onset of corneal ulceration represents an emergency as the initially sterile ulcer may be vulnerable to infection.

In class 6, the extraocular muscles become so enlarged at the apex of the oribit that they can literally squeeze the optic nerve to death. This complication occurs in approximately 5% of patients. The visual loss may be either unilateral or bilateral but typically is bilateral at its onset. Congestive signs and symptoms always precede visual loss, but compressive optic neuropathy is more common *without* obvious proptosis. The visual loss may be gradual; however, it can be quite rapidly progressive in some patients. Typically, the visual loss is cecocentral; however, any combination of an arcuate defect or altitudinal defect suggests that the nerve fiber layer is compromised and appropriate treatment is mandatory.

B. Laboratory Evaluation

The laboratory evaluation of TRO consists of the evaluation of the systemic thyroid status. This usually involves screening the patient for T_3, T_4, and thyroid-stimulating hormone (TSH). In cases where Hashimoto's thyroiditis is suspected, obtaining antimicrosomal antibodies is helpful. More sophisticated evaluation of the thyroid status, including thyrotropin-releasing hormone (TRH) suppression tests, should be done at the discretion of the internist or endocrinologist taking care of the patient. The interpretation of serum thyroid abnormalities is a "black hole" that is wise to avoid. Innumerable factors may influence the status of serum thyroid studies and the interpretation of these numbers is best left up to the internist or endocrinologist expert in this area.

The most common error that I see is missing the diagnosis of TRO based on the lack of any abnormal thyroid studies. It is generally assumed, although incorrectly, that a patient with signs and symptoms typical for TRO must have concomitant laboratory abnormalities. It is further assumed that treatment of any thyroid abnormalities will prevent the onset of or reverse any signs or symptoms of TRO. Studies have clearly shown that there is no necessary correlation between any definable serum thyroid abnormalities and the presence or degree of TRO. Further, normalization of serum thyroid abnormalities has little effect on the course of TRO.

C. Radiological Studies

Once the clinical constellation of symptoms suggests TRO as a possible diagnosis, the first test that I usually order is a computed tomography (CT) of the orbits. This CT is usually obtained with and without contrast and in my opinion requires *direct* coronal studies whenever possible. Although reconstructions may in some cases be adequate, I find direct coronal imaging far more sensitive to orbital compression. With direct coronal imaging all of the muscles may be compared simultaneously without slice angle interpretation being required. Also, the optic nerve shadow disappears at the orbital apex in patients with severe TRO with concomitant optic neuropathy and this feature is more easily seen with direct coronal imaging. The use of magnetic resonance (MR) scanning in TRO is not as well demonstrated. Although, clearly the MR scan is capable of beautiful delineation of tissue structures within the brain, its use within the orbit is limited by motion artifact and a bright signal return from fat that obscures orbital detail. The advent of sophisticated computer programs that have a fat-saturation capability that suppresses the fat signal has greatly added to the utility of the MR for orbital disease; however, its increased costs, increased acquisition times, and eye motion signal degradation limit its use at this time for all patients.

D. Ultrasound

The usefulness of orbital ultrasound in TRO is limited; it is best utilized to document enlargement of extraocular muscles where in the right hands it may be more sensitive than CT or MR in early TRO. Likewise the delineation of orbital fat accentuation may nonspecifically indicate an orbital inflammatory process. There are no specific ultrasonographic tissue characteristics that are characteristic of TRO. As with all ultrasound, it is ultimately technician and interpretation sensitive, and care should be exercised in diagnosing TRO with ultrasound alone, as other disorders such as dural shunts may mimic TRO on ultrasound. This modality should always be used in combination with other imaging studies.

II. MANAGEMENT

A. Medical Therapy

1. Symptomatic Therapy

Since many of the symptoms of TRO are secondary to corneal exposure from lid retraction with decreased or inadequate blinking, lubricating drops during the day and ointments at night will provide temporary relief for some patients. It has been suggested that sleeping with one's head elevated may reduce some of the periorbital edema experienced in the morning by some patients. Diuretics have not been efficacious in decreasing the interstitial edema of thyroid eye disease; however, an occasional patient reports relief with this modality. Most commonly, simple observation of patients who neither have corneal exposure nor optic neuropathy is justified. A detailed explanation of their disease process frequently helps the patients to "wait it out." I explain that the disorder may last between 6 months and 5 years in unusual cases; however, in almost all cases, the disorder eventually stabilizes. Recurrence of TRO is distinctly unusual. Periodic evaluation of these patients on a biannual basis along with warning them of symptoms of corneal exposure and optic neuropathy is essential. I also warn them of the possibility of diplopia from thyroid muscle involvement and encourage their return if this occurs.

2. Anti-inflammatory Agents

Anti-inflammatory agents such as ibuprofen have little, if any, benefit in patients with TRO. Since their ability to interfere with cellular immune reactions is minimal, anti-inflammatories do not seem to aid in the therapy of TRO.

3. Corticosteroid Therapy

Corticosteroids are the most commonly used agents used to treat TRO. A minority of patients, perhaps 30%, will respond well and for prolonged periods to low or moderate doses of prednisone in the range of 5–40 mg per day. If a patient is very symptomatic, I typically begin with 20 mg twice or three times a day and use this dosage for 10 days. If the patient experiences dramatic relief of symptoms, then I decrease this dose slowly to approximately 5–10 mg a week and will try to eventually taper them off steroids in 6 months. If there is little or no response, I simply stop the steroids (with under 2 weeks of therapy adrenal suppression is not a factor). The most logical use of steroids is for the feared, but unusual, complication of thyroid optic neuropathy that only occurs in approximately 5% of patients with TRO. Typical doses are in the range of 60–100 mg/day of prednisone. Patients are observed for a beneficial clinical response to the steroids and tapered slowly over several months. Unfortunately, as with many people, complications usually ensue in patients treated with long-term corticosteroids, and these medications are rarely a long-term solution in any type of TRO. Recently, megadose corticosteroid therapy, using between 2–4 g per day in divided of intravenous SoluMedrol, has been proposed as a short-term therapy for compressive optic neuropathy (i.e., 3–5 days) followed by tapering oral therapy for several months. In most cases, patients requiring such therapy will also require definitive surgical therapy.

4. Cytotoxic Agents

Although little has been written about cytotoxic agents and TRO, I have had some experience with this modality. This modality is especially useful in patients who develop steroid complications. I have routinely used methotrexate in a dose of 12 mg per week (five 2.5-mg pills once a week). This therapy has been used very successfully by our rheumatology department for the treatment of rheumatoid arthritis and other disorders with very little toxicity. Since methotrexate requires 6–8 weeks to reach full effectiveness, steroids should only be withdrawn after this period of time. I have no personal experience with other cytotoxic agents.

B. Radiotherapy

Low-dose orbital radiation is an effective treatment for TRO. The older literature is replete with reports of damage induced by older modes of radiotherapy that were inappropriately directed. This damage included radiation-induced optic neuropathy and radiation-induced retinopathy. Even brain necrosis was noted in rare cases from poorly aimed x-rays. The advent of modern x-ray equipment with the ability to very specifically target and deliver radiation has made this mode of therapy very beneficial. Radiation has the ability to reduce the congestive signs and symptoms of TRO and usually begins to show its beneficial effects in 6–8 weeks. We typically use a dose of 2000 rads in divided doses of 200 rads per fraction. For mild to moderate orbitopathy, mild corneal exposure, and mild optic neuropathy, this mode of therapy seems to provide much more long-lasting relief. Patients with optic neuropathy being treated with this modality should be covered medically (usually with steroids) for this period of time, as radiation will usually cause more edema and congestion before it has a beneficial effect.

C. Surgical Therapy

1. Orbital Decompression

Orbital decompression for TRO is used in several circumstances. All of the procedures described have the goal of increasing orbital volume by removing bone on either one, two, three, or four walls of the orbit (inferior, medial, lateral, or superior) (Fig. 1). In patients with long-standing TRO and exophthalmos, orbital decompression may produce an impressive cosmetic result. However, the attendant risks of neural damage and strabismus must be considered before performing orbital decompression for this indication. The use of orbital decompression for severe exposure keratopathy from TRO is well accepted. Typically, only the inferior and the medial walls need to be decompressed in order to protect

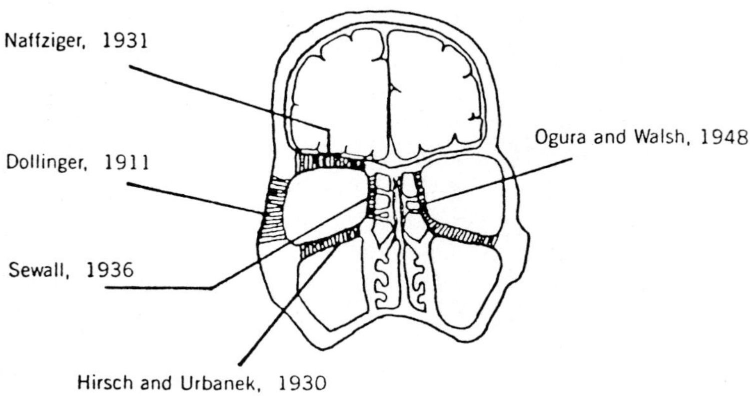

Figure 1 Various bony decompresive approaches for TRO.

the cornea. In this case, a direct ophthalmic approach through a transconjunctival incision with infracture of the inferior and/or medial walls is usually quite satisfactory. Optic neuropathy secondary to TRO is the most feared complication of thyroid eye disease. In severe cases of compressive optic neuropathy, decompression of one or more walls of the orbital cavity must be performed. In these cases, the more posterior approach to decompress the optic nerve, usually through the transantral route, is most efficacious. Typically, patients are first tried on corticosteroids; however, in severe cases of compressive optic neuropathy, I prefer initially to try steroids for several days and then proceed to surgery if the vision does not respond immediately to steroid therapy.

2. *Strabismus*

Strabismus is a rather common complication of TRO. The diagnosis of strabismus is usually straightforward. However, in some patients, it is intermittent at first, which makes it a challenging diagnostic dilemma in the differential diagnosis of transient diplopia. One should be aware of the unusual association of myasthenia gravis, another autoimmune disease with TRO, and should not hesitate to embark on a workup for concomitant myasthenia if signs and symptoms suggest this disorder. I usually obtain an acetylcholine receptor antibody assay and a blocking antibody if I am suspicious of myasthenia gravis. Although a positive result is diagnostic of myasthenia a negative antibody result does not exclude myasthenia. Ptosis, which would be unusual with TRO, is a clue to the presence of myasthenia gravis. If there is extraocular motility weakness and an equivocal forced duction, I perform a Tensilon test and only accept unequivocal strengthening (as opposed to paradoxical weakening or ambiguous changes in prism measurements) as an indicator of true myasthenia gravis. Typically, patients with TRO-related strabismus initially present with dysfunction of the inferior rectus, which means that their first symptom may be in the reading position. A careful evaluation of ocular motility in all gaze positions is essential in the diagnosis of this complication. The inferior rectus is the muscle most frequently involved in thyroid orbitopathy followed in order by the medial rectus, superior rectus, and then lateral rectus. The oblique muscles although obviously involved on imaging studies, are not typically a clinically important factor, although in some patients they can be clinically significant. The use of a forced duction test to evaluate restriction is very useful in patients with TRO.

The surgical repair of thyroid strabismus is very challenging. The clinical course of thyroid strabismus is that it is a continually changing process; therefore, strabismus surgery should only be performed after prism measurements become stable for at least 4 months. Once the disorder has "burned out," a reasonable plan for strabismus surgery may be formulated. During surgery, the muscles are found to be extraordinarily stiff, and in fact one may be operating in a deep hole in order to cut the muscle off the globe, as it cannot be pulled forward to be operated on. I prefer to use an adjustable suture technique in patients with TRO, as it seems to be the most reasonable approach to these patients, who may present with large angles of deviation and incomitant strabismus. Recession of conjunctiva and Tenon's capsule also is as these tissues are usually scarred and aggravate the motility defect.

3. *Lids*

The most common complication of lid involvement in TRO is corneal exposure secondary to lid retraction. Mueller's muscle is typically infiltrated and scarred in TRO, which produces lid retraction. The levator complex may also be involved with cicatrization and secondary foreshortening of the aponeurotic tendon with secondary lid retraction. The scarring process may be quite severe leading to lid lag and in some cases a frank inability to close the eyes completely. A lid traction test will demonstrate the inelasticity of the upper lid. Numerous procedures, including muellerectomies and various types of aponeurogenic surgeries, have been proposed and are routinely employed to achieve a more normal lid position for cosmesis and comfort. The most important thing to keep in mind here, once again, is that patients should not be operated on for this problem while they are "hot." Not only may upper lid procedures be helpful in hiding exophthalmos, but scleral or ear cartilage grafts into the inferior lid that also undergoes lid retraction with inferior corneal exposure may be carried out to elevate the lower lids.

In severe cases of corneal exposure, a tarsorrhaphy may be extremely helpful. Any number of procedures, including temporary or permanent approaches, may be utilized.

III. CONCLUSIONS

The diagnosis of TRO is usually not difficult. A history of serum thyroid abnormalities is helpful but not necessary for the diagnosis of TRO. There is no good correlation between the treatment of serum thyroid abnormalities and the clinical course of TRO.

Symptomatic treatment includes observation, ocular lubricants, and reassurance. The medical therapy of TRO usually involves the use of corticosteroids; however, these should be used only on a short-term basis where possible to avoid steroid dependency and its attendant complications. Only a minority of patients will respond to chronic steroid administration and reserving this modality for more severe cases of TRO seems appropriate. High-dose intravenous SoluMedrol may be beneficial in the short term for severe corneal exposure and optic neuropathy.

The surgical therapy of TRO requires the removal of bone by various procedures to create more orbital volume and thereby relieve orbital pressure. Surgical correction of lid malposition is usually carried out for cosmetic reasons but occasionally must be used to treat corneal exposure (Fig. 2).

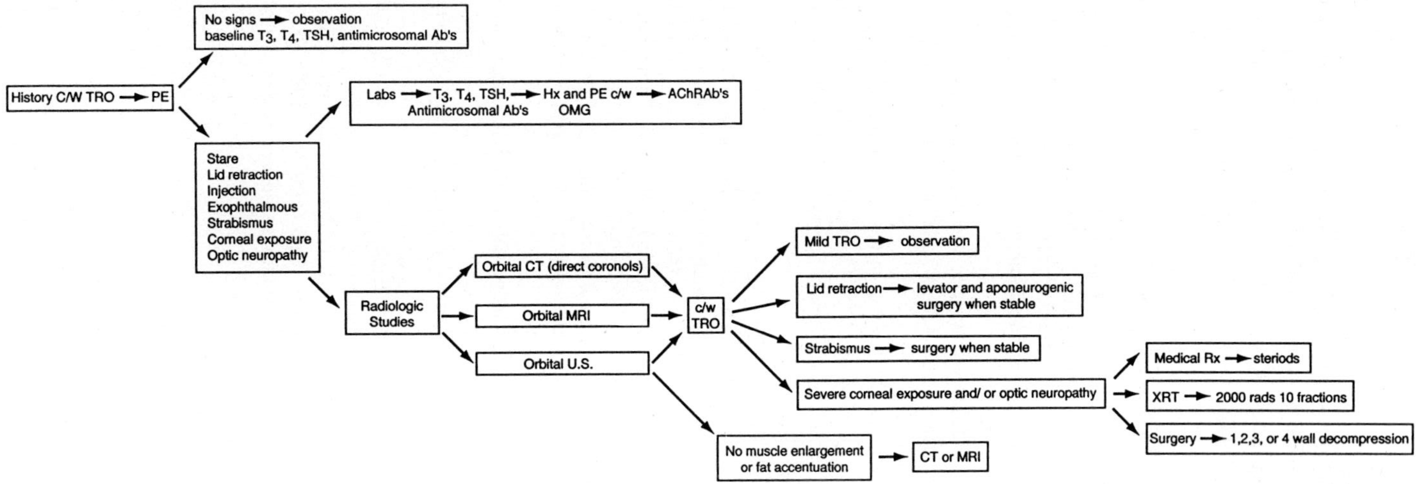

Figure 2 An algorithm for the evaluation and treatment of TRO.

The cooperation of an internist or endocrinologist is very helpful in TRO. These patients have a chronic disease with multiple complications and this must be carefully explained to each patient. Diligent follow-up and patience are required for the best possible result for both the physician and patient.

SUGGESTED READINGS

1. Anderson RL, Tweeten JP et al. Dysthyroid optic neuropathy without extraocular muscle involvement. Ophthalmic Surg 2 1989; 20:568.
2. Char DR. *Thyroid eye disease*. Baltimore: Williams and Wilkins, 1985.
3. Felberg NT et al. Lymphocyte subpopulations in Graves' ophthalmopathy. Arch Ophthalmol 1985; 103:656.
4. Feldon SE et al. Quantitative computed tomography of Graves' ophthalmopathy: extraocular muscle and orbital fat in development of optic neuropathy. Arch Ophthalmol 1985; 103:213.
5. Feldon SE et al: Clinical classification of Graves' ophthalmology, identification of risk factors for optic neuropathy. Arch Ophthalmol 1984; 102:1469.
6. Frueh BR et al. Lid retraction and levator aponeurosis defects in Graves' eye disease. Ophth Surg 1986; 17(4):216.
7. Glaser JS. Graves' ophthalmopathy. Arch Ophthalmol 1984; 102:148.
8. Hudson HL, Levin L, Feldon SE. Graves' exophthalmos unrelated to extraocular muscle enlargement. Superior rectus muscle inflammation may induce venous obstruction. Ophthalmology 1991; 98:1495.
9. Hufnagel TJ et al. Immunohistochemical studies on the exenterated orbital tissues of a patient with Graves' disease. Ophthalmology 1984; 91:1411.
10. Leone CR. Management of ophthalmic Graves' disease. Ophthalmol 1984; 91:770.
11. Neigel JM, Rootman J et al. Dysthyroid optic neuropathy. Ophthalmology 1988; 95:1515.
12. Sergott RC, Galser JS. Graves' ophthalmopathy. A clinical and immunologic review. Survey Ophthalmol 1981; 26:1.
13. Shammos HJF et al. Ultrasound in early thyroid orbitopathy. Arch Ophthalmol 1980; 98:277.
14. Sho'rr N, Seiff S. The four stages of surgical rehabilitation of the patient with dysthyroid ophthalmopathy. Ophthalmology 1986; 93:476.
15. Spierer A, Eisenstein Z. The role of increased intraocular pressure on upgaze in the assessment of Graves' ophthalmopathy. Ophthalmology 1991; 98:1491.
16. Symposium: Extraocular muscle problems associated with Graves' disease. Ophthalmology 1979; 86:2051.

IV

TECHNOLOGICAL ADVANCES IN NEURO-OPHTHALMOLOGY

26

Magnetic Resonance Angiography Relevant to Neuro-Ophthalmology

David I. Kaufman, James E. Siebert, and Joseph R. Pernicone
Michigan State University, East Lansing, Michigan

Angiography has long been an important part of the diagnostic evaluation of patients with neuro-ophthalmological disorders. Egos Moniz in the 1920s first developed the technique to visualize the brain's blood vessels using x-ray and various x-ray–dense salts. In 1931, he published his experience with 90 human cases (reporting only two deaths). Radiological investigation of extracranial and intracranial vasculature since then has traditionally required catheterization of the arterial circulation, with the exception of the brief popularity of venous digital subtraction angiography (DSA) during the late 1970s and early 1980s (1). Regrettably, venous DSA proved inadequate despite the fact it was initially thought to be an excellent, nearly noninvasive replacement for contrast angiography. Magnetic resonance angiography (MRA) has now emerged as the "latest" noninvasive method to study cerebral vasculature in patients with neuro-ophthalmological disorders and appropriately is being used "cautiously" (1).

The limitations of modern x-ray contrast angiography do include a small but important rate of morbidity and mortality. Patients complain of pain and discomfort. Severe nausea and extreme headache at the time of contrast injection are a few of the more common side effects. Although contrast angiography is excellent for detecting aneurysms and stenotic blood vessels, it is a two-dimensional method with some technical limitations. Typically, it shows only the anteroposterior (AP), lateral, or oblique view of a vessel. It is limited in its ability to show thrombi around the walls of an aneurysm. In addition, the position of lesions relative to surrounding structures is less apparent than on other imaging techniques such as computed tomography (CT) and magnetic resonance imaging (MRI). Contrast angiography is expensive, and it is frightening to many patients. However, it remains the "gold standard" to detect and evaluate abnormalities such as aneurysms, AVM, high-grade artery stenosis, or occlusion in symptomatic patients.

Contrast angiography presents essentially anatomical data along with some important information on the physiology of blood flow. MRA, in essence, represents only the physiology of flowing blood that is indirectly being used to demonstrate anatomy. If the clinician remembers that MRA demonstrates phenomena of physiological flow only and realizes its limitation, it appears to have some very useful clinical application.

I. BACKGROUND

Introduction of MR angiography for routine clinical use began in the mid-1980s (1–5). Since that time it has demonstrated its theoretical ability to revolutionize noninvasive evaluation of the body's vasculature. For the first time, contrast angiogram–like images can be obtained, with good reference to surrounding tissue, in minutes.

Clinical MRA development usually is traced to Singer. He demonstrated an "in-flow" experiment on blood flow rates using NMR published in the journal *Science* in 1959. In this set of experiments, it was shown that protons could continuously enter the detected region of a mouse tail and thereby enhance the detected signal (6). The velocity of blood could be inferred from the apparent reduction in the observed T_1 relaxation time.

Other experiments with clinical relevance were performed during the 1960s and 1970s (7–14), particularly on velocity of flow measurement. Then, Valk et al. (15) and Hale et al. in 1985 (16) showed how blood vessel–like images could be obtained using NMR. Their reformated images were very promising but technically poor because of resolution compromises that had to be made. Wedeen et al. (17) and Macovski (18) began solving this problem by using rudimentary phase contrast techniques and subtraction to produce direct, projective imaging of pulsatile flow.

Dumoulin and Hart further evaluated the known ability of MRI selectively to detect and analyze flow in a system of moving spins. They presented clinically important work and coined the term *phase contrast*, which enabled quantitative measurement and visualization of blood flow directly in a projected angiographic format. They also showed that venous and arterial flow can be measured at any point in the cardiac cycle (2) allowing for better use in human vasculature (2,19–22).

Dumoulin and Hart also overcame the serious problem of suppressing signals from stationary protons allowing vessels with lesser signal to be detected. Their article in the journal *Radiology* entitled "Magnetic Resonance Angiography" showed excellent AP and oblique images of the head and neck blood vessels in a normal volunteer (2). Considering the time of publication in 1986, these images were stunning to clinicians used to subjecting their patients to catheters and iodinated contrast agents. Other important clinical advances occurred quickly (23–73). In 1988, the first three-dimensional MRA results incorporating computer projection images became available (31,38). Norbert Pelc improved on Dumoulin's technique for phase contrast by introducing better encoding strategies allowing for a more efficient collection of data and precise flow quantification (33). In addition, the method explicitly reveals the direction of flow in a vessel.

Further development of techniques in time-of-flight–type acquisition were developed by Gerhardt Laub in the late 1980s (31). Useful information on the use of "black blood" technique was provided by Edelmann et al. in 1991 (32). Other improvements included the important step of development of MOTSA technique (34,35) by Parker, Blatter, and associates. MOTSA is a time-of-flight MRA technique using *m*ultiple *o*verlapping *t*hin *s*lab *a*cquisition. This enables time-of-flight MRA to be used more effectively and will be discussed below (34–35). Further review of the history of MRA and as in-depth understanding of the technique in general is available (1,36,39).

II. METHODOLOGY

Two major MRA techniques are useful: phase contrast and time-of-flight. Both techniques demonstrate flowing blood usually as bright and stationary tissue as dark. Generally, MRA methods that rely on the effect of flow on MR signal *phase* are called phase contrast. Methods depending on signal *magnitude* are called time-of-flight. A full understanding of methodology is essential if a clinician is correctly to apply MRA. Without this background, inappropriate interpretation of MRA studies will be common.

A. Phase Contrast

Phase contrast (PC) technique uses flow-velocity encoding to produce a signal. Stationary tissue (such as the brain) cannot contribute a velocity signal. Only a moving tissue, such as blood, will contribute a signal related to its speed and direction of movement. The faster the velocity, the higher (brighter) the signal image pixel or voxel value up to a certain point. This velocity encoding can be accomplished with the use of bipolar flow-encoding gradient pulses (23). Movement during the bipolar pulse causes phase shift proportional to speed given by $\phi_1 = \gamma$ VT A_γ, where γ = gyromagnetic ratio, V = speed of flow in the direction of the gradient, T = time separation of the center of bipolar lobes, and A_g is the area under one lobe (2,23). Figure 1 depicts these variables.

A working knowledge of MRI physics is essential to understand this technique fully. The smallest possible data volume (voxel) is assigned a digital value of

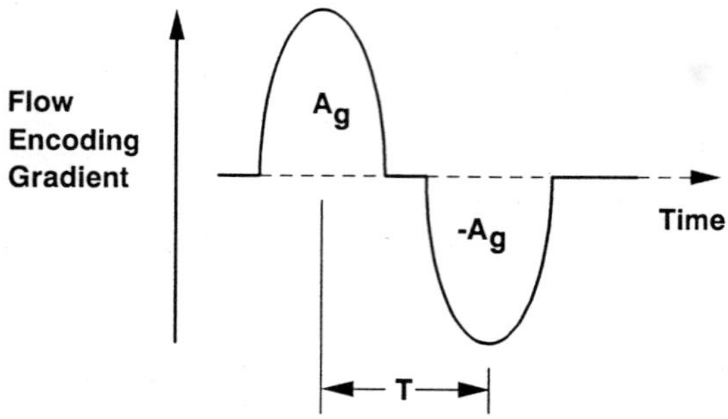

Figure 1 Flow-induced phase shift: $\phi = \gamma VTA_g$; V: velocity component along gradient; A_g: gradient lobe area. Bipolar gradient pulses can encode flow velocity on to the MR signal. A shift in the signal phase (ø) is proportional to the flow velocity component along that gradient direction (V) and the gradient pulse lobe area ($T \cdot A_g$). For stationary spins, no net phase change occurs for the bipolar pulse. A phase shift occurs for moving spins because the precessional frequency changes with position as the spin moves along the gradient direction during the bipolar pulse. The total phase accumulation during a positive lobe will not then be perfectly reversed during the application of the negative lobe.

brightness. It is proportional to the directional or vector difference in average transverse magnetization of two MR acquisitions. Only moving tissue produces a bright (nonzero velocity) signal intensity, since both bipolar lobe polarities cause a net zero phase shift for stationary tissue (23). The contribution to signal intensity will increase for moving tissue to a given maximum, which is predetermined by the strength of the bipolar flow-encoded gradient (TA_g). The higher the speed of flow, the brighter the image to the maximum intensity possible (36).

Despite the risk of overgeneralizing, to obtain a PC-MRA two MRIs are recorded. Volumes of brain not having substantial movement cancel each other's signal by using the elegant computer subtraction technique described above. Only flowing blood produces significant signal, which is recorded as the PC-MRA.

Clinically, small vessels and artery wall details can be enhanced by using a higher degree of flow encoding. However, artifacts can arise. Information may be obtained as either a two-dimensional (2-D) slab or three-dimensional (3-D) (volume) acquisition (Fig. 2).

2D phase contrast obtains the signal from a slab of "excited tissue," the spatial orientation of which is selected prior to the study. It projects the acquired signal onto a 2-D image plane. The signal for overlapping vessels is added in a vectorial fashion. The image intensity is determined by the amount of constructive or destructive interference. This implies that signal intensity at

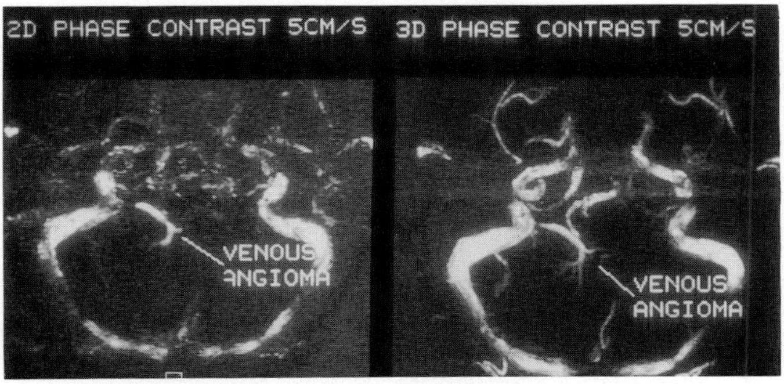

Figure 2 Venous angioma imaged with MRA phase contrast technique. Two-dimensional phase contrast is left and 3-D phase contrast is right. Note the better resolution with 3-D PC.

overlapping vessel crossings could be essentially meaningless. Slabs as small as 3 mm may be obtained in the 2-D PC method.

The advantage of the 2-D PC technique is that on an average, images useful for localization can be produced in as little as 27s for three different directions of flow encoding (23). Diagnostic-quality 2-D PC MRA of the brain can be obtained in about 5 min. Often it is used as a "scout" to allow for better localization of a 3-D acquisition. It also can address clinical questions involving flow in major vessels (such as ruling out superior sagittal sinus thrombosis) or achieve time resolution in a dynamic study.

The disadvantage is that 2-D PC acquires only a single view angle projection across the excited slab thickness. There also is decreased spatial resolution in the slab-select direction from the large elongated voxel. Complex flow, a phenomenon that causes loss of signal in all types of MRA, can be a problem, particularly with stenosis, aneurysms, or at bends in vessels. It is essential that the clinician be certain 2-D PC is not the only MRA technique being used to rule out significant pathology (such as aneurysm) in a symptomatic patient.

3-D phase contrast typically gives better resolution when compared with 2-D PC (see Fig. 2). Unfortunately, it typically takes roughly 30–40 min to perform. Patient motion may be a problem but can be minimized with coaching and restraint. There is great flexibility in image display as with all methods that give 3-D data. Images can be computed from any view by projecting selected 3-D PC image data into a 2-D–type display image (Fig. 3).

B. Time-of-Flight

Time-of-flight (TOF) techniques rely on fully relaxed proton spins flowing into the excited volume being imaged. A volume of brain can be saturated by constant

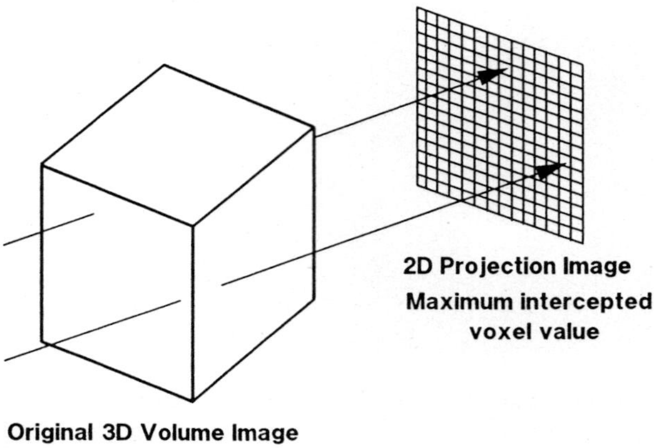

Figure 3 Projection images are 2-D representations of the information contained in 3-D volume images. Three-dimensional acquisitions enable the later computation of many 2-D images from any viewing angle, selected portion of the volume data, or thin slice orientations. The clinical practice of MRA makes extensive use of projection images.

radio frequency (RF) signal to a steady state so that it produces only low signal (23,26). Unsaturated blood flowing into this volume, like from the internal carotid artery, can have detectably higher signal compared with stationary brain tissue, a phenomenon called *flow-related enhancement*. Blood flowing into the excited area has not yet been saturated by the RF pulses. If flow is fast enough, signal strength will be maintained so that a blood vessel can be imaged throughout the course of the excited volume. However, a point along the course of a longer vessel may be reached where even the signal from normally flowing blood will not be distinguished from brain, because prolonged RF pulse exposure will cause even blood to reach a steady state (36) (Fig. 4).

TOF techniques also are 2-D or 3-D. The volume being "excited" equals the volume being imaged with single volume 3-D TOF. With 2-D TOF, the excited volume equals only a single thin (typically 1.5–2.0 mm) slice of the entire imaged volume. The 2-D TOF individual slices are acquired individually and sequentially and then "stacked" to form the volume image for presentation minimizing loss of signal with flow in longer vessels (2,4,27,31,36–39) (Figs. 5–7). TOF typically allows shorter acquisition times than 3-D PC.

A main disadvantage of 3-D TOF is that signal from slow flow may not be separated from brain in a longer vessel. This is because in 3-D TOF slow flow may become just as saturated by RF pulses as the brain around it making a blood vessel seem as though it "disappears." To a naive observer this normal 3-D TOF physiological phenomenon might be misinterpreted as an occlusion of the artery.

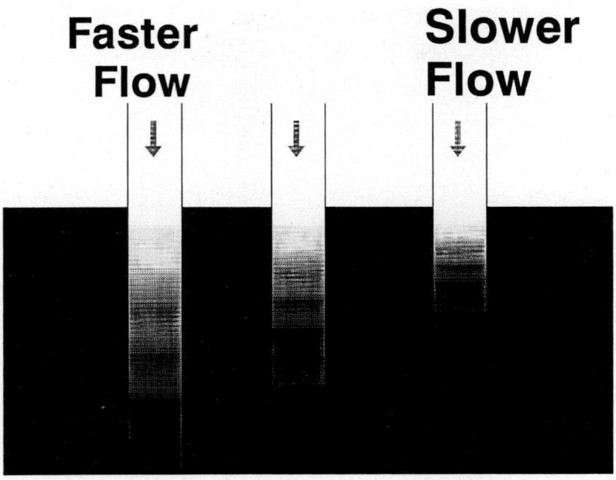

Figure 4 Flow-related enhancement provides the image contrast in the TOF methods. TOF acquisitions apply a gradient-recalled sequence using a small to moderate flip angle (10°–60°) excitation, short repetition time (TR, 30–100 ms), and very short echo times (TE, 2–20 ms). A gradual loss of flow-to-stationary tissue contrast occurs with the time blood has occupied the excitation slab as the blood approaches the steady state. So for given acquisition parameters (TR, flip angle), the faster the flow velocity, the brighter the blood signal and the deeper the effective penetration. The slower the flow, the shorter the distance traversed before loss of contrast.

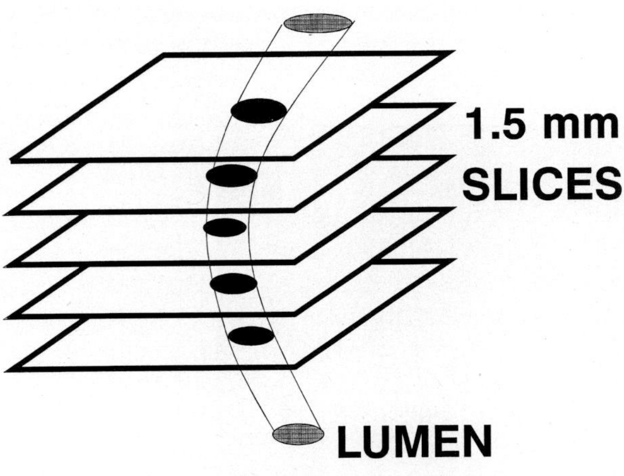

Figure 5 The 2-D TOF method employs thin slices acquired quickly, one at a time, and successively spaced. The individual images are stacked to form the 3-D image data. Two-dimensional TOF is exquisitely sensitive to slow flow and used commonly in the peripheral areas. Voxels are elongated as per the slice thickness.

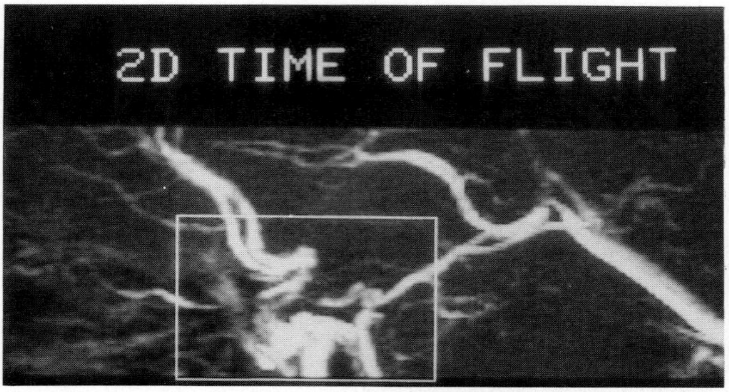

Figure 6 Two-dimensional time-of-flight through the carotid siphon. Notice the abundance of detail available.

Also, subacute thrombus (formed by methemoglobin) appears bright on all types of TOF and may therefore be difficult to distinguish from flowing blood (if using only TOF) (Fig. 8). Further disadvantages of 3-D TOF compared with PC are the former's inability reliably to detect slow flow in smaller vessels using standard techniques. TOF collects little information about relative flow direction, cannot make flow quantitative measurement, and cannot suppress brain tissue background like with PC.

The largest problem with 3-D TOF (loss of signal in a longer vessel) has been helped by the advent of multiple overlapping thin slab angiography (MOTSA)

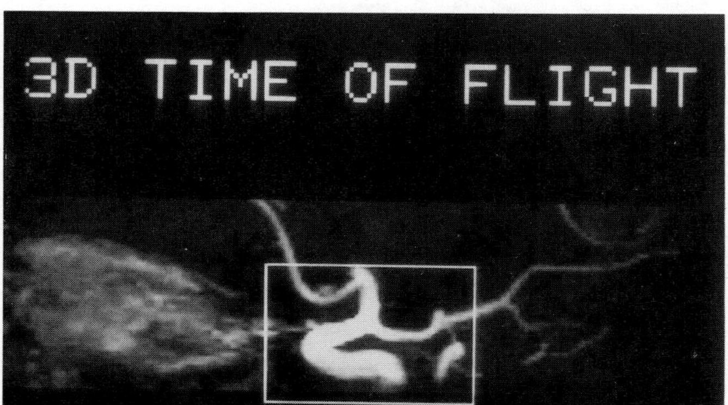

Figure 7 Three-dimensional time-of-flight through the carotid siphon. Notice loss of vessel detail compared with Figure 6.

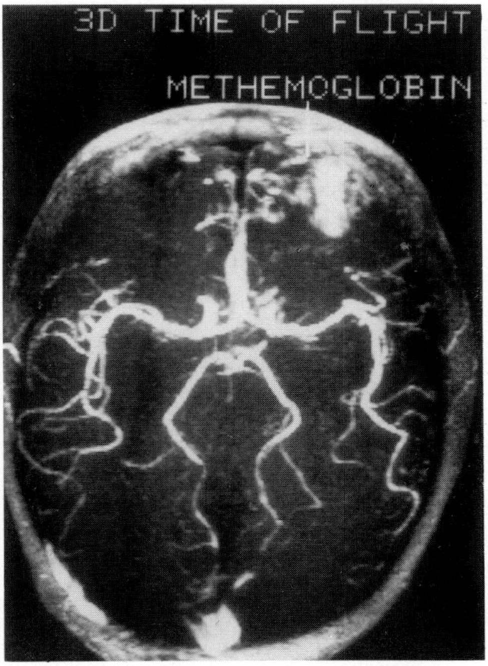

Figure 8 Three-dimensional time-of-flight of brain in a patient with a hemorrhagic stroke. Notice how subacute hemorrhage (methemoglobin) has increased signal intensity with this type of acquisition. Methemoglobin can be mistaken for patent blood vessels if only this technique is used.

(34,35). MOTSA (also called 3-D TOF multislab technique) is a hybrid of the best aspects of 2-D TOF and regular single volume 3-D TOF (34,35) (Fig. 9).

With MOTSA the desired image is obtained by two or more overlapping slabs that are excited *separately*. This avoids loss of signal in long vessels, which is a serious problem with 3-D TOF. Each slab is acquired as a thin 3-D TOF volume of 16 or 32 small slices. Adjacent slabs are usually overlapped by 25–50% on both sides (36,70). After acquisition of the slabs, overlapping slices are combined. Redundant slice pairs are compared and the higher valued signal at each location is automatically selected by computer processing to form the slice for that position in the volume. Acquisition time can be shortened by using optional techniques (interleaved slabs) (34–36,70) (Fig. 10).

The advantage of MOTSA is that this technique improves image quality and reliability of TOF by reducing the signal drop off common with single volume 3-D TOF due to saturation effect deep in the imaged volume (at the end of

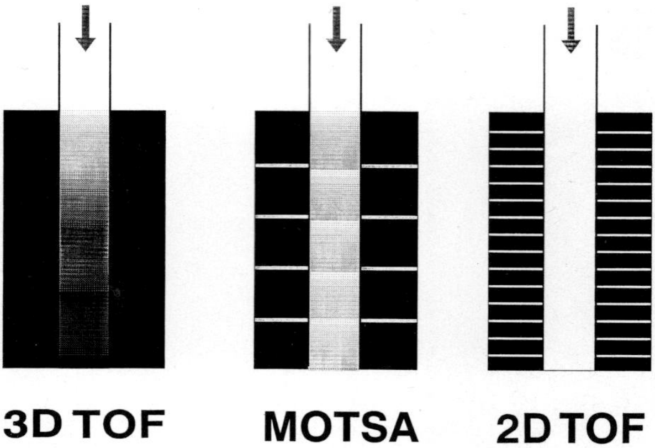

Figure 9 Flowing-to-static tissue contrast behavior of the three TOF methods. Contrast reduces with the approach to a steady state. Three-dimensional TOF is most susceptible to the loss of contrast due to this saturation effect. Two-dimensional TOF provides the maximum contrast for situations where flow is slow and orthogonal to the acquisition plane. MOTSA provides a compromise approach by combining the advantages of the other two methods.

blood's "flight" through a vessel). The technique preserves the small well-defined voxels of 3-D acquisition (36). MOTSA also enables effective TOF imaging in larger fields of view. In short, MOTSA takes the best virtues of both 2-D and 3-D TOF, while avoiding their deficiencies (see Fig. 9). In many situations, MOTSA TOF may represent the best practical compromise among 2-D and 3-D TOF and PC. It will become a routinely applied sequence in clinical MRA protocols (36) (Figs. 11A,B and 12).

C. Black Blood

Black blood methods are designed to avoid the consequences of signal loss inside vessels. The main difference from TOF is that with black blood, flowing tissue appears dark. It does this by creating a signal void for all flowing spins while maintaining a moderate signal from stationary tissues. It can also be used to label explicitly a volume of blood to see the direction it goes (36). A variety of black blood techniques have been tried (32,39–43). Acquisition parameters are usually chosen to boost stationary tissue (brain) signal. A saturation band slab is applied, usually outside of the area to be imaged, so that the inflowing blood has very low signal. Black blood is hampered by the fact that low-intensity perivascular signal from soft tissue and the regaining of signal in vessels far into the excited volume may yield insufficient contrast.

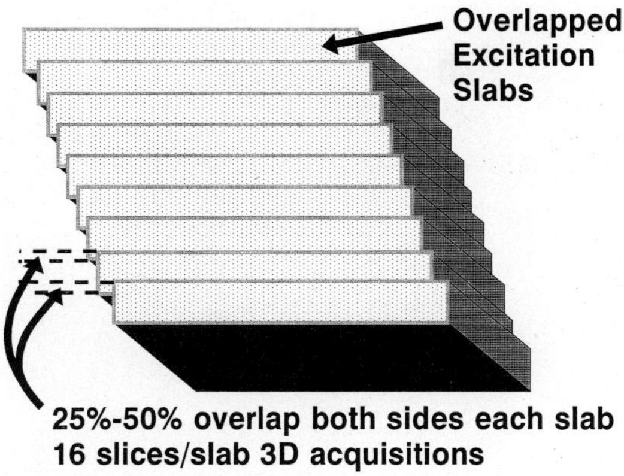

Figure 10 MOTSA acquisition scheme (also called 3-D multislab). Individual thin slabs, typically 10–40 mm thick, are acquired one at a time as thin 3-D acquisitions of 16–32 slice partitions each. Each successive slab overlaps the neighboring slab by ~50%. The overlap reduces banding artifacts ("venetian blind" artifact) caused by non-rectangular slice profile and slow flow effects. MOTSA represents a compromise scheme to reduce the loss-of-contrast saturation effects relative to 3-D TOF single volume while providing small well-defined acquisition voxels unachievable with 2-D TOF.

D. Comparison with Contrast Angiography

In comparing MRA with traditional contrast angiography, it is important to remember than MRA techniques use blood vessel flow physiology phenomena to demonstrate anatomy. It is not a pure "anatomical" display. The diameter of vessels will tend, to varying degrees, to appear smaller with MRA techniques because of the nature of this flow physiology. This is due to slow-flow characteristics near walls of vessels or complex (nonlaminar) flow causing some loss of signal. Aneurysms, ulcerations, and plaques may not always be well visualized on MRA to varying degrees. This is primarily due to complex flow phenomena causing signal loss in a vessel at an aneurysm, stenosis, or ulceration. These phenomena may cause MRA, if not properly interpreted, to overestimate vessel stenosis, make some aneurysms appear smaller than they actually are, or miss some pathology altogether.

The advantage of MRA, of course, is that it is noninvasive. The data can be manipulated better with good reference to surrounding tissue and can be obtained in minutes. There also is the ability to quantify flow (with phase contrast) and obtain total vascular information at once.

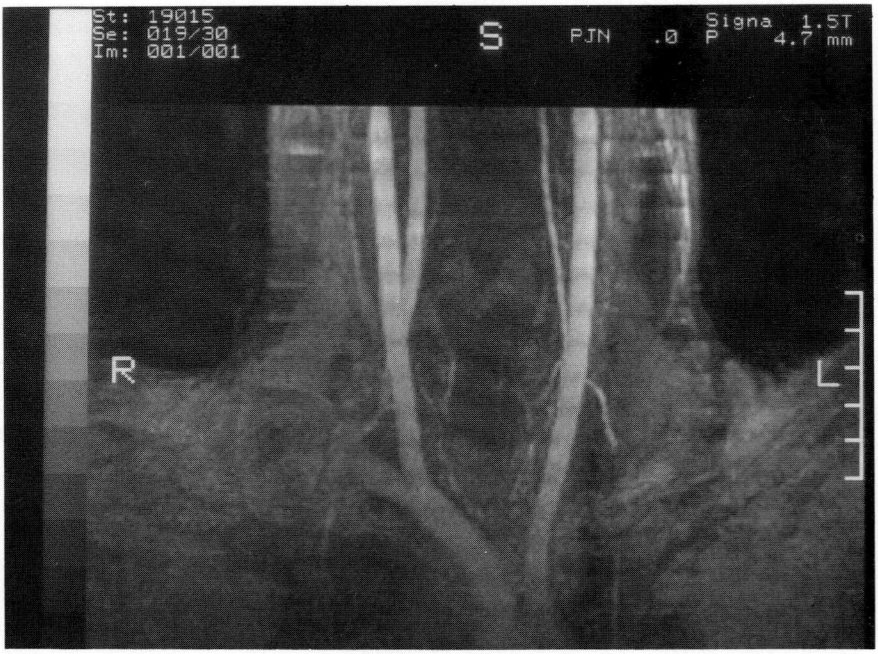

(A)

Figure 11 (A) Multiple overlapping thin slab angiography (MOTSA) technique in a 34-year-old with a small left vertebral artery. Note the ability to see the aortic arch, both carotids, the normal right vertebral, and the small left vertebral artery as they go through the neck. (B) Higher neck view of the same patient using MOTSA technique.

III. IMAGE PRESENTATION

The accurate interpretation of MRA requires dedication on the part of the radiologist to search the huge volume of data available in order to find features perhaps only a few millimeters in size that are germane to the clinical problem (36). It is essential to highlight that the accuracy of MRA is highly dependent on the radiologist, the method of acquisition, the method of display, and the time taken for image analysis (29). Image processing and presentation comprise an intrinsic step in efficacious clinical application of MRA.

A. Maximum Intensity Projections

MRA examinations produce a large number of images that must be analyzed scrupulously. To aid the process, projection images are computed from the

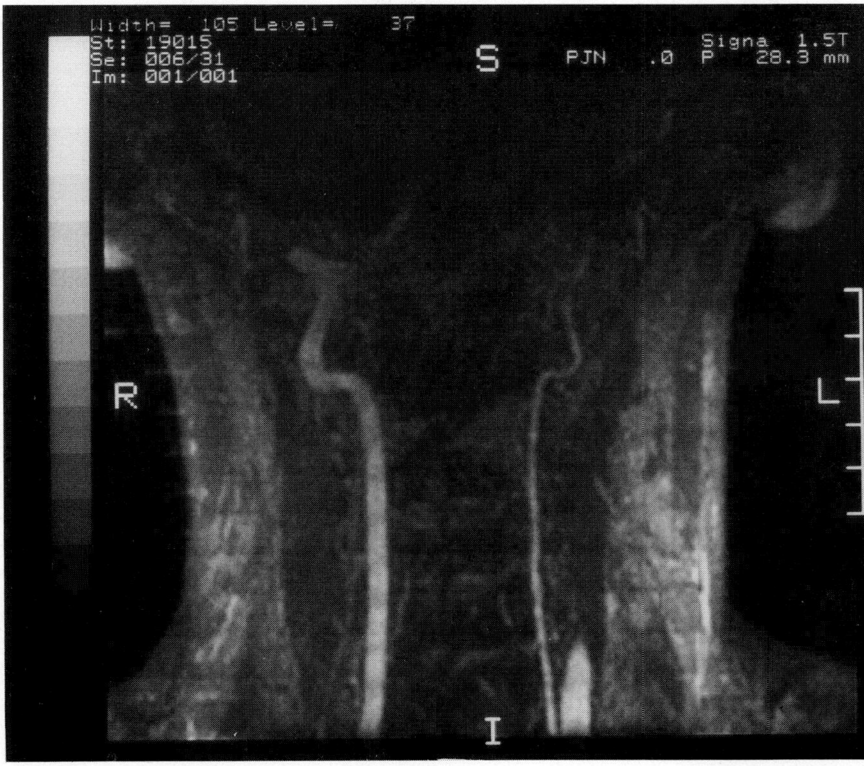

(B)

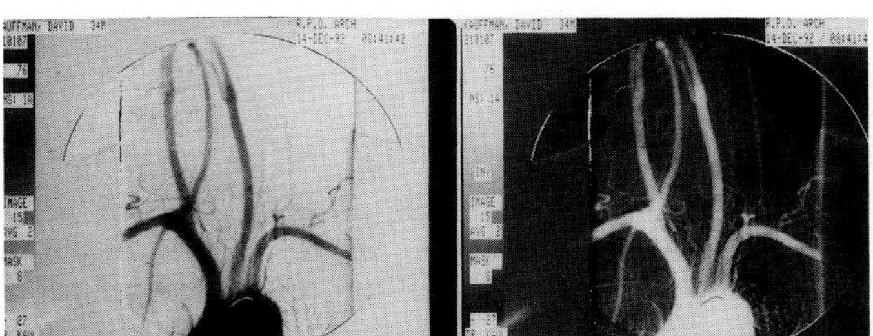

Figure 12 Compare conventional contrast angiography in the same patient as described in Figure 11.

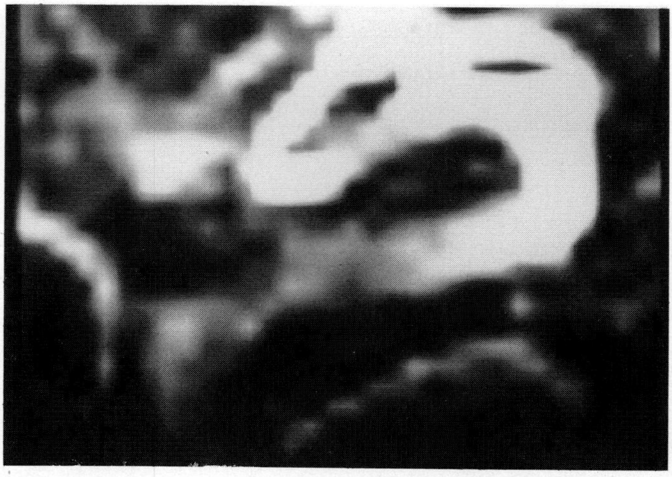

(A)

Figure 13 Maximal intensity projection (MIP) in a patient suspected of an aneurysm. Notice in the figure on the left (A) how only a large area of high-valued bright signal is displayed. This technique may obscure aneurysms (as detected in B). (B) An actual subvolume slide taken of the artery in A. It is important that thin subvolumes are used for MRA analysis (see Figs. 14 and 15).

original volume image. Three dimensions of information are compressed onto the 2-D display format (see Fig. 3). Projection images thus provide efficient representations of the volume image information and serve an important role in the MRA modality.

The projection method routinely used for MRA is called maximum intensity projection (MIP). A remarkably simple process, the algorithm casts a ray from each new projection image pixel through the image volume and selects the highest valued (brightest) intercepted voxel (1,6,24,31,36,70). This value is assigned to the projection image pixel as depicted in Figure 14. Images are computed for several projection angles to reveal 3-D details and to limit overlapping structures. Generally, the most useful MIP images for MRA interpretation are those computed for specific selected subvolumes of the original volume image. Advantages of MIP are that data is reduced in an efficient portrayal, it is reliable and automatic with a high contrast of vessel to background ratio, and it has a simple intuitive basis (1,39,44,45).

MIP, however, will display any high-valued bright signal. Nonvascular structures such as fat or subacute clot will be displayed indiscriminately instead of eliminating them from the display process (see Fig. 8). Conversely, low-val-

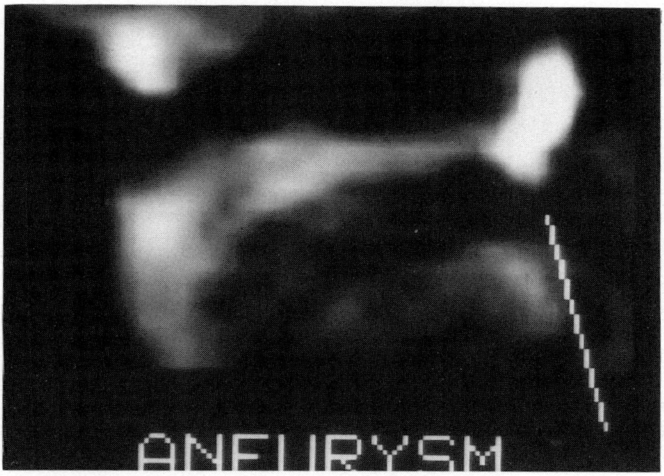

(B)

ued–low-signal flow features may be "edited out" such as, for example, regions of complex flow around stenosis or aneurysms with slow flow. Other problems include the fact that overlapping high-intensity features (such as from a normal vessel) may obscure any lower valued feature, such as an aneurysm, regardless of clinical significance (44–49). Information about the depth position of individual vessels is lost (50). Also, this method of display is insensitive to some differences in cross-sectioned shape (51). MIP also makes image right/left orientation ambiguous. Since only one voxel value contributes to the projection image pixel, MIP also severely reduces data relative to the original volume image (49).

All this makes it imperative that thin subvolumes are used in MRA interpretation. These "subvolume projection images," also called "targeted MIP," are projection images made from a subset of the full data set at various angles. Subvolume selection usually simplifies presentation of the vessels of interest, while eliminating overlapping features and reducing noise contribution. The smaller the subvolume that includes the area of interest, the better the ability to detect vessel signal over background (36) (Figs. 14 and 15).

B. Cine Display

Cine display is useful for panning through volume images slice-by-slice and for inducing 3-D visualization which is based on the repetitious display of projected images computed at incremental angles of 5–15 degrees about a primary axis. These images are displayed sequentially as a closed-loop movie.

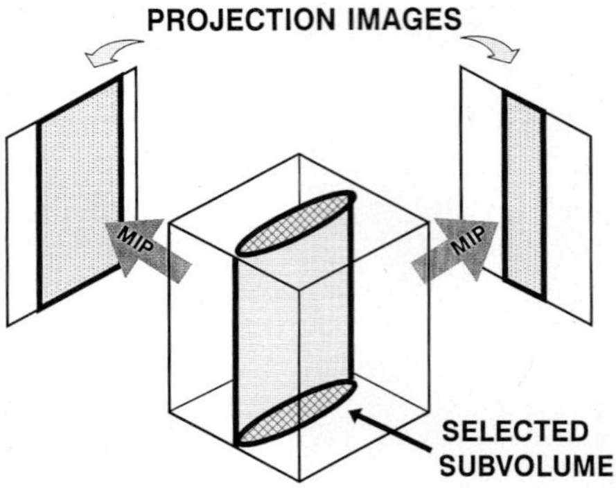

Figure 14 Maximum-intensity projection images computed for selected subvolumes (also called "targeted MIP") comprise the routine postprocessing technique for clinical MRA interpretation. The highest-valued voxel within the subvolume along the projection direction is selected as the new projection image pixel value. Subvolume projections provide clear views of the structure(s) of interest while also reducing the background noise contribution in the new image (see Figs. 13 and 15).

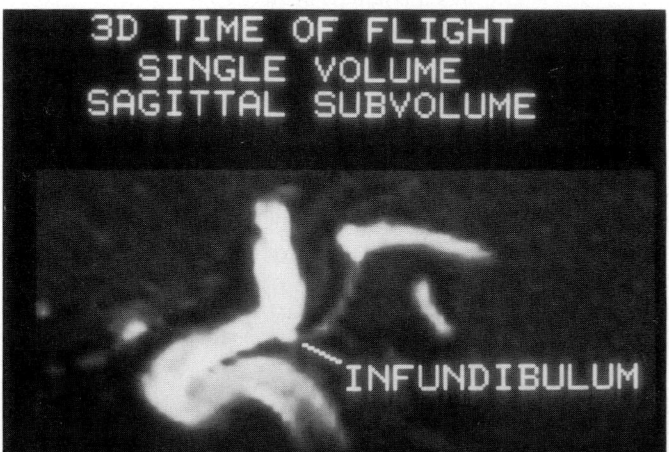

Figure 15 Three-dimensional time-of-flight subvolume. Note how targeted MIP with subvolume analysis helps find structures as small as this 2-mm infundibulum if the technique is used correctly.

The observer naturally integrates information frame-to-frame and interprets the relative motions of features in the series. The viewer thus visualizes these separate images as a spinning 3-D vascular structure.

C. Slice-by-Slice Analysis

It is essential to remember that the "compromised" projection process causes information from the original data acquisition to be lost. Complete information can be obtained by inspection of volume images as individual slices rather than compressing large volume of interest into a single "observation slice" (36,52) (see Figs. 13 and 15).

The volume image can be reformated into sagittal, axial, coronal, or oblique slices for best display of the features of interest. It is essential to review individual thin slices through suspicious areas. Individual slice analysis best demonstrates fine detail (45,51,52). When critical detail is lost or "missed" by MRA, in reality it is many times due to radiologists viewing only projections of volumes that are too large to "save time" (see Fig. 13).

Because so much data are available by MRA technique, a strong understanding of image presentation is essential to avoid missing critical detail. Image presentation and the importance of slice-by-slice analysis will be more readily appreciated as MRA experience expands.

IV. CLINICAL EXAMPLES

Well-designed examination protocols and display methods, in addition to meticulous review by the radiologist, are the key to efficacious evaluation of the intra- and extracranial vessels by MRA. However, as with any radiographic study, MRA analysis is at its best when the clinician and radiologist are together when the study is reviewed. Clinical correlation always improves a radiologist's analysis.

A. Aneurysms

In a series of autopsy studies, it was estimated that over 10 million people in the United States (5% of the population) have one or more clinically silent intracranial aneurysms (53). About 25,000–30,000 people per year will have a subarachnoid hemorrhage due to aneurysm rupture. About two thirds will die or be disabled with or without therapy. About one third survive without significant disability (54–61). It is obvious that a noninvasive means to detect unruptured aneurysms would be a significant advance in medicine. In neuro-ophthalmology, the main clinical symptom is a complete third nerve palsy including pupil involvement or less often an atypical optic neuropathy. However, painful, progressive, partial third nerve palsy, rare fourth and sixth nerve palsies, and atypical eye pain may all on occasion be the presenting feature of intracranial aneurysm.

Flow in aneurysms may be slow or complex. In our experience, the clinically significant aneurysms (3 mm or greater) and even infundibulum usually can be easily seen with MRA, but in some cases, only if proper acquisition parameters and display techniques are used (36,52) (see Figs. 13–15). Complex flow can lead to signal loss, and slower flow can lead to contrast loss due to saturation effect (52). Since MRA detects blood flow physiology instead of anatomy, aneurysms can be, and at some centers have been, missed. However, with correct technique MRA holds great promise for very sensitive, noninvasive, reliable detection of aneurysms. This is particularly true given the remarkable amount of research underway in this area of radiology (1,36,39) (Fig. 16).

1. Suggested MRA Protocol

At present, two acquisitions are the core of accurate aneurysm detection protocol (Table 1). First a 3-D TOF single-volume technique with a 4.8-cm axial slab excitation about the circle of Willis is performed. This is followed with a 3-D TOF multislab (MOTSA) technique (34,35) through the entire head (36,39,52).

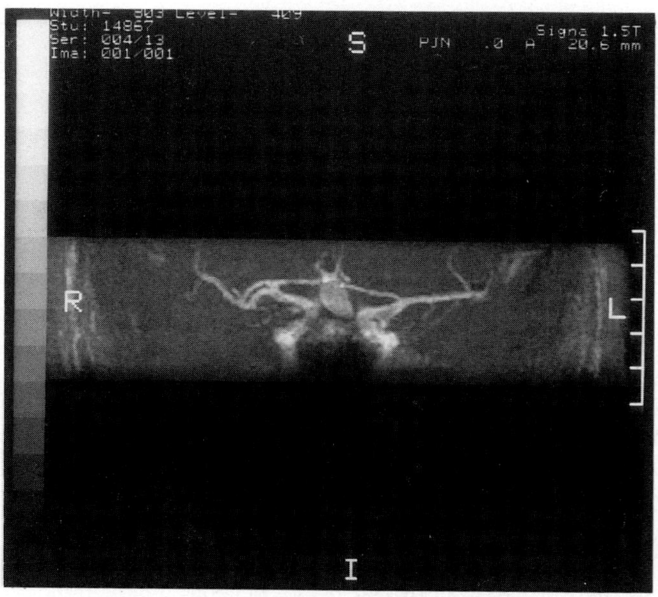

Figure 16 Large aneurysm around the chiasm easily detected using coronal phase contrast MRA. MRA tends to underestimate the size of aneurysms.

Table 1 Intracranial MR Angiographic Examination.

When searching for aneurysms or other intracranial pathology, our standard protocol currently consists of the following:

1. A 3-D TOF single volume study, with a 4.8-cm axial slab about the circle of Willis with the inferior aspect of the volume just inferior to the cavernous segment of the internal carotid artery. Acquisition parameters: 256 X 256 X 64 matrix isotropic 0.7 mm voxels, 40 to 50 ms TR, minimum TE, 15 to 20 degree flip angle.

2. A 3-D TOF multislab study of the entire head with 16 slices per slab and 25% slab overlap, 256 X 192 X 16 matrix over 12-mm excitation slab, TR 26 ms, minimum TE, 25 degree flip angle, using two-slab interleaved acquisition (effective slab TR is thus 52 ms). If there is a known or discovered vascular malformation, or if there is a question of infundibulum versus aneurysm, then additional acquisitions are performed.

3. If stenotic or occlusive disease is anticipated or found, then a 3-D PC study about the circle of Willis and/or through the abnormal vessel is obtained. Acquisition parameters: 256 X 192 X 64 matrix, minimum TR and TE, 15 degree flip angle, 5 to 25 cm/s V_{enc} reconstruct all five possible image types.

In order to best detect aneurysms, the following image presentation strategy has been developed. It takes into account the most likely projection direction of aneurysms in different locations. For the 3-D TOF data the following images are computed and filmed: (1) six images at incremental angles about the supero-inferior axis from subvolumes through each carotid siphon separately. The subvolume is made as small as possible to include the relevant structures. These images are viewed in cine format and individually; (2) reformatted sagittal and coronal slices through each carotid siphon; (3) a coronal subvolume through the bifurcations of the internal carotid artery; (4) an axial subvolume through the circle of Willis; and (5) a coronal subvolume through the anterior communicating artery. For the 3-D TOF multislab data the following images are obtained: (1) three images from a subvolume that includes the distal anterior cerebral arteries in sagittal and 45 degree oblique views; (2) six views about the superior inferior axis from a subvolume through the vertebral basilar system from the anteroposterior to the lateral view; (3) six images about a right left axis from the coronal to the axial plane to better display the middle cerebral branches; (4) sagittal subvolumes through each internal carotid artery siphon; and (5) a coronal subvolume through the anterior communicating artery. Finally, mandatory for the sensitive detection of aneurysms in the carotid siphons and circle of Willis, the single-volume 3-D TOF data must be inspected in reformatted sagittal and coronal slices.

Whenever suspicions are aroused during the interpretation process, single slice images (original or reformatted orientations) through the region of interest are inspected to obtain the final diagnostic conclusions. The original slice data serves as a primary basis for interpretation, while the projection images provide efficient representation of volumes of interest. Similarly, other pathology is studied by viewing individual slices and subvolumes in the appropriate planes (52).

A slice-by-slice postacquisition analysis (using the 0.7-mm slices and subvolume projections) is then undertaken in axial, sagittal, and at times coronal views through the most relevant areas (see Fig. 15).

3-D TOF single volume has the properties that best prevent signal loss from complex flow so necessary to image aneurysms accurately. However, it is not optimal away from the circle of Willis in the more peripheral zones, since saturation effects decrease flow signal contrast significantly (52,62). MOTSA *at times* will detect aneurysms better around the circle of Willis than 3-D TOF single volume owing to MOTSA's decreased saturation of spins (52). Also, MOTSA nicely detects peripheral aneurysms that may be too far into the excited volume if only 3-D TOF single volume acquisition was used. This combination is the best we have found in minimizing the possibility of "missed" aneurysms.

3-D PC, with parameters that might be used for overall intracranial image quality, may unfortunately be insensitive to the slow flow seen in many aneurysms, usually making it less reliable than a relatively small 3-D TOF single volume (52). 2-D TOF also is not good at aneurysm detection due to the limited spatial resolution related to slice thickness and its susceptibility to complex flow signal loss (52).

Although the recent advent of the MOTSA technique has improved the aneurysm detection protocol, in the past the combination of a circle of Willis 3-D TOF single-volume study and 3-D PC study through the entire head still proved very effective at aneurysm detection. It is important for the clinician to realize that relying on techniques such as only a simple 2-D TOF to eliminate an aneurysm may well be inadequate. The protocol used at each institution must be carefully reviewed by the clinician prior to using MRA as the only means to rule out an aneurysm, particularly in suspicious clinical presentations.

There is disagreement about the value of MRA with aneurysms. In a study by Ross et al., MRA demonstrated only 14 of 21 aneurysms (67%). When MRA was combined with a routine spin-echo study, as well as individual partitions from the MRA, sensitivity increased to 86% compared with contrast angiography (62). However, in a later study, Sevick et al. found six out of six (100%) aneurysms with 3-D TOF MRA (63).

It is obvious that comparisons of success between contrast angiography and MRA in detecting aneurysms vary in the literature. However, MRA success seems clearly dependent on the techniques used (1,52,62,63,70).

At our institution, 40 aneurysms or infundibula discovered on contrast angiography were seen using the above MRA techniques retrospectively. However, on two occasions, an occult aneurysm was missed prospectively. Both were in patients with "multiple aneurysms," where at least one or more other aneurysms were visualized and reported on the initial MRA reading. When these two examinations were reanalyzed with slice-by-slice presentation analysis, the "missing aneurysms" were clearly visible in the MRA data (see Fig. 13) (52).

Other investigators suggest the use of simultaneous MRI scanning may be beneficial (70). If the MIP images, individual MRA slice-by-slice analysis, and the routine MRI are all normal, aneurysms of 3 mm in diameter or greater should be excluded, except in the most unusual of circumstances (1,52,64,73) (Figs. 13–17). Naturally, if clinical correlation strongly suggests an aneurysm despite a normal, well-performed and well-analyzed MRA, contrast angiography should be performed.

MRA has progressed with recent research to the point where a major difficulty is actually distinguishing a normal 2-mm infundibulum from an aneurysm. Determining the exact size of an "aneurysm" versus an infundibulum is challenging (see Fig. 15). MRA tends to underestimate slightly the size of such structures as signal is lost with complex and slow flow, as might occur in or around an aneurysm (52,62,64). Nevertheless, it is our experience that structures above 2 mm are rarely missed with properly performed MRA.

Vessels filled with subacute hemorrhage (methemoglobin) may appear to have a patent lumen on TOF MRA owing to a short T_1 relaxation time (see Fig. 8). In TOF images, substances with short T_1, like methemoglobin, will appear bright in addition to bright flow features. This represents a potential pitfall in MRA interpretation; that is, mistaking a thrombosed aneurysm or vessel lumen as containing normal flow. Phase contrast methods are not affected by T_1 effects and can be applied to resolve such clinical questions.

B. Arterial Venous Malformations

Arterial venous malformations (AVMs) can have a variety of clinical presentations. Rarely is there mass effect or papilledema unless there is an acute intracranial hemorrhage. Homonymous hemianopsia or cranial and orbital bruits may be found incidentally. Visual hallucinations due to seizure are another interesting presentation.

MRA can be useful in both detecting AVMs and evaluating them before and after therapy. However, there is a problem with MRA resolution limits. In addition there is a lack of time sequence of flow information making assessment of feeder vessels difficult (Fig. 18). There is also signal loss due to complex flow (52).

In general, all standard MRA techniques in AVMs do not give absolutely complete information. The use of black blood may help with sensitivity and discrimination (40,52). The use of different velocity encoding values (speed of flow preselected for maximum signal acquisition, usually called venc) in phase contrast technique may also help with detection and evaluation (39).

Spin-echo MR also provides a valuable adjunct to MRA in evaluation of AVMs (65). The anatomy of arterial feeders is best evaluated with 3-D TOF

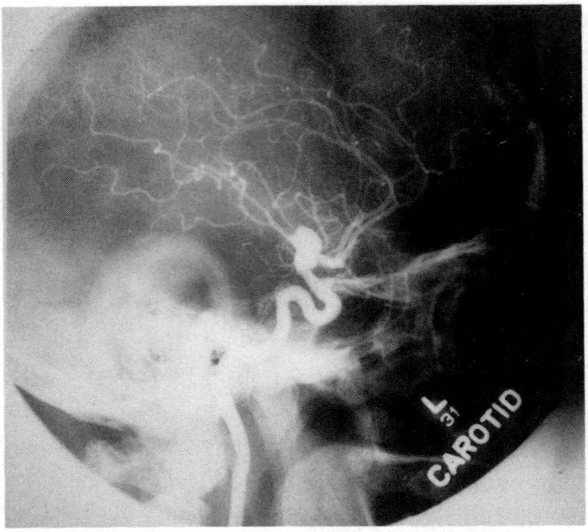

(A)

Figure 17 Conventional contrast angiogram performed in patient with clinical evidence of an aneurysm (A). MRA in same patient using sagittal (B) and axial time-of-flight technique (C). Notice that this patient's aneurysm is visualized well on both techniques.

single volume. The venous portion is best studied with 2-D TOF. 2-D PC may also be useful (65).

MOTSA may be able to show feeder vessels missed by the above technique. However, experience with this is limited at present (52). It may be a good screening test for AVMs, and once they are detected, more specific testing can be done, including black blood.

C. Stenosis of Extracranial and Intracranial Vessels

Atherosclerotic lesions predominate in the distal portion of the common carotid, at the bifurcation, and in the proximal 2 cm of the posterior wall of the internal carotid (53,57). Plaques can cause high-grade stenosis. Neuro-ophthalmological sequelae include transient monocular blindness (TMB), central or partial retinal artery occlusion (CRAO), or stroke with homonymous hemianopsia. Transient ischemic attacks (TIAs) or cerebral vascular accidents of the posterior cerebral circulation usually involve ocular motility or homonymous visual field defects. Atherosclerosis can affect intracranial vessels in addition to the extracranial circulation (53,57).

MRA can depict the luminal contour of the extracranial and intracranial

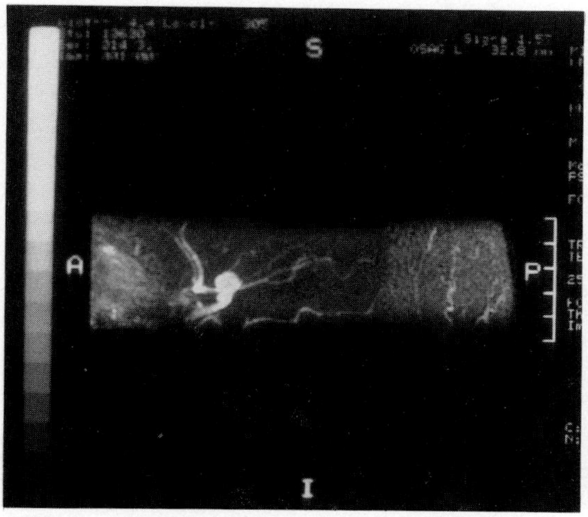

(B)

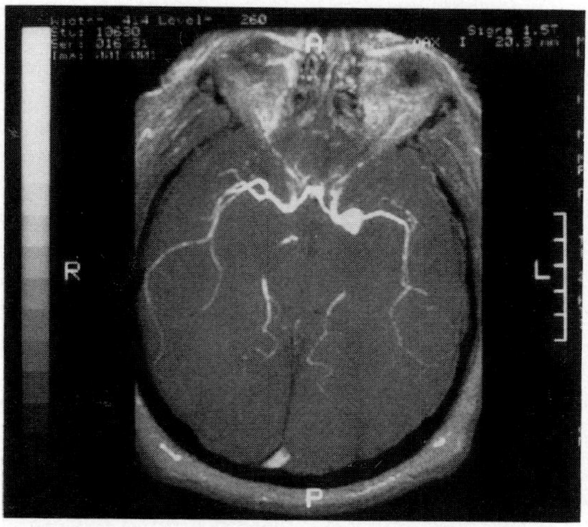

(C)

arteries (Figs. 11 and 19–21). Detecting mild stenosis can be a challenge. Moderate stenosis is often detected but overestimated because of loss of signal caused by complex and slow flow. Ulcerations may be missed (70). Severe stenosis can be characterized by complete signal loss in the area in question with signal recovery in a distal part of the vessel (Fig. 20). With complete occlusion there is usually no distal vessel recovery unless supplied via collateral circulation (Fig. 21). In short, the physiology of blood flow obtained by MRA does not

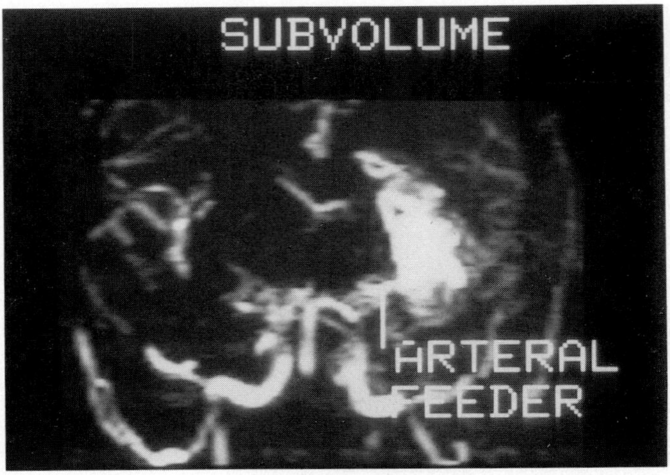

Figure 18 Phase contrast MRA performed in a patient with an orbital bruit. Notice arterial feeder going to this arterial-venous malformation.

always equal anatomical reality. These principles of signal loss with slow flow must be constantly borne in mind with MRA evaluation. However, MRA has good value in noninvasive evaluation of patients with expected cerebral vascular disease. A normal MRA, essentially all but eliminates significant vessel stenosis extracranially.

Warach et al. (66) reported on 24 patients with cerebrovascular accident (CVA). Intracranial occlusion or severe stenosis on MRA was noted in 16 (67%). Infarcts of 2 cm or less were not reliably shown. Small branch occlusions were not shown, probably related to insufficient spatial resolution. Masaryk, however, found excellent correlation in 21 of 22 carotid arteries evaluated by contrast angiography and MRA [27]. Other studies show varying results (1).

PC technique can be used to assess collateral flow pattern around the circle of Willis (67). In order to obtain direction of flow with TOF technique, black blood is useful (68,69). It is believed 3-D TOF multislab (MOTSA) will eventually prove to be the most reliable at demonstrating stenosis and occlusions and hopefully minimizing "overreading" of stenosis by MRA (34,35,52).

In analysis of patients with TIAs, relatable to the posterior circulation or the specific areas of the carotid or aortic arch in which Doppler analysis might be inadequate, MRA provides an excellent noninvasive means of eliminating significant stenosis (see Figs. 11, 20, and 21). It may well be these areas of the brain's circulation (not well studied by Doppler) that MRA will prove invaluable in eliminating significant disease.

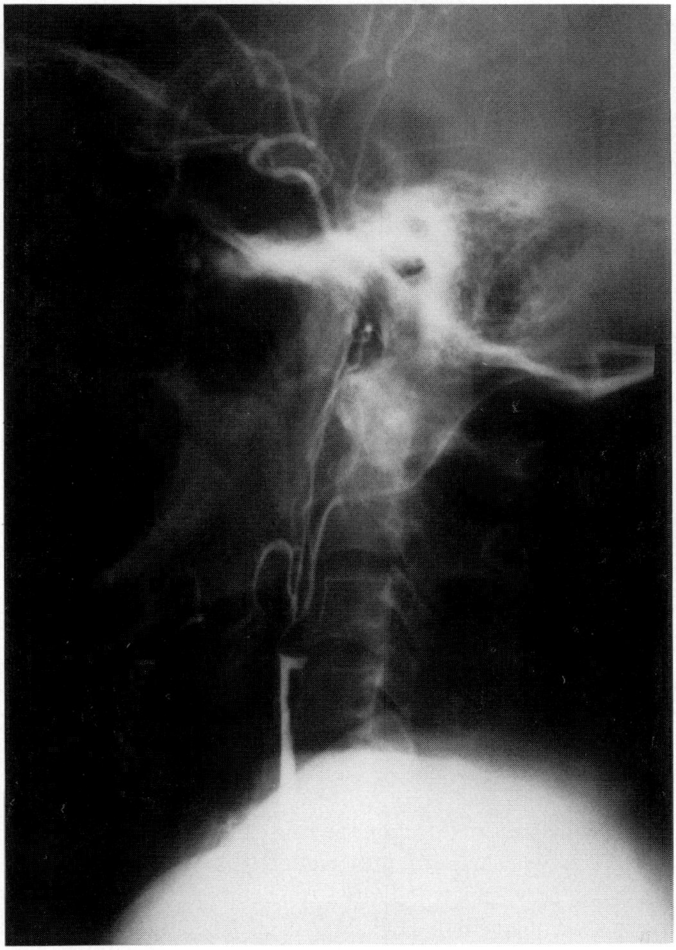

(A)

Figure 19 Severe widespread cerebral vascular disease in a 62-year-old man. Conventional contrast cerebral angiogram (A) shows occlusion of the left internal carotid and high-grade stenosis of the external carotid. Compare this with MOTSA time-of-flight MRA image (B).

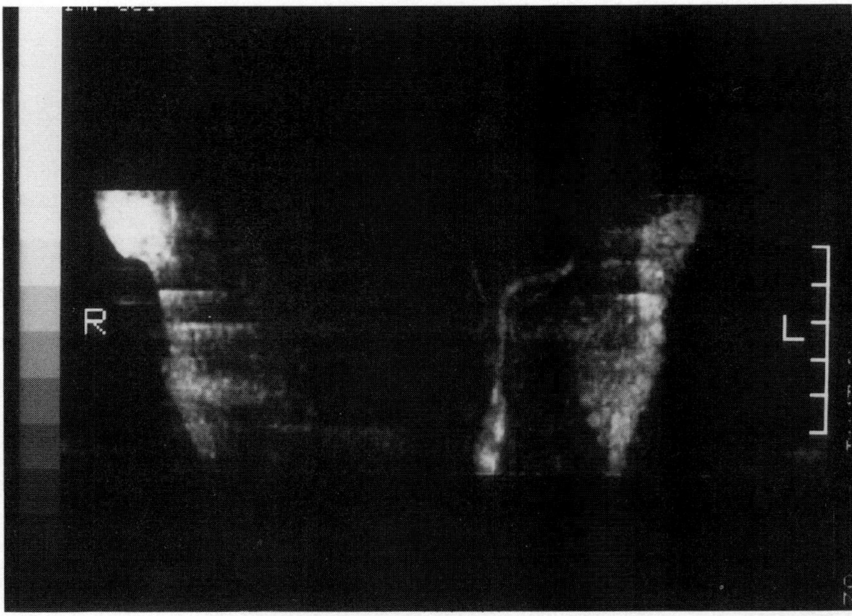

(B)

Figure 19 (***Continued***)

D. Venous Sinus Thrombosis

Hypercoagulation, adjacent masses, or infection can cause thrombosis of the cerebral venous vasculature. The typical clinical presentation includes headache, seizure, papilledema, and sixth nerve palsy. PC MRA can demonstrate lack of flow in such vessels in a very specific fashion. TOF alone is inadequate, because subacute clot may appear bright and masquerade as normal flowing vessel. In idiopathic intracranial hypertension (pseudotumor cerebri) presenting in a clinically atypical fashion, careful elimination of occult cerebral venous thrombosis is essential (Fig. 22). MRA has proven useful in this regard, not only in diagnosis but in longitudinal analysis of the treatment strategy being used for such thrombosis.

E. Preoperative Evaluation

Neurosurgeons at some centers are now using MRA to evaluate patients with brain tumors preoperatively instead of contrast angiography. It is believed that large anomalous vessels or occult (but significant) aneurysms will be detected by the combination of spin-echo MR and MRA. The opportunity to avoid contrast

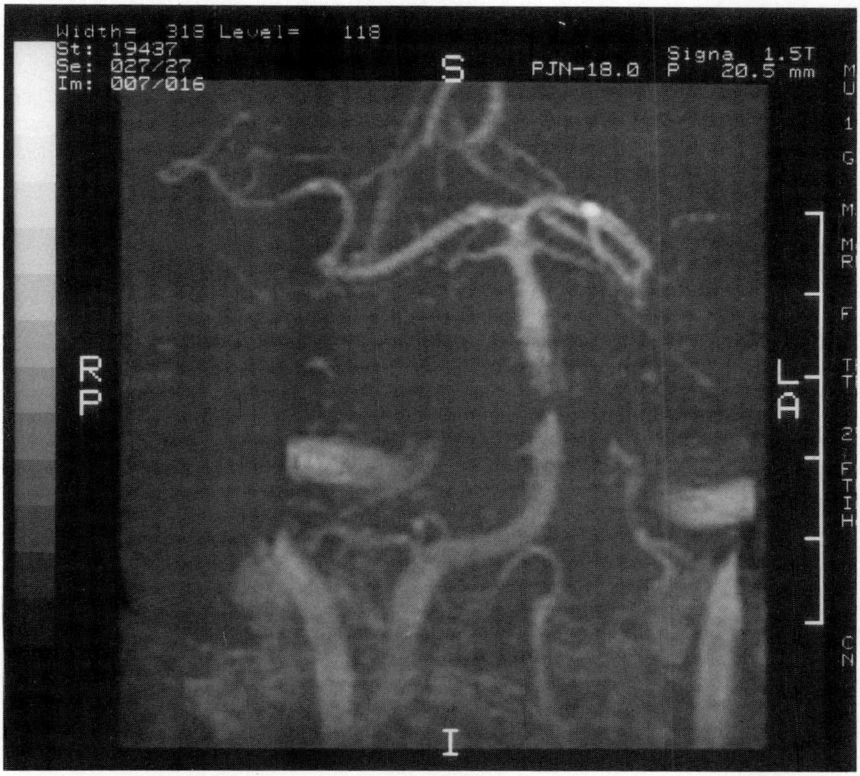

Figure 20 Transient ischemic attack referable to the posterior circulation in a 54-year-old man. Note the apparent occlusion (or very high level stenosis) in the basilar artery on this MOTSA time-of-flight image. Conventional contrast cerebral angiography showed moderate grade stenosis. MRA tends to overestimate the degree of stenosis.

angiography preoperatively reduces a small but real risk of morbidity in neurosurgical procedures.

F. Orbit Vasculature

Evaluation of the ophthalmic artery using MRA in regard to anatomy, direction of flow, and speed of flow may now be possible with emerging techniques (30). The potential clinical importance of this is identified in the emerging work regarding color Doppler and the ophthalmic artery. Blood flow velocity and direction of flow in the ophthalmic artery may theoretically provide prognostic indicators for the

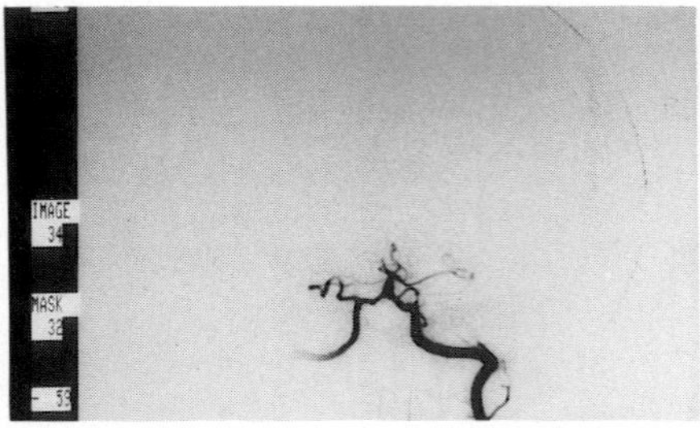

(A)

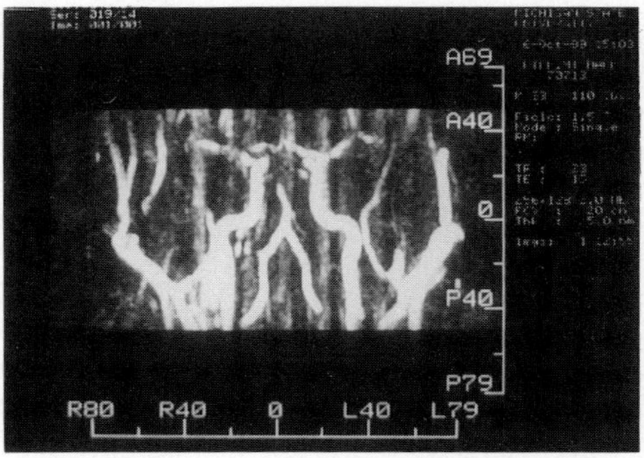

(B)

Figure 21 A 33-year-old male had sudden onset of coma during a racketball game. Conventional contrast angiogram shows basilar artery occlusion (A). MRA demonstrates patent carotids bilaterally. Note the vertebral-basilar circulation (wishbone-shaped structure between the carotids) also ends abruptly, consistent with the contrast angiogram (B). Patient did regain consciousness but had bilateral rostral interstitial medial longitudinal fasiculus strokes on CT (C). Residual gaze palsy included a skew deviation and reduced down gaze with absent saccades but retained slow pursuit (D). MRA is an excellent way noninvasively to follow such lesions over time.

success of optic nerve sheath fenestration in diseases like anterior ischemic optic neuropathy. However, Doppler has some limitations in its ability to demonstrate 3-D vascular anatomy along the entire ophthalmic artery (30), especially near the carotid take-off. MRA may be useful in demonstrating the anatomy around the carotid and ophthalmic arteries and also to help quantitate flow in these structures.

In imaging the orbital vasculature, 3-D TOF multislab (MOTSA) and PC are useful. The former can show excellent 3-D "anatomy," including the vessel take-off from the carotid artery and (when present) ophthalmic artery stenosis

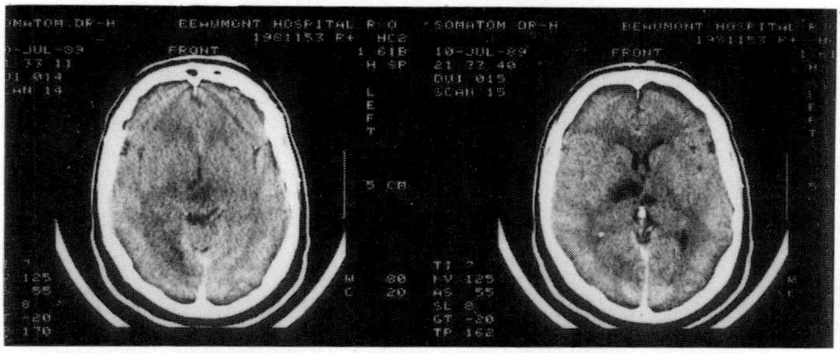

(C)

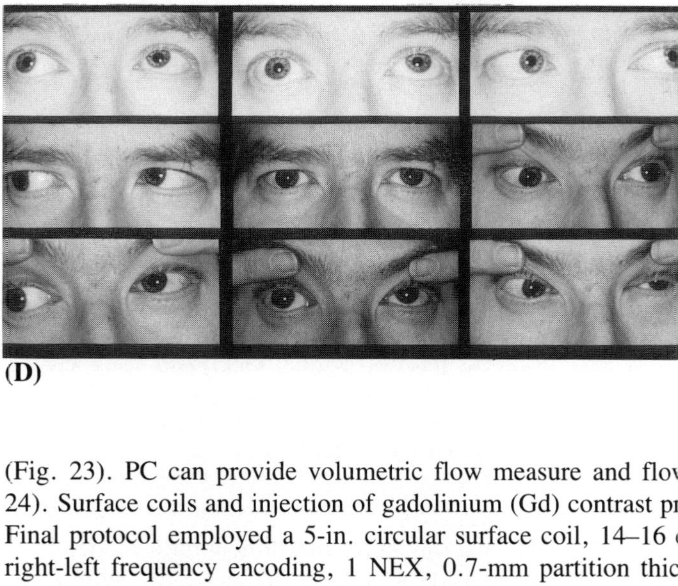

(D)

(Fig. 23). PC can provide volumetric flow measure and flow dynamics (Fig. 24). Surface coils and injection of gadolinium (Gd) contrast proved useful (30). Final protocol employed a 5-in. circular surface coil, 14–16 cm field of view, right-left frequency encoding, 1 NEX, 0.7-mm partition thickness (1.5 T GE Signa). MOTSA parameters: coronal 256 × 192 × 32, 40/3.7–4.5/30° (TR/TE/FA). 3-D PC parameters: axial 256 × 192 × 32, 25/9–4/25°, 25 cm/s velocity encoding. Gd-diethylenetriaminepentaacetic acid (DTPA) 0.1 mmol/kg was used. With these parameters, six of seven patients (86%) with visual loss thought to be due to ophthalmic artery disease clinically were noted to have decreased or absent blood flow with orbital MRA (30).

V. FUTURE DEVELOPMENTS

A significant amount of research is underway to further refine MRA. Larger matrix size (smaller acquisition voxels) may eventually help with some resolution problems. In addition, injecting gadolinium-DTPA helps decrease 3-D TOF saturation effects increases vessel contrast, and can make high-resolution MRA

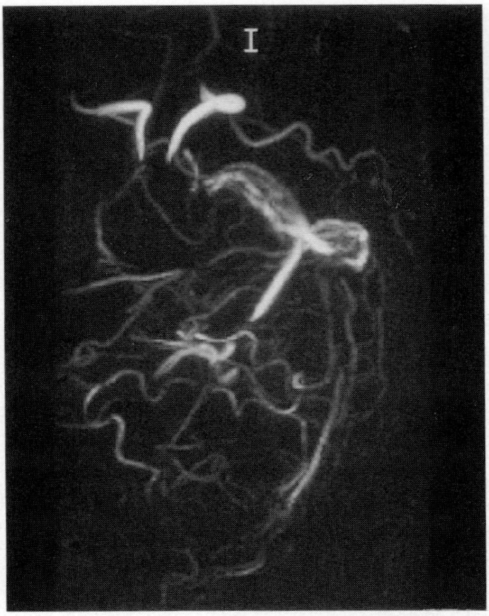

Figure 22 Phase contrast MRA in a 35-year-old thin man with headache, seizure, papilledema, bilateral sixth nerve palsy, and a normal CT scan. Cerebral spinal fluid opening pressure was 560 mm H_2O. Referring diagnosis was atypical pseudotumor. Occipital lobe circulation is to the left. Notice the straight sinus emptying into the torcula (on left of figure). There is no flow in the superior sagittal sinus consistent with superior sagittal sinus thrombosis.

practical (1). New contrast agents that stay intravascular may further extend the clinical applications and sensitivity of MRA in the future (1,63,70). With these new substances, vessels will be able to be studied independent of flow and thereby reduce the imaging problems currently caused by slow and complex flow.

VI. CONCLUSIONS

MRA is an emerging but complex physiological technique that can indirectly provide anatomical imaging of cerebral vasculature and specific vascular lesions. The limitation of using physiology to demonstrate anatomy must be kept in mind at all times by the clinician. A thorough understanding of the properties of the MRA acquisition techniques, the use of optimal display methods, and careful interpretation for each type of clinical entity under question is essential. Many times it is best to acquire data by two separate acquisition techniques. It also is

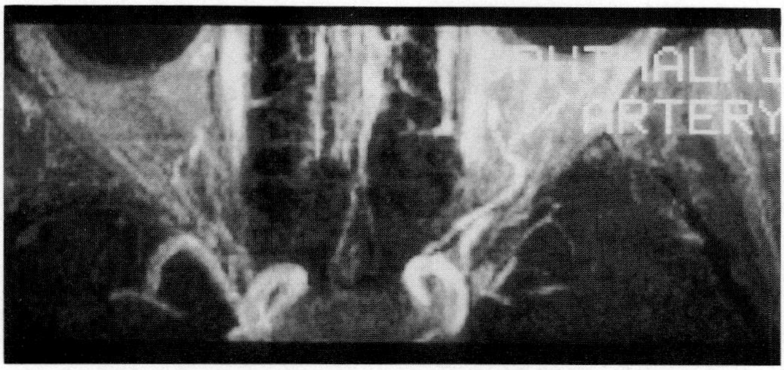

(A)

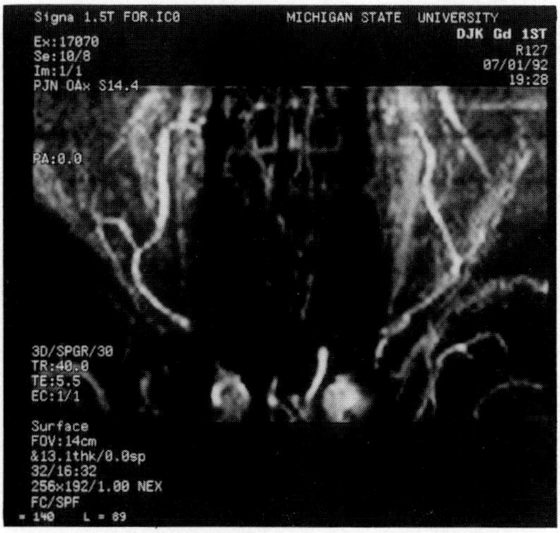

(B)

Figure 23 MOTSA time-of-flight study of the ophthalmic arteries. Note both carotid siphons at the bottom of A. Take off of the ophthalmic is well seen on the right. The optic canal may obscure parts of the ophthalmic artery. Note good acquisition of the ophthalmic artery and its major branches in both orbits in B. These acquisitions were gadolinium enhanced.

very important that the clinician be familiar with the wide variety of scanning techniques and review those used by their department of radiology to be certain optimal methods are in use for the patient.

For intracranial aneurysms, the use of slice-by-slice analysis of data acquired by 3-D TOF single volume through the circle of Willis and whole-head MOTSA technique seems optimal. MRA does tend to underestimate slightly the size of

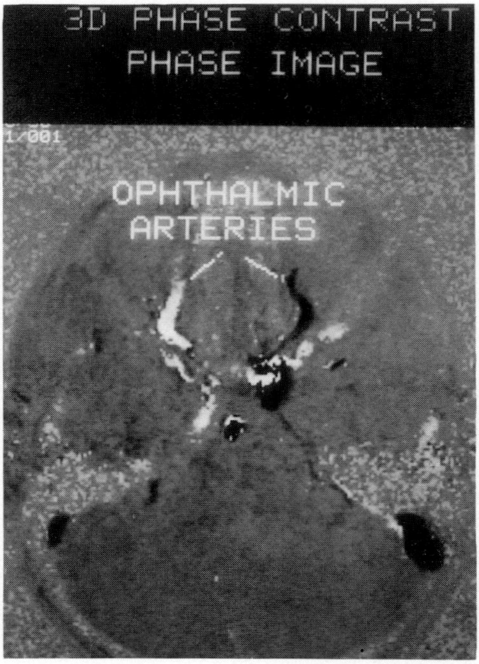

(A)

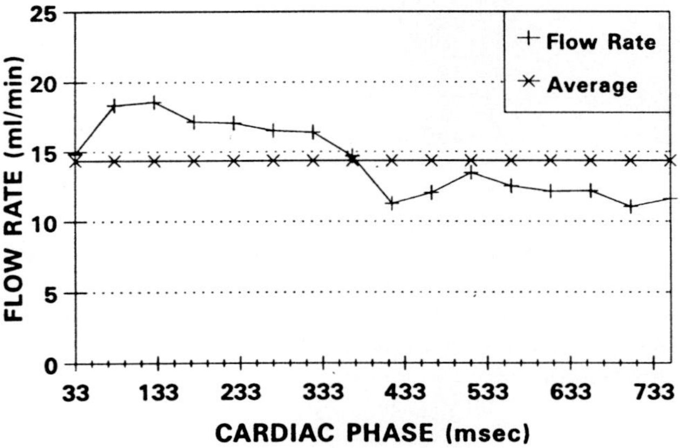

(B)

Figure 24 Noninvasive quantification of blood flow in a human ophthalmic artery using cine 2-D phase contrast MRA (A). Note how actual volumetric flow values and changes with the cardiac cycle can be calculated using this technique (B).

aneurysms. For intra- or extracranial artery stenosis or occlusions, MRA tends to overestimate the amount of artery stenosis. The MOTSA technique appears to be an improvement over previous techniques. If a vessel lumen appears absolutely normal on MRA, there is very little chance of a significant stenosis in our experience.

Continued orderly and careful evaluation of MRA with clinical correlation remains necessary as its usefulness and potential technical flaws are investigated. However, MRA appears to have promise as a potential noninvasive alternative to contrast angiography in several circumstances relevant to neuro-ophthalmology.

REFERENCES

1. Keller PJ, Drayer BP, et al., eds. Magnetic resonance angiography. Neuroimag Clin North Am 1992; 2(4):623–835.
2. Dumoulin CL, Hart HR. Magnetic resonance angiography. Radiology 1986; 161(3):717–20.
3. Ruggieri PM, Laub GA, Masaryk TJ, et al. Intracranial circulation: pulse sequence considerations in three-dimensional (volume) MRA. Radiology 1989; 171:785–91.
4. Masaryk TJ, Modic MT, Ross JS, et al. Intracranial circulation: preliminary clinical results with three-dimensional (volume) MR angiography. Radiology 1989; 171:793–9.
5. Alfidi RJ, Masaryk TJ, Haacke EM, et al. MR angiography of peripheral, carotid, and coronary arteries. AJR 1987;149:1097–1109.
6. Singer JR. Blood flow rates by nuclear magnetic resonance. Science 1959; 130:1652–3.
7. Crooks LE, Mills CM, David PL, et al. Visualization of cerebral and vascular abnormalities by NMR imaging: the effects of imaging parameters on contrast. Radiology 1982; 144:843–52.
8. Morse OC, Singer JR. Blood velocity Measurements in intact subjects. Science 1970; 170:440–1.
9. Feinberg DA, Crooks L, Hoenninger J, et al. Pulsatile blood velocity in human arteries displayed by MRI. Radiology 1984; 153:177–80.
10. Wehrli FW, Shimakawa A, MacFall JR, et al. MR imaging of venous and arterial flow by a selective saturation-recovery spin echo (SSRSE) method. J Comput Assist Tomogr 1985; 9:537–45.
11. Hahn EL. Detection of sea-water motion by nuclear precession. J Geophys Res 1960; 65:776–7.
12. Grover T, Singer JR. NMR spin-echo flow measurements. J Appl Phys 1971; 42:938–40.
13. O'Donnell M. NMR blood flow imaging multiecho, phase contrast sequences. Med Phys 1985; 12:59–64.
14. Bryant DI, Payn JA, Firmin DN, et al. Measurement of flow with NMR imaging using a gradient pulse and phase difference technique. J Comput Assist Tomogr 1984; 8:588–93.

15. Valk PE, Hale JD, Kaufman L, et al. MR imaging of the aorta with three-dimensional vessel reconstruction: validation by angiography. Radiology 1985; 157:721–5.
16. Hale JD, Valk PE, Watts JC et al. MR imaging of blood vessels using three-dimensional reconstruction: methodology. Radiology 1985; 157:727–33.
17. Wedeen VJ, Reto AM, Edelman RR, et al. Projective imaging of pulsatile flow with magnetic resonance. Science 1985; 230:946–8.
18. Macovski A. Selective projection imaging: applications to radiology and NMR. IEEE Trans Med Imaging 1982; 1:42–7.
19. Dumoulin CL, Souza SP, Hart HR. Rapid scan magnetic resonance angiography. Magn Reson Med 1987; 5:238–245.
20. Walker MF, Souza SP, Dumoulin CL. Quantitative flow measurement in phase contrast MR angiography. J Comput Assist Tomogr 1988; 12(2):304–13.
21. Dumoulin CL, Souza SP, Walker MF, et al. Three dimensional phase contrast angiography. Magn Reson Med 1989; 9:139–49.
22. Dumoulin CL, Cline HE, Souza SP, et al. Three-dimensional time-of-flight magnetic resonance angiography using spin saturation. Magn Reson Med 1989; 11: 35–46.
23. Pernicone JR, Siebert JE, Potchen EJ, et al. Three-dimensional phase-contrast MR angiography in the head and neck: preliminary report. AJNR 1990; 11:457–66.
24. Rossnick S, Kennedy D, Laub G, et al. Three dimensional display of blood vessels in MRI. Proceedings of IEEE Computers in Cardiology Conference. Piscataway, NJ, 1986:193–6 (abstract).
25. Keller PJ, Drayer BP, Fram EK, et al. MR angiography via 2D-acquisition but yielding a 3D-display: a work in progress. Radiology 1989; 173:527–32.
26. Masaryk TJ, Modic MT, Ross JS, et al. Intracranial circulation: preliminary clinical results with three-dimensional (volume) MR angiography. Radiology 1989; 171:793–9.
27. Masaryk TJ, Modic MT, Ruggieri PM, et al. Three-dimensional (volume) gradient-echo imaging of the carotid bifurcation: preliminary clinical experience. Radiology 1989; 171:801–6.
28. Gale KL, Kaufman DI, Pernicone J. Two MRI advances relevant to neuro-ophthalmology. Invest Ophthal Visual Sci 1989 ;30(Suppl.):246.
29. Kaufman DI, Pernicone JR. Advances in MRI and their impact on neuro-ophthalmology. Semin Ophthalmol 1992; 7(1):2–23.
30. Kokinakis DJ, Siebert JE, Kaufman DI, et al. Evaluation of ophthalmic arteries is possible using MRA. Invest Ophthal Visual Sci 1993; 34;4(Suppl.):1123.
31. Laub GA, Kaiser WA. MR angiography with gradient motion refocusing. J Comput Assist Tomogr 1988; 12:377–82.
32. Edelman RR, Chien D, Kim D. Fast selective black blood imaging. Radiology 1991; 181:655–60.
33. Pelc NJ, Bernstein MA, et al. Encoding strategies for three-direction phase-contrast MR imaging of flow. J Magn Reson Imaging 1991; 1:405–13.
34. Blatter DD, Parker DL, Robison RO. Cerebral MR angiography with multiple overlapping thin slab acquisition. Part I. Quantitative analysis of vessel visibility. Radiology 1991; 179:805–11.

35. Parker DL, Yuan C, Blatter DD. MR angiography by multiple thin slab 3D acquisition. Magn Reson Med 1991; 17:434–51.
36. Siebert JE, Pernicone JR, Potchen EJ. Physical principles and application of magnetic resonance angiography. Seminar Ultrasound CT MRI 1992; 13(4):227–45.
37. Ross JS, Masaryk TJ, Modic MT, et al. Magnetic resonance angiography of extracranial carotid arteries and intracranial vessels: A review. Neurology 1989; 39:1369–76.
38. Groen JP, de Graaf RD, van Dijk P. MR angiography based on inflow. In: Book of Abstracts, 7th Annual Meeting of the Society of Magnetic Resonance in Medicine, 1988:906.
39. Potchen EJ, Haacke EM, Siebert JE, et al., eds. Magnetic resonance angiography concepts and application. St. Louis: Mosby–Year Book 1993.
40. Edelman RR, Wentz KU, Mattle HP, et al. Intracerebral arteriovenous malformations: Evaluation with selective MR angiography and venography. Radiology 1989; 173:831–7.
41. Edelman RR, Mattle HP, O'Reilley GV, et al. Magnetic resonance imaging of flow dynamics in the circle of Willis. Stroke 1990; 22:56–65.
42. Pernicone JR, Siebert JE, Potchen EJ. Demonstration of an early draining vein by MR angiography. J Comput Assist Tomogr 1991; 15:829–31.
43. Edelman RR, Mattle HP, Wallner B, et al. Extracranial carotid arteries: evaluation with black blood MR angiography. Radiology 1990;177:45–50.
44. Cline HE, Dumoulin CL, Lorensen WE, et al. Volume rendering and connectivity algorithms for MR angiography. Magn Reson Med 1991; 18:384–94.
45. Brown DG, Reiderer SJ. Contrast-to-noise ratios in maximum intensity projection images. Magn Reson Med 1992; 23:130–7.
46. Anderson CA, Saloner D, Tsuruda JS, et al. Artifacts in maximum-intensity-projection display of MR angiograms. Am J Roentgen 1990; 154:623–9.
47. Siebert JE, Rosenbaum TL. Projection algorithm imparting a consistent spatial perspective. In: Book of abstracts, society of magnetic resonance in medicine, 9th Annual Meeting, New York, 1990:60.
48. Lin W, Haacke EM, Smith AS. Lumen definition in MR angiography. Magn Reson Med 1991; 1:327–36.
49. Keller PJ, Wilkenfeld M, Abrahams E. SIMP: An integrative combination with MIP. In: Book of abstracts, society of magnetic resonance medicine, 10th Annual Meeting, San Francisco, 1991:201.
50. Laub G. Displays for MR angiography. Magn Reson Med 1990; 14:222–9.
51. Saloner D, Hanson WA, Tsuruda JS, et al. Application of a connected-voxel algorithm to MR angiographic data. Magn Reson Med 1991; 1:423–30.
52. Pernicone JR, Thorp KE, Ouimette MV, et al. Magnetic resonance angiography in intracranial vascular disease. Semin Ultrasound CT MRI 1992; 13(4):256–73.
53. Kistler JP, Ropper AH, Martin JB. Cerebrovascular disease. In: Harrison's Principles of Internal Medicine. 12th ed. New York: McGraw-Hill, NY 1991:1998–2000.
54. Barnett HJM. Spontaneous intracranial hemorrhage. In: Cecil textbook of medicine. 18th ed. Philadelphia: Saunders, 1988:2173–86.
55. Osborn AO. Introduction to cerebral angiography. Philadelphia: Harper & Row, 1980:154–9.

56. Locksley HB. Report on the cooperative study of intracranial aneurysms and subarachnoid hemorrhage. Section V. Natural history of subarachnoid hemorrhage, intracranial aneurysms and arteriovenous malformations, based on 6368 cases in the cooperative study. J Neurosurg 1966; 25:219–36, 321–69.
57. Mohr JP, Fisher CM, Adams RD. Cerebrovascular diseases. In: Harrison's principles of internal medicine. 9th ed. New York: McGraw-Hill, 1980:1935–7.
58. Rhoton AL. Jr. Microsurgical anatomy of saccular aneurysms. In: Wilkins RH, Rengachary SS, eds. Neurosurgery. New York: McGraw-Hill, 1985:1330–40.
59. Allcock JM. Radiology of the skull and brain. In: Newton TH, Potts DG, eds. Angiography. Medibooks, Great Neck, NY: 1974:2435–3489.
60. Wirth FP, Laws ER, Piepgras D, et al. Surgical treatment of incidental intracranial aneurysms. Neurosurgery 1983; 12:507–11.
61. Sabiston Jr DC. Essentials of surgery. Philadelphia: Saunders, 1987:865–6.
62. Ross JS, Masaryk TJ, Modic MT, et al. Intracranial aneurysms: evaluation by MR angiography. Am J Neurorad 1990; 11:448–55.
63. Sevick RJ, Tsuruda JS, Schmalbrook P. Three dimensional time-of-flight MR angiography in the evaluation of cerebral aneurysms. J Comput Assist Tomogr 1990; 14:874–81.
64. Pernicone JR. Intracranial aneurysms. In: Potchen EJ, Haacke EM, Siebert JE, et al., eds. Magnetic resonance angiography: concepts and applications. St. Louis: Mosby–Year Book, 1992.
65. Turski PA, Korosec F, Graves VB, et al. Magnetic resonance angiography of vascular malformations. In: Potchen EJ, Haacke EM, Siebert JE, et al., eds. Magnetic resonance angiography: concepts and applications. St. Louis: Mosby–Year Book, 1992.
66. Warach S, Wei L, Ronthal M, et al. Acute cerebral ischemia: evaluation with dynamic contrast-enhanced MR imaging and MR angiography. Radiology 1992; 182:41–7.
67. Pernicone JR, Siebert JE, Laird TA, et al. Determination of blood flow direction using velocity-phase image display with 3D phase contrast MR angiography. Am J Neurorad 1992; 13:1435–38.
68. Edelman RR, Mattle HP, O'Reilley GV, et al. Magnetic resonance imaging of flow dynamics in the circle of Willis. Stroke 1990; 22:56–65.
69. Edelman RR, Mattle HP, Kleefield J, et al. Quantification of blood flow with dynamic MR imaging and presaturation bolus tracking. Radiology 1989; 171:551–6.
70. Bradley WG. MRA abets visualization of intracranial aneurysms. Diagnostic Imaging. 1992; November: 122–128.
71. Carr HY, Purcell EM. Effects of diffusion on free precession in NMR experiments. Phys Rev 1954; 94:630–88.
72. Torrey HC. Bloch equations with diffusion terms. Phys Rev 1956; 104563.
73. Groen JP, deGraaf RG, van Dijk P. MR angiography based on inflow. Soc Magn Reson Med Book of Abstracts 1988:906.

27

Color Doppler Imaging of the Eye and Orbit

Wolfgang E. Lieb
Johannes Gutenberg-University, Mainz, Germany

Real-time A-mode and B-mode ultrasonography have been used for the diagnostic evaluation of ophthalmic disorders since the early 1960s. Modern digital high-resolution equipment has improved diagnostic imaging and made it an essential part of many ophthalmological evaluations. Doppler ultrasound detects changes in the frequency of sound reflected from flowing blood allowing estimation of flow velocity. Doppler ultrasonography of the carotid arteries and the periorbital vessels is frequently employed in patients with ischemic ocular disease. The technology of duplex scanning allows for simultaneous B-mode imaging and Doppler spectral analysis. Since the diameters of the vessels in the eye and orbit are too small to be imaged with conventional duplex scans, Doppler spectra are obtained without precise localization and without knowledge of the Doppler angle. The latest technology change in the character of diagnostic ultrasound is color Doppler imaging (CDI). To facilitate localization of vascular structures, the two-dimensional flow information in CDI is encoded in color and superimposed on the gray scale structural image. Since the sensitivity of detecting Doppler shifts is not limited by the resolution of the gray scale image, Doppler shifts in very small vessels can be detected that depict the course of the vessels (1–4).

This technology started out in echocardiography, but new developments point to several portions of the vascular system throughout the entire human body.

The three major areas of application of color Doppler imaging can be described as primarily organ perfusion, tumor neovascularity, and vascular evaluation.

I. ORGAN PERFUSION

CDI can be utilized to visualize the perfusion of the liver, kidneys, spleen, placenta, and brain. In this area, CDI can be used as a guide to obtain selective Doppler information, which allows better assessment of the hemodynamics in these organs. The major indication of that category is the assessment of perfusion in kidney transplants (5,6).

II. TUMOR NEOVASCULARITY

CDI adds a new dimension to the ultrasound evaluation of mass lesions (7,8). This technique is already being successfully used to differentiate some benign from malignant tumors of the liver (9), tumors of the female breast, and the testicles, as well as tumors of other regions.

III. VASCULAR EVALUATION

Application of CDI includes the detection and measurement of arterial stenosis and flow-restricting or flow-disturbing abnormalities. This can be performed at the large abdominal vessels, aorta, iliac, femoral, and popliteal arteries and other peripheral arteries, and of course at large vessels of the head and neck, the carotid bifurcation, and the vertebral arteries (2,10).

There has been recently an increasing number of reports on applications of CDI in the study of the ocular and orbital vasculature in the literature (11–13). CDI and duplex-Doppler have also been used to demonstrate flow in intraocular and orbital tumors (12,14–17). We and others have shown the value of CDI in the noninvasive diagnosis of an orbital varix (18,19) and in the diagnosis of cavernous sinus fistulas (20). Recent reports addressed the application of CDI in the assessment of ocular and orbital vascular changes, such as the ocular ischemic syndrome (21), arterial and venous occlusions of the retinal vessels (22–24), diabetic retinopathy (25), glaucoma (26), and retinitis pigmentosa (27).

IV. EXAMINATION TECHNIQUE

The examination using color Doppler imaging can be separated into two parts:

Color-coded display of the orbital vessels
Selective analysis of the Doppler spectrum using the color as a guide to the vessels of interest

The ultrasound transducer is applied to the closed eyelids using sterile ophthalmic methylcellulose as a coupling agent. During the examination, the patient is in a supine position and care is taken not to apply pressure to the eye to avoid artifacts. As has been shown by Williamson (28), the increase in intraocular pressure caused by the transducer placed on the eyelids is negligible in skilled hands. Horizontal and vertical scans through the eye and orbit are performed. Depending on the direction of flow with respect to the transducer, the blood flow data displayed is either in red or blue. The colors can be arbitrarily assigned, but in the orbit flow toward the transducer is usually depicted as red and away from the transducer as blue. The color saturation in the image represents the average frequency (first moment average) from a spectral analysis performed at each sample site. These frequencies can be turned into velocities by solving the Doppler equation for velocity.

When examining the eye and orbit through the eyelids, the ultrasound beam is essentially parallel to the orbital and ocular vessels; thus most arterial flow is depicted in red. Arteries can usually be distinguished from veins by noting the pulsatility of the former. Pulsed Doppler spectral analysis also helps to distinguish between pulsatile arterial and the usually more continuous or minimally pulsatile venous flow and allows for the quantification of data. When the ultrasound beam is at an angle of 90 degrees to a vascular structure or if a vessel contains only stagnant blood, no Doppler flow information is obtained and the structure is shown in gray scale display only.

All examinations are performed in a "low"- or "medium"-flow setting to allow for optimal detection of low to medium Doppler frequency shifts of the slow-flowing blood in the small orbital vessels. For the ophthalmic artery, medium- to high-flow settings are applied, since flow in this vessel is faster. Color threshold levels are adjusted to minimize artifacts by lid and involuntary eye movements. To obtain Doppler spectra, a sample volume of approximately 1.2 mm is chosen within the selected vessel. The proximal and distal portions of the vessel are imaged to facilitate determination of the Doppler flow angle for estimation of velocity. From the frequency-time display, the peak systolic velocity (V_{syst}), the mean velocity (V_{mean}), and the end-diastolic velocity can be measured, when the Doppler angle is known (Fig. 1). These parameters can be used to calculate the so-called Pourcelot's index (RI) (29), which is a measure for the vascular resistance.

$$RI = \frac{(V_{syst} - V_{diast})}{V_{syst}}$$

The scan images can be recorded on video tape and later reviewed with the benefit of cine-loop and frame-by-frame analysis of selected segments. Images

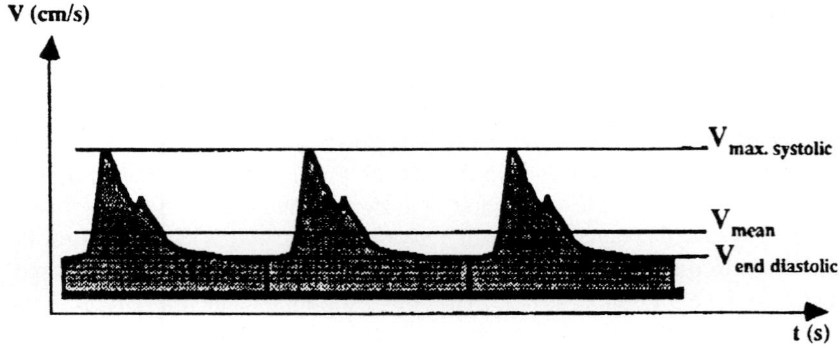

Figure 1 Schematic display of the Doppler spectrum (frequency-time-display) from an arterial vessel. From the Doppler spectrum the peak systolic, the mean and the end diastolic velocity can be measured when the Doppler angle is known.

can be photographed directly from an isolated on-board color monitor during cine-loop replay using a 35-mm camera. The duration of the examination ranges from 20 to 40 min for both eyes (11,12,30).

V. SAFETY CONSIDERATIONS

As in any diagnostic tests, there may be some risk in diagnostic ultrasound. The American Institute of Ultrasound in Medicine (AIUM) has reviewed reports of bioeffects in ultrasound and has issued a statement in respect to ultrasound bioeffects on in vivo mammalian tissue.

According to the AIUM, there is in the low megahertz frequency range (0.5–10.0 MHz) no independently confirmed significant biological effect in mammalian tissue exposed in vivo to unfocused ultrasound with intensities below 100 mW/cm^2 or focused ultrasound with intensities of 1000 mW/cm^2 [31]. Currently, in the United States, the Food and Drug Administration (FDA) has established guidelines of ultrasound intensity limits for various clinical applications. The basis for these limits was linked to the measured output level of machines sold for ophthalmic and other particular applications prior to the enactment of the 1976 Medical Device Amendment. These parameters have not been based on the assessment of risks published today.

For the instrument used in our studies (QAD 1 and QAD 2000, Siemens-Quantum, Inc., Issaquah, WA), the estimated in situ spatial peak temporal average intensity (SPTA) in the color imaging mode is 5–55 mW/cm^2 for the 7.5-MHz transducer. During spectral analysis, the in situ peak temporal average intensity is approximately 56–476 mW/cm^2 (Siemens-Quantum, Inc.), which exceeds the currently approved FDA upper guidelines of 17 mW/cm^2. The SPTA is the highest intensity within the ultrasound field average over an entire scan frame period.

Depending on the device settings for commercially available color Doppler units, the acoustic intensity values dated in the AIUM bioeffect statements and in the FDA guidelines is exceeded especially during pulsed Doppler spectrum analysis. According to studies by Lizzi et al. (31) and Coleman et al. (32), who performed numerous experiments on ultrasound bioeffects to ocular tissues, intensities used for diagnostic imaging are significantly lower than those that would be expected to cause unwanted ocular side effects, especially chorioretinal lesions and cataract formation. Nevertheless, the time of spectrum analysis should be kept short to minimize potential risks. In more than 2000 examinations, we have not seen any side effects.

VI. NORMAL VASCULATURE OF THE EYE AND ORBIT

A horizontal scan through the eye and orbit at the level of the optic nerve allows the depiction of the central retinal artery (CRA) and vein (CRV). Those vessels can be identified within the anterior portion of the optic nerve shadow (Fig. 2). The central retinal artery can be traced during its course deep into the orbit and in most cases its entrance into the optic nerve, about 10 mm behind the disc, can be seen. The CRV can be easily identified, not only because of its blue color code, but also during spectrum analysis. The CRV usually runs in close proximity to the CRA and the spectrum of both vessels usually overlaps. In contrast to the arterial spectrum with high systolic velocities in the central retinal artery (Fig. 2), the central retinal vein shows a continuous flow with only minimal fluctuations during diastole and systole. On either side of the optic nerve, the posterior ciliary arteries (PCA) can be shown. In some cases, even a differentiation between a short (PCAs) and long posterior ciliary artery (PCA1) is possible. In comparison with the CRA, the spectrum of the posterior ciliary vessels shows a slightly higher systolic velocity and also a higher end diastolic velocity indicating a low resistance vascular system (choroid) distal to the sample area. Deep into the orbit the ophthalmic artery (OA) can be depicted, which usually enters the orbit temporal to the optic nerve and crosses over the nerve in the mid orbit (Fig. 3). The peak systolic flow velocity of the ophthalmic artery (37 cm/s) is significantly higher than the velocities measured in the CRA (9.5 cm/s) and posterior ciliary arteries (Table 1). On the venous side, superior nasally, the

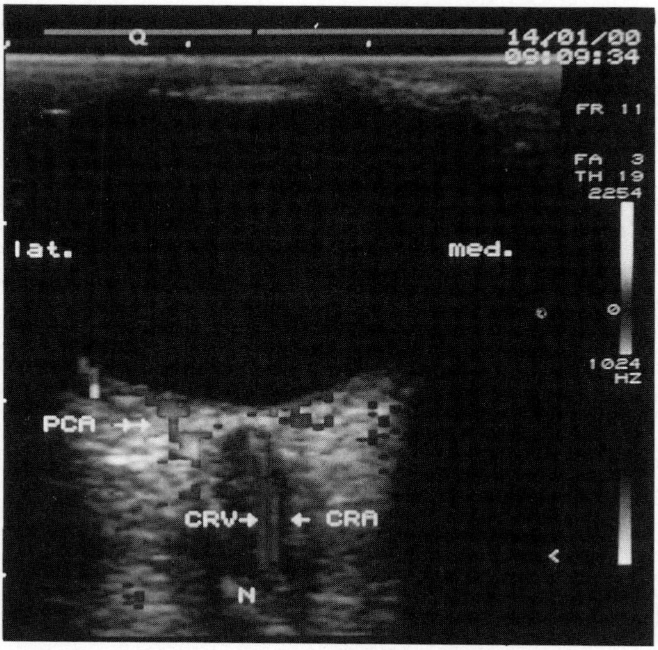

Figure 2 Depiction of the central retinal artery (CRA) and accompanying central retinal vein (CRV) within the optic nerve echo (N) in the color-encoded B-scan image. Lateral (lat) to the optic nerve a segment of a short posterior ciliary artery is displayed (PCA).

course of the superior ophthalmic vein (SOV) can in some cases be shown. In most instances, however, it is possible to depict all the four vortex veins in the superior and inferior quadrants of the eye. As a baseline for further investigations, we have measured the peak systolic and end diastolic velocities of the small orbital vessels in 187 normal volunteers (Table 1). These values lie well within the range of velocities measured by other investigators (Table 2) using CDI or other Doppler techniques (11,30,33–38).

VII. APPLICATIONS IN OPHTHALMOLOGY

Color Doppler imaging combines both anatomical and velocity data and displays the information in a format that can be easily comprehended. Blood flow velocity information can be obtained quantitatively within the entire two-dimensional gray

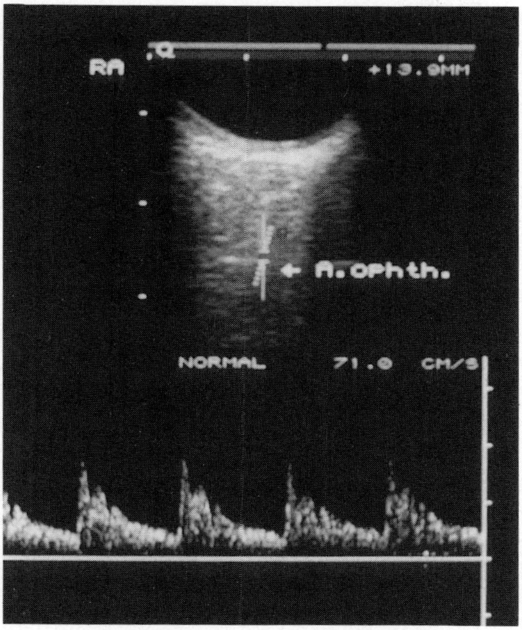

Figure 3 Analysis of the Doppler spectrum of the ophthalmic artery. A cursor is placed on the vessel, and the angle is corrected according to the vessel course. The spectrum of the ophthalmic artery (A. ophth) has higher velocities than the central retinal artery and the posterior ciliary vessels.

scale image. Various applications of CDI have evolved over a 3-year period working with this technique. As we and others have shown, CDI is able to localize small vessels in the eye, the orbit, and the optic nerve. By coding the Doppler shifts in color CDI allows for the first time reproducible noninvasive imaging and selective Doppler information of the small orbital vessels. At present, it is not likely that CDI will not allow blood volume measurements, since accurate diameters of the vessels cannot be assessed. The analysis of selectively obtained Doppler spectra from the different vessels, that is, the CRA, CRV, posterior ciliary arteries, and branches of the ophthalmic artery, might however allow some insight into the hemodynamics of the eye and its supplying vessels. This technique allows measurement of flow velocities in the CRA and ophthalmic artery with good accuracy. In addition to measuring the velocities, the analysis of the shape of the waveforms using indices, such as the Pourcelot's index, provides information about the vessel and the vascular system proximal and distal to it. Besides fluorescein angiography, there is so far no accepted

Table 1 Flow Velocities in Normal Orbital Vessels Measured by Color Doppler Imaging

Variable	Mean	STD	Median	Min	Max
CRA–Vsyst (cm/s)	9.55	1.37	9.56	5.26	13.06
CRA–Vdiast (cm/s)	2.31	0.74	2.17	0.86	4.03
CRA–RI	0.76	0.07	0.76	0.59	0.90
CRV–Vmax (cm/s)	−4.21	0.73	−4.16	−6.66	−2.54
PCAs–Vsyst (cm/s)	10.74	2.70	10.94	3.92	19.91
PCAs–Vdiast (cm/s)	3.24	1.17	3.24	0.98	7.00
PCAs–Vmean (cm/s)	4.75	1.62	5.00	1.00	10.00
PCAs–RI	0.70	0.08	0.70	0.47	0.90
PCAl–Vsyst (cm/s)	11.03	1.87	11.07	6.25	15.96
PCAl–Vdiast (cm/s)	3.44	1.24	3.56	0.67	7.24
PCAl–Vmean (cm/s)	5.38	1.29	5.21	2.37	7.96
PCAl–RI	0.69	0.09	0.68	0.53	0.93
OA–Vsyst (cm/s)	37.33	6.80	36.61	19.03	58.28
OA–Vdiast (cm/s)	8.32	2.82	7.97	2.46	17.14
OA–Vmean (cm/s)	15.18	3.87	15.00	5.50	27.00
OA–RI	0.78	0.06	0.78	0.60	0.93
SOV–Vmax. (cm/s)	−7.37	2.69	−7.00	−18.00	−2.00

Group of 187 normal volunteers examined with color Doppler sonography (Q 2000, Siemens-Quantum Issaquah, WAT, USA). Spectrum analysis with angle correction was used to establish reference values. Displayed are the flow velocities during systole and diastole in centimeters per second and the Pourcelot's index (RI) calculated for the different orbital vessels. Central retinal artery (CRA) and vein (CRV), short and long posterior ciliary arteries (PCAs and PCA1), the ophthalmic artery (OA), and the superior ophthalmic vein (SOV).

clinical method available to study the ocular and orbital vasculature. Although CDI provides only velocity information, it has several advantages over other techniques. It is noninvasive and easily repeatable, there is minimal patient cooperation necessary, and it can be used in patients with opaque optical media, where other techniques requiring direct visualization of the fundus fail.

A. Retinal and Retinal Vascular Disease of the Eye

The study of retinal vascular disorders is a domain of fluorescein angiography. However, CDI is capable of adding valuable information about the circulation in the central retinal artery (CRA) and the posterior ciliary circulation by looking at these vessels posterior to the retina and choroid. Patients with central retinal artery occlusions (CRAO), when examined with CDI, revealed either absence

Table 2 Literature Review of Flow Velocities in Orbital Vessels

Author (Doppler technique)	N	CRA (cm/s) V_{syst}	CRA (cm/s) V_{diast}	OA (cm/s) V_{syst}	OA (cm/s) V_{diast}
Lieb 1993 (CDI)	187	9.5 ± 1.4	2.3 ± 0.7	37.3 ± 6.8	8.3 ± 2.8
Guthoff 1991 (Duplex-sonography)	72	9.5 ± 3.1	3.1 ± 1.6	31.6 ± 9.0	8.2 ± 3.7
Lieb 1990 (CDI)	40	10.3 ± 2.1	—	31.4 ± 4.2	—
Cesarone 1992 (Duplex-sonography)	200	12.5 ± 6.0	5.5 ± 3.0	—	—
Galassi 1992 (CDI)	20	13.4 ± 2.4	2.0 ± 1.8	41.3 ± 3.4	9.5 ± 2.0
Bucci 1992 (CDI)	20	9.73	—	28.37	—
Michelson 1992 (pw-Doppler)	206	—	—	38.8 ± 8.6	12.0 ± 3.1
Rojanapongpun 1993 (pw-Doppler)	60	—	—	45.1 ± 7.7	11.9 ± 3.4

Maximum systolic (V_{syst}) and end diastolic (V_{diast}) flow velocities (cm/s, mean ± STD) of the central retinal artery (CRA) and ophthalmic artery (OA) measured with various Doppler techniques: color Doppler imaging (CDI), pulsed wave (pw) Doppler, and duplex-scan.

or markedly decreased flow in the central retinal artery compared with normal controls. The maximum systolic amplitude is low and flow during diastole is also decreased. In central retinal artery occlusions, massive calcifications of the vessel walls as well as calcific plaques can also be detected. The technique can in addition be used to study the extracranial vascular system, which might be a source of emboli to the retina.

In patients with arterial occlusions of the retinal vessels, CDI allows us to determine if there are:

- Emboli along the course of the CRA behind the optic disc
- Reduced flow velocities in the ophthalmic, central retinal, and ciliary arteries
- Collaterals from the external carotid circulation
- Arteriosclerotic disease of the carotid and vertebral artery system

The *ocular ischemic syndrome* (OIS), which characteristically presents with peripheral ocular retinal hemorrhages, dilated nontortuous retinal veins, iris neovascularizations, cataract, and neovascular glaucoma, is sometimes difficult to diagnose. Color Doppler imaging of the carotid artery reveals in these patients a high-grade ipsilateral carotid artery stenosis ranging from a 70% stenosis to total occlusion. Color Doppler imaging demonstrates a markedly reduced central retinal artery peak systolic blood flow velocity in all eyes with OIS. Peak systolic velocity ranges from 1.3 to 6.0 cm/s with a mean of 3.5 cm/s. It also documents a reversal of ophthalmic artery blood flow, being an indicator for collateralization by branches of the external carotid artery system. The flow patterns in those collaterals are quite different from the normal ophthalmic artery. Because of the pressure gradient, there is very low resistance (Fig. 4). In the posterior ciliary arteries, the flow velocity is either nondetectable or significantly decreased. The specific finding of the posterior ciliary artery hypoperfusion may explain why patients with the OIS and similar degrees of carotid stenosis and retinal findings can have very different levels of visual function.

In patients with *central retinal vein occlusions* (CRVO), a characteristic Doppler spectrum pattern can be seen. Flow velocity in the central retinal artery during systole is decreased, the peak systole waveform is blunted, and there is absent or massively decreased flow in diastole, which is also an indication for

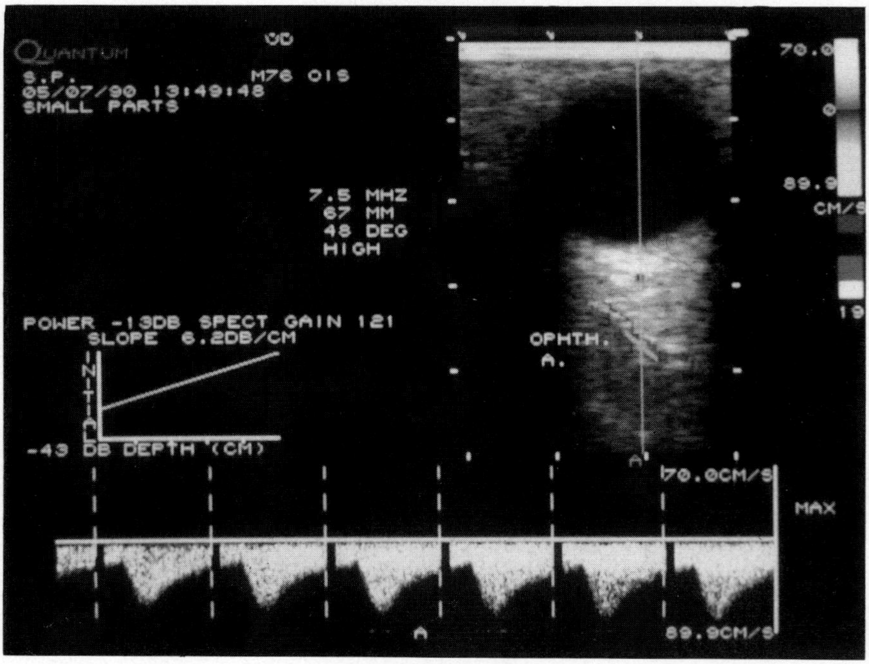

Figure 4 Doppler spectrum of flow reversal in the ophthalmic artery via a collateral from the external carotid artery circulation. Note the relatively high end diastolic flow of the ophthalmic artery indicating a low vascular resistance.

the high resistance caused by the blockage of venous outflow in CRVO (Fig. 5).

We found in a group of patients with proliferative *diabetic retinopathy* a significant decrease of the peak systolic and end-diastolic flow velocity of the CRA. The blood flow velocities in the PCA and OA were almost unchanged compared with age-matched controls (Goebel and Lieb, 1992, unpublished data).

Although the posterior ciliary circulation can be difficult to assess, there are reports indicating decreased flow velocities in patients with anterior ischemic optic neuropathy.

B. Intraocular Tumors

Doppler signals as an indicator for *tumor vessels* can be detected in the majority of intraocular neoplasias. In a collective of 44 patients with intraocular tumors, we found Doppler signals in 38 of these lesions (90.5%). In contrast to that, we were unable to detect flow in all three cases of tumorlike lesions (age-related maculopathy). In those tumors studied pre- and postradiotherapy, the detectable Doppler shifts significantly decreased after successful plaque radiotherapy [15]. Similar results were reported by other investigators [14,17,39].

Histopathologically, tumor vessels are often primitive vascular channels lacking smooth muscle consisting of an endothelial layer and connective tissue alone. Low resistance to flow is expected, since in most neoplasms the vessels lack normal arteriolar smooth muscle, the recognized site of peripheral vascular resistance. High sensitivity in detecting even minimal flow is necessary to allow detection of fine tumor vascularity. Lesions that can simulate uveal melanomas,

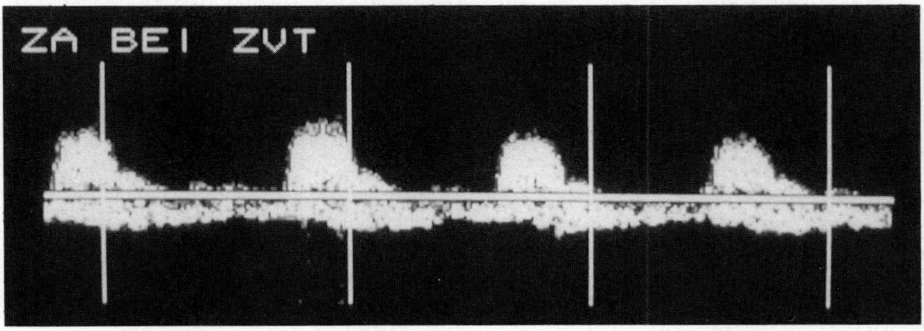

Figure 5 Doppler signal of the central retinal artery (CRA) in a patient with ischemic central retinal vein thrombosis (CRVO). The Doppler signal demonstrates a plump peak in systole and no flow in diastole. This pattern is characteristic for a high vascular resistance. The Pourcelot's index is 1,0.

such as large subretinal hemorrhages, usually do not have a distinctive blood supply. Therefore, they can be differentiated from melanomas on the basis of the absence of Doppler flow. The vascularity patterns of uveal melanomas, choroidal metastases, and choroidal hemangiomas are, however, quite similar and thus do not permit differentiation on the basis of the Doppler signals.

C. Orbital Vascular Disorders and Tumors

In the orbit, Doppler signals can be detected in most *orbital tumors*. In cavernous hemangiomas, however, the speed of flowing blood is usually so low and stagnant that the flow velocities are below the detection level. In other lesions, especially malignant tumors, significant vascularity with high arterial flow velocities and large feeding vessels can be seen within the tumor. CDI also is able to evaluate the vascular compromise to the retinal and ciliary circulation through compression by a mass lesion. In most cases, the affected vessels show decreased or normal systolic flow but low or absent flow during diastole. In patients with *optic nerve sheath meningioma* (OSM), CDI demonstrates the progressive compression of the optic nerve and its vasculature. In advanced stages, a high-resistance flow pattern is found in the CRA (Fig. 6). Vascular abnormalities, such as carotid-cavernous-sinus-fistulas (CCSF), orbital varices and arteriovenous malformations are easily diagnosed with CDI. Patients with CCSF all had a markedly dilated superior ophthalmic vein with reversed arterialized blood flow in the vein (Fig. 7). Several studies have shown that CDI was able to demonstrate the dilated arterialized superior ophthalmic vein (SOV) with high-velocity blood flow toward the transducer. CDI further depicts the dilated preseptal high blood flow shunts and the secondary extraocular enlargement of muscles characteristic of this entity (20,40). In some cases, the retrograde arterial filling of the venous outflow system of the vortex veins explains the mechanisms, which leads to the increase of intraocular pressure. One report (41) confirmed our findings and stressed the point that this technique can be used to monitor CCSFs noninvasively and to assess their spontaneous course or effects of embolization and balloon occlusions. Absent flow in a dilated superior ophthalmic vein, together with the characteristic clinical findings, can support the diagnosis of a *superior ophthalmic vein thrombosis*. In *orbital varices*, color Doppler imaging shows the dynamic changes throughout a Valsalva maneuver; that is, the active filling and distension of the orbital varix during inspiration, the stagnant flow during maximum filling, and the flow directed into the depth of the orbit during expiration (18).

D. Other Applications

Color Doppler imaging might also be used in cases where *retinal detachments* and dense *vitreous membranes* cannot be distinguished by routine A- and B-scan ultrasonography (42,43). In most cases, CDI allows depiction of flow in the

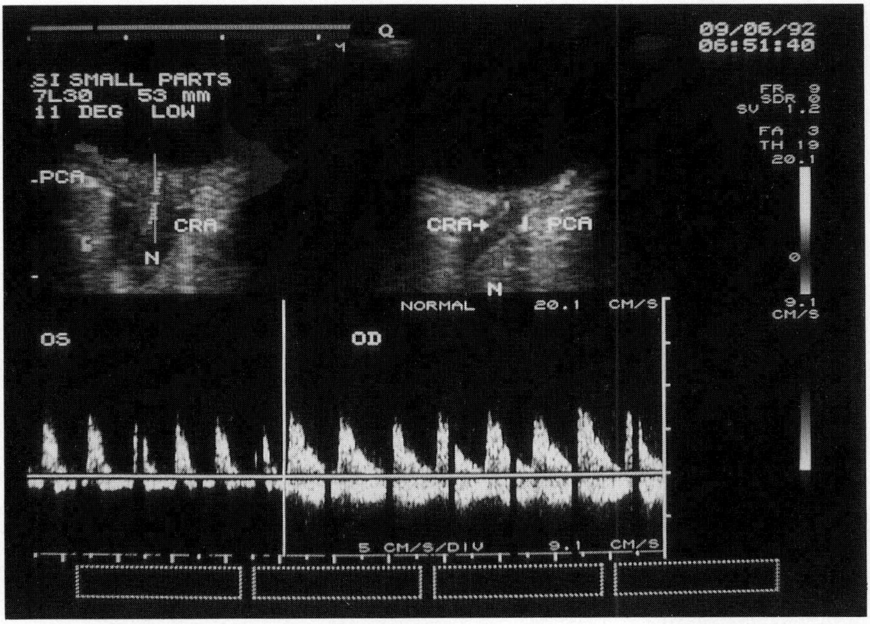

Figure 6 Doppler spectrum of the central retinal artery (CRA) is an optic nerve (N) with a large optic sheath meningioma on the left (OS). The normal fellow eye (OD) shows higher flow velocities and a lower Pourcelot's index in the CRA.

retinal vasculature, being an indicator for retinal detachment rather than dense vitreous membranes. In several patients with *drusen of the optic nerve* and visual field defects, we could demonstrate highly turbulent flow with extremely high Doppler shifts and a high-resistance flow pattern within the central retinal artery. This supports the fact that there is direct compromise of the vasculature in the optic nerve head in addition to the mechanical compression of the nerve fibers.

In patients with *primary open angle glaucoma* (POAG), we and others found decreased flow velocities in the long and short posterior ciliary vessels supporting the thinking of vascular changes in the ciliary and choroidal vascular system (26). *Pharmacological influence* on the flow parameters have been investigated by Belfort (44) and Baxter et al. using CDI (45). In the first study, the investigators were able to detect a significant reduction in pulsatility and Pourcelot's index of the CRA and PCA in a group of preeclamptic women, which was treated with magnesium sulfate. Baxter studied the effect of posture and topical β-blockers on the hemodynamics of the orbital vessels. He found no effect of posture; however, there was a fall in Pourcelot's index. Since the identification of the orbital vessels

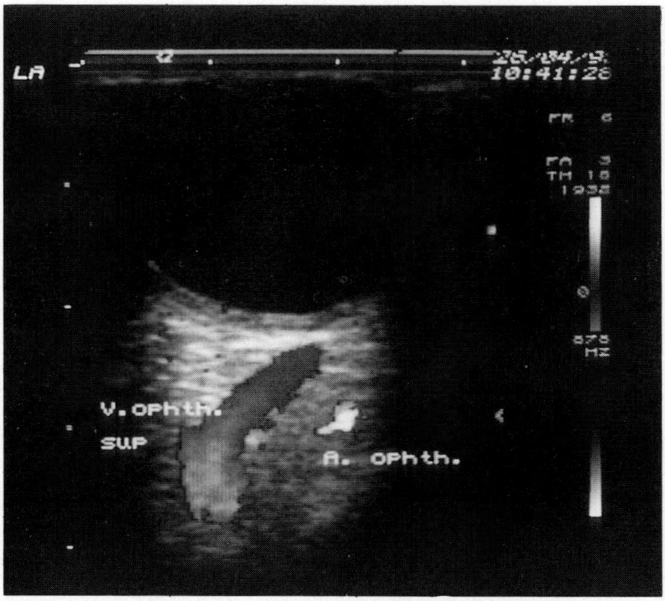

Figure 7 Large superior ophthalmic vein (V. ophth.sup) with reversal of blood flow (red color code) to the right is a cross section of the ophthalmic artery (A. ophth.).

was difficult to reproduce in their study, caution should be used when interpretating this information as an indication that CDI is capable of demonstrate subtle pharmacological effects on orbital hemodynamics. Large effects, such as the marked peripheral vasodilatation caused by nitroglycerine, can be shown to increase end-diastolic flow velocity in the central retinal artery.

E. Outlook

Advances in Doppler and conventional B-scan ultrasound systems improve their ability to acquire and detect ultrasonic signals and to analyze them in terms of a spatial and frequency distribution. Nevertheless, the fundamental physical restrictions of ultrasonography and Doppler will always remain the same. Since CDI allows for the first time a noninvasive assessment of the retrobulbar vasculature in a clinical setting, we think that many more applications of this technology will develop for ophthalmology. Most available color Doppler instruments are still very expensive, which limits their use in ophthalmology to large academic centers. We hope that less expensive color Doppler systems with specifically designed ophthalmic probes, improved two-dimensional resolution, and Doppler spectrum acquisition will become available. The use of ultrasound contrast agents may further improve the imaging and acquisition of Doppler spectra from the small orbital vessels.

REFERENCES

1. Grant E, Tessler F, Perella R. Clinical Doppler Imaging. AJR 1989; 152:707–17.
2. Merrit C. Doppler color-flow imaging. J Clin Ultrasound 1987; 15:591–7.
3. Mitchell DG. Color Doppler imaging: principles, limitations, and artifacts. Radiology 1990; 177:1–10.
4. Powis R. Color flow imaging. Understanding its science and technology. J Diagno Med Sonogr 1988; 4:234–45.
5. Becker CD, Cooperberg PL. Sonography of the hepatic vascular system. AJR 1988; 150:999–1005.
6. Lewis BD, James EM. Current applications of duplex and color Doppler ultrasound imaging: abdomen. Mayo Clin Proc 1989; 64:1158–69.
7. Taylor K, Ramos I, Carter D, Morse S, Snower D, Fortune K. Correlation of Doppler ultrasound tumor signals with morphologic features. Radiology 1988; 166:57–62.
8. Orr NM, Taylor KJW. Doppler detection of tumor vascularity. Clin Diagnostic Ultrasound 1990; 26:149–63.
9. Goldberg BB, Hilpert PL, Burns PN, Liu JB, Newman LM, Merton DA, Witlin LA. Hepatic tumors: signal enhancement at Doppler US after intravenous injection of a contrast agent. Radiology 1990; 177:713–7.
10. Erickson SJ, Mewissen MW, Foley WD, Lawson TL, Middleton WD, Quiroz FA, Macrander SJ, Lipchik EO. Stenosis of the internal carotid artery: assessment using color Doppler imaging compared with angiography. AJR 1989; 152:1299–305.
11. Lieb WE, Cohen SM, Merton DA, Shields JA, Mitchell DG, Goldberg BB. Color Doppler imaging of the eye and orbit. Technique and normal vascular anatomy. Arch Ophthalmol 1991; 109:527–31.
12. Lieb WE, Flaharty PM, Ho A and Sergott RC. Color Doppler imaging of the eye and orbit. A synopsis of a 400 case experiment. Acta Ophthalmol 1992; 204:(Suppl.):50–4.
13. Erickson SJ, Hendrix LE, Massaro BM, Harris GJ, Lewandowski MF, Foley WD, Lawson TL. Color Doppler flow imaging of the normal and abnormal orbit. Radiology 1989; 173:511–6.
14. Guthoff RF, Berger RW, Winkler P, Helmke K, Chumbley LC. Doppler ultrasonography of malignant melanomas of the uvea. Arch Ophthalmol 1991; 109:537–41.
15. Leib E, Shields JA, Cohen SM, Merton DA, Mitchell DG, Shields CL, Goldberg BB.
16. Wolff-Korman PG, Korman B, Hasenfratz GC, Spengal FA. Duplex and color Doppler ultrasound in the differential diagnosis of choroidal tumors. Acta Ophthalmol 1992; 204(Suppl.):66–7.
17. Wolff-Kormann PG, Kormann B, Riedel KG, Hasenfratz GC, Stefani FH, Spengel FA, Lund O-E. Quantitative Color Doppler Imaging in untreated and irradiated choroidal melanoma. Invest Ophthalmol Vis Sci 1992; 33:1928–33.

18. Lieb W, Merton D, Shields J, Cohen S, Mitchell D, Goldberg B. Color Doppler imaging in the demonstration of an orbital varix. Br J Ophthalmol 1990; 74:305–8.
19. Wildenhain P, Lehar S, Dasturr K, Dodd III G. Orbital varix: color flow imaging correlated with CT and MR studies. Comput Assist Tomogr 1991; 15:171–3.
20. Flaharty PM, Lieb WE, Sergott RC, Bosley TM, Savino PJ. Color Doppler imaging. A new noninvasive technique to diagnose and monitor carotid cavernous sinus fistulas. Arch Ophthalmol 1991; 109:522–6.
21. Ho AC, Lieb WE, Flaharty PM, Sergott RC, Brown GC, Bosley TM, Savino PJ. Color Doppler Imaging of the ocular ischemic syndrome. 1991; 99:1453–62.
22. Williamson T, Baxter G, Dutton G. Color Doppler velocimetry of the optic nerve head in arterial occlusion. Ophthalmology 1993; 100:312–7.
23. Lieb WE, Flaharty PM, Sergott RC, Brown G, Bosley T, Savino P, Shields J. Color Doppler Imaging in patients with central retinal artery obstructions and normal controls. Ophthalmology 1990; 97:114 (abstract).
24. Williamson T, Baxter G. Retinal blood flow measurement by color Doppler imaging in patients with central retinal vein occlusion. Invest Ophthalmol Vis Sci 1993; 34:841 (abstract).
25. Goebel W, Lieb W, Ho A, Sergott R, Farhoumand R, Grehn F. Die Farb-Duplex Sonographie als neues Verfahren zur Untersuchung der orbitalen Gefäβe bei Retinopathiia diabetica. Der Ophthalmol 1993;
26. Trible J, Sergott R, Spaeth G, RP W, Katz L, Moster C, Schmidt C. Color Doppler analysis of hemodynamic alterations in glaucoma patients after trabeculectomy. Invest Ophthalmol Vis Sci 1993; 34:1286 (abstract).
27. Bucci M, Quaranta L, Giogagnorio F, Fazio V, Semeraro F, Quaranta M, Nascimbeni G. Orbital blood flow assessment by Color Doppler imaging in retinitis pigmentosa. Invest Ophthal Vis Sci 1993; 34:1369 (abstract).
28. Williamson T, Baxter G, Dutton G. Colour Doppler velocimetry of the arterial vasculature of the optic nerve head and orbit. Eye 1993; 7:74–70.
29. Pourcelot L. Applications cliniques de l'examen Doppler transcutane. INSERM 1974; 34:213–40.
30. Guthoff RF, Berger RW, Winkler P, Helmke K, Chumbley LC. Doppler ultrasonography of the ophthalmic and central retinal vessels. Arch Ophthalmol 1991; 109:532–6.
31. Lizzi F, Coleman D, Driller J, Franzen L, Leopold M. Effects of pulsed ultrasound on ocular tissue. Ultrasound Med Biol 1981; 7:245–52.
32. Coleman DJ, Lizzi LF, Chang S, Driller J. Applications of therapeutic ultrasound in ophthalmology. Progr Med Ultrasound 1981; 2:
33. Bucci M, Quaranta L, Ripandelli G, Manni G, Giovagnorio F, Cavallo V. Orbital blood flow assessment by color Doppler imaging in normal human subjects. Invest Ophthalmol Vis Sci 1992; 33:807 (abstract).
34. Cesarone MR, Laurora G, Steigerwalt R and Belcaro G. Retinal duplex scanning in cerebrovascular disease and hypertension. Vasa 1992; 21:163–6.
35. Galassi F, Nuzzaci G, Sodi A, Casi P, Vielmo A. Color Doppler imaging in evaluation of optic nerve blood supply in normal and glaucomatous subjects. Int Ophthalmol 1992; 16:273–176.
36. Michelson G, Gierth K, Priem R, Laumer R. Blood velocity in the ophthalmic artery

in normal subjects and patients with endophthalmitis. Invest Ophthalmol Vis Sci 1990; 31:1919–23.
37. Rojanapongpun P, Drance SM, Morrison B. Ophthalmic artery flow velocity in glaucomatous and normal subjects. Br J Ophthalmol 1993; 77:25–9.
38. Rojanapongpun P, Drance SM. Velocity of ophthalmic arterial flow recorded by Doppler ultrasound in normal subjects. Am J Ophthalmol 1993; 15:174–80.
39. Falco L, Esente S, Fantani S, Pasarelli N, Utari S. Our experience in the diagnosis of intraocular tumors by a B-scan system and angiodynography (Doppler). Preliminary results. Acta Ophthalmol 1992; 204(Suppl.):76–80.
40. Kotval PS, Weitzner IJ, Tenner MS. Diagnosis of carotid-cavernous fistula by periorbital color Doppler imaging and pulsed Doppler volume flow analysis. J Ultrasound Med 1990; 9:101–6.
41. Soulier-Sotto V, Beaufrere L, Laroche JP, Dauzat M, Bourbotte G, Bourgeois JM, Janbon C, Arnaud B. Diagnostic par écho-Doppler-couleur d'une fistul durale de la loge caverneuse à révélation ophthalogique. J Fr Ophthalmol 1992; 15:38–42.
42. Wong AD, Cooperberg PL, Ross WH, Araki DN. Differentiation of detached retina and vitreous membrane with color flow Doppler. Radiology 1991; 178:429–31.
43. Wells RG, Miro P, Brummond R. Color-flow Doppler sonography of persistent hyperplastic primary vitreous. J Ultrasound Med 1991; 10:405–7.
44. Belfort MA. The effect of magnesium sulphate on blood flow velocity in the maternal retina in mild pre-eclampsia: a preliminary colour flow Doppler study. Br J Obstet Gynaecol 1992; 99:641–5.
45. Baxter GM, Williamson TH, McKillop G, Dutton GN. Color Doppler ultrasound of orbital and optic nerve blood flow: effects of posture and Timolol 0.5%. Invest Ophthalmol Vis Sci 1992; 33:604–10.

28

Pupil Perimetry

Randy H. Kardon
University of Iowa and Department of Veterans Affairs, Iowa City, Iowa

An automated form of "pupil perimetry" has been devised to obtain objective information about the sensitivity of the perimetric field in normal subjects and in patients with visual pathway damage. The timing and amplitude of pupillary contractions to focal light stimuli were recorded using a computerized infrared pupillometer linked to a Humphrey automated perimeter. Pupillomotor and visual sensitivity are compared at the same 76 locations across a 30-degree field of view. Pupil perimetry and standard threshold perimetry showed corresponding defects in the visual field of patients with ischemic and anterior compressive optic neuropathy, but poor correspondence in primary open-angle glaucoma and optic neuritis. Patients with isolated occipital strokes showed matching homonymous visual and pupillary fields suggesting a suprageniculate influence on the pupillary light reflex. Pupil perimetry is a useful objective form of perimetry and can be used to compare the effect of disease on the visual and pupillary pathways.

Perimetry has changed considerably in the last 10 years since the introduction of automated, computerized methods of visual field examination. Most clinical visual field evaluation is now performed using computerized static, threshold determination. Testing is usually confined to the central 30-degree field. More recently it has been confined to the central 24-degree field in order to shorten testing time. The major driving force for switching from tangent screen and Goldmann kinetic perimetry to automated, static threshold examination has been the desire to standardize perimetric testing.

Modern computer-run testing strategies make use of stair step and bracketing algorithms quickly to determine threshold. This has enabled visual sensitivity and its variability to become quantified within a testing time tolerated by most patients. Perimetric sensitivity can then be statistically compared with age-matched normative data to provide an objective guide for determining whether a visual field is abnormal or has significantly changed from previous examinations.

Any clinician who has tried to use the results of automated perimetry for clinical decision-making knows that the information obtained is not always trustworthy. Some patients do not understand the test well enough to provide reliable results, some cannot maintain the level of concentration necessary to perform the test, and some have a high level of anxiety that can cloud their judgment. Often the perimetric results are inconsistent with the clinical findings, and the clinician is left wondering what the patient really did see.

Even with better ergonomic design and faster testing strategies, automated threshold perimetry will always require a subjective response that may not reflect the true functioning of the visual system. A number of studies comparing threshold perimetry to loss of optic nerve fibers has shown that a considerable amount of damage can occur before any visual field abnormalities become apparent. Perimetric testing is needed that would bypass the subjective responses now required of the patient and that would reflect damage at an earlier time.

A number of candidate tests have been tried (1–4). These include evoked potentials from either the retina (focal or pattern ERG) or the visual cortex (VEP). The focal ERG has a low signal to noise ratio and is difficult to perform on even the most cooperative of patients. The stray light can be suppressed with a background light surrounding the stimulus light, but even the averaged signal is difficult to obtain outside of the central 15 degrees, unless much larger areas of retina are stimulated (1). Time constraints also limit the testing of multiple locations. Another type of focal ERG has also been derived using time averaged signals from multiple square array locations stimulated simultaneously but in randomly changing combinations. This type of visual field ERG takes approximately 15 min per eye and yields a perimetric ERG map that shows a steep rise in electrical potential at the center of the visual field (2). These maps provide information about the working of the inner retina but not the ganglion cells. Optic nerve damage would be expected to have no effect on the perimetric ERG map. Pattern ERG responses have been obtained outside of the macular area using a scanning laser ophthalmoscope (3), but the weak signals are highly dependent on macular function.

Averaging of visual evoked potentials from focal stimuli has also been tried (4), but the results did not yield a high enough signal to noise ratio to be of clinical use. The signals were too weak, especially outside of the central 5 degrees, partly because the potentials measured from visual cortex are primarily from macular representation of the occipital pole.

One promising technique for obtaining objective visual field information involves monitoring of the pupillary light reflex to focal perimetric light stimuli. Use of the pupillary light reflex to objectively monitor the sensitivity of the visual field is not new. Previous investigators have attempted pupil perimetry in both normal subjects and in patients with homonymous field loss (5–22). Early studies have been summarized by Loewenfeld (23,24). Unfortunately, most previous studies have only collected information along one meridian of the visual field (usually the horizontal axis) and most of this information has been obtained in only a limited number of normal subjects. This is because previous attempts at pupil perimetry involved the manual presentation of focal light stimuli and the associated pupil responses had to be estimated with the unaided eye or with the use of a magnifying telescope. In more quantitative studies using an electronic pupillograph, the recorded pupil contractions had to be measured by hand from chart recordings, a process that was very time consuming and labor intensive. In addition, many of the studies used lighting conditions and adapting states that were not conducive to collecting focal responses due to the effect of scattered light.

Our initial goal was to gain experience with pupil perimetry and assess its potential in evaluating patients with visual field loss due to optic nerve disease. We were interested in whether areas of visual perceptual loss corresponded to the same areas of "pupil perimetry" loss. In early studies, we used a Canon infrared fundus photoperimeter simultaneously to view and perimetrically stimulate the fundus through an undilated pupil. A second infrared video camera and telephoto lens was pointed at the fellow eye to monitor the consensual pupil response to focal spots of light presented to the fundus under direct visual guidance (Fig. 1A). The fundus photoperimeter also had a built-in marking system allowing us to place marks on the image of the fundus that could not be seen by the subject in order to delineate the borders of the retina where pupillary contractions to light stimuli were not obtained.

These results were encouraging. In patients with glaucoma demonstrating nerve fiber–related absolute defects, the borders of the retina showing no pupil contractions to focal light stimuli corresponded closely with the borders of the absolute visual field defect (Fig. 1B–1C). This technique of fundus pupil perimetry was advantageous because the location of the retina stimulated by the 1.7-degree light could be confirmed during video recording under direct visual guidance. The consensual pupil movement could be simultaneously observed by combining its video image with the fundus image on the same television screen. Although this method of fundus pupil perimetry had certain advantages, it still lacked features that were needed for standardized clinical testing and more rigorous evaluation of the technique.

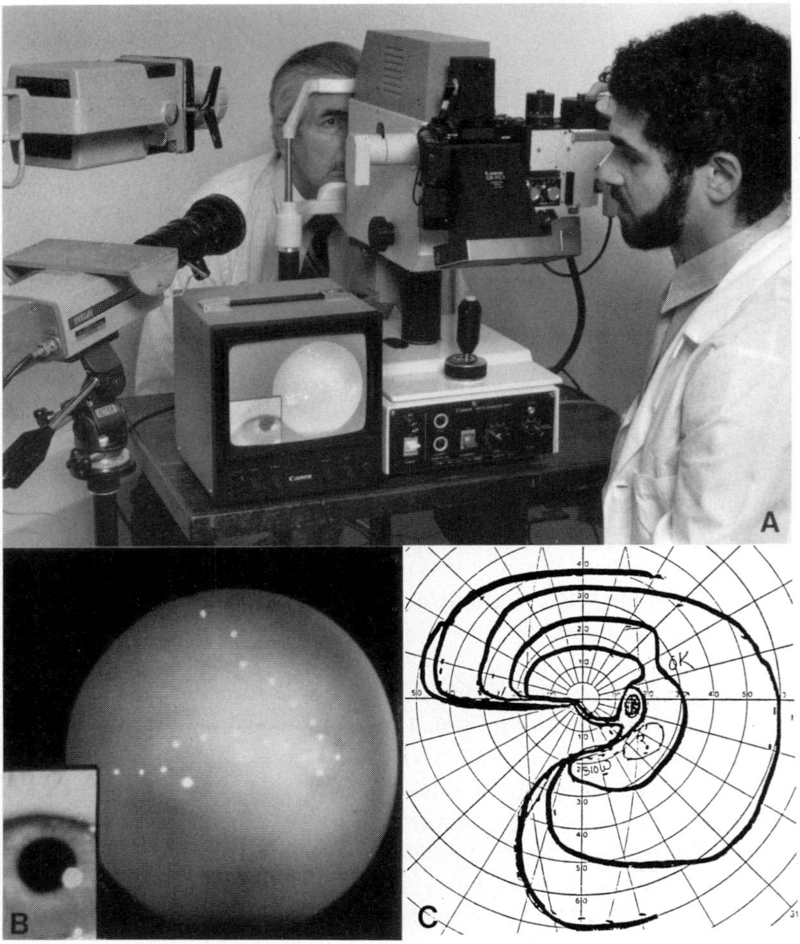

Figure 1 (A) The instrumentation used in initial studies for fundus pupil perimetry included a fundus photoperimeter (center), infrared video camera, and infrared light source (left). A spot of light is placed on the retina of the patient under direct visualization of the fundus and the consensual pupil movement is monitored at the same time by combining the images on the same television screen (foreground). (B) Photograph of the infrared video image of the right retina of a patient with low-tension glaucoma. The optic nerve border was outlined by four white marks. The other marks define an arcuate and temporal area of the retina where spots of light had no affect on pupil movement (pupil blindness). The image of the pupil is seen at the lower left. (C) Corresponding Goldmann visual field from the same patient showing an absolute arcuate and nasal step visual deficit which matched the area of retina defined by the absence of pupillary light reflexes.

What was needed was an automated method for presenting the stimulus light, computer recording of the pupil movement, and a software algorithm for determining the contraction amplitude of each pupillary light reflex. This would allow a more systematic, quantitative evaluation of pupil perimetry and its relation to visual threshold perimetry.

We (25,26) and others (27,28) have attempted to bring current technology to bare on these problems in hopes of using the pupillary light reflex as a means to answer important clinical and scientific questions. In the last 6 years, my colleagues and I have been able to automate the process of pupil perimetry by linking a commercially available static threshold perimeter (Humphrey Field Analyzer) with a computerized infrared pupillograph (Fig. 2). Software analysis of the recorded pupillary contractions (Fig. 3) had allowed us objectively and rapidly to monitor the pupillary response to perimetric light stimuli in health and disease (25,26) and compare it with visual threshold values obtained at the same location using the same perimeter. The specific details of this automated form of pupil perimetry have been previously reported (26). There are two differences in stimulus conditions between standardized visual threshold perimetry and pupil

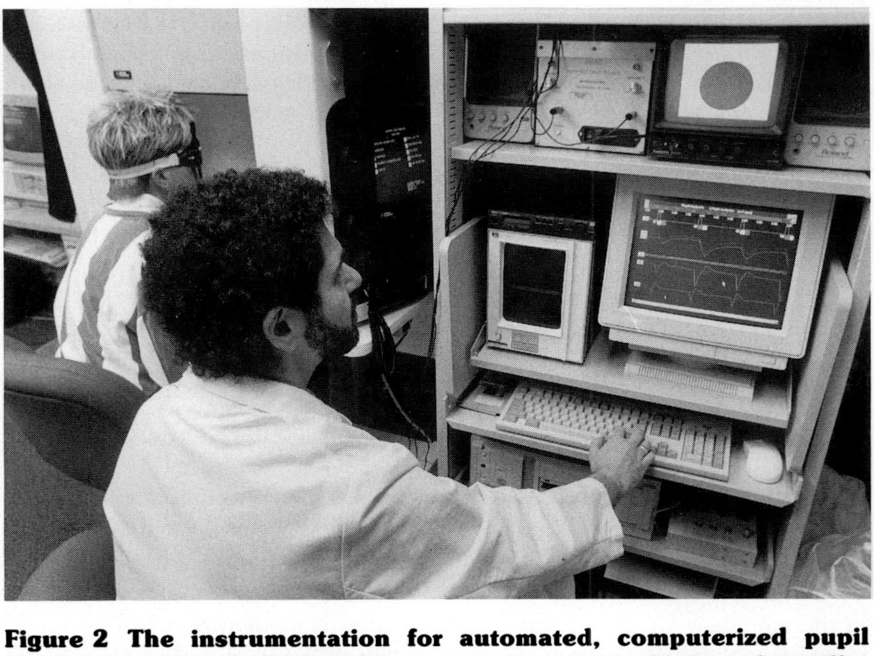

Figure 2 The instrumentation for automated, computerized pupil perimetry is shown. To the right is the computerized infrared pupillometer that continually records pupil area at 60 times/s from an infrared video camera placed behind the Humphrey perimeter bowl shown at left.

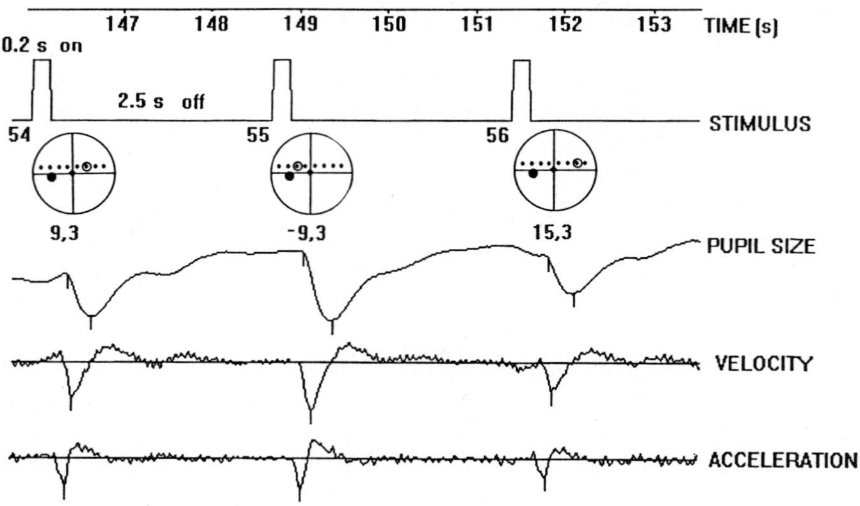

Figure 3 Example of sequence of pupil recordings from a pupil perimetry test as analyzed by a customized software program. The time scale (in seconds) is at the top, the stimulus tracing is next, followed by circles signifying the visual field location of the stimulus light and then the tracing of pupil area. The velocity and acceleration tracings are shown consecutively below the pupil area tracing. The beginning of each pupil reaction is marked at the time when maximum acceleration takes place. The peak of the contraction is defined by the point at which velocity changes sign.

perimetry. First, in order to keep the steady-state pupil size within its optimal operating range, the mesopic background illumination is reduced from 31.5 apostilbs to 3.15 apostilbs. Second, the size of the stimulus light used in pupil perimetry is 1.7 degrees (Goldmann size V).

Unlike visual perceptual responses, the pupillary light reflex is a graded response, and its magnitude is proportional to stimulus light intensity. When log stimulus intensity is graphed as a function of pupil contraction amplitude, the response curve is sigmoidal in shape (Fig. 4). The shape of this curve is steeper at more peripheral locations but basically retains the same general shape over the visual field in normal subjects. Within the linear portion of the curve, changes in the amplitude of pupil contractions are directly proportional to changes in retinal sensitivity. We have taken advantage of this proportionality indirectly to estimate retinal sensitivity over the visual field. This is done by using the same stimulus intensity, 1000 apostilb (–1.0 log stimulus attenuation), at each location—a level well within the linear portion of each location's response curve.

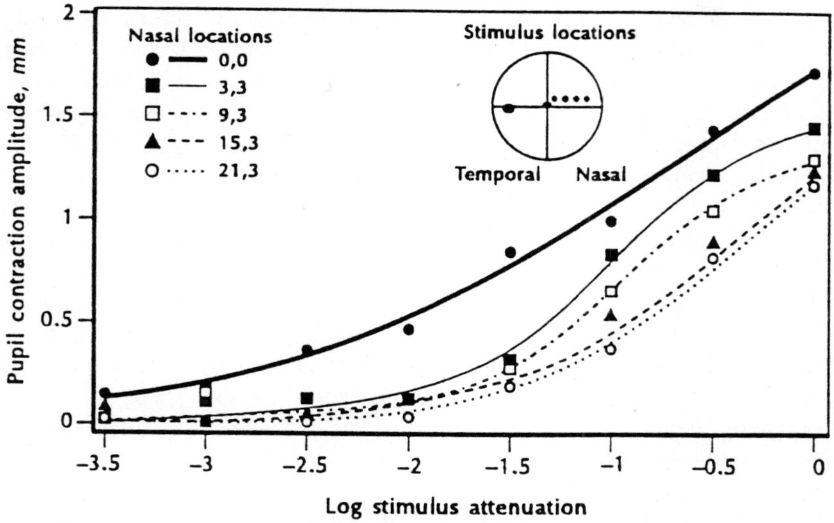

Figure 4 Plot of stimulus intensity versus pupil contraction amplitude for nasal locations along the horizontal meridian illustrating the response curve as a function of eccentricity in the field. Note that the curve for the fovea is more sensitive (shifted to the left), has a more shallow slope, and has a greater maximum response. The pupil response is fairly linear over the majority of the range of stimulus light intensity. Each point shown is the mean of 10 responses at a given intensity for that location.

When the same stimulus intensity is used, a map of the pupil contraction amplitude at each location reflects the retinal sensitivity in terms of the pupillomotor system. It is important that the stimulus light not be too bright, as scatter of light can become significant and result in loss of a focal pupil response.

Our initial studies using automated pupil perimetry have been directed toward comparing visual threshold with pupillomotor sensitivity at the same locations in normal eyes and in eyes exhibiting visual field deficits. When visual threshold is compared with pupil threshold in normal eyes under low mesopic background conditions (3.15 apostilbs) using a 1.7-degree 1000 apostilb stimulus light, the pupil "hill of vision" shows a steep rise toward the center and the sensitivity falls off more in the nasal field compared with the temporal field. In contrast, the visual hill is much flatter, with little difference between the nasal and temporal field.

The magnitude of difference between visual and pupil threshold varies between individuals. This is partly explained by individual differences in the level of supranuclear inhibition of the Edinger-Westphal nucleus. This can produce differences in pupillary contraction independent of retinal sensitivity. An excited individual may exhibit more central inhibition resulting in large pupils that react less to light. A fatigued, sleepy subject will show central disinhibition causing the pupils to become small and resulting in mechanical limitations imposed on the amplitude of contractions to light stimuli (29). Therefore, steady-state pupil size is important in the interpretation of pupil perimetry, because it reflects not only the retinal sensitivity to the background illumination, but it also gives an indication of the level of central inhibition of the midbrain pupillomotor center.

We have had an opportunity to test over 300 subjects with visual field defects due to damage to the retina, optic nerve, chiasm, optic tract, visual radiation, and visual cortex. Differences between the visual and pupil fields in some cases have forced us to rethink some of the concepts relating pupillomotor input and visual perception. The following examples serve to illustrate some of the similarities and differences between the two pathways when pathology is present.

In general, eyes exhibiting visual deficits due to outer retinal damage show a remarkable correspondence between visual and pupillomotor sensitivity. This is not surprising, since the pathway for visual light perception and the pupillary light reflex share the same rod and cone input (23). The patient in Figure 5 initially presented with a constricted visual field but a normal-appearing fundus. Pupil perimetry confirmed a pathological constriction of the field and an electroretinogram confirmed the presence of retinitis pigmentosa. In contrast, the patient in Figure 6 also presented with constriction of the visual field, but unlike the first patient, pupil perimetry revealed normal retinal sensitivity. This led to the suspicion of functional field loss, which was later substantiated with further clinical testing. We have found pupil perimetry very useful in differentiating functional field loss from pathological visual field deficits.

Patients with various causes of pregeniculate visual field loss vary in the degree of correspondence with pupil field deficits. Most patients with ischemic optic neuropathy show a high correlation between the pupil and visual fields (Fig. 7). This also seems to hold true for damage due to compression of the optic nerve near the globe. Compression more distal to the globe, toward the chiasm, may show differences between the visual and pupil fields. One possible explanation may be differences in the anatomical location of the visual and pupillary axons as they travel further in their course toward the brain.

Differences in susceptibility to damage of the visual and pupillary nerves may also help to explain differences in the pupil and visual field. We have observed such differences in patients with glaucomatous nerve damage and in patients with optic neuritis. In patients with glaucoma, there were often more deficits in the pupil field than in the visual field (Fig. 8). This took the form of more focal deficits as well as more generalized loss. In patients with optic neuritis, the pupil

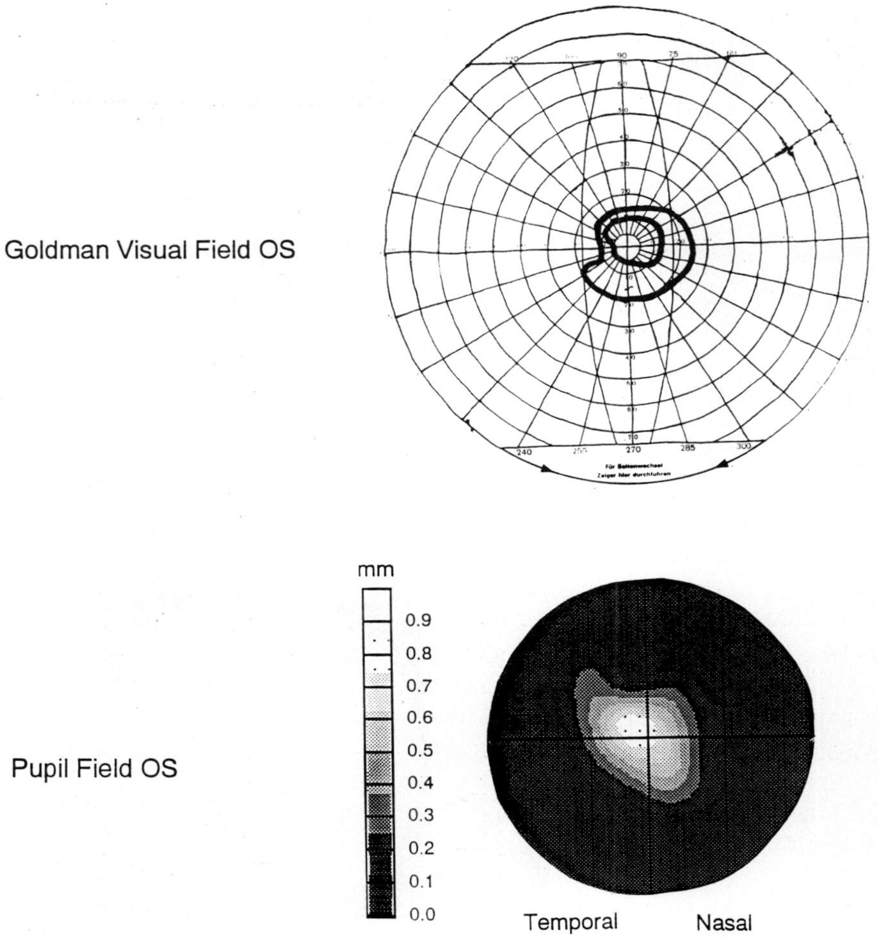

Figure 5 Comparison of visual and pupil fields from the left eye of a patient with retinitis pigmentosa. Initially, the constricted visual field (top) was thought to be functional, but the matching constricted pupil field (bottom) also showed no pupil responses outside of 15 degrees leading to the correct diagnosis. The absence of pupil response in the periphery also demonstrates that the responses are focal, with little significant scatter of light. Pupil field gray scale is in units of millimeters (mm) of contraction amplitude to a 1000 apostilb stimulus light (Goldmann size V, 1.7 degrees).

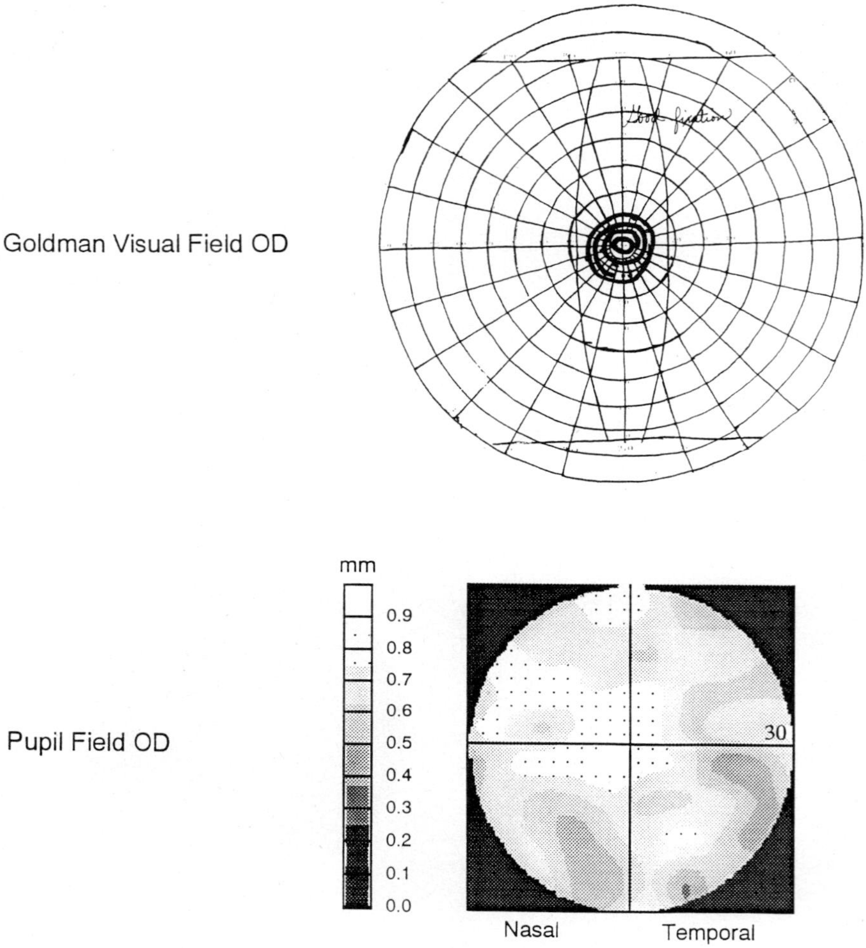

Figure 6 A patient also demonstrating a constricted visual field (top) but with normal pupil contraction amplitudes (in mm) across the same area of field, which indicates functional visual loss.

field deficits were often not located in the same area as the visual field deficits. The patient shown in Figure 9 had extensive visual threshold loss in the superior nasal field but no defects on pupil perimetry. Lack of correspondence between the visual and pupil fields in these patients may reflect demyelination within an area of the nerve where the visual fibers are separated from the pupil fibers or differential susceptibility of the two pathways to damage.

Finally, patients with isolated damage to the visual cortex have been found

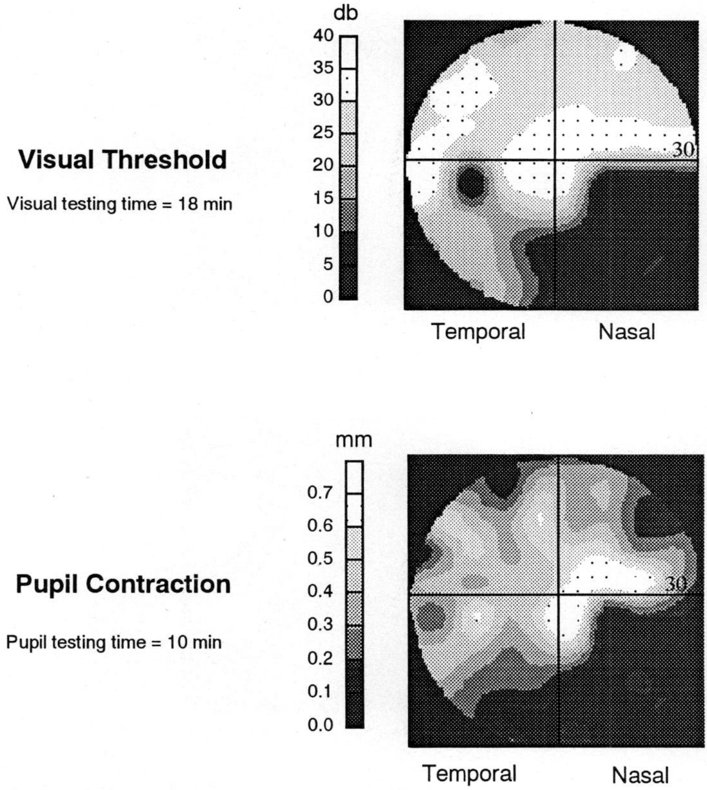

Figure 7 Shown are the gray scales of visual threshold (top) and pupillary contraction amplitude (bottom) for the left eye of a patient with anterior ischemic optic neuropathy. Note that there was a high degree of correspondence between the visual and pupil response in the area of the inferior nasal field defect.

to exhibit homonymous pupil field defects that parallel the visual homonymous fields (Fig. 10). This has been reported previously by other investigators (9–16) and has been referred to as "pupillary hemiakinesia." Some investigators have postulated a separate cortical pupillary pathway to explain the results. Loewenfeld has discussed this issue (30) and has proposed that some of the patients may not have had isolated lesions of visual cortex, since vascular ischemic events can often lead to more than one site of damage (i.e., optic tract and radiation). Retrograde degeneration affecting pregeniculate pupil fibers also was suggested. Many of our patients were tested within the first few weeks of their damage, which makes classic retrograde degeneration less likely.

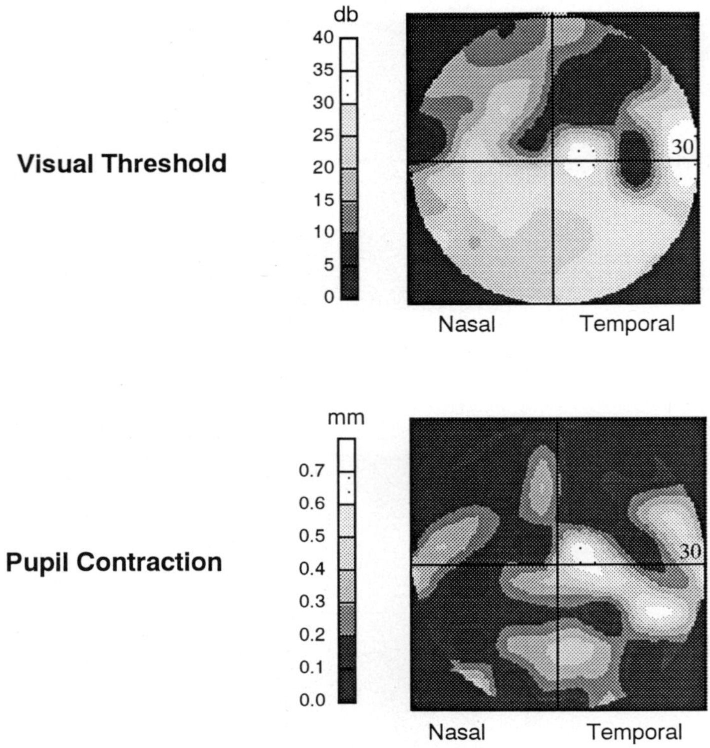

Figure 8 Comparison of visual threshold (top) and pupil contraction amplitude (bottom) of the right visual field of a patient with glaucoma (not on miotics). Note the superior arcuate and nasal visual threshold loss. The pupil contraction amplitude (in millimeters) shows similar deficits but also shows much more extensive nasal and arcuate pupil field loss inferiorly as well as superiorly. In addition, there appears to be diffuse, generalized loss.

However, it is possible that cortical damage may affect the function of pregeniculate fibers before retrograde degeneration has taken place. We also believe that many of our cases did represent isolated cortical lesions based on magnetic resonance imaging (MRI) and the lack of clinical and pupillary signs of a tract lesion. More work needs to be done in this area in order to better understand this unexpected finding.

In summary, our present experience comparing pupil perimetry with visual threshold perimetry has raised a number of questions. What is the anatomical pathway for afferent input to the pupillomotor system and how closely do the afferent pupil and visual nerve fibers travel within the pregeniculate system? Do

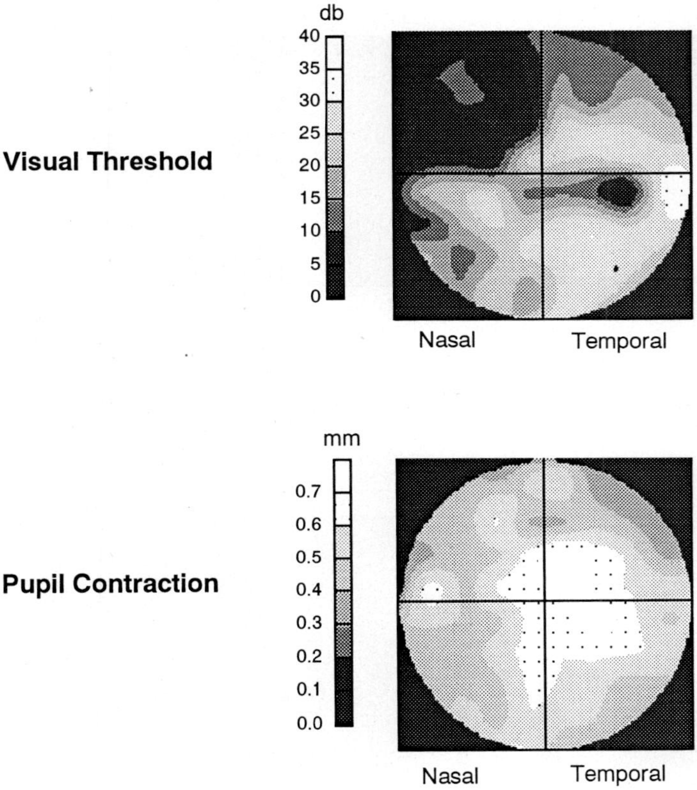

Figure 9 In this young woman, demyelination of the right optic nerve caused acute optic neuritis resulting in visual threshold loss primarily in the superior field (top). However, pupil perimetry performed on the same day (bottom) showed no corresponding deficit.

the two pathways have the same susceptibility to damage and will differences help to diagnose the etiology and location of the damage? What influence does visual cortex have on the pupillary light reflex pathway in health and in disease? Addressing these questions is anticipated to lead to a greater understanding of how pupil perimetry can be used to help prevent blindness.

ACKNOWLEDGMENTS

This work was supported in part by an unrestricted grant to the Department of Ophthalmology from Research to Prevent Blindness, in part by a Fight For

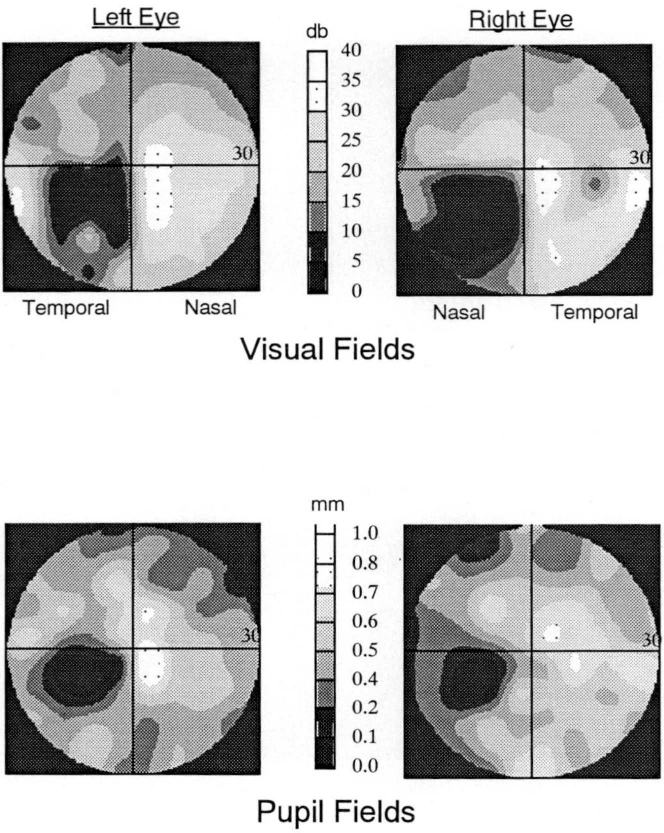

Figure 10 Comparison of visual threshold (top) and pupil contraction amplitude (bottom) from the right and left fields of a patient with a 1-month-old right occipital infarct. This resulted in a left homonymous scotoma. The pupil responses show the same homonymous deficit, even though there was no clinically discernible relative afferent pupillary defect using the swinging flashlight test and no MRI evidence of extraoccipital involvement.

Sight–Prevent Blindness Grant-in-Aid Fellowship (GA90063), and in part by a grant from Zeis-Humphrey corporation.

I would like to acknowledge the expert assistance of Paula Moore in performing pupil perimetry testing and in preparation of the accompanying figures. I am also grateful for the help of Drs. Pinar Aydin-Kirkali, Stanley Thompson, and Irene Loewenfeld and Roger Anderson, Chad Denison, Stacy Thompson, and Chris Haupert.

REFERENCES

1. Hamazaki S, Matsuo H. Quantitative perimetry and local ERG in the diseases of macular area and bjerum area. In: Proceedings of the Second International Visual Field Symposium, Tubingen, 1976. Doc Ophthalmol Proc Series 1977; 14:173–87.
2. Sutter EE. The field topography of ERG components in man. I. The photopic luminance response. Vision Res 1992; 32:433–46.
3. Katsumi O, Van de Velde FJ, Mehta MC, Hirose T. Topographical analysis of peripheral vs central retina with pattern reversal visual evoked response and the scanning laser ophthalmoscope. Acta Ophthalmol 1991; 69:596–602.
4. Van Lith GH. Perimetry and electrophysiology. In: Proceedings of the Second International Visual Field Symposium, Tubingen, 1976. Doc Ophthalmol Proc Series 1977; 14:169–71.
5. Wernicke G. Uber hemiopische pupillenreaktion. Fortschr Med 1883; 1:49–53.
6. Walker C. Further observations on the hemianopic pupillary reaction obtained with a new clinical treatment. JAMA 1914; 63:846–51.
7. Harms H. Grundlagen, Methodik und Bedeutung der Pupillenperimetrie fur die Physiologie und Pathologie des Schorgans. Albrecht von Graefes Arch Klin Exp Ophthalmol 1949; 149:1–44.
8. Bresky R, Charles S. Pupillomotor perimetry. Am J Ophthalmol 1969; 68:108–12.
9. Cibis G, Campos E, Aulhorn E. Pupillary hemiakinesia in suprageniculate lesions. Arch Ophthalmol 1975; 93:1322–7.
10. Hellner K, Jensen W, Muller-Jensen A. Video-processing pupillography as a method for objective perimetry in pupillary hemiakinesia. In: Proceedings of the Second International Visual Field Symposium, Tubingen, 1976. Doc Ophthalmol Proc Series 1977; 14:221–6.
11. Hellner KA, Jensen W, Muller A. Video processing pupillographic perimetry in hemianopsia. Klin Mbl Augenheik 1978; 172:731–5.
12. Alexandridis E, Krastel H, Reuther R. Disturbances of the pupil reflex associated with lesions of the upper visual pathway. Albrecht von Graefes Arch Klin Exp Ophthalmol 1979; 209:199–208.
13. Reuther R, Alexandridis E, Krastel H. Disturbances of the pupil reflex associated with cerebral infraction in the posterior cerebral artery territory. Arch Psychiatr Nervenkr 1981; 229:249–57.
14. Reuther R, Krastel H, Alexandridis E. Disturbances of the pupil reflex associated with homonymous hemianopic paracentral scotoma. Arch Psychiatr Nervenkr 1981; 229:259–66.
15. Hamann K, Hellner K, Muller-Jensen A, Zschocke S. Videopupillographic and VER investigations in patients with congenital and acquired lesions of the optic radiation. Ophthalmologica 1979; 178:348–56.
16. Barbur JL, Forsyth PM. Can the pupil response be used as a measure of the visual input associated with the geniculo-striate pathway? Clin Vision Sci 1986; 1:107–11.
17. Burke DW, Ogle K. Comparison of visual and pupillary light thresholds in perimetry. Arch Ophthalmol 1964; 71:400–8.
18. Narasaki S, Kawai K, Kubota S, Noguchi J. Videopupillographic perimetry and its clinical application. Jpn J Ophthalmol 1974; 18:253–74.

19. Yoshitomi M. The examination of pupillary light reflex with a specific pupillary paralysis. Acta Soc Ophthalmol Jpn 1955; 9:853.
20. Ishikawa S, Naito M, Inaba K. A new Videopupillography. Ophthalmologica 1970; 60:248–59.
21. Jensen W. A description of a method for objective perimetry. Albrecht von Graefes Arch Klin Exp Ophthalmol 1976; 201:183–91.
22. Aoyama T, Kani K. Pupillographic perimetry. In: Proceedings of the Second International Visual Field Symposium, Tubingen, 1976. Doc Ophthalmol Proc Series 1977; 14:207–12.
23. Loewenfeld IE. Pupillary movements associated with light and near vision. In: Whitcomb A, ed. Recent developments in vision research. Washington, DC: National Academy of Sciences, Publication 1272, 1966:17–105 (Tables 5 and 10).
24. Loewenfeld, I. The pupil. Wayne State and Iowa State University Press, Ames, Iowa, 1993: 110–12.
25. Kardon RH, Haupert C, Thompson HS. Automated pupil perimetry. Noninvasive assessment of the visual system, 1990 Technical Digest Series. Vol. 3. Optical Society of America, 1990:44–7.
26. Kardon RH, Aydin-Kirkali P, Thompson HS. Automated pupil perimetry. I. Pupil field mapping in patients and normal subjects. Ophthalmol 1991; 98:485–96.
27. Frankhauser F, Flammer J. Puptrak 1.0—a new semiautomated system for pupillometry with the Octopus perimeter: a preliminary report. Doc Ophthalmol 1990; 73:235–48.
28. Alexandridis E, Krastel, H. New equipment for pupillographic perimetry. Neuro-ophthalmology 1990; 10:331–6.
29. Loewenfeld IE, Newsome, D. Iris mechanics I. Influence of pupil size on dynamics of pupillary movement. Am J Ophthalmol 1971; 71:347–62.
30. Loewenfeld, I. The pupil. Wayne State and Iowa State University Press, Ames, Iowa, 1993:211–20.

29

Radiation-Induced Optic Neuropathy

John Guy
University of Florida, Gainesville, Florida

Norman J. Schatz
University of Miami, Miami, Florida

Radiation-induced optic neuropathy (RON) is an uncommon, rapidly progressive disorder resulting in visual loss that occurs months to years after completion of radiation therapy (1–46). The visual loss of RON may be reversible provided treatment is instituted within days of the onset of visual loss (16,45). Consequently, it is important for all internists, neurologists, neurosurgeons, ophthalmologists, and radiation oncologists involved in the treatment of cancer patients to be able to recognize this disorder and promptly refer patients for treatment. Patients must also be made aware of the need to seek immediate medical attention should they lose vision. It is the aim of this chapter to provide these physicians with the knowledge they will need to diagnose and treat RON by providing answers to the following questions.

I. WHAT IS RADIATION-INDUCED OPTIC NEUROPATHY (RON)?

Radiation-induced optic neuropathy is an ischemic disorder of the optic nerve and/or optic chiasmal vasculature that usually results in irreversible devastating visual loss months to years after radiation therapy to the cranium and/or orbit (1–46). Pathological specimens of the optic nerves and/or optic chiasm obtained at autopsy or by surgical biopsy of the anterior visual pathways have shown ischemic demyelination, obliterative endarteritis, and fibrinoid necrosis (18,19,

34,35,38). Although the damaging effects of ionizing radiation to the cerebral vasculature have been well documented (12,16,18,19), the mechanism for this delayed effect of radiation on the vasculature of the central nervous system (CNS) is unclear (19).

II. WHO IS AT RISK FOR RON?

All patients who have had the orbital optic nerve, intracranial optic nerve, or optic chiasm in the field of therapeutic CNS irradiation are potentially at risk for delayed visual loss from RON. In the past, RON had a higher incidence with large doses of radiotherapy (RT) delivered over comparatively short time spans (40). A complete summary of doses of RT and the visual complications associated with RON from the medical literature are listed in Table 1. The cumulative doses of RT reported in patients with RON ranged from 2400 (39) to 12,500 rads (40). Although no dose of RT is risk free, the risk of development of RON climbs steeply with cumulative doses greater than 5000–5500 rads, which is considered to be the tolerance level of the optic nerves (33). Parsons found RON developed in 8% of patients who received daily doses of 165–190 rads with total doses ranging from 6000 to 7300 rads (22). The risk of RON rose sharply to 41% with daily doses ≥195 rads, within the same total dose range of 6000–7300 rads (22). Goldsmith and associates found that a cumulative dose of 5400 rads delivered at 180 rads/day had a very low risk of RON (23).

Patients who have received chemotherapy in conjunction with RT and patients with acidophilic pituitary adenomas who have received RT appear to have a greater risk for the development of RON even at "safe" doses of RT (4,25,28).

It must be emphasized that the dose of RT delivered to the optic nerves may be higher than actually desired. Equipment may not be frequently calibrated or it may malfunction, which among other reasons may result in a higher dose of ionizing radiation than set by the operator. Consequently, do not be led away from the possibility of RON as the cause of visual loss, even when inquiries to the radiation oncologist seem to indicate the tolerance dose (either cumulative or daily) of the optic nerves was not exceeded!

III. WHAT ARE THE PRESENTING SIGNS AND SYMPTOMS OF RON?

Rapid and progressive visual loss in one or both eyes is the predominant presenting symptom associated with RON. Initial visual loss may occur in one or both eyes and is usually rapidly progressive leading to irreversible blindness if untreated[1–46] (see Table 1). Transient episodes of visual loss indistinguishable from amaurosis fugax may occur weeks prior to the onset of RON (16). Unlike recurrent tumors producing compression of the anterior visual pathways where

Table 1 Radiation-Induced Optic Neuropathy Reported in the Literature

Authors	No. of cases	Dose RT	OD	OS	Comment
Crompton and Layton (35)	2	4500	20/200	20/200	
		6250	20/60	20/200	
Schatz et al. (28)		5000	CF	20/20	
		5000	CF	20/20	
Fitzgerald et al. (12)	5	8060	Blind		Shrinkage of VF
		7680	20/20	20/25	
		7950	20/20	CF	
		5000	20/20	LP	Retinopathy
		7200	20/20	20/20	
Harris and Levene (37)	6	4500	Blindness		
		7000	Blindness		
		5000	Bitemporal hemianopsia		
		4500	Blindness		
		4500	Blindness		
		4500	Tunnel vision		
Martins et al. (20)	2	6738	LP	Not given	
		6580	Blind	20/30	
Brown et al. (9)	1	3600–7000	20/20	20/40	Not case-by-case report. Hyperbaric O2 given as treatment in an unidentified case
	3	3600–7000	20/50	20/100	
	1	3600–7000	20/200	CF	
		3600–7000	NLP		

Table 1 (*Continued*)

Authors	No. of cases	Dose RT	OD	OS	Comment
Hammer (17)	4	4250	CF	LP	
		4250	20/20	20/200	
		4250	CF	CF	
		4250	20/200	NLP	
Ghatak and Whitel (38)	1	7995	Complete loss of vision		
Aristizabal et al. (1)	4	4000–5000	All 4 blind		Vision not reported
Fishman et al. (39)	2	2400	20/20	LP	Total right temporal hemianopsia
		Initially 2400 followed by mother 2500	NLP	NLP	Both patients received chemotherapy
Atkinson et al. (4)	4	4240	HM	HM	Became totally blind
		4380	HM	Blind	
		4520	HM	Blind	
		4240	HM	Blind	Became blind OD
Boys and Kerns (40)	2	7000 followed by 6000	NLP	NLP	
		12,500	CF	NLP	
Rosengren (41)	2	2700 followed by 3250	0.7	LP	
		6000	1.0	NLP	
Egbert (42)	1	4700 followed by 4900	LP	NLP	
Shukovsky and Fletcher (43)	1	7330	NLP	NLP	
Tomsak and Smith (44)	1	3300	20/20	CF retinopathy OD	Had radiation

Guy and Schatz (16)	4	5400	20/70	20/50	
		4500–6500	CF3'	20/25	
		5000	LP	20/800	
		6000	CF1'	CF4'	
Borruat et al. (45)	1	5000	NLP	20/20	Lt temporal hemianopia
Hudgins et al. (31)	3	5400	Not given		Lt optic neuropathy
		6600–7500	Not given		Rt optic neuropathy
		5040	Not given		Bilateral optic neuropathy
Tachibana et al. (32)	1	5860	Not given		Bilateral optic neuropathy
Zimmerman et al. (30)	3	5040	HM	20/25	Tx HBO
		5040	20/25	20/20	Tx HBO
		7000	20/200	NLP	
Young et al. (33)	2	5940	20/20	20/20	
		5940	Not given		Junctional syndrome
Goldsmith et al. (23)	1	5670	5/200	HM	
Kline et al. (19)	4	5000	20/20	20/400	
		5000	20/20	20/400	
		4600	20/25	LP	
		5000	2/200	20/20	
Martins et al. (46)	1	6500	Blind	20/30	
DiLorenzo et al. (36)	1	5000	3/10	Blind	

Table 1 (*Continued*)

Authors	No. of cases	Dose RT	OD	OS	Comment
Guy et al. (14)	6	6000	NLP	20/20	
		4500	20/70	20/30	
		5340	CF1'	20/25	
		4450	NLP	20/50	
		6400	CF2'	20/25	
		5228	20/25	LP	
Parsons et al. (22)	9	5000–6500			Disc edema
Urdaneta et al. (27)	1	?	Not given		
Roden et al. (2)		5000	20/20	20/400	
		5000	HM	CF	
		6000	20/70	NLP	
		5000	CF	20/100	
		5142	HM	NLP	
		4500	20/100	20/200	
		4500	20/25	20/25	
		5600	20/200	20/200	
		4500	HM	20/20	
		4500	20/30	LP	
		6500	20/50	20/40	
		6400	CF	20/20	
		7200	CF	CF	

NLP = no light perception; LP = light perception; CF = counting fingers; OS = left eye; OD = right eye; HM = ha the onset of visual loss may be insidious and slowly progressive over months to years, the visual loss of RON is rapid in onset and progresses over days to weeks to blindness. Moreover, initial visual loss in one eye may rapidly occur in the contralateral eye.

Visual loss associated with RON may have its onset as early as 2 months after radiation therapy. On the other hand, patients may do well for as long as 7 years after completion of radiotherapy before the onset of visual loss associated with RON (2,5,13,14,19,30). The great majority of patients with RON develop visual loss within 3 years after radiation therapy (1–46).

Most patients with RON present as a "posterior" ischemic optic neuropathy in which optic disc edema is absent (19). Neuro-ophthalmological findings in such patients usually include an afferent pupillary defect, visual field defect, dyschromatopsia, and an initially normal optic nerve head. The optic disc may become atrophic within a few weeks. The visual field of such patients may be an altitudinal, nerve fiber bundle defect, or central scotoma. Some patients with RON can present with a junctional syndrome; that is, an optic neuropathy and contralateral temporal hemianopsia (45). Other patients with RON may present with a bitemporal hemianopsia mimicking recurrence of a tumor involving the chiasm (16,30). In these patients, the intracranial optic nerves and chiasm were included in the field of RT.

Patients with RON may mimic an anterior ischemic optic neuropathy, with optic disc edema, peripapillary hemorrhages, and exudates (9,22). These patients frequently have a coincident radiation retinopathy and the globe and/or retrobulbar optic nerve was usually included in the field of RT.

IV. HOW DO I MAKE THE DIAGNOSIS OF RON?

The clinical signs and symptoms of RON are similar to those of an anterior ischemic optic neuropathy, retrobulbar optic neuropathy, or junctional or chiasmal syndrome. Consequently, the neuro-ophthalmological findings in RON are not exclusive, and in and of themselves do not make the diagnosis of RON.

The first step in the diagnosis of RON is a history of RT usually in cumulative doses exceeding 2400 rads or a daily dose greater than 180 rads. Visual loss is usually sudden and progresses rapidly to blindness over days to weeks, particularly in those with posterior signs (19). The neuro-ophthalmological signs of anterior, posterior, junctional, or chiasmal syndromes are usually present.

Recurrence of the primary tumor or development of a secondary tumor must be excluded as the cause of visual loss before diagnosis of RON. Neuroimaging has made this task less daunting (13,14,30–33). In patients with lymphoma or carcinoma, lumbar puncture with cytological examination should be performed to exclude seeding of the leptomeninges.

Patients with RON usually have no abnormality on computed tomographic (CT) scanning to explain the recent visual loss and may even have a normal CT scan (19). Cerebral angiography is usually normal (19).

Magnetic resonance imaging (MRI) with contrast gadolinium-diethylenetriaminepentaacetic acid, (Gd-DTPA) appears to show the greatest promise in the diagnosis of RON (13,14,30–33,45). Unlike recurrence of tumor where precontrast T_1- and T_2-weighted MRI is usually abnormal, after administration of contrast, patients with acute RON have marked Gd-DTPA enhancement of the optic nerves and/or optic chiasm (13,14,30,31,32,33,45). In most cases of RON, enhancement is usually apparent in one or both of the intracranial segments of the optic nerves, although enhancement of the optic chiasm can be seen in those

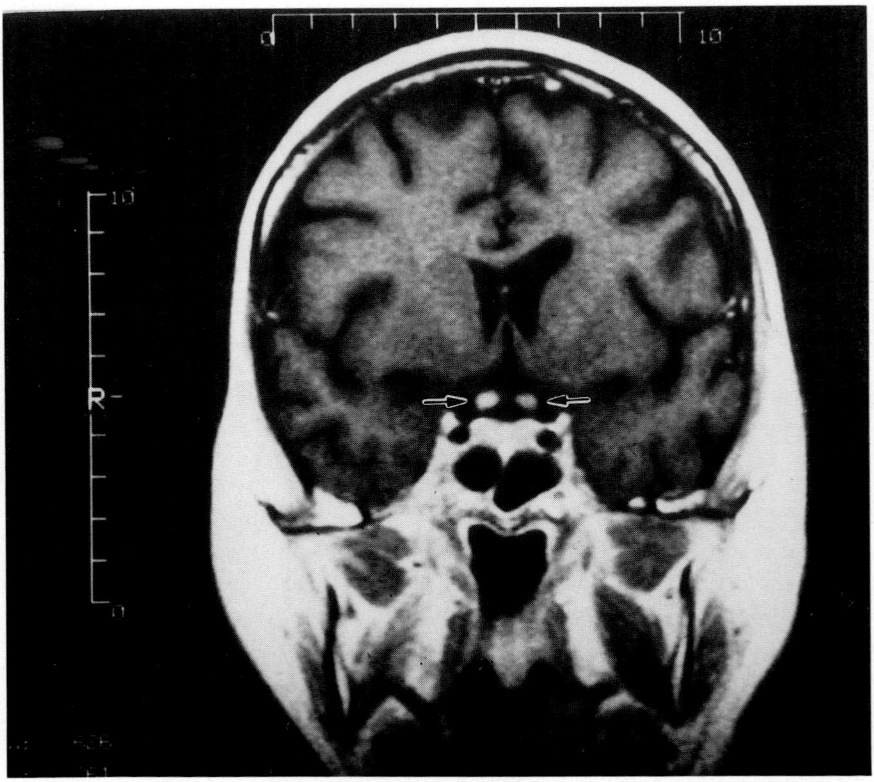

Figure 1 Coronal magnetic resonance imaging showing Gd-DTPA enhancement of the optic nerves (arrows) (patient of James Carl, M.D.).

with junctional or bitemporal hemianopsia. Figure 1 illustrates the Gd-DTPA enhancement of the optic nerve in a patient with RON.

Do not be misled by a "normal" MRI of the "brain"! Be sure to order a contrasted chiasmal MRI study with axial and coronal views. The field of view should include the orbital and intracranial optic nerves along with the optic chiasm. If available, fat suppression, preferably with a frequency selective saturation pulse, should be utilized to visualize lesions of the intraorbital optic nerve.

There may be patients in whom the neuroradiologist cannot exclude recurrence of tumor on the basis of the MRI findings of Gd-DTPA enhancement of the optic nerve. One does not immediately have to resort to neurosurgical exploration to exclude recurrent tumor. An option would be to repeat the MRI 1–3 months later (14). If RON is the cause of the Gd-DTPA enhancement of the optic nerves, this will resolve, although vision may not improve. In contrast, recurrent tumor will still show Gd-DTPA enhancement and a mass lesion that may be even larger than initial MRI.

Be aware that contrast-enhanced CT is usually normal in patients with RON (19). Consequently, CT can not be substituted for MRI in this disorder! A normal CT may aid in the exclusion of recurrent tumor in patients with RON with Gd-DTPA enhancement of the optic nerves visualized on MRI but does not exclude RON.

Occasionally, the cause of recurrent visual loss may still be unclear as the initial tumor was not totally eradicated by previous RT, surgery, or chemotherapy. Such patients may require a neurosurgical exploration for a definitive diagnosis. However, the pitfalls in such exploration are emphasized by the experience of Newman, whose patient expired after failure of a radiation necrotic carotid artery resulted in death from exsanguination but pathological examination confirmed RON (34).

Beware, RON is not exclusively the etiology of recent visual loss in patients without recurrent tumor directly involving the visual pathways. Cancer associated retinopathy (CAR), a remote effect of neoplasia, may be a cause of delayed visual loss in patients with cancer. If MRI does not show Gd-DTPA enhancement characteristic of RON, then an electroretinogram (ERG) and serum for CAR antigen should be obtained to exclude CAR as the etiology of visual loss. Patients with CAR may have neuro-opthalmological signs indistinguishable from a posterior optic neuropathy of RON but will have an extinguished ERG.

The diagnostic workup for RON that includes the neuro-ophthalmological examination and contrast-enhanced MRI (LP if necessary) must be obtained quickly; usually within 24–48 hours after initial visual loss.

V. WHAT CAN I DO FOR MY PATIENT WITH RON?

Now that the diagnosis of RON has been made, what now? Prior to 1986, there was no proven treatment for RON. Guy and Schatz described the first successful management of two patients with RON utilizing hyperbaric oxygen (HBO) (16). In their first patient, vision improved from 20/50 to 20/20 on the second day of HBO treatment. After 14 treatments, this improvement was maintained for the 9 months of follow-up reported. In the second patient, HBO was instituted 3 days after visual loss from RON. After 2 days of HBO, vision improved from counting fingers at 3 feet to 20/200. After 14 days of treatment, vision improved to 20/40. Two weeks later, vision had dropped to 20/300. Reinstitution of HBO for another 14 sessions resulted in no improvement. Treatment with HBO was ineffective in two other patients when instituted more than two weeks after the onset of visual loss.

The efficacy of HBO in the treatment of RON was challenged 4 years later. In 1990, Roden and colleagues found no improvement in vision after HBO (2). All the patients in Roden et al.'s series were treated 2–12 weeks after the onset of visual loss from RON. This poor result was predictable based on the results of Guy and Schatz, in whom successful reversal of visual loss occurred only when treatment began within 2–3 days after visual loss. Consequently, the results of Roden and associates support those of Guy and Schatz; that is, HBO is not effective when treatment is administered late (2 weeks or longer after the onset of visual loss).

It was not until recently that this point was brought home. In 1993, Borruat and colleagues initiated HBO 2 weeks after complete loss of vision in the left eye to NLP and 20/20 in the left eye with a dense left temporal hemianopsia (45). After HBO, the hemianopsia resolved completely and vision in the right eye improved slightly to LP. This one patient illustrated that treatment after 2 weeks of visual loss in the left eye had little effect. On the other hand, HBO administered after 2 days of onset of a complete temporal hemianopsia promptly reversed the defect (Fig. 2). This case emphasizes that in order to be effective, treatment with HBO must be prompt and instituted within 2–3 days of the onset of visual loss.

We suggest the following guidelines for HBO treatment:

1. In order to reverse the visual loss of RON, HBO must be instituted within 2–3 days of visual loss.
2. Treatment with HBO is expensive and may not be indicated if 2 or more weeks have lapsed between the onset of visual loss.
3. The indications for treatment between 4 and 14 days are currently unclear. Successes or failures during this time point have not yet been reported.
4. The duration of treatment should be at least 14 sessions at 2.4–2.8 atmospheres of hyperbaria with 2 sessions a day for the first 2 days if possible. Longer treatments may be necessary depending on the extent of radionecrosis. We have performed HBO for as long as 8 weeks (with a 1-2-day rest period every 14 sessions) in a patient with multiple myeloma

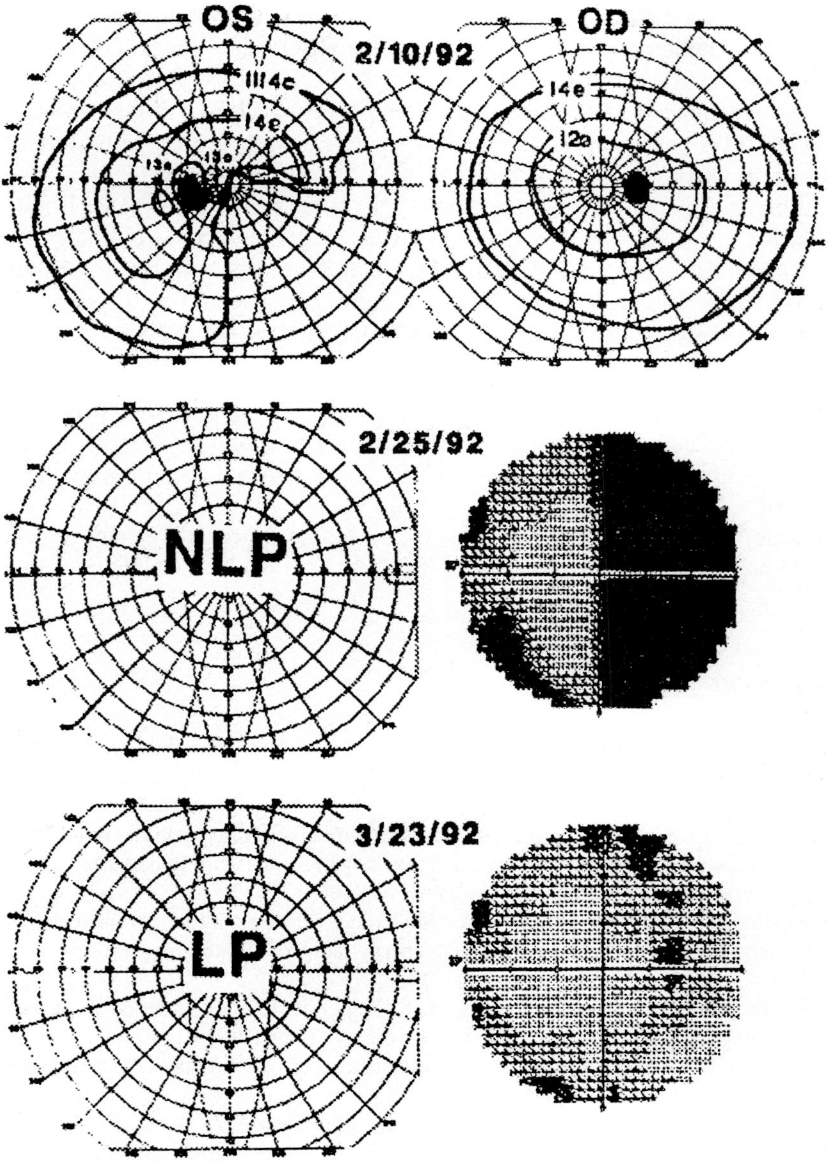

Figure 2 Showing initial visual field loss of left eye (top). After complete visual loss in the left eye, a dense temporal hemianopsia developed in the right eye (middle). After HBO the temporal hemianopsia resolved completely (bottom). (From Ref. 45.)

who received both chemotherapy and RT. This patient had progression of bilateral optic neuropathy after cessation of HBO. He eventually elected to stop HBO after 2 months and was NLP OU.

5. We recommend MRI be repeated after 2 weeks of HBO. If resolution of Gd-DTPA enhancement of the optic nerve occurs, there may be no further risk to vision.
6. Although methylprednisilone alone is not effective in RON (16), it may have a synergistic effect when added to HBO (45). Consequently, methylprednisilone at a dose of 250–500 mg intravenously every 6 hs for 3–5 days followed by 1 mg/kg of oral prednisone for 2 weeks is recommended while the patient is receiving HBO.

In our experience, adverse effects of HBO were minor. Some of our patients required auricular intubation, since they were unable to equalize the changes in pressure associated with hyberbaria. Although seizures and pulmonary edema are known complications of HBO, none of our patients experienced these problems.

Beware! The window between success and failure in the HBO management of RON is narrow. Do not miss it!

REFERENCES

1. Aristizabal S, Caldwell WL, Avila J. The relationship of time-dose fractionation factors to complications in the treatment of pituitary tumors by irradiation. Int J Radiat Oncol Biol Phys 1977; 2:667–73.
2. Roden D, Bosley TM, Fowble B, et al. Delayed radiation injury to the retrobulbar optic nerves and chiasm: clinical syndrome and treatment with hyperbaric oxygen and corticosteroids. Ophthalmology 1990; 97:346–51.
3. Arnold A, Bailey P, Harvey RA. Intolerance of the primate brainstem and hypothalamus to conventional and high energy radiations. Neurology 1954; 4:575–85.
4. Atkinson AB, Allen IV, Gordon DS, et al. Progressive visual failure in acromegaly following external pituitary irradiation. Clin Endocrinol 1979; 10:469–79.
5. Warman R, Glaser JS, Quencer RM. Radionecrosis of optico-hypothalamic glioma. Neuro ophthalmology 1989; 9:219–26.
6. Benson EP. Radiation injury to large arteries. Radiology 1973; 106:195–7.
7. Brant-Zawadzki M, Anderson M, DeArmond SJ, et al. Radiation-induced large intracranial vessel occlusive vasculopathy. AJR 1980; 134:51–5.
8. Brasch RC, Weinmann HJ, Wesbey GE. Contrast-enhanced NMR imaging: animal studies using gadolinium DTPA complex. AJR 1984; 142:625–30.
9. Brown GC, Shields JA, Sanborn G, et al. Radiation optic neuropathy. Ophthalmology 1982; 89:1489–93.
10. Conomy JP, Kellermeyer R. Delayed cerebrovascular consequences of therapeutic

radiation: a clinicopathologic study of a stroke associated with radiation-related carotid arteriopathy. Cancer 36: 1702–8, 1975.
11. Dooms GC, Hecht S, Brant-Zawadzki M, et al. Brain radiation lesions: MR imaging. Radiology 1986; 158:149–55.
12. Fitzgerald CR, Enoch JM, Temme LA: Radiation therapy in and about the retina, optic nerve, and anterior visual pathway. Psychophysical assessment. Arch Ophthalmol 1981; 99:611–23.
13. Guy J, Mancuso A, Quisling RG, et al. Gadolinium-DPTA-enhanced magnetic resonance imaging in optic neuropathies. Ophthalmology 1990: 97:592–600.
14. Guy J, Mancuso A, Beck R, et al. Radiation-induced optic neuropathy: a magnetic resonance imaging study. J Neurosurg 1991; 74:426–32.
15. Glaholm J, Bloom HJG, Crow JH. The role of radiotherapy in the management of intracranial meningiomas: the Royal Marsden Hospital experience with 186 patients. Int J Radiat Oncol Biol Phys 1990; 18:755.
16. Guy J, Schatz NJ. Hyperbaric oxygen in the treatment of radiation-induced optic neuropathy. Ophthalmology 1986; 93:1083–8.
17. Hammer HM: Optic chiasmal radionecrosis. Trans Ophthal Soc UK 1983; 103:208–11.
18. Husain MM, Garcia JH. Cerebral "radiation necrosis" vascular and glial features. Acta Neuropathol 1976; 36:381–5.
19. Kline LB, Kim JY, Ceballos R. Radiation optic neuropathy. Ophthalmology 1985; 92:1118–26.
20. Kuharik MA, Edwards MK, Farlow MR, et al. GDenhanced MR imaging of acute and chronic experimental demyelinating lesions. AJNR 1988; 9:643–8.
21. Mikhael MA: Radiation necrosis of the brain. Correlation between computerized tomography, pathology, and dose distribution. J Comput Assist Tomogr 1978; 2:71–80.
22. Parsons J, Fitzgerald CR, Hood Cl, et al. The effects of irradiation on the eye and optic nerve. Int J Radiat Oncol Biol Phys 1983; 9:609–22.
23. Goldsmith BJ, Rosenthal SA, Wara WM, Larson DA. Optic neuropathy after irradiation of meningioma. Radiology. 1992 185(1):71–6.
24. Murros KE, Toole JF. The effect of radiation on carotid arteries. A review article. Arch Neurol 1989; 46:449–55.
25. Peck FC Jr, McGovern ER. Radiation necrosis of the brain in acromegaly. J Neurosurg 1966; 25:536–42.
26. Rosengren B: Two cases of atrophy of the optic nerve after previous roentgen treatment of the chiasmal region and the optic nerves. Acta Ophthalmol 1958; 36:874–7.
27. Urdaneta N, Chessin H, Fischer JJ. Pituitary adenomas and craniopharyngiomas: analysis of 99 cases with radiation therapy. Int J Radiat Oncol Biol Phys 1976; 1:895–902.
28. Schatz NJ, Lichtenstein S, Corbett JJ. Delayed radiation necrosis of the optic nerves and chiasm. In: Glaser JS, Smith JL, eds. Neuro-Ophthalmology. Vol. 8. Symposium of the University of Miami and the Bascom Palmer Eye Institute. St. Louis: Mosby, 1975: 131–9.
29. Tindall GT, Barrow DL. Disorders of the pituitary. St. Louis: Mosby, 1986.

30. Zimmerman CF. Schatz NJ, Glaser JS. Magnetic resonance imaging of optic nerve meningiomas: enhancement with gadolinium-DTPA. Ophthalmology 1990; 97:585–91.
31. Hudgins PA, Newman NJ, Dillon WP, Hoffman JC Jr. Radiation-induced optic neuropathy: characteristic appearance on gadolinium-enhanced MR. AJNR 1992; 13(1):235–8.
32. Tachibana O, Yamaguchi N, Yamashima T, Yamashita J. Radiation necrosis of the optic chiasm, optic tract, hypothalamus, and upper pons after radiotherapy for pituitary adenoma, detected by gadolinium-enhanced, T1-weighted magnetic resonance imaging: case report. Neurosurgery. 1990; 27(4):640–3.
33. Young WC, Thornton AF, Gebarski SS, Cornblath WT. Radiation-induced optic neuropathy: correlation of MR imaging and radiation dosimetry. Radiology. 1992; 185:904–7.
34. Newman NJ. Contralateral optic neuropathy following adenoid cystic carcinoma. Presented at the Walsh Society. Salt Lake City, Utah, 1991.
35. Crompton MR, Layton DD. Delayed radionecrosis of the brain following therapeutic x-radiation to the pituitary. Brain 1961; 84:85–101.
36. DiLorenzo N, Nolletti A, Palma L. Late cerebral necrosis. Surg Neurol 1978; 10:281–90.
37. Harris JR, Levene MB. Visual complications following irradiation for pituitary adenomas and craniopharyngiomas. Radiology 1976; 120:167–71.
38. Ghatak NR, White BE. Delayed radiation necrosis of the hypothalamus; report of a case simulating recurrent craniopharyngioma. Arch Neurol 1969; 21:425–30.
39. Fishman ML, Bean SC, Cogan DG. Optic atrophy following prophylactic chemotherapy and cranial irradiation for acute lymphocytic leukemia. Am J Ophthalmol 1976; 82:571–6.
40. Buys NS, Kerns TC Jr. Irradiation damage to the chiasm. Am J Ophthalmol 1957; 44:483–6.
41. Rosengren B. Two cases of atrophy of the optic nerve after previous roentgen treatment of the chiasmal region and the optic nerves. Acta Ophthalmol 1958; 36:874–7.
42. Egbert PR, Donaldson SS, Moazed K, Rosenthal AR. Visual results and ocular complications following radiotherapy for retinoblastoma. Arch Ophthalmol 1978; 96:1826–30.
43. Shukovsky LJ, Fletcher GH. Retinal and optic nerve complications in a high dose irradiation technique of ethmoid sinus and nasal cavity. Radiology 1972; 104:629–34.
44. Tomsak RL, Smith JL. Radiation retinopathy in a patient with lung carcinoma metastatic to brain. Ann Ophthalmol 1980; 12:619–22.
45. Borruat F-X, Schatz NJ, Glaser JS, Feun LG, Matos L. Visual recovery from radiation-induced optic neuropathy. The role of hyperbaric oxygen therapy. J Clin Neuro Ophthalmol 1993; 13(2):98–101.
46. Martins A, Johnston JS, Henry JM, et al. Delayed radiation necrosis of the brain. J Neurosurg 1977; 47:336–45.

30

Oculinum Therapy: Its Use in Neuro-Ophthalmology

Joseph A. Mauriello, Jr., Rudolph S. Wagner, Ramin Mostafavi, and Larry P. Frohman
University of Medicine and Dentistry of New Jersey, Newark, New Jersey

This chapter discusses the use of botulinum A toxin for the therapy of motility disturbances, including nystagmus and facial dyskinesias.

The pharmacological treatment of strabismus was pioneered by Alan Scott beginning in the late 1970s (1,2). He experimented with the direct injection of vari- ous neurotoxins into the extraocular muscles. Scott correctly theorized that the tem- porary paralysis of an extraocular muscle produced by chemodenervation could result in a change in the relative alignment of the eyes. During a 10-year investiga- tional period under Food and Drug Administration (FDA) regulation, over 8000 injections of botulinum toxin type A were administered in human subjects (3). In 1990, botulinum toxin type A (Oculinum, Allergan Pharmaceuticals, Irvine, CA) was granted FDA approval and removed from investigational status. Approved indications for the toxin include the treatment of strabismus and abnormal facial movements, including hemifacial spasm and blepharospasm associated with dysto- nia in patients 12 years of age and above. Based on the accumulated data from over 200 investigators treating over 4000 patients during the investigational period, the true role of chemodenervation in the treatment of strabismus and facial dyskinesias is now established.

I. CLINICAL PHARMACOLOGY

Botulinum toxin type A (Oculinum) is a large protein molecule (150,000 daltons) that following intramuscular injection is irreversibly bound at the receptor sites on motor nerve terminals within 24 h. The toxin enters and remains at the nerve terminal for several days to weeks. Here it inhibits the release of the neurotransmitter acetylcholine, which functionally denervates the muscle. It is not known for certain how this comes about, but it is probably related to some effect on intraneuronal calcium (4). When injected in therapeutic doses, the effect remains localized to the injected region. This results in a chemical denervation paresis with the onset 2–5 days after injection. Although an irreversible binding occurs when the muscle is chemically denervated, extrajunctional acetylcholine receptors may develop in the atrophied muscle. The nerve, therefore, can reinnervate the muscle with a reversal of the paralysis and eventual recovery. The dose-related extraocular muscle paralysis usually lasts from 2 to 8 weeks. Toxin-induced paralysis lasting for several weeks can result in permanently changed ocular alignment as the injected muscle lengthens and its antagonist contracts (1).

Botulinum toxin type A is prepared for clinical use in units. The lyophilized drug is supplied in 100-U vials and is reconstituted with nonpreserved saline solution (0.9% sodium chloride injection) resulting in doses from 1.0 U 0.1 ml to 12.0 U 0.1 ml. The dose can be increased or decreased to modify the effect. The estimated systemic toxic dose is 40 U/kg body weight. Two nanograms (2×10^{-9} g), an amount frequently used in treating strabismus, is 1/1000 of the lethal dose (LD_{50}) in the macaque monkey (11,20). No systemic paralytic effect has been seen or suspected in any patient treated with the small doses used for strabismus or with the larger doses for facial dyskinesis. Antibodies to the toxin have not been detected in patients given small doses for ocular use, so repeat injections can be given when necessary (3). Botulinum toxin is not approved for use during pregnancy.

II. THERAPEUTIC TECHNIQUE FOR STRABISMUS AND NYSTAGMUS

The injection technique involves transconjunctival injection under topical anesthesia performed in an outpatient setting. Topical vasoconstrictors are administered to help avoid local hemorrhaging at the injection site. An electromyography (EMG) electrode needle is attached to a 1-ml syringe containing 0.1 ml of toxin. The needle is connected to an audible EMG amplifier.

The needle is passed along the surface of the globe posteriorly into the belly of the extraocular muscle. The tip is approximately 2.5 cm into the muscle from its insertion. This approximates the location of the motor endplate, which is the desired injection site for minimal diffusion into adjacent structures. Once the needle is in the muscle, the patient is asked to perform a version to cause the muscle to contract. For example, when the needle is in the medial rectus muscle, the patient is told to adduct the eye.

A characteristic noise from the amplifier is heard as the muscle contracts and the injection is given. This technique involves minimal discomfort to the patient but necessitates a certain level of cooperation. There is a minimal recovery period (minutes) in most patients, and they can resume normal activities on the day of injection.

Some children can be nurtured through the same injection procedure as described here for adults (5). Younger children and those less cooperative need to be injected in the operating room. In such cases, intravenous ketamine (0.1–1.0 mg/kg) is administered. This is approximately one fifth the usual dose of ketamine but produces a suitable hypnotic state for injection without eliminating the EMG response that is essential to the procedure. In these cases, topical proparacaine provides anesthesia, and the ketamine provides sedation (5).

III. THERAPY OF STRABISMUS

Treatment of horizontal forms of strabismus with botulinum toxin comprises the bulk of clinical experience(s) (3). The injection can reduce but does not usually eliminate larger deviations and all results were better for smaller angles of strabismus (<40 prism diopters) (Table 1). Two hundred sixty-one patients with esotropia were injected by Scott, with a 68% reduction of the deviation was achieved. Sixty-eight percent of patients had a final deviation of 10 prism diopters or less after a follow-up of 6–65 months (mean = 27 months). One hundred fifteen (44%) of these patients required more than one injection to obtain this result (3).

Biglan et al. injected 32 patients for the primary treatment of comitant esotropia (6). Only 11 patients (34%) were controlled with the drug. Eleven patients required additional injections to improve alignment.

Lingua injected 33 patients for esotropia and found an early recurrence of the strabismus in nine patients (37.4%) (7). He defined early recurrence as a return of the original strabismus (at least 15 prism diopters with full ductions) within 3 months of having attained alignment with one to four injections. In 19 patients

Table 1 Selected Indications for Botulinum Toxin Injection for Strabismus

1. Treatment of the antagonist muscle in paralytic strabismus
2. Postoperative adjustment of residual small-angle strabismus or overcorrections
3. Esotopia of <40 prism diopters in poor surgical candidates
4. Strabismus following retinal detachment surgery in patients with fusion

injected for esotropia, Wagner had an 87% reduction of the strabusmus after 8 weeks but in 2 years had only a 47% reduction (unpublished data).

Results for treatment of exotropia have not been as good as for esotropia. Scott found a 50% reduction of the angle of exotropia in 95 patients injected, with 49% achieving a final deviation of 10 prism diopters or less. Twenty-nine patients in this group required more than one injection (3).

In the study of Biglan et al. 15 patients received botulinum toxin for the primary treatment of comitant exodeviations either intermittent or constant (6). Five (33%) patients required one or more reinjections. Twelve (79%) required traditional strabismus surgery to achieve satisfactory alignment. Only two patients (13%) were well controlled with the injections alone. The mean reduction in the magnitude of the deviation was only 15 prism diopters in their study. Similarly, Lingua found an early recurrence of exotropia in 12 of 22 patients (55%) (7). As with esotropia, large strabismus angles tended to return to preinjection position and required repeat injections more frequently than smaller angles.

It is evident that better results have been obtained with injection of the medial rectus muscle for esotropia, although the lateral rectus muscle can be injected to treat exotropia. Scott attributes the increased success with esotropia to the greater concentration of global layer singly innervated fibers in the medial rectus muscle, which are singularly and profoundly affected by botulinum (5).

Vertical strabismus can be corrected or improved with botulinum toxin injection in some cases, particularly hypotropias treated with injection of the inferior rectus muscle (8). In Dunn's study, vertical strabismus associated with thyroid ophthalmopathy was treated with injection of the inferior rectus muscle in 27 patients. Eleven patients achieved satisfactory results with multiple injections in some cases.

Sixteen patients, however, eventually required surgery. It is very difficult to selectively inject the superior rectus muscle or the superior oblique muscle. Frequently when injection of these muscles is attempted, a marked ptosis is produced as the toxin diffuses into the levator muscle. It is also very difficult to inject the inferior oblique muscle using present techniques.

A. Paralytic Strabismus

If a lateral rectus muscle remains totally paralyzed for more than 4–6 weeks, increasing esotropia occurs as the medial rectus muscle shortens. A limitation of passive abduction of the eye can be demonstrated on traction testing. In addition to this shortening, there is a reduction in elasticity of the medial rectus muscle. The combination of shortening and increased stiffness constitutes the clinical condition of contracture. In cases where paralysis is incomplete and return of function anticipated, contracture is less likely to occur. It remains, however, difficult to predict which cases of acute sixth nerve palsy will fully recover (Fig. 1).

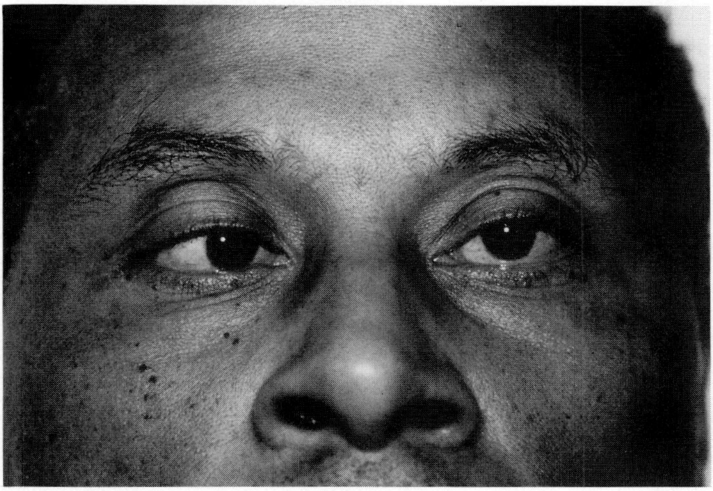

(A)

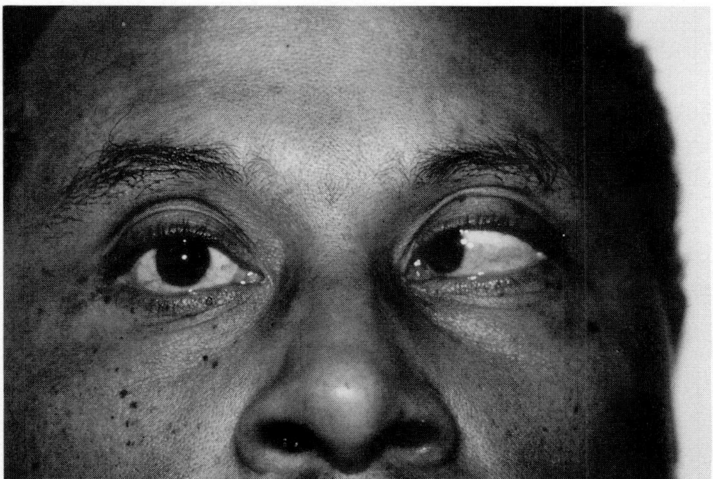

(B)

Figure 1 **(A) Patient with right sixth nerve palsy and prism diopters of esotropia. (B) Abduction to midline only in right eye. (C) Orthophoria and mild ptosis of the right eye 2 weeks following 5 U botulinum injected into right medial rectus muscle. (D) Toxin-induced adduction paresis as shown in left gaze. (E) Orthophoria and resolution of ptosis 8 months following injection. (F) Resolution of abduction deficit as shown in right gaze.**

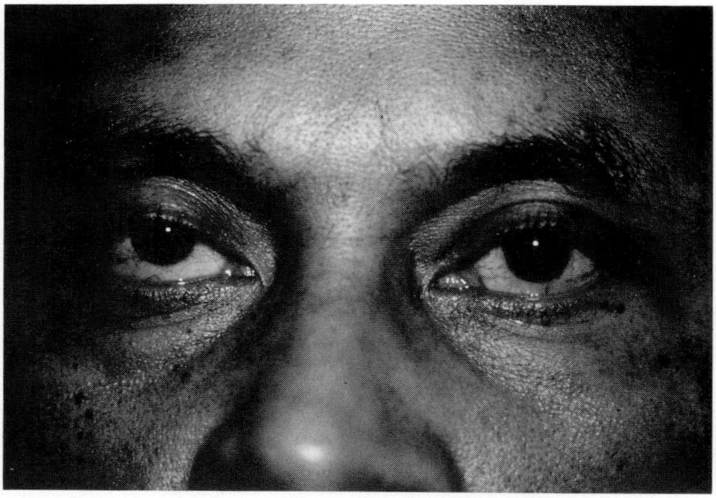

(C)

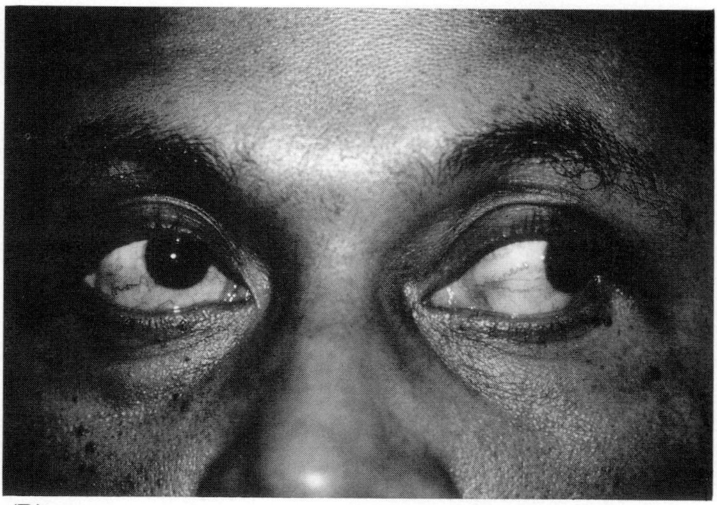

(D)

Figure 1 (***Continued***)

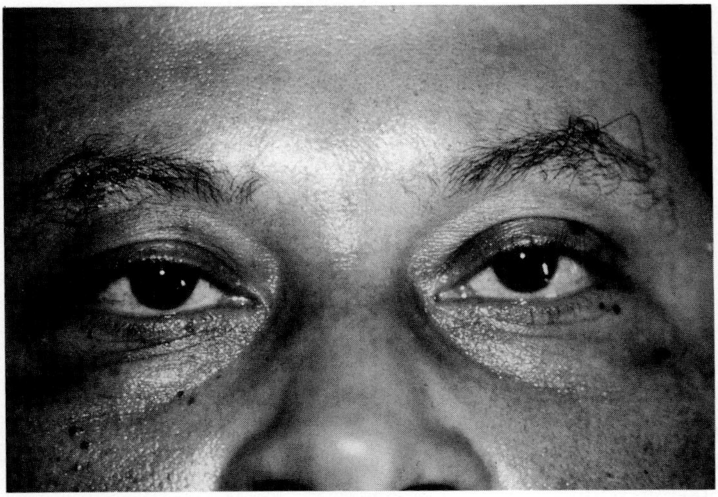

(E)

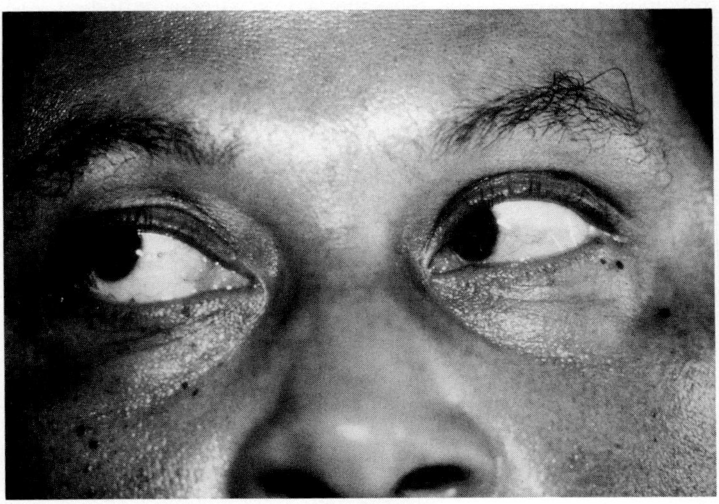

(F)

Metz and Mazow prospectively followed 45 patients with acute unilateral sixth nerve palsy and seven patients with acute bilateral sixth nerve palsy for 6 months after the onset of the palsy (9). The majority of these patients had traumatic sixth nerve palsies, although other etiologies included cerebrovascular disease, tumor, and two patients were thought to have diabetic sixth nerve palsies. Of the 45 patients with unilateral palsy, only 13 (30%) recovered spontaneously, whereas 32 patients (70%) maintained an esotropic deviation large enough to require therapy. In the group of seven patients with bilateral sixth nerve palsy, three recovered spontaneously and four required surgery.

Perhaps the best indication for the use of botulinum toxin is for the treatment of esotropia resulting from a sixth cranial nerve palsy (6,9–11). In these cases, the antagonist medial rectus muscle is injected in the eye with the palsy. This can balance the paralysis and straighten the eye to correct primary gaze diplopia while simultaneously preventing secondary contracture of the medial rectus muscle. Future surgery may be obviated in such cases if significant recovery of lateral rectus function returns.

Eustis and Parks have shown that newly acquired constant strabismus in adults can result in irreversible loss of single binocular vision after a period of 2–3 months (12). Injection during the acute period, even in patients expected to recover lateral rectus muscle function, might help to prevent this occurrence.

Injection of botulinum toxin into the antagonist medial rectus muscle in cases of lateral rectus muscle palsy and paresis has been shown to be effective in relieving secondary contracture (13). In acute sixth nerve palsies, Scott and Kraft were able to prevent secondary contracture of the medial rectus muscle in three of four cases injected within 2–8 weeks of the onset of the palsy (10). Metz was able to avoid surgery in 16 of 20 patients treated for acute lateral rectus palsy (9,14). Wagner and Frohman treated eight patients with sixth nerve palsies secondary to intracranial disease with botulinum toxin to the ipsilateral medial rectus muscle (15). Five of six patients injected within 12 weeks of the onset of the palsy achieved orthophoria, whereas one patient later required a modified Jensen procedure without a recession of the medial rectus muscle. In all studies, best results have occurred in patients who had some recovery of lateral rectus function.

Patients with acute sixth nerve palsies can be effectively treated with botulinum toxin injections within weeks of the onset of the palsy. The dose is titrated according to the deviation but is usually 2.5–5.0 U for the initial injection. Best results are obtained when a transient overcorrection with exodeviation is produced. Ideally, as the deviation is reduced or eliminated, the patient will obtain fusion in or near primary gaze. If recovery of lateral rectus function occurs, fusion may be maintained and the field of single binocular vision enlarged as the effects of the toxin abate. Patients must be informed that a vertical deviation may be induced following injection due to the diffusion of the toxin into the vertical rectus or oblique muscles. A toxin-induced vertical deviation may preclude fusion and interfere with recovery of lateral rectus function.

In patients undergoing strabismus surgery for sixth nerve palsies, botulinum injection to the ipsilateral or contralateral medial rectus muscle can be used in combination with a transposition procedure. Rosenbaum and Kushner reported on the use of botulinum toxin injection in conjunction with strabismus surgery for lateral rectus palsies in 10 patients (16). Patients with sixth nerve palsy without recovery of function after at least 8 months were included in their study. Total transposition of the superior rectus muscles and inferior rectus muscles to the insertion of the lateral rectus muscle was supplemented by botulinum toxin injection of the ipsilateral medial rectus muscle. Most patients were injected intraoperatively, although four were injected within 15 days of surgery. The patients developed a mean diplopia-free field of 51 degrees. By comparison, Cline and Scott were able to achieve a mean diplopia-free field of 44 degrees with a Jensen procedure combined with medial rectus recession (17). Botulinum injections also decrease the risk of anterior segment ischemia by protecting the anterior ciliary arteries of the medial rectus muscle.

Some patients with sixth nerve palsies may develop a comitant esotropia following partial or full recovery of lateral rectus muscle function (Fig. 2). If they continue to experience diplopia and have demonstrated potential for fusion, they may benefit from botulinum toxin injection into one medial rectus muscle even though they are beyond the "acute" period. We have corrected the strabismus and eliminated diplopia in such patients. This therapy may be offered to these patients as an alternative to strabismus surgery.

We have treated patients in whom the etiology of the palsy was known and documented (such as tumors of the cavernous sinus) and who were poor candidates for spontaneous recovery of lateral rectus function (15,18). Often these patients were poor surgical candidates, with a low life expectancy. Such individuals are often anxious to have their diplopia improved or eliminated. In these cases, 6 months may be an inordinate period of time to await recovery. Since side effects are few and the procedure is associated with minimal morbidity, we recommend botulinum toxin injection for acute and some chronic cases of lateral rectus palsy of known etiology.

Metz reported on injecting the lateral rectus muscle with botulinum for patients with acute third nerve palsies (14). All of the eight patients had recovery of medial rectus function with fusion horizontally in primary gaze following injection. Vertical rotations did not improve in most cases. It has been our experience that many cases of acquired third nerve palsy spontaneously recover medial rectus function but often have a residual vertical strabismus secondary to a lack of recovery of the superior rectus, inferior rectus, and inferior oblique muscles or development of aberrant regeneration. Unfortunately, these patients are less amenable to botulinum toxin treatment.

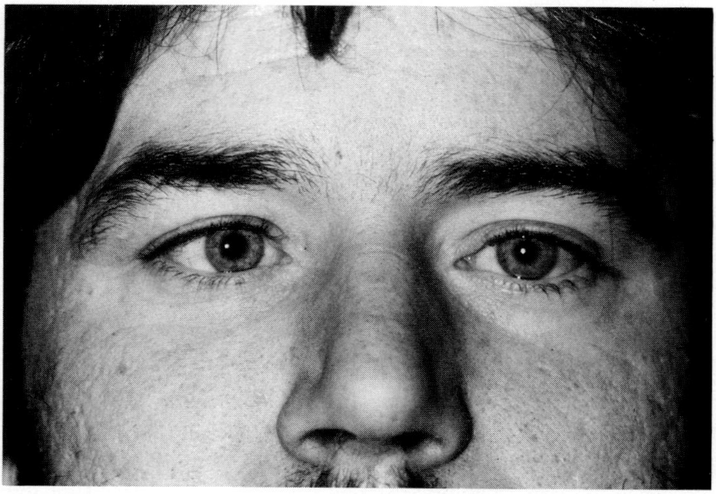

(A)

Figure 2 (A) Patient with 30–prism diopter right esotropia secondary to chronic sixth nerve palsy. (B) Same patient showing esotropia remaining even though lateral rectus function recovering. (C) Small exotropia right eye following injection of 5 U Oculinum to right medial rectus muscle. (D) Toxin-induced adduction deficit 10 days post-injection. (E) Orthotropia 12 weeks following injection. (F) Full abduction right eye. (G) Full adduction right eye.

IV. NYSTAGMUS

Surgical management of nystagmus-producing oscillopsia has been disappointing. Attempts have been made to treat this condition with recessions of all four rectus muscles beyond the limits of usual recession with modest success. The limitations of such procedures were probably related to the contractibility of the muscles being unchanged because the recessions were not large enough. Furthermore, many of these patients have horizontal, vertical, and rotary components to their nystagmus and would thus potentially require dampening the effects of all of the extraocular muscles.

Botulinum toxin has been injected into all four horizontal rectus muscles in an attempt to decrease or eliminate nystagmus and oscillopsia (19). This can be of some benefit in the short term, but the effect wears off and transient strabismus is frequently induced. Helveston and Pogrebniak injected the toxin into the retrobulbar space in one eye each in two patients with vertical, horizontal, and rotary components to their nystagmus and oscillopsia (20). They injected 25 U, which is a very large dose, and were able to demonstrate improved visual acuity

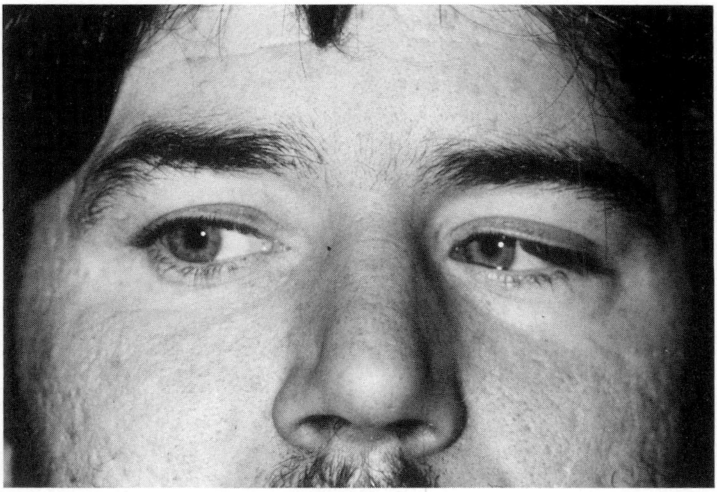

(B)

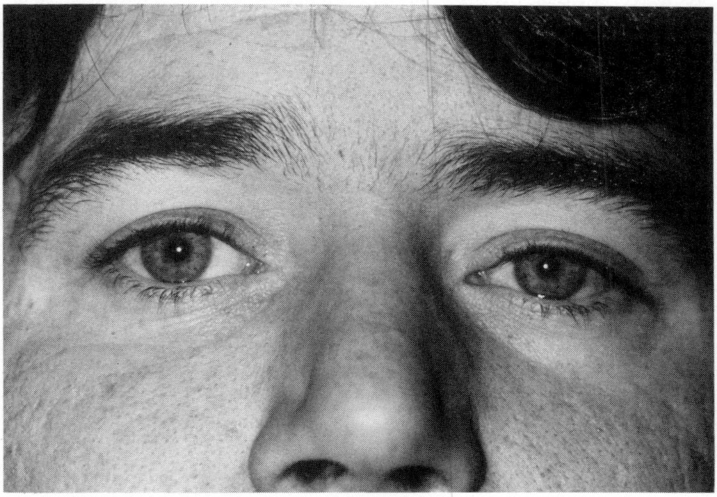

(C)

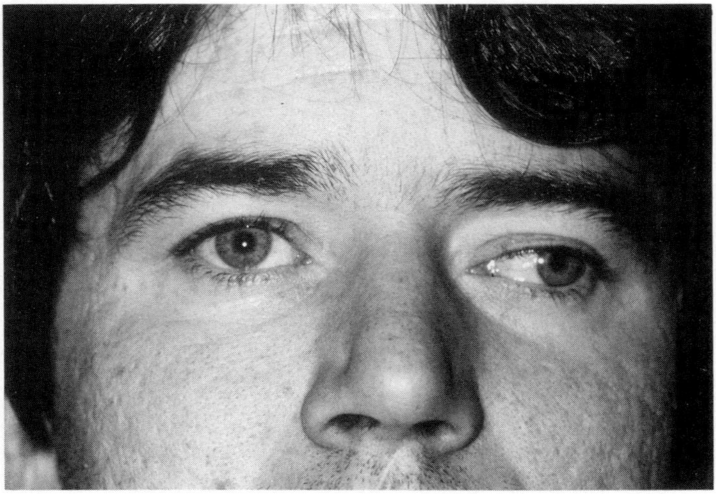

(D)

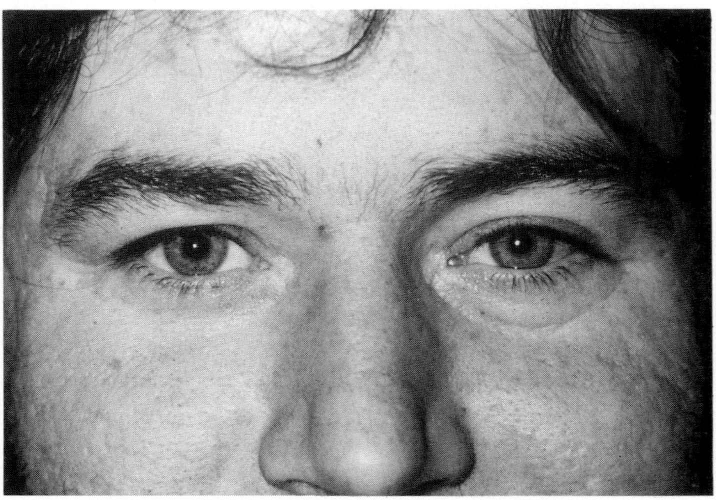

(E)

Figure 2 (***Continued***)

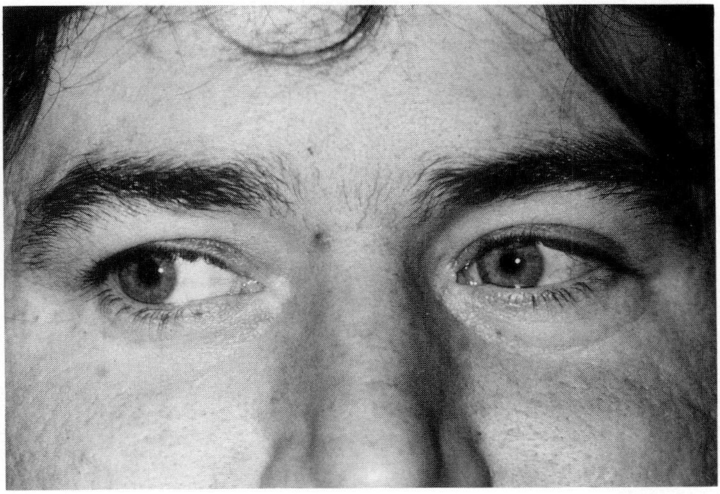

(F)

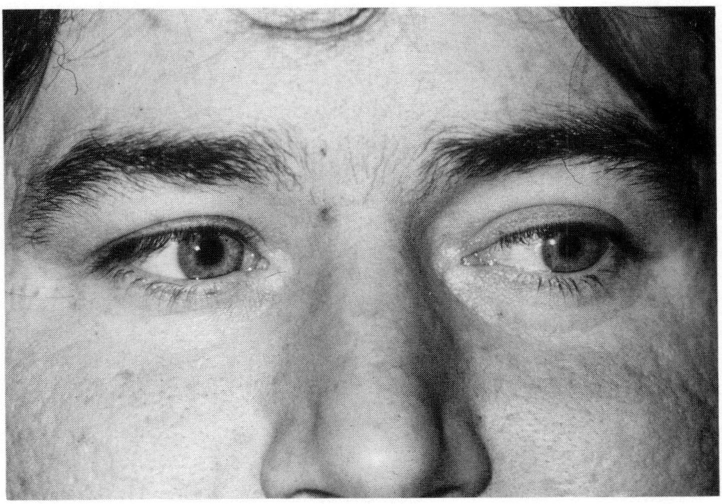

(G)

accompanying the reduced nystagmus. The effect lasted from 5 to 13 weeks. They observed no adverse side effects. We have treated a patient with oscillopsia and nystagmus secondary to multiple sclerosis with 25 U of botulinum injected into the retrobulbar space. The nystagmus was significantly reduced as was the oscillopsia compared with the nontreated eye. A significant ptosis was produced, however, which lasted for 6–8 weeks and resolved as the nystagmus returned.

Injecting botulinum into the retrobulbar space can be an effective, although temporary, therapeutic modality for patients with this disabling condition. It has been suggested by Helveston that ptosis may be avoided by having the patient sit up immediately after administering the injection to avoid contact with the levator muscle within the superior orbital apex (personal communication). Considering the potential for spread within the orbit, this may not be completely protective.

V. COMPLICATIONS—SIDE EFFECTS OF THERAPY OF STRABISMUS AND NYSTAGMUS

Botulinum toxin is a relatively safe drug. No systemic paralytic effect has been seen or suspected in any patient treated with the doses used for treating strabismus. Antibodies to the drug have been detected in a few patients who received large experimental doses for spasmodic torticollis but not in patients injected for strabismus. This accounts for the continued effect in patients injected more than once (3).

The most common side effects or complications of the toxin are ptosis, which is usually partial and occurs in about 16% of adults and 25% of children (3,20,22). Ptosis is more likely to occur following injection of the medial rectus muscle and usually resolves by 6 weeks following the injection. A second significant untoward effect is induced vertical strabismus (22). Induced vertical deviations have been reported to occur in as many as 17% of patients injected (3). This is a particular problem in patients with fusion, as diplopia may be bothersome. Furthermore, the vertical deviation may prevent fusion and result in a recurrence of the initially corrected horizontal deviation. Some investigators think that with increased experience in injection techniques diffusion of toxin into adjacent muscles is less likely, although there are no data to support this observation.

Scleral perforation has occurred in 9 of 8300 injections (0.11%) (3). This tended to occur in large myopic eyes. If there is doubt about needle position, the retina should be examined following withdrawal of the needle. Retrobulbar hemorrhage occurred in 16 cases (0.2%) and cleared without residual effect. Local, subconjunctival hemorrhage occurs frequently and is only a cosmetic problem.

Patients with binocularity frequently experience diplopia, past pointing, and spatial disorientation following injection. It is important to understand that the best results following injection often initially have an overcorrection of the strabismus. Patients must be prepared that diplopia may accompany this temporary overcorrection and last for several weeks.

Although not considered a complication, patients must be told that the effect of the toxin may not be permanent and that the strabismus may not be totally corrected. Some patients may then require additional injections or strabismus surgery. Patients with restrictive strabismus and those having an overrecessed antagonist or ineffective antagonist as in Duane's retraction syndrome are poor candidates for botulinum therapy (Table 2) (6).

VI. FACIAL DYSKINESIAS: DIAGNOSIS OF BLEPHAROSPASM, MEIGE'S SYNDROME, AND HEMIFACIAL SPASM

Benign essential blepharospasm is a clinical syndrome that usually presents as increased frequency of blinking and progresses to involuntary prolonged muscular contractions. It may start unilaterally and over a period of weeks to months develop bilaterally. Similarly, eyelid involvement may predate or follow midfacial, oral, mandibular, laryngeal, or pharyngeal involvement as in Meige's syndrome. Associated involuntary motions include facial grimacing, frowning, head titubation, torticollis and spastic dysphonia.

Hemifacial spasm, a synkinetic contraction of the muscles of one side of the face, is usually due to compression of the seventh nerve by a tortuous branch of the basilar artery. Infrequently, other mass lesions such as aneurysm of tumor may be responsible. A neurological examination should exclude other possible cranial nerve of brainstem findings. An MRI with gadolinium should exclude a tumor or aneurysm. Over a 10-year period at the University of Medicine and Dentistry of New Jersey–New Jersey Medical School, over 350 patients with blepharospasm, Meige's syndrome, and hemifacial spasm have been treated with botulinum toxin type A according to the principles outlined below (23–25).

Table 2 Relative Contraindications to Botulinum Injection for Strabismus

1. Restrictive strabismus
2. Strabismus secondary to an over recessed or slipped muscle
3. Antagonist muscle not intact or functioning (e.g., Duane's retraction syndrome)
4. Horizontal deviation >40 prism diopters (partial correction may result)

VII. THERAPEUTIC TECHNIQUE: FACIAL DYSKINESIAS—DRUG PREPARATION

Once reconstituted in nonpreserved saline, the drug must be used within 4 h in order to maintain its biological effect and is stored in a refrigerator at between 2° and 8° C. On the day of injection, the 100 U of toxin is diluted with 4 ml of nonpreserved saline such that 0.1 ml of drug is equivalent to 2.5 U. The diluted drug is drawn into a tuberculin syringe with a 25-gauge needle and is injected into the patient with a 30-gauge needle. If a patient receives more than 1 ml of drug, a fresh tuberculin syringe is used to withdraw the appropriate amount of drug. In this manner, sterility is maintained, and a vial of drug may be used for more than one patient. According to the package insert from the manufacturer, Allergan, a vial of Botox should not be used for more than one patient because the product and diluent do not contain a preservative.

VIII. BLEPHAROSPASM AND MEIGE'S SYNDROME—INITIAL TREATMENT

The initial treatment of blepharospasm with botulinum toxin type A consists of the following regimen. A dose of 5.0 U is injected into two divided doses of 2.5 U (total of 5.0 U) into the medial and lateral aspects of the pretarsal orbicularis muscle of the upper eyelids; similarly, a total of 5 U is injected into the corresponding medial and lateral portions of the lower eyelids. An additional 2.5 U is injected in the lateral canthus. The total dose in the eyelids on one side is 12.5 U (Fig. 3).

Patients with significant brow spasms receive 5 U into two injections sites (2.5 U in each site) into the procerus and corrugator supraciliaris muscles above the medial aspect of the eyebrows (Fig. 3). Injections above the lateral eyebrow, which is anatomically more fixed than the medial eyebrow, may also be given in the same doses as those given above the medial eyebrow. In general, however, injections above the lateral eyebrow are avoided in order to preserve frontal muscle function that may serve to break the orbicularis muscle spasms.

Because the orbicularis muscle is just below the skin, injections are easily given into the muscle in the orbital region without electromyographic guidance. Care is taken not to perforate the underlying tarsus. In the facial areas other than the eyelids, there is a layer of fat above the musculature, and therefore the injections are given deeper in these locations than in the eyelid area. Aspiration of the syringe prior to injection is helpful in the facial area in order to avoid injection into a blood vessel.

Midfacial and mandibular spasms may be treated with relatively little risk, although the doses necessary to control such contractures may be two to five times greater than the dose needed to control eyelid spasms. In general, 5 U is

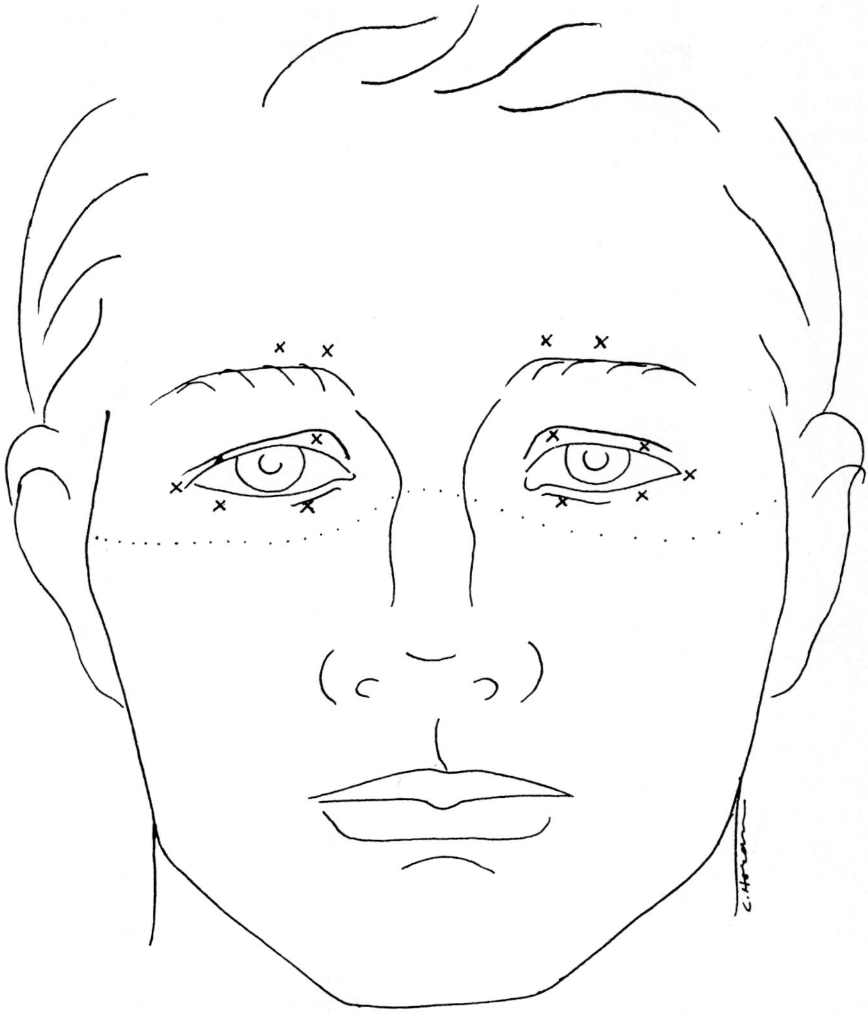

Figure 3 Drawing with sites of injections in the eyelid and above the medial brow at a dose level of 2.5 U of botulinum toxin per site "X" for treatment of blepharospasm.

given in two separate locations in the upper face in the area of the malar eminence and just medial the mid aspect of the inferior orbital rim (see Fig. 4). Five units may be given at the angle of jaw in the muscle just above the condyle of the jaw (below the zygomatic arch) but not into the joint space. Five to 7.5 U may be given in two to three sites along the ramus of the jaw, respectively (see Fig.

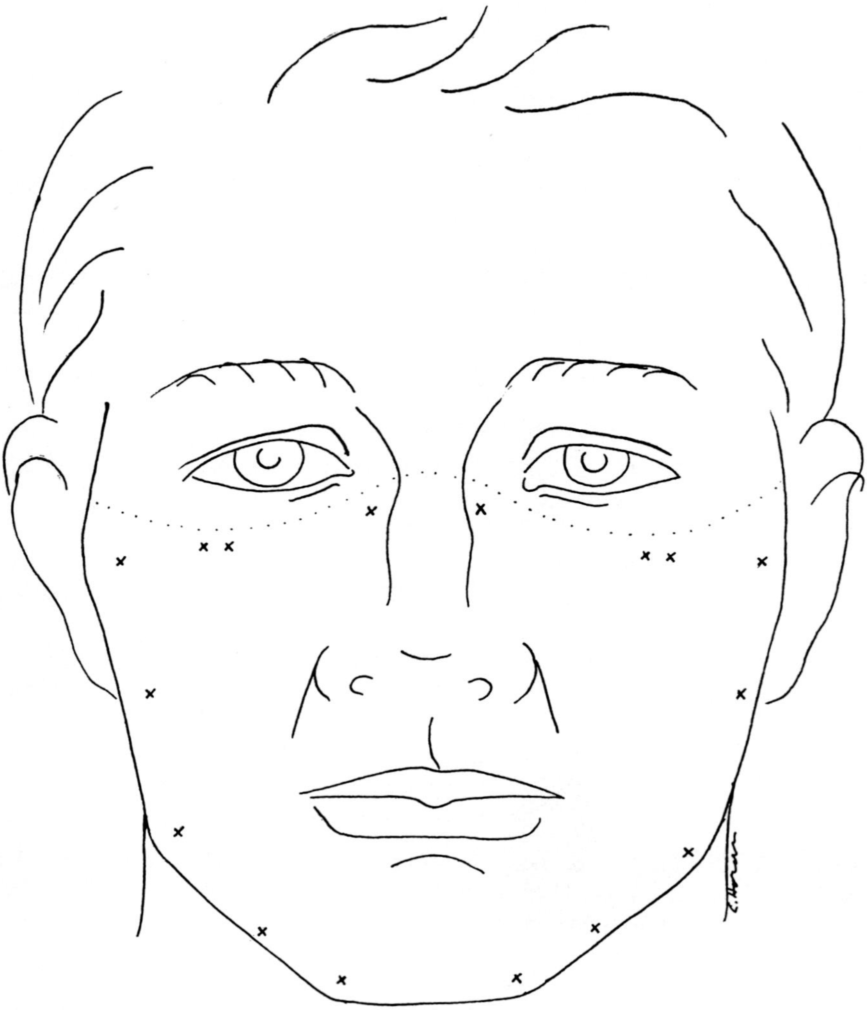

Figure 4 Drawing with sites of injections in the face and jaw at a dose level of 2.5 U of botulinum toxin per site "X" for treatment of facial dyskinesias (5- to 7-U injections may be given per site, especially in the jaw).

4). Injections adjacent to the corner of the mouth or above the upper lip are generally not given, since drooling, slurred speech, and biting of the flaccid buccal mucosa may result.

IX. BLEPHAROSPASM AND MEIGE'S SYNDROME—TREATMENT AT 2-WEEK FOLLOW-UP

Two weeks after injection, the patients are asked to assess their subjective percentage of improvement as compared with pretreatment. On examination, the relative weakness of the eyelids on forced closure is graded on a scale from +1 to +4, where +1 is the least generated forced closure. The patients are objectively observed for evidence of residual spasm.

If the patients are satisfied with their responses and there are few involuntary eyelid contractions, they return for reinjection in several months once the spasms become moderate to severe. They are reminded not to return for reinjection until the spasms are at least 50% as severe as when they first received treatment. The goal of treatment is effectively to control symptoms with the lowest dose and least frequency of injections to minimize complications.

If the patients are not satisfied with their result, injections above the medial eyebrows (5 U in two sites above the medial aspect of the brow) may be given, especially if eyebrow spasms are noted. Additional drug may be given in the upper lid (5 U in each lid) but should not be given in the upper lid if there is evidence of ptosis or superior rectus weakness. Generally, doses of drug injected above the eyebrow, in the lower lid, and in the lateral canthus do not need to be increased. Occasionally, residual spasms in the temporal brow area just above the lateral canthus are treated with 2.5 to 5.0 U depending on their severity.

Patients with a less than satisfactory initial response to treatment are examined again in 2 weeks (4 weeks after the initial injection). At this time, eyelid injections (an additional 5 U in each upper lid) may be repeated a third and even a fourth time 2 weeks later. Once the successful dose is determined, the cumulative dose of the previous weeks' injections is given on reinjection several months later after the effect of the last injection has dissipated. For example, if repeat upper eyelid injections (5 U in each eyelid) are necessary 2 weeks after the initial injection, a total of 10 U is given in each lid on reinjection (since 5 U was given in each eyelid on the first injection and 5 U was injected 2 weeks later).

Ideally, for higher than "standard" doses, the drug is diluted with 50% less saline (to double its potency) to minimize the amount of fluid injected into the eyelid. This technique decreases the risk of diffusion of drug into the levator and orbital tissues associated with increasing volumes of fluid. Doses of the drug vary with different dilutions in the following manner. If the vial of drug is diluted with 2 ml of saline, there will be 100 U in 2 ml, or 50 U in 1 ml or 5 U in each

0.1-ml injection. This dilution would double the standard dose. Diluting the drug with 1.0 ml of saline quadruples the dose in the upper lid if 0.1 ml of diluted drug was injected at each site in the upper lid. Patients who fail to respond to quadruple doses in the upper eyelids (20 U in each upper lid) are considered failures and probably should not be reinjected. The manufacturer's package insert for the drug does not recommend injecting more than 5 U per site and indicates that no more than 200 U should be given within a 1-month period.

X. HEMIFACIAL SPASM—INITIAL TREATMENT

Patients with hemifacial spasm receive the same eyelid dose as patients with blepharospasm on the involved side only. Approximately 40% of patients will have relief of midfacial and lower facial spasms, including oral spasms, with this technique.

XI. HEMIFACIAL SPASM—TREATMENT AT 2-WEEK FOLLOW-UP

It has not been necessary to increase the dose in the eyelids in patients with hemifacial spasm. However, approximately 40% of patients require two injections of 2.5 U in the cheek area (Fig. 5). Injections adjacent to the corner of the mouth or above the upper lip may cause drooling, slurred speech, biting of the flaccid buccal mucosa, and facial asymmetry even more commonly in patients with hemifacial spasm than in patients with Meige's syndrome, since facial nerve weakness accompanies hemifacial spasm. Potential asymmetrical facial movement may be addressed by injections on the opposite normal side to equalize the lack of facial animation. This effect must be carefully explained to the patient prior to treatment. Rarely, patients complain of facial asymmetry after injections in the malar eminence and just below the orbital rim (Fig. 5).

XII. TORTICOLLIS

The treatment of torticollis is beyond the scope of this chapter. The major complication of treatment of torticollis with botulinum toxin is dysphagia. Borodic et al. believe that limiting the dose in the sternomastoid muscle to 100 U or less significantly reduces the incidence of this complication. All aspects of torticollis—pain, postural deformity, range of motion, activity, hypertrophy, and tremor—were improved better with multiple rather than single injections (26–28). In one series of patients with torticollis treated with botulinum toxin, circulating antibodies were detected in three of five patients who no longer responded to botulinum treatment (29).

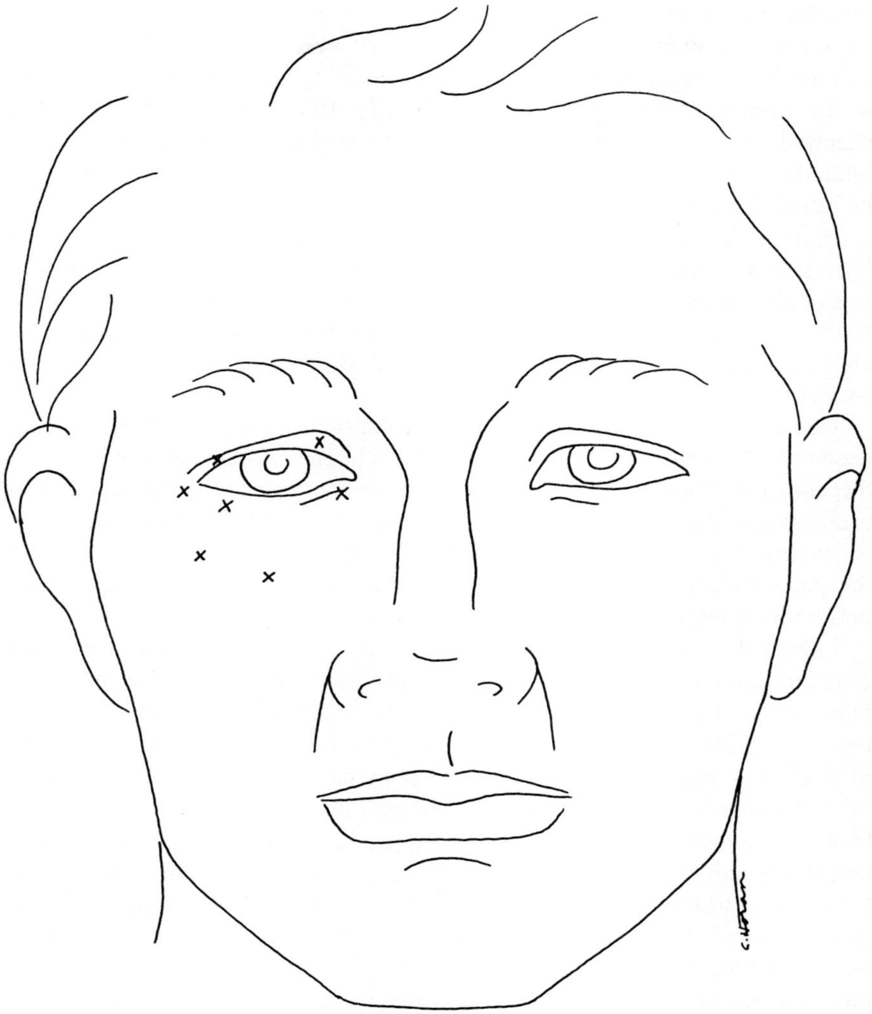

Figure 5 Drawing with sites of injections in eyelid and cheek with 2.5 U of botulinum toxin per site "X" in the treatment of hemifacial spasm.

XIII. COMPLICATIONS–SIDE EFFECTS OF THERAPY OF FACIAL DYSKINESIAS

Systemic toxicity in the doses utilized to treat facial dyskinesias has not been reported. The entire vial (100 U) is below the dose for systemic toxicity in humans weighing 6 kg or greater. For this reason, the drug is not recommended for administration to patients less than 12 years of age. The intramuscular LD50 for juvenile monkeys (*Macaca fascicularis*) has been reported to be 39 mouse units/kg by intravenous injection, which is much higher than those doses given in the treatment of facial dyskinesias (30,31). Rare allergy to the drug has occurred. Two sedentary patients with cardiac disease suffered myocardial infarctions after treatment presumably from an increased activity level allowed by relief of blepharospasm.

In our series, transient headaches developed in two patients on two separate injections in each patient. The headaches did not recur in either patient on reinjection. Medical evaluation was negative. Localized transient eyelid edema lasting 3–4 weeks has rarely occurred in our series without associated systemic effects. A generalized hivelike rash necessitated cessation of treatment in one patient.

Pain on injection occurs to some extent in all patients, although a fine 30-gauge needle is utilized to inject the drug into the skin and the pain lasts only during the injection. Should eyelid hemorrhage occur, the physician may apply local pressure and even ice over the eyelids immediately before and after injection. Ice both lessens the pain of injection and also decreases bleeding, especially if the patient receives anticoagulants or platelet inhibitors such as aspirin and nonsteroidal anti-inflammatory agents.

Lagophthalmos results from incomplete involuntary as well as weakened forced eyelid closure. Mild to severe transient symptoms of dry eye, including burning, itching, irritative tearing, foreign body sensation, conjunctival injection, photophobia, and blurred vision. In our series, corneal erosion occurred in 2 of 354 patients (0.5%); one of whom had previous failed orbicularis muscle extirpation that probably contributed to the poor lid closure after botulinum injection. Both patients required patching at bedtime, and one patient required a soft contact lens, because topical lubricants, including ointments, failed to control the persistent corneal epithelial defect. Patients are instructed to start using a topical lubricating drop four times a day in both eyes should any symptoms of dry eye develop. In addition, forced closure may help to maintain eye lubrication. In potentially severe cases of dry eye, patients are asked to come into the office for a slit lamp examination.

Owing to a decreased lacrimal pump and an increased tear meniscus without dry eye, there may be transient tearing and blurred vision that is again improved by increased forced blinking. These symptoms tend to lessen after 2–4 weeks as the maximum drug effect dissipates. Decreasing the total lower lid dose from 5.0 U (in two sites) to 2.5 U per lid on subsequent injections may cause less weakening of the lacrimal pump. In addition, concentrating the drug in the lateral aspect of the lower lid away from Horner's muscle may diminish tearing (32).

Mild, transient ptosis of 2–4 weeks' duration occurs in 14% of patients, whereas severe ptosis that obscures vision for the duration of the drug has occurred three times in over 1000 injections (25). Unfortunately, there is no treatment for this complication other than reassurance to the patient that the ptosis is temporary (33). A preexisting levator dehiscence or ptosis may be missed on preinjection examination because of severe eyelid spasms. It also is possible that long-term severe orbicular spasm may increase the incidence of levator dehiscence. In such rare cases, ptosis surgery may later be necessary (23–24).

Lower lid ectropion and entropion each occurred in one patient (2%); both tend to occur in patients with preexisting lower lid laxity (25). Lower lid ectropion is avoided by decreasing the lower lid dose to 2.5 U, whereas entropion may require surgical repair.

Double vision due to superior rectus, inferior rectus, or inferior oblique weakness is extremely rare (2%) (25). One patient with double vision received a double dose of botulinum in the upper lids (a total of 10 U in each upper lid in two sites) and had temporary diplopia in up gaze in four of eight injections. This complication is minimized by the injecting over the tarsus and massaging the injected drug toward the lid margin. This technique applies to both upper and lower lid injections.

XIV. DURATION OF EFFECT

It is important to stress to patients that the injections are palliative and need to be repeated at anticipated intervals based on the response to the initial injections. Clinical response to treatment may last between 6 weeks and 1 year, with a median duration of 12–14 weeks for blepharospasm control and 16–18 weeks for hemifacial spasm. The patient needs to understand that a small percentage of patients may obtain little or no relief in from 6.9% (33) to 3% (24). Less commonly, in approximately 3% of our patients, there is an initial response to one or more injections and then little response to subsequent injections. We have found that one subset of patients, who often have received antidepressants or major tranquilizers and note the onset of blepharospasm after the administration of such drugs, may not respond well to botulinum injections.

XV. RESULTS OF TREATMENT—LONG-RANGE PERSPECTIVE

Although the relatively short-term efficacy of botulinum toxin in treating facial dyskinesias has been demonstrated in the literature (23,24,34–39), long-term acceptance of this treatment has not been as well documented (25,40,41). Our review of 50 patients initially treated between September 1983 and June 1984 and followed for 7 years included 34 patients with blepharospasm, 13 with hemifacial spasm, and 4 with Meige's syndrome (25). The cohort of patients received a total of 520 injections. Of the original 50 patients, 26 (52%) continued to return for periodic injections and included 18 of 33 patients with blepharospasm, 7 of 13 with hemifacial spasm, and 1 of 4 with Meige's syndrome.

In this study, the mean duration of action was 14.9 weeks for 18 patients with blepharospasm, 16.3 weeks for 7 patients with hemifacial spasm, and 11 weeks for the patient with Meige's syndrome. Three patients no longer received injections, since they failed to respond. One such patient was unusual in his response in that he received 10 treatments with good to excellent response that lasted 14–18 weeks, respectively. The last three injections lasted 10, 7, and 4 weeks, respectively. He later underwent retromastoid craniotomy for microvascular decompression of the seventh nerve with a good result. Another patient with blepharospasm received one injection and did not improve.

Six patients were treated until they died of causes unrelated to facial dyskinesia or its treatment (Table 3). Six patients were treated elsewhere because of the geographical convenience of treatment. Six patients continued to be treated but had excision of excess skin and plication of the levator aponeurosis. As stated previously, complications were minimal and well tolerated. Clinically significant antibodies rarely developed to the toxin at least over a 7-year period in this study. Patients who responded to two or more injections rarely developed tolerance to the drug (25).

The established bioassay for antibodies to botulinum toxin, the mouse assay, requires mixing the patient's serum with a standardized test doses of toxin. Neutralizing antibodies if present within the patient's serum mix with the

Table 3 Follow-up Data of 50 Patients with Facial Dyskinesias Treated Over 7 Years

Treatment status	Blepharospasm	Hemifacial spasm	Meige's syndrome	Total (%)
Still treated	19	6	1	52
Treatment no longer required	3	0	0	6
Treatment failures	1	1	1	6
Treatment until deceased	1	4	1	12
Treatment elsewhere	4	1	1	12
Lost to follow-up	5	0	0	10
Good response but no longer treated	0	1	0	2

Source: Modified from Mauriello JA, Aljian J. The natural history of treatment of facial dyskinesias with botulinum toxin: a study of fifty consecutive patients over seven years. Br J Ophthalmol 1992; 76:349–52.

botulinum test dose, and the mouse survives the injection of predetermined lethal quantity of toxin. In one study, the amount of toxin necessary to elicit antibodies was greater than the lethal dose to humans in one study (less than 300 U per treatment) (42). Antibodies have not been found in a small number of patients treated for blepharospasm (43). Theoretically, toxin that is incorrectly formulated, dried, or rehydrated may form inactive, antigenic toxin (toxoid).

Orbicularis muscle weakness did not develop from repeated injections over a 7-year period to the extent that lower doses of toxin were effective. Histological examination of muscle biopsies from patients who have been treated with botulinum toxin showed no originally significant evidence of muscle or other degenerative changes (44,45).

XVI. TREATMENT OF PATIENTS UNRESPONSIVE TO BOTULINUM A TOXIN

Various neuroleptic medications include anticholinergic trihexyphenidyl (Artane) and clonazepam (Clonopin). Cyproheptadine (Periactin) may be a beneficial adjunct to the toxin (46–47).

In the past 2 years, we have combined preseptal and pretarsal muscle excision with botulinum toxin injections in five patients. Such patients obtain a greater duration of action and appear to respond better to the drug with an overall subjective improvement of 50–70% greater than with toxin injection alone. In 10 years, one upper lid myectomy combined with browplasty was performed with an excellent result without need for botulinum toxin injections with 1-year follow-up.

In all patients with hemifacial spasm, the alternative of posterior fossa decompressive surgery is discussed at the initial visit before botulinum injection and is especially considered in young patients of 40 years or less (3). All patients to date have opted for injections as the initial treatment, yet the surgery is a viable modality for those who fail injections. Microvascular decompression offers the only effective potential cure.

REFERENCES

1. Scott AB. Botulinum toxin injection of eye muscles to correct strabismus. Trans Am Ophthalmol Soc 1981; 79:734.
2. Scott AB, Rosenbaum A, Collins CC. Pharmacologic weakening of extraocular muscles. Invest Ophthalmol 1973; 12:924.
3. Scott AB. Botulinum toxin treatment of strabismus. American Academy of Ophthalmology Clinical Modules for Ophthalmologists 1989; 7:1.
4. Flynn JT, Bachynski B. Botulinum toxin therapy for strabismus and blepharospasm: Bascom Palmer Eye Institute Experience. In: Pediatric Ophthalmology and Strabismus: Transactions of the New Orleans Academy of Ophthalmology. New York: Raven Press, 1986:73.

5. Scott AB, Magoon EH, McNeer KW, et al. Botulinum treatment of childhood strabismus. Ophthalmology 1990; 97:1434.
6. Biglan AW, Burnstine RA, Rogers GL, et al. Management of strabismus with botulinum A toxin. Ophthalmology 1989; 96:935.
7. Lingua RW. Sequelae of botulinum toxin injection. Am J Ophthalmol 1985; 100:305.
8. Dunn WJ, Arnold AC, O'Conner PS. Botulinum toxin for the treatment of dysthyroid ocular myopathy. Ophthalmology 1986; 93:470.
9. Metz HS, Mazow M. Botulinum toxin treatment of acute sixth and third nerve palsy. Graefe's Arch Clin Exp Ophthalmol 1988; 226:141.
10. Scott AB, Kraft SP. Botulinum toxin injection in the management of lateral rectus paresis. Ophthalmology 1985; 92:676.
11. Wagner RS. The role of botulinum for strabismus. Ophthalmol Clin N Am 1992; 5:105.
12. Eustis HS, Parks MM. Acquired monofixation syndrome. J Pediatr Ophthalmol Strabismus 1989; 26:169.
13. Elston JS, Lee JP. Paralytic strabismus: The role of botulinum toxin. Br J Ophthalmol 1985; 69:891.
14. Metz HS. Botulinum toxin treatment of acute third and sixth nerve palsies (ARVO abstract). Invest Ophthalmol Vis Sci 1987; 28:153.
15. Wagner RS, Frohman LP, Litecky RJ. Prevention of secondary contracture of the medial rectus muscle by botulinum toxin chemodenervation in sixth nerve palsies (ARVO abstract). Invest Ophthalmol Vis Sci 1987; 28:34.
16. Rosenbaum AL, Kushner BJ, Kirschen D. Vertical rectus muscle transposition and botulinum toxin (Oculinum) to medial rectus for abducens palsy. Arch Ophthalmol 1989; 107:820.
17. Cline RA, Scott WE. Long-term follow-up of Jensen procedure. J Pediatr Ophthalmol Strabismus 1988; 25:264.
18. Wagner RS, Frohman LP. Long-term results: Botulinum for sixth nerve palsy. J Pediatr Ophthalmol Strabismus 1989; 26:106.
19. Crone RA, deJong PJ, Notermans G. Behandlung des nystagmus durch injektion von Botulinum toxin in die augenmuskeln. Klin Monatsbl Augenheilkd 1984; 184:216.
20. Helveston EM, Pogrebniak AE. Treatment of acquired nystagmus with botulinum A toxin. Am J Ophthalmol 1988; 106:584.
21. Burns CL, Gammon JA, Gemmill MC. Ptosis associated with botulinum toxin treatment of strabismus and blepharospasm. Ophthalmology 1986; 93:1621.
22. Shippman S, Weseley AC, Cohn KR, et al. Secondary vertical deviations after oculinum injection. Am Orthopt J 1986; 36:120.
23. Mauriello JA: Blepharospasm, Meige syndrome, and hemifacial spasm: treatment with botulinum toxin. Neurology 1985; 35:1499–1500.
24. Mauriello JA, Coniaris H, Haupt EJ: Use of botulinum toxin in the treatment of one hundred patients with facial dyskinesias. Ophthalmol 1987; 94:976–979.
25. Mauriello JA, Aljian J. The natural history of treatment of facial dyskinesias with botulinum toxin: a study of fifty consecutive patients over seven years. Br J Ophthalmol 1992; 76:349–52.
26. Borodic GE, Mills L, Joseph M. Botulinum A toxin for the treatment of adult-onset spasmodic torticollis. Plast Reconstruc Surg 1991; 87:285–9.

27. Borodic GE, Pearce LB, Mith K, et al. Botulinum A toxin for spasmodic torticollis: multiple vs single injection points per muscle. Head Neck 1992; 12:33–7.
28. Anderson TJ, Rigvest J, Stel R, et al. Botulinum toxin treatment of spasmodic torticollis. J R Soc Med 1992; 85:524–9.
29. Greene P, Kang U, Fahn S, et al. Double-blind, placebo-controlled trial of botulinum toxin injections for the treatment of spasmodic torticollis. Neurology 1990; 40:1213–1318.
30. Scott AB, Suzuki D. Systemic toxicity of botulinum toxin by intramuscular injection in the monkey. Mov Disord 1988; 3:333.
31. American Academy of Ophthalmology: botulinum toxin therapy of eye muscle disorders. Safety and effectiveness. Ophthalmology 1989; 51:767–72.
32. Borodic GE. Involuntary eyelid closure and orbicularis paralysis. Curr Opin Ophthalmol 1990; 1:463–8.
33. Kraft SP, Long AE. Botulinum toxin injections in the treatment of blepharospasm, hemifacial spasm, and eyelid fasciculations. Can J Neurol Sci 1988; 15:276–80.
34. Scott AN, Kennedy RA, Stubbs HA. Botulinum A toxin injections as a treatment for blepharospasm. Arch Ophthalmol 1985; 103:347–50.
35. Frueh BR, Musch DC: Treatment of facial spasm with botulinum toxin: an interim report. Ophthalmology 1986; 93:917–23.
36. Shorr N, Seiff RS, Kopelman J. The use of botulinum toxin in blepharospasm. Am J Ophthalmol 1985; 99:917–23.
37. Jankovic J, Ford J. Blepharospasm and orofacial-cervical dystonia: clinical and pharmacologic findings in 100 patients. Ann Neurol 1983; 13:402–11.
38. Savino PJ, Sergott RC, Bosley TM et al. Hemifacial spasm treated with Botulinum A toxin injection. Arch Ophthalmol 1985; 103:1305–6.
39. Cohen DA, Savino PJ, Stern MB, et al. Botulinum injection therapy for blepharospasm: a review and report of 75 patients. Clin Neuropharmacol 1986; 9:415–29.
40. Elston JS. Long-term results of treatment of idiopathic blepharospasm with botulinum toxin injections. Br J Ophthalmol 1987; 71:664–8.
41. Dutton JJ, Buckley EG. Long-term results and complications of botulinum A toxin in the treatment of blepharospasm. Ophthalmology 1988; 95:1529–34.
42. Borodic GE, Pearce LB, Johnson E, et al. Clinical and scientific aspects of botulinum A toxin. Ophthalmol Clin North Am 1991; 4:491–503.
43. Gonnering RS. Negative antibody response to long term treatment of facial spasm with botulinum toxin. Am J Ophthalmol 1988; 105:313.
44. Borodic GE, Ferrante R. Effects of repeated botulinum toxin injections on orbicularis oculi muscle. J Clin Neuro Ophthalmol 1992; 12:121–7.
45. Harris CP, Alderson K, Nebeker J, et al. Histologic features of human orbicularis oculi treated with botulinum A toxin. Arch Ophthalmol 1991; 109;393–5.
46. Fasanella RM, Aghajanian GK. Treatment for benign essential blepharospasm with cyproheptadine. N Engl J Med 1990; 322:778 (letter).
47. Mauriello JA. Treatment of benign essential blepharospasm and hemifacial spasm with botulinum toxin: a preliminary study of 68 patients. In: Bosniak SL, Smith BC, eds. Blepharospasm advances in Ophthalmol Plast Reconstruc Surg. New York: Pergamon Press, 1985: 283–90.

V

PATHOLOGY

31

Neurosarcoidosis

Barney J. Stern
Sinai Hospital and Johns Hopkins University, Baltimore, Maryland

Cherie J. Sewell
Sinai Hospital, Baltimore, Maryland

I. SARCOIDOSIS

Sarcoidosis, a multisystem disorder of uncertain etiology, typically afflicts adults between the ages of 20 and 40 years. The most frequent manifestations include bilateral hilar lymphadenopathy, pulmonary infiltrates, and eye, liver, and skin disease. Ocular pathology is the most frequently documented extrathoracic manifestation of sarcoidosis, occurring in 50% of patients. Ocular and orbital involvement include the anterior and, to a lesser extent, the posterior uvea; conjunctiva; lacrimal glands; cornea; sclera; retina; lens; optic nerve: and rarely orbital contents. Clinical features of ocular and orbital disease are outlined in Table 1. Sarcoidosis accounts for approximately 25% of granulomatous disease of the eye. When ocular disease is the initial symptom of sarcoidosis, an investigation for systemic disease is warranted.

II. NEUROSARCOIDOSIS

Neurological complications of sarcoidosis develop in approximately 5% of patients. Almost one half of patients with neurosarcoidosis present with neurological disease. Manifestations include cranial nerve palsies; meningeal disease with aseptic meningitis or dural masses; hydrocephalus; central nervous system (CNS) parenchymal disease with neuroendocrinological disorders, mass lesions, seizures, or a vasculopathy/encephalopathy; peripheral neuropathy; and myopathy.

Table 1 Ocular Sarcoidosis

Area of involvement	Clinical features	Primary symptoms	Complications
Anterior segment anterior uveitis (iritis)	Unilateral or bilateral Acute: ciliary flush, keratic precipitates, aqueous cell and flare, inflammatory iris Chronic: fatty nodules, synechiae	Photophobia, ocular injection, decreased corneal sensation	Band keratopathy (secondary to calcium deposits), glaucoma, cataracts, blindness
Posterior segment	Retina: vascular sheating "candle-wax drippings," large granuloma in fundus, vascular occlusions, disseminated chorioretinitis, hemorrhages Optic disc: papilledema, nodules, granulomas, atrophy. Vitreous: opacities	Floaters, diminished visual acuity; minimal/no pain; painful if associated with anterior uveitis (dull aching and photophobia)	Retinal and disc neovascularization
Skin lesions (lids and periorbital skin)	Lupus pernio, subcutaneous nodules, macules, plaques, palpable masses	Cosmetic disfigurement	Scarring, hypopigmentation, ectropion, entropion
Conjunctiva	Injection	Itching	Dry eye, corneal ulceration
Lacrimal gland	Swelling: superior temporal orbit	Mild to moderate pain, dry eyes	Dry eye
Orbit granulomas	Palpable mass, decreased eye movement	Orbital pain, visual loss	Optic nerve compression

III. NEURO/OPHTHALMOLOGICAL SARCOIDOSIS

Neuro-ophthalmological manifestations associated with sarcoidosis include optic neuropathy, disorders of ocular motility, and pupillary abnormalities.

Optic nerve involvement may occur in up to 5% of patients with sarcoidosis and can be unilateral or bilateral. The optic nerve is the second most common cranial nerve to be targeted by sarcoidosis. When sarcoidosis-associated optic nerve disease is the initial clinical feature of sarcoidosis, it can be several years before other systemic manifestations appear. Optic neuropathy can remain an isolated finding.

Optic disc edema, the most common optic nerve abnormality related to sarcoidosis, can be secondary to increased intracranial pressure or inflamed meninges enveloping the optic nerve.

Papilledema can occur from an intracranial mass effect, hydrocephalus, or basal granulomatous meningitis involving the optic nerve sheath and blocking cerebrospinal fluid (CSF) resorption. The diagnosis of CNS sarcoidosis should be especially entertained for a patient with rapidly developing papilledema accompanied by facial weakness or other cranial nerve palsies.

Papillitis or retrobulbar optic neuritis can be due to sarcoidosis. This inflammation is usually unilateral but can be bilateral. Visual loss associated with optic neuritis can range from a small central scotoma to blindness and often reaches a maximum deficit within 1–2 days.

Granulomatous nodules can compress the optic nerve and extend intraocularly from the optic disc causing "cauliflower" discs. These optic nerve granulomata commonly appear in association with other evidence of ocular inflammation. Without uveitis or other stigmata of sarcoidosis, the disc lesion may be confused with a tumor.

Optic nerve atrophy can result from retinal degeneration, papilledema, or optic nerve granulomas or develop de novo. Ischemic damage to the optic nerve also is a possible consequence of inflammation compromising the microvasculature. If optic atrophy develops, varying degrees of visual loss can be experienced.

A chiasmatic syndrome can be a sequel of meningeal inflammation or a parasellar granulomatous mass.

Vision can also be affected by mass lesions or an encephalopathy/vasculopathy that compromises the optic tracts, optic radiations, or the occipital cortex.

Disorders of ocular motility can be the presenting sign of sarcoidosis or develop later in the disease. In our experience, sixth nerve palsies are the most common cause of diplopia. Increased intracranial pressure or a granulomatous meningitis can compromise the abducens nerve. Intra-axial or meningeal inflammation can compromise oculomotor pathways and lead to altered motility. Even an internuclear ophthalmoplegia (INO) can develop.

Nystagmus can result from brainstem or cerebellar inflammation. Ocular flutter can be an early sign of a sarcoidosis-associated aseptic meningitis.

Pupillary dysfunction is associated with third nerve or sympathetic nervous system lesions. The parasympathetic pathway can be compromised by midbrain inflammation or a third nerve lesion secondary to increased intracranial pressure or meningeal inflammation. A Horner syndrome can result from an intra-axial inflammatory process in the brain or cervical spinal cord as well as compromise of the ascending sympathetic pathway by enlarged lymph nodes.

IV. DIAGNOSTIC EVALUATION

A specific test or battery of tests to confirm the diagnosis of sarcoidosis is not available. We are most confident of a diagnosis of sarcoidosis if we demonstrate evidence of multisystem disease and histological confirmation, if feasible, of noncaseating granulomas. An ophthalmological evaluation may reveal ocular findings supportive of a diagnosis of sarcoidosis (see Table 1). The presence of skin lesions or enlarged lymph nodes should be sought. A chest roentgenogram can demonstrate pulmonary disease or intrathoracic adenopathy in 85–90% of patients. Pulmonary function tests, including a diffusing capacity, and a thorax computed tomographic (CT) scan can also reveal disease. Other findings that suggest a diagnosis of sarcoidosis include abnormal liver function tests, an increased serum angiotensin-converting enzyme (ACE) assay (elevated in approximately 50% of patients), hypercalcemia, hypercalciuria (a 24-h urine sample), hypergammaglobulinemia, and anergy on skin testing. A gallium scan can highlight inflammation of abdominal and thoracic structures and parotid, lacrimal, and salivary glands. A muscle MRI can demonstrate abnormalities amenable to stereotactic biopsy.

V. NEURODIAGNOSTIC ASSESSMENT

The diagnosis of CNS sarcoidosis presents a complex task because histological confirmation is rarely available. Furthermore, neurodiagnostic tests can yield suggestive, but not pathognomonic, results. We are most secure of a diagnosis of CNS sarcoidosis if there is multisystem disease and the CNS findings are consistent with the well-known manifestations of CNS sarcoidosis. If disease is confined to the CNS, examination of local tissue is necessary to document noncaseating granulomas. If granulomatous CNS inflammation is found, a search for systemic disease should ensue. Such a search can be futile, however, since concurrent corticosteroid therapy, which may have been prescribed for a variety of reasons (i.e., perioperative management), can cause resolution of systemic inflammation.

Because of the proximity of the anterior visual pathways to the hypothalamus and pituitary gland, symptoms of a diencephalic syndrome or neuroendocrinological disturbance should be sought (thirst disturbance, somnolence, altered appetite or libido, amenorrhea, or galactorrhea). A comprehensive neuroendocrinological evaluation can reveal hyperprolactinemia, hypothyroidism, hypocortisolism, hypoganodism, or disorders of antidiuretic hormone secretion.

Examination of the CSF can be helpful in lending support to a diagnosis of sarcoidosis. However, the CSF findings of CNS sarcoidosis are nonspecific and include, in various combinations, increased pressure, elevated total protein, hypoglycorrhachia, a predominantly mononuclear pleocytosis, elevated immunoglobulin G index, and oligoclonal bands. Innovative assays include determination of the CSF CD4:CD8 ratio and an ACE assay; the specificity and the utility of these tests is not well defined.

Imaging studies are very helpful in the evaluation and management of CNS inflammation. CT, especially contrast-enhanced CT, has proved useful in defining meningeal disease, hydrocephalus, and mass lesions. However, gadopentetate dimeglumine–enhanced magnetic resonance imaging (MRI) is the preferred CNS imaging modality because of its exquisite ability to demonstrate meningeal disease and lesions at the base of the brain, periventricular sites, and posterior fossa. Enhancement and thickening of the optic nerves and chiasm are well documented by MRI. Parasellar masses and inflammation can be visualized and their relationship with the visual pathways defined.

Visual evoked potentials (VEPs) can detect the presence of an optic neuropathy. VEPs can highlight optic nerve dysfunction in patients with neurological disease with visual symptoms and occasionally in patients without visual symptoms. VEPs can help monitor the clinical course of patients with a sarcoidosis-related optic neuropathy; we have found that the P100 latencies can change depending on the clinical status. We have not found a high proportion of VEP abnormalities in patients with systemic sarcoidosis and no visual or neurological complaints.

VI. THERAPEUTIC CONSIDERATIONS

The mainstay of treatment for sarcoidosis is corticosteroid therapy. Corticosteroids suppress the inflammatory process and relieve acute symptoms. Whether corticosteroids change the natural history of neurosarcoidosis has not been critically defined. We always remain alert to the possibility that clinical deterioration might be due to intercurrent conditions, such as infection or neoplasia, or an incorrect diagnosis of sarcoidosis.

For neurological complications of sarcoidosis, we usually treat with prednisone, 40–60 mg daily for 2–4 weeks and then taper by 5-mg decrements every 2 weeks or so while the clinical status is monitored until a dose of 10 mg daily is reached. At this low dose, we usually taper by 1-mg decrements every 1 to 4 weeks with careful attention to any exacerbation of symptoms. If there is a recurrence of symptoms at any corticosteroid dosage level, we recommend doubling the dose for 2–4 weeks, assessing the clinical response, and then attempt to taper the medication again. If the patient is doing well, we may try to use alternate-day corticosteroid dosing to spare long-term medication complications.

For severe disease unresponsive to moderate corticosteroid doses, a 3-day course of methylprednisolone, 20 mg/kg/day, or dexamethasone, 100 mg/day IV, followed by prednisone 40–80 mg daily may yield improvement. In patients with progressive visual loss despite aggressive therapy, a biopsy of the optic nerve may be warranted to confirm the diagnosis of sarcoidosis.

With the long-term use of corticosteroids, several issues need to be addressed. Females with impaired estrogen activity are at high risk for osteoporosis. Hormonal therapy replacement and vitamin D and calcium supplements may help avoid this complication. Since hypercalcemia and hypercalciuria are associated with sarcoidosis, serum and urine calcium should be monitored if vitamin D and calcium supplements are utilized. Dietary counseling can help patients cope with the weight gain and sodium retention associated with corticosteriod therapy. We work closely with endocrinologists to ensure optimal osteoporosis treatment.

If inflammation continues in spite of high-dose corticosteroid treatment, or if the patient experiences serious corticosteroid side effects, alternative therapies can be considered. Immunosuppressive therapy, radiation treatment, and surgical resection of mass lesions are adjunctive treatment modalities.

Immunosuppressive agents include azathioprine, cyclosporine, cyclophosphamide, methotrexate, and chlorambucil. These drugs offer the opportunity to decrease inflammation, stabilize function, and lower the dose of corticosteroids. The guidelines we use to initiate immunosuppressive therapy include a deteriorating clinical status in spite of "optimal" corticosteroid therapy, undue side effects of corticosteroid treatment, or documentation of disease progression by appropriate ancillary studies in spite of "optimal" corticosteroid therapy. Occasionally, we will try immunosuppressive treatment if ancillary studies alone demonstrate continuing disease activity in spite of aggressive corticosteroid use. We are not aware of studies documenting the superiority of any one alternate therapy over another. Rarely is an immunosuppressive agent alone sufficient to treat severe disease; usually we use these agents in conjunction with corticosteroids.

There are reports of successful treatment of CNS sarcoidosis with radiation therapy. We usually recommend radiation therapy only in life-threatening situations, although its use to try to prevent blindness may be necessary at times. Radiation can also be considered if the patient fails adjunct immunosuppresive treatment.

Surgical resection is rarely recommended as primary treatment for a mass lesion. A deteriorating patient with a granulomatous mass unresponsive to corticosteroids may benefit from surgical decompression. If a CNS mass thought to be due to sarcoidosis does not respond to a trial of corticosteroids, or if the lesion increases in size despite aggresive therapy, a biopsy of the lesion is helpful to confirm the diagnosis. Surgical intervention with a ventriculoperitoneal shunt can control symptomatic hydrocephalus.

VII. COURSE AND PROGNOSIS

The clinical course of neurosarcoidosis varies with each patient and can be characterized by remissions and exacerbations. Patients with CNS parenchymal disease and hydrocephalus are most likely to have a chronic course.

Neuro-ophthalmic sarcoidosis can cause varying degrees of disability and progressive deterioration, including blindness. On the other hand, substantial symptom resolution and preservation of sight may result from optimal therapy.

Inflammation about the optic nerves and chiasm can be self-limited, but in our experience, there is often slowly progressive visual loss. Vision can also deteriorate in a step-wise fashion in spite of aggressive management. We have found the optic neuropathy and chiasmal syndromes associated with sarcoidosis particularly refractory to treatment.

Sixth nerve palsies, fortunately, are often quite responsive to treatment.

VIII. CONCLUSIONS

The diagnosis of neuro-ophthalmological sarcoidosis can present a diagnostic challenge, particularly if ocular problems are the initial presentation of the disease. A comprehensive evaluation is warranted for each patient. Early diagnosis and treatment of sarcoidosis may help decrease the symptoms of acute inflammation and minimize complications. Patients can benefit from support, counseling, and an ongoing therapeutic relationship with a cohesive team of practitioners.

IX. EDUCATION FOR THE PATIENT WITH NEURO-OPHTHALMOLOGICAL SARCOIDOSIS

The focus of patient education is often dependent on the specific problem at hand but a general approach can alleviate patient anxieties:

1. Provide information concerning the inflammatory process, the impact on the involved area, course of the disease, and possible complications.
2. Patients respond most favorably to a proposed treatment plan and review of therapeutic options.
3. We are available to patients to monitor their status and answer any questions. We recommend frequent contact, especially when lower doses of corticosteroids are being used or there are any changes in symptoms.

4. We are not aware of any information that concurrent sarcoidosis and pregnancy are adversely affected by the other. There is the possibility of remission of systemic sarcoidosis during pregnancy. A relapse of symptoms during the puerperium may occur.
5. Since sarcoidosis can affect multiple systems, a coordinated team approach is recommended to provide optimal patient care. Often, an ophthalmologist, internist, neurologist, and pulmonologist combine their efforts to establish the diagnosis and treatment plan.
6. We encourage patients to be active participants in their care. Often support groups can provide patients with information and general guidance concerning their disease.

Patient Resources

Sarcoidosis Family Aid and Research Foundation
760 Clinton Avenue
Newark, NJ 07108
(201)676–7901

Sandra Frazier
437 Rivercrest Drive
Piscataway, NJ 08854

Pacific Northwest Sarcoid Association
656 NW 54th Street
Seattle, WA 98107
(206)784–9365
1–800–998–8660

Northern Virginia Sarcoidosis Self-Help Group
Alexandria Hospital
Dudley Conference Room
4320 Seminary Road
Alexandria, VA 22304
Group Leader: Cindy Flynn
(703)591–4131

SELECTED READINGS

Caplan L, Corbett J, Goodwin J, Thomas C, Shenker D, Schatz N. Neuro-ophthalmologic signs in the angiitic form of neurosarcoidosis. Neurology (Cleveland) 1983; 33:1130–1135.

Cornblath WT, Elner V, Rolfe M. Extraocular muscle involvement in sarcoidosis. Ophthalmology 1993; 100:501–505.

Engelken JD, Yuh WTC, Carter KD, Nerad JA. Optic nerve sarcoidosis: MR findings. AJNR 1992; 13:228–230.

Gelwan MJ, Kellen RI, Burde RM, Kupersmith MJ. Sarcoidosis of the anterior visual pathway: successes and failures. J Neurol Neurosurg Psychiatry 1988; 51:1473–1480.

Mayers M. Ocular sarcoidosis. Int Ophthalmol Clinics 1990; 30:257–263.

Stern BJ, Krumholz A, Johns C, Scott P, Nissim J. Sarcoidosis and its neurological manifestations. Arch Neurol 1985; 42:909–917.

Stern BJ, Schonfeld SA, Sewell C, Krumholz A, Scott P, Belendiuk G. The treatment of neurosarcoidosis with cyclosporine. Arch Neurol 1992; 49:1065–1072.

Walker FO, McLean WT, Elster A, Stanton C. Chiasmal sarcoidosis. AJNR 1990; 11:1205–1207.

32

Internuclear Ophthalmoplegia

David S. Zee
Johns Hopkins Hospital, Baltimore, Maryland

Internuclear ophthalmoplegia (INO) is one of the classic ocular motor syndromes. The cardinal clinical features—a failure of adduction with conjugate movements but spared convergence, and a dissociated horizontal nystagmus, greater or only in the abducting eye—are well known to all neurologists. Early descriptions of INO appear in the late nineteenth and early twentieth centuries (45,38). Spiller (48) suggested a localization of the lesion to the medial longitudinal fasciculi (MLF) based on pathological examination of a patient with a bilateral INO. For unilateral INO, the anatomical locus was only clearly established relatively recently (10,8,25). Not only does the recognition of INO allow precise anatomical localization of the responsible lesion, but analysis of the ocular motor disorder in INO offers insight into basic mechanisms of ocular motor control. In this chapter, we review INO, with an emphasis on recognition and interpretation of the clinical findings using current ideas of the physiological and anatomical organization of central ocular motor pathways.

I. OCULAR MOTOR CONTROL SIGNALS

A. Pulse-Step of Innervation

One basic concept that can help one to understand the pattern of eye movement abnormalities in INO is that for normal eye motion the ocular motoneurons

This chapter is based on material published in Bailliere's Clinical Neurology, Vol 1, No 2, pp 455–470 and entitled "Internuclear ophthalmoplegia: Clinical and pathophysiological considerations," U. Buttner and T. Brandt, eds. London: Saunders, 1993.

require both a *velocity*- and a *position*-coded signal; the first to rotate the eye from one location to another at the correct speed and the second to hold the eye steady in the correct position at the end of the movement. For saccades, these velocity and position signals have been called, respectively, the *pulse* and *step changes* in innervation.

B. Velocity-Position Integration

The position-coded signal is probably derived from the velocity-coded signal by the process of *integration*, in the mathematical sense. A neural network or neural integrator has been hypothesized to perform such an integration. For horizontal rotations, this neural integrator probably lies in an area in the rostral medulla between and including adjacent portions of the medial vestibular nucleus and the nucleus prepositus hypoglossus (NPH) (6). For vertical and torsional rotations of the eyes, the integration is probably performed, in a distributed fashion, within rostral portions of the vestibular nuclei (and possibly the NPH) and more cephalad within the interstitial nucleus of Cajal (INC) (16,12). The INC and the vestibular nuclei are interconnected by the MLF. The cerebellar flocculus also plays a role in velocity-to-position integration both by improving the fidelity of integration (increasing the time constant of the integrator so that the eyes can be held in eccentric positions of gaze) and by matching the size of the output of the integrator (the step) with the velocity command (the pulse), so that the eyes stop abruptly, without drift, at the end of every conjugate eye movement (55).

II. ANATOMICAL CONNECTIONS OF THE MLF

The MLF are a pair of conduits extending through the pons and mesencephalon where they lie near the midline, just under the fourth ventricle. The MLF carry pathways that mediate both ascending and descending control of structures involved in the generation of both conjugate and vergence eye movements.

For horizontal gaze, the important projections that coarse through the MLF arise in the abducens nucleus. The abducens nucleus contains both motoneurons, with axons that innervate the lateral rectus muscle, and internuclear neurons, with axons that cross the brainstem and ascend in the MLF to impinge on medial rectus motoneurons within the contralateral oculomotor nucleus. The projections from the abducens internuclear neurons convey signals for adduction during all types of conjugate eye movements. Abducens internuclear neurons also carry an "inappropriate" signal for vergence; producing an increase of activity of medial rectus motoneurons when divergence is called for and a decrease of activity when convergence is called for (see Sec. III.C) (17).

The MLF also carries ascending projections from the vestibular nuclei and

NPH destined for the third and fourth cranial nerve nuclei and for more rostral structures including the interstitial nucleus of Cajal (INC). There also are descending pathways from the INC to the vestibular nuclei. These ascending and descending pathways convey velocity- and position-coded signals that help to generate vertical (and torsional) slow-phase movements in response to vestibular and visual (optokinetic and pursuit) stimuli and to hold eccentric positions of up and downward gaze. Other ascending vestibular projections within the MLF probably mediate static otolith-ocular reflexes that occur in response to tilt of the head.

The MLF also carries descending projections to the abducens nucleus; some probably arise from interneurons within the oculomotor nucleus (29). Their function is unknown, although it has been suggested that they play a role in vergence.

Intermingled among the MLF fibers are the cell groups of the paramedian tracts (5). They receive afferents from the vestibular nuclei, the pontine and mesencephalic reticular formation, the NPH, the INC, and probably other areas. They project in turn to the cerebellar flocculus. The effect of damage to these neurons of the paramedian tracts, or to their afferent or efferent fibers, is not known.

III. PATHOPHYSIOLOGY OF OCULAR MOTOR ABNORMALITIES IN INO (Table 1)

A. Disorders of Adduction

The adduction weakness of INO is readily explained by interruption of the ascending axons that arise from the internuclear neurons in the abducens nucleus.

Table 1 Clinical-Anatomical Correlations in INO

Abnormality	Projections
Adduction paresis	Abducens internuclear neurons
Skew deviation	Vestibular nuclei (otolith-ocular reflexes)
Vertical gaze-evoked nystagmus	Vestibular nuclei (and nucleus prepositus hypoglossi)
Vertical pursuit deficit	Interstitial nucleus of Cajal
Vertical vestibuloocular reflex	Vestibular nuclei (canal-ocular reflexes)
Dissociated vertical-torsional nystagmus	

When the lesion is complete, the loss of both the velocity and the position-coded information necessary for adduction during conjugate eye movements prevents the eye from adducting beyond the midline. When the lesion is partial, the attenuation of velocity and position-coded information reduces the speed and limits the range of adduction. In most respects, these abnormalities of horizontal eye movements are comparable with those produced by a peripheral medial rectus palsy, with the exception, of course, that adduction during convergence is usually spared in INO.

1. Postsaccadic Drift

In INO, as well as with medial rectus palsies, there is horizontal postsaccadic drift of the affected eye after both adducting and abducting saccades. The drift is always directed nasally. This pattern of postsaccadic drift can be explained by the fact that the step component of innervation for saccades arises from both an increase in the activity of the agonist muscle and a decrease in the activity of the antagonist muscle, whereas the pulse component of innervation during saccades arises primarily from a large increase in the activity of the agonist muscle (24,37). Therefore, saccades made in the direction of action of the paretic muscle will be slow and undershoot the target (because of the loss of the pulse generated by the agonist) but will be followed by postsaccadic drift onwards (because of the relative preservation of the step). Likewise, saccades made opposite to the direction of action of the paretic muscle will be rapid and arrive nearly on target (because of sparing of the pulse made by the agonist) but will be followed by backward postsaccadic drift (because of the relative loss of the step). Put in another way, postsaccadic drift is always in the direction of action of the paretic muscle because of the relative sparing of the step of innervation that comes from the relaxation of the strong muscle when it is acting as the antagonist, and because of the change in innervation secondary to the relative loss of the step of innervation that comes from the relaxation of the weak muscle when it is acting as the antagonist.

2. Adduction Lag

During horizontal saccades, some patients with INO have prominent slowing of adduction, so-called adduction lag, but no limitation in the range of motion of that eye. This pattern of abnormality differs from that in patients with, for example, a partial medial rectus palsy in which there is usually a clinically obvious limitation in the range of motion by the time that saccades appear slow. Patients with INO who show "adduction lag" often have multiple sclerosis. The dissociation between saccade speed and range of motion probably reflects the inability of demyelinated fibers to sustain high-frequency discharges but with preservation of their ability faithfully to carry low-frequency discharges. Thus, the saccadic pulse of innervation is deficient causing adduction to be slow. The saccadic step, though, is spared, which allows the range of adduction to be full.

Another explanation for slow adduction without a limitation in range in INO would be the existence of pathways outside the MLF, which could also convey tonic commands to medial rectus motoneurons. Kommerell (22) has studied, with ocular electromyography (EMG), a patient with a unilateral INO and total paralysis of adduction. In the affected medial rectus, this patient showed a complete loss of burst activity but there was still some modulation of tonic activity. Whether this residual modulation is due to some of the tonic signal being carried by pathways outside the MLF (e.g., coming from the vestibular nucleus as the ascending tract of Dieters), due to the relative sparing of the ability of MLF fibers to carry low frequency (tonic) signals, or due to the sparing and modulation of vergence inputs (see Sec. III.C) is unsettled.

B. Disorders of Abduction

1. Abduction Nystagmus

A horizontal, dissociated nystagmus, greater or only in the abducting eye, is the other cardinal feature of INO. A number of mechanisms have been invoked to account for the nystagmus; they are not mutually exclusive and in each individual patient one or a combination of mechanisms may be responsible.

2. Abduction Nystagmus as an Adaptive Response

One explanation for the abduction nystagmus in unilateral INO is that it reflects an adaptive response to overcome the weakness of the contralateral medial rectus (3,54). The abnormality of abduction in the strong eye would then reflect an increase in the sizes of both the saccadic pulse and step of innervation. Because, as discussed above, the pulse portion of the saccade is created primarily by the agonist muscle and the step portion by more nearly equal contributions of the agonist and antagonist muscles, the increase in the pulse would have to be relatively greater than the increase in the step. This change in innervation would have to go to both eyes; that is, be a conjugate change, because of Hering's law of equal innervation. Thus, the conjugate adaptive response, although improving the accuracy and speed of the weak eye, would cause abnormalities of the pulse and step of innervation to the strong eye. The combination of an increase in size of the saccadic pulse and the change in the match between the sizes of the pulse and step would be reflected in the abducting eye as saccadic overshoot (hypermetria) followed by a brief (lasting several hundred milliseconds), backward, postsaccadic drift. Presumably, such a conjugate adaptive mechanism would only be invoked if a patient preferentially fixated with the paretic eye, and so opted to optimize the pattern of innervation to the paretic eye at the expense of disturbing the pattern of innervation to the strong eye.

Effects of Patching. A prediction of the adaptation hypothesis is that if one patched the nonparetic eye of a patient with a unilateral INO, ensuring *habitual viewing with the paretic eye*, there would be an increase in any abduction nystagmus, with overshooting of saccades made by the abducting eye. On the other hand, patching of the paretic eye, ensuring *habitual viewing with the nonparetic eye*, would lead to a diminution in the abduction nystagmus and the disappearance of the saccadic overshoot. Indeed, these changes are the case in some patients with INO, which confirms a role for adaptation in the genesis of the abduction nystagmus of INO (54). An additional finding in INO that is compatible with the adaptation hypothesis is that overshoot on abduction is more likely to be observed when the degree of the contralateral paresis of adduction is large (50).

There is other evidence that the abduction nystagmus of INO may be a response to the adduction weakness per se and not due to a direct central effect of the lesion. Medhorn (31) reported dissociated nystagmus, similar to that of INO, in patients with peripheral ocular motor palsies. Von Noorden and colleagues (52) reported bilateral abduction nystagmus in a group of strabismic patients who had weakness of adduction of both eyes due to a surgically induced recession of the medial recti. In one patient, patching of one eye for 4 days caused the abduction nystagmus in the other eye to diminish suggesting that it may have reflected an adaptive response. Finally, monkeys with experimental lesions of the MLF frequency show no or only a transient abduction nystagmus, even when the adduction paresis is profound (7,14,18). Likewise, patients with INO and marked adduction weakness occasionally have no or little abduction nystagmus (22,33). These findings imply that the MLF lesion itself does not produce abduction nystagmus.

Adaptation in Bilateral INO. In patients with bilateral INO who have bilateral abduction, nystagmus patching also may alter their abduction nystagmus. This finding implies that conjugate adaptive mechanisms also play a role in the pattern of nystagmus in bilateral INO [54]. The presence, however, of bilateral abduction nystagmus indicates that preferred fixation with one eye can not explain the nystagmus in its entirety. If that were the case, abduction nystagmus would only be apparent in one eye, the one not preferred for fixation. Conceivably, the eye preferred for fixation could alternate, so that the adducting eye was always made the preferred one. If this were the case, the conjugate adaptive mechanism would also have to be able to make direction-specific changes in innervation. In fact, such a capability does seem to exist; it has been demonstrated in other types of saccade adaptation paradigms (13). Even so, for the majority of patients with bilateral INO, it seems unlikely that such a complicated pathophysiology accounts for their abduction nystagmus.

On other grounds, too, the actions of conjugate adaptive mechanisms do not explain all facets of the abduction nystagmus of INO (54). Not all patients with

INO show a change in abduction mystagmus following patching. Other, probably disconjugate, adaptive mechanisms likely can alter abduction nystagmus following habitual *binocular* viewing.

3. Other Mechanisms for Abduction Nystagmus in INO

Increase in Convergence. An increase in convergence tone has been invoked as a cause of abduction nystagmus in INO (49). Although convergence may exacerbate an already present abduction nystagmus, and even produce an abduction nystagmus in, for example, patients with extreme convergence spasm (23), it is unlikely that an increase in convergence is the major cause of abduction nystagmus in INO. Indeed, monkeys with an experimental INO do have an increase in convergence but no abduction nystagmus (18) (see Sec. III.C).

Loss of Descending Excitation Inputs to the Abducens Nuclei. A loss of excitatory inputs traveling down the MLF to the abducens nucleus lying contralateral to the side of the lesion has also been proposed as a mechanism for abduction nystagmus in INO (39). Again, the lack of abduction nystagmus in some patients with INO, and in experimental models of INO, are against this hypothesis. There is, however, a descending projection in the MLF originating in internuclear neurons located within the oculomotor nucleus (29). Its function is unknown.

Failure of Inhibition of Medial Rectus Motoneurons. A failure of inhibition of medial rectus motoneurons lying contralateral to the side of the MLF lesion has also been hypothesized as a cause of the abduction nystagmus in INO (40). Although there is some electromyographic (EMG) evidence that is compatible with this hypothesis (27,20), in one well-studied patient with a complete unilateral INO, EMG did not show any failure of inhibition of the medial rectus (22). This patient, however, had little abduction nystagmus, so the issue is not totally resolved. (See also Sec. III.B.4.)

It should be emphasized that although many mechanisms can be invoked to explain the postsaccadic drift of the abducting eye in INO, only the adaptation hypothesis readily accounts for abduction overshoot. Of course, patients with INO may have saccadic overshoot because of involvement of other structures, such as the cerebellum, that function in the control of saccadic accuracy. Thus, saccadic overshoot in itself does not prove the adaptation hypothesis. Only demonstration of a goal-directed change in saccadic innervation that alters the nystagmus, such as with patching experiments, conclusively points to an adaptive mechanism.

Horizontal Gaze-Evoked Nystagmus in INO. Patients with INO may have a horizontal, "conjugate," gaze-evoked nystagmus superimposed on their adduction weakness. The gaze-holding difficulty could be due to a variety of causes: involvement of adjacent structures in the brainstem, such as the medial vestibular nuclei or the NPH; involvement of the cerebellar flocculus; or perhaps involvement of the cell bodies of the paramedian tracts that are intermingled among the fibers of the MLF. In the case of INO, any associated gaze-evoked nystagmus would be more obvious in the abducting eye owing to the damping effect of the weakness of the medial rectus on the adducting saccades (and quick phases) made by the paretic eye.

The abduction nystagmus associated with a gaze-evoked nystagmus differs from that caused by the pulse-step mismatch of an adaptive response. The former appears on attempting to hold eccentric gaze, has a relatively linear slow-phase waveform (due to a relatively large time constant of decay), and is relatively sustained. The latter appears after saccades to a wide range of orbital positions, including the primary one, has a rapid, exponentially decaying waveform, and dies away after a few beats. Individual patients with INO can probably show either, or in some cases both, of these patterns of abduction nystagmus.

To summarize, there are a number of possible reasons for abduction nystagmus in INO, and which one(s) accounts for the findings in an individual patient may not be readily deciphered without sophisticated testing procedures and specific behavioral paradigms. Nevertheless, whenever a dissociated horizontal nystagmus is detected on clinical examination, the syndrome of INO must be kept in mind.

4. *Abducting Saccades in INO*

Apart from abduction nystagmus, abnormalities of abducting saccades per se have been reported both in patients with unilateral and with bilateral INO (15,50,4). There may be a slowing of the *abducting* eye during saccades, with a decrease in the peak velocity-amplitude relationship, or abducting saccades may be "fractionated," with brief discrete decelerations. The slowing is usually greater on the side of the adduction paresis (in unilateral INO) and need not be accompanied by any evidence of a concomitant horizontal gaze paresis. The more prominent the INO, and the larger the lesion (on MRI), the more likely there will be slowing of abduction (4). Such abnormalities of abduction, however, are not invariable in INO; they may be absent even when the paresis of adduction is profound (22). Likewise, in experimental INO abducting saccades are normal (14,18).

A paresis of abduction with saccades but with normal abduction in response to a vestibular stimulus has been termed posterior INO (of Lutz) (28). This entity is as yet poorly substantiated. Coexistent peripheral involvement, possibly with relative sparing of one or another class of ocular motor nerve fibers or muscles, must be ruled out in such cases.

What might be the explanation for the abnormalities of saccades by the abducting eye when they do occur with an otherwise typical INO? A small degree of abduction slowing might be expected in a complete paralysis of the medial rectus because of the loss of the contribution, albeit relatively small, of the "off-pulse" of innervation when the affected muscle is acting as an antagonist (24). A failure of inhibition of the medial rectus, on the side of the adduction paresis, has also been proposed as the cause for the slowing of abducting saccades in INO (15). As indicated above, in one well-studied patient with a complete unilateral INO (22), there was no failure of inhibition of either medial rectus.

These findings raise the question as to how activity in medial rectus motoneurons, when the medial rectus is acting as the antagonist, is decreased under normal circumstances. On the one hand, disfacilitation of activity of medial rectus motoneurons can take place by virtue of inhibition of abducens internuclear neurons that project to (contralateral) medial rectus motoneurons. There is also evidence for a direct, ipsilateral projection from the pontine paramedian reticular formation to the oculomotor nucleus (43). Whether or not this pathway mediates inhibition on medial rectus motoneurons is unsettled. Thömke and Hopf (50), however, have used the idea of interruption of such an inhibitory pathway running close to, but not in, the MLF to explain slowing of abduction saccades made by the eye on the side of an MLF lesion.

Taking these findings together, it may be that abnormalities of abducting saccades only occur in INO when the lesion extends into the adjacent reticular formation, and thereby also involves fibers that mediate direct inhibition on medial rectus motoneurons.

C. Vergence and the MLF

The main difference between the paresis of adduction with an oculomotor nerve palsy and that with an INO is that in the latter adduction induced by vergence is spared. Likewise, preservation of vergence tone is probably the explanation for the lack of exotropia in most patients with INO (9). Recent work in monkeys has shown that not only is vergence spared with an MLF lesion but that it actually may be increased, as reflected in an increase in the relative amount of convergence induced by an accommodative stimulus (18). This increased vergence can be related to the electrophysiological finding that during symmetrical convergence, abducens internuclear neurons *decrease* their discharge rate leading to an "inappropriate" vergence signal (for a decrease in activity) being sent to the medial rectus motoneurons (17). In intact animals, an appropriate signal, probably arising from cells lying close to and projecting to the oculomotor nucleus, presumably compensates for this incorrect signal. Hence, one would predict that after a unilateral MLF lesion there would be an excessive vergence signal reaching ipsilateral (on the side of the lesion) medial rectus motoneurons. This appears to be the case (18).

It should be reemphasized that in spite of an increase in vergence produced by experimental lesions of the MLF, there is no abduction nystagmus or slowing of abducting saccades. Thus, the increase in vergence with an isolated MLF lesion does not readily account for the abnormalities of abduction seen in patients with INO.

D. Disorders of Vertical Eye Movements in INO

1. Bilateral INO

Both human beings and experimental animals with bilateral INO show a characteristic pattern of abnormalities of *vertical eye movements*: disturbances of gaze holding and inadequate vestibuloocular and optokinetic and pursuit responses (14,41). These findings reflect interruption of connections between the vestibular nuclei (and the NPH), the trochlear and the oculomotor nuclei, and the INC. Note that vertical saccades and quick phases are spared in INO.

Ranalli and Sharpe (41) have studied in detail the vertical eye movements in patients with INO. They found, in addition to the above-described abnormalities, that the ability to cancel the vertical vestibulo-ocular reflex (by fixing on an object rotating with the head) was less impaired than was vertical smooth pursuit with the head still. This dissociation between the ability to cancel the vestibulo-ocular reflex and to pursue targets with the head still implies a difference in the mechanisms by which these two processes are accomplished.

During testing of the vertical vestibulo-ocular reflex, Ranalli and Sharpe (41) also found a change in the phase relationships between head and eye velocity (more phase lag at higher frequencies). This finding was attributed to a sparing of position-coded signals (from the vertical neural integrator) relative to velocity-coded signals during vestibular stimulation. Ranalli and Sharpe (41) further suggested that the spared position-coded signal could be carried in fibers outside the MLF. On the other hand, just as for slowing of adduction during saccades, but with a full range of motion, there could also be a relative sparing of the ability of fibers within the MLF to carry signals discharging at lower rates during vestibular stimulation. In other words, the abnormal phase relationships of the vertical vestibulo-ocular reflex at high frequencies (and hence velocities) of stimulation could be the equivalent of the adduction lag during horizontal saccades in INO. Both would be due to a decrease in the velocity command relative to the position command.

One puzzling aspect of bilateral INO is why patients do not more frequently show a downbeating nystagmus in the primary position of gaze. Such a nystagmus is what one would expect from a preponderance of activity from pathways mediating excitation from the anterior semicircular canals. (Projections mediating anterior semicircular responses probably ascend outside the MLF via the ventral tegmentum and the brachium conjunctivum (42). It may be that adaptive mechanisms quickly restore vestibular balance after an MLF lesion, so that any spontaneous nystagmus in the primary position is promptly nullified. Nevertheless, patients with bilateral INO frequently have vertical nystagmus on extremes of vertical gaze as part of their gaze-holding disturbance.

2. Unilateral INO

The effects of unilateral INO on vertical eye movements are less consistent and more evanescent, probably because considerable adaptation to unilateral lesions can be accomplished by altering signals carried by the intact MLF on the other side. Acutely, however, in the monkey, Gamlin and colleagues (18) have reported a monocular, vertical nystagmus, with slow phases directed upwards, in the eye on the side of the lesion. No abnormalities were reported in the other eye, although torsion was not measured and the animals could well have had a torsional nystagmus in the other eye. Indeed, a dissociated pattern of vertical-torsional nystagmus has been reported in patients with a unilateral INO (36,30). There was a downbeating nystagmus in the eye on the side of the lesion and a torsional nystagmus (quick phases such that the upper pole of the eye beat toward the nose) in the eye contralateral to the side of the lesion. Such a pattern of nystagmus is similar to that arising from stimulation of an anterior semicircular canal and is what one would predict from the interruption, on the side of the lesion, of the three pathways in the MLF that carry signals mediating responses from the vertical semicircular canals. Normally, each MLF carries signals mediating inhibition from the anterior and posterior canals on the same side and excitation from the posterior canal on the opposite side. A loss of these inputs would lead to a dissociated nystagmus of the pattern described above.

Conversely, we recently examined a patient who initially had an INO with a dissociated mixed vertical-torsional nystagmus that beat upwards in the eye contralateral to the adduction weakness and counterclockwise (upper pole away from the nose) in the eye with the adduction weakness. Such a pattern of nystagmus suggests a lesion involving the anterior semicircular canal pathways from the labyrinth contralateral to the eye with the adduction weakness after they have crossed so as to be on the same side as the eye with the adduction weakness.

Human beings with a unilateral INO occasionally show a skew deviation (a vertical misalignment between the two visual axes) with the eye usually being higher on the side of the lesion (9). There may also be a head tilt directed opposite to the side of the lesion. These abnormalities probably reflect interruption of ascending projections from the vestibular nuclei, which mediate utricular-ocular reflexes that occur when the position of the head with respect to gravity is altered. The normal response to a lateral head tilt is ocular counterroll (contralateral cyclorotation but without any vertical deviation of the visual axes). With lesions in a variety of locations, including the labyrinth, the dorsolateral medulla (Wallenberg's syndrome), and the midbrain, the so-called ocular tilt reaction may appear: skew deviation, ocular counterroll, and head tilt. Note that with Wallenberg's syndrome, the eye is lower on the side of the lesion (and the head is tilted toward the side of the lesion), whereas in INO, the eye is usually higher on the side of the lesion (and the head is tilted away from the side of the lesion).

IV. ETIOLOGY OF INO

A number of processes can affect the fibers of the MLF and cause INO (46,9,26). Perhaps the two most common are multiple sclerosis and ischemic vascular disease. Although classic teaching has the etiology of unilateral INO as vascular and of bilateral INO as demyelinating, a large number of patients with a unilateral INO on clinical examination have multiple sclerosis. Quantitative measures of eye movements in such patients, though, often show evidence of bilateral involvement. Bilateral INO, when marked and without signs of involvement of adjacent structures related to ocular motor control (e.g., that might produce a concomitant gaze palsy), is more commonly due to multiple sclerosis than to vascular disease, although the presence of other ocular motor signs by no means rules out a demyelinating lesion. Occasionally, patients with coma due to metabolic disturbances or to drug intoxications show the pattern of INO during reflex vestibuloocular testing. The INO disappears when a normal metabolic state is restored. Naloxone has reversed INO in a patient with a drug overdose (44).

V. DIAGNOSIS OF INO

A. Symptoms

The main symptoms of INO are diplopia, blurred vision, and oscillopsia. Vertigo also frequently occurs but in most cases probably reflects involvement outside the MLF (25). The cause of the diplopia (if mild it may be described simply as visual blurring) can be due to the adduction paralysis and/or to the skew deviation. Because of the sparing of convergence, and consequent fusional capabilities, there may be little horizontal diplopia when the eyes are near the primary position of gaze. Patients with persisting symptomatic diplopia may be treated with botulinum toxin (35). Oscillopsia in INO can be due to the abduction nystagmus (in which case it is monocular), due to the decreased vestibulo-ocular response during head motion (both vertically and also horizontally and due to the adduction paresis), or due to any spontaneous vertical nystagmus. In the case of adduction lag, the visual disturbance (often described as visual blurring) may be transient and only apparent during and immediately after the saccade when the eyes are disconjugate.

B. Clinical Examination

Slowing of adduction is the hallmark of INO and should be explicitly tested for as part of the routine neurological examination. Ask the patient to make rapid horizontal refixations between two, relatively widely spaced targets and look for a slowing or a decrease in the amplitude of the adducting relative to the abducting eye. An optokinetic tape may also be used to reveal the disconjugate nature of horizontal saccades (quick phases) when made in the direction of the adduction weakness (47). A dissociated nystagmus, greater in the abducting eye is a common, although not invariant, finding in INO and should also be carefully looked for.

In patients with a limitation of adduction, convergence should be elicited to see if it improves the range of motion. It is often difficult to elicit convergence in patients with a marked unilateral or with a bilateral INO. A large stimulus, with features to focus upon, should be moved slowly toward the patient and the patient instructed carefully to fix on a specific aspect of the target. The patients may need to be strongly encouraged, and it sometimes helps if they themselves move the vergence target. Even when convergence does not seem to improve adduction, a diagnosis of INO is still likely if there are no other signs of an oculomotor nerve palsy. In some patients in whom convergence does not improve adduction, it has been suggested that the lesion may extend from the MLF into the third nerve complex and involve medial rectus motoneurons (Cogan's anterior INO versus Cogan's posterior INO, in which convergence is spared (9). Such a process has also been invoked to account for the marked exotropia, with each eye deviated temporally, that appears in some patients with bilateral INO. This is called wall-eyed bilateral internuclear ophthalmoplegia (WEBINO syndrome).

Remember that INO may be mimicked by abnormalities in the ocular motor periphery, such as myasthenia gravis, demyelinating neuropathies (Fisher's syndrome), and restrictive processes (19). In these patients, there may be "quiver" eye movements—saccades that start out quite fast but then markedly slow down or terminate abruptly before reaching the target (53).

Patients with a possible INO should also be examined for a skew deviation (with the eye usually higher on the side of the lesion) and for a head tilt (away from the side of the lesion). A skew deviation and adduction paresis may be confused with a partial (inferior division) third nerve palsy, although the sparing of the pupillary reflex and the sparing of adduction during convergence usually establishes the supranuclear location of the lesion. The skew deviation of INO must also be distinguished from a fourth nerve palsy. In weakness of the superior oblique muscle, the characteristic influence of orbital position and of head posture (Bielschowsky's test) on the pattern of ocular misalignment points to the correct diagnosis.

Vertical eye movements must also be examined in INO to look for a pattern of dissociated vertical-torsional nystagmus in unilateral INO and for the characteristic deficits in gaze holding and pursuit and vestibuloocular responses in bilateral INO. Vertical saccades are spared in INO.

C. Laboratory Testing

Although the diagnosis of INO is largely based on the clinical examination, magnetic resonance imaging (MRI) may be helpful in confirming the diagnosis, although all patients with INO do not have abnormal MRI scans (2,21,34,1). One must not be confused by the slight increase in intensity in the midline of the brainstem on T_2-weighted images that occurs in normal individuals. Quantitative testing of eye movements may reveal subtle degrees of adduction slowing (often best revealed by comparing the ratio of adduction with abduction velocities) (11,32,51), and may also demonstrate abnormalities such as the suprafast saccades that are characteristic of peripheral ocular motor involvement as in myasthenia gravis (53).

VI. CONCLUSIONS

1. The main findings in unilateral INO are paresis of adduction in the eye on the side of the lesion (for conjugate not vergence eye movements) and abduction nystagmus in the eye on the side opposite to the lesion. A skew deviation (eye usually higher on the side of the lesion) or a dissociated, mixed vertical-torsional nystagmus with the eye beating down on the side of the lesion may also occur.
2. The main findings in bilateral INO are paresis of adduction in both eyes, bilateral abduction nystagmus, and in the vertical plane, impaired gaze-holding, vestibular responses, and smooth tracking.
3. Abduction nystagmus in INO may have a number of causes; probably most common are a gaze-evoked nystagmus superimposed on adduction weakness and adaptation to adduction weakness.
4. Most of the findings in INO can be explained by interruption of projections from abducens internuclear neurons, mediating adduction, and from the vestibular nuclei, mediating both canal and otolith induced reflexes, as well as vertical gaze holding and pursuit. Extension of the lesion to structures near but outside the MLF or involvement of cell bodies intermixed with MLF fibers may also be important in the pathogenesis of the abduction nystagmus and the occasional slowing of abducting saccades.

ACKNOWLEDGMENT

We acknowledge the support of the National Institutes of Health (EY01849).

REFERENCES

1. Alexander JA, Castillo M, Hoffman JC. Magnetic resonance findings in a patient with internuclear ophthalmoplegia. Neuroradiological-clinical correlation. J Clin Neuro Ophthalmology 1991; 11:58–61.
2. Atlas SW, Grossman RI, Savino PJ, et al. Internuclear ophthalmoplegia: MR-anatomic correlation. Am J Neuroradiol 1987; 8:243–7.

3. Baloh RW, Yee RD, Honrubia V. Internuclear ophthalmoplegia. I. Saccades and dissociated nystagmus. Arch Neurol 1978; 35:484–9.
4. Bronstein AM, Rudge P, Gresty MA, Du Boulay G, Morris J. Abnormalities of horizontal gaze. Clinical, oculographic and magnetic resonance imaging findings. II. Gaze palsy and internuclear ophthalmoplegia. J Neurol Neurosurg Psychiatry 1990; 53:200–7.
5. Büttner-Ennever JA, Horn AKE, Schmidtke K. Cell groups of the medial longitudinal fasciculus and paramedian tracts. Rev Neurol (Paris) 1989; 145:533–9.
6. Cannon SC, Robinson DA. Loss of the neural integrator of the oculomotor system from brain stem lesions in monkey. J Neurophysiol 1987; 5:1383–1409.
7. Carpenter MG, Strominger NL. The medial longitudinal fasciculus and disturbances of conjugate horizontal eye movements in the monkey. J Comp Neurol 1965; 125:41–66.
8. Christoff N, Anderson PJ, Nathanson M, Bender MB. Problems in anatomic analysis of lesions of the medial longitudinal fasciculus. Arch Neurol 1960; 2:293–304.
9. Cogan DG. Internuclear ophthalmoplegia, typical and atypical. Arch Ophthalmol 1970; 84:583–9.
10. Cogan DG, Kubik CS, Smith SL. Unilateral internuclear ophthalmoplegia: report of eight clinical cases with one post mortem study. Arch Ophthalmol 1950; 44:783–96.
11. Crane TB, Yee RD, Baloh RW, Hepler RS. Analysis of characteristic eye movement abnormalities in internuclear ophthalmoplegia. Arch Ophthalmol 1983; 101:206–10.
12. Crawford JD, Cadera W, Vilis T. Generation of torsion and vertical eye position signals by the interstitial nucleus of Cajal. Science 1991; 252:1551–3.
13. Deubel H. Adaptivity of gain and direction in oblique saccades. In: O'Regan JK, Levy-Schoen A, eds. Eye movements: from physiology to cognition. Amsterdam: Elsevier, 1987:181–90.
14. Evinger LC, Fuchs AF, Baker R. Bilateral lesions of the medial longitudinal fasciculus in monkeys: effects on the horizontal and vertical components of voluntary and vestibular induced eye movements. Exp Brain Res 1977; 28:1–20.
15. Feldon SE, Hoyt WF, Stark L. Disordered inhibition in internuclear ophthalmoplegia. Analysis of eye movement recordings with computer simulations. Brain 1980; 103:113–37.
16. Fukushima K, Fukushima J, Harada C, Ohashi T, Kase M. Neuronal activity related to vertical eye movement in the region of the interstitial nucleus of Cajal in alert cat. Exp Brain Res 1990; 79:43–64.
17. Gamlin PDR, Gnadt JW, Mays LE. Abducens internuclear neurons carry an inappropriate signal for ocular convergence. J Neurophysiol 1989a; 62:70–81.
18. Gamlin PDR, Gnadt JW, Mays LE. Lidocaine-induced unilateral internuclear ophthalmoplegia: effects on convergence and conjugate eye movements. J Neurophysiol 1989b; 62:82–95.
19. Glaser JS. Myasthenic internuclear ophthalmoplegia. Arch Ophthalmol 1966; 75:363–6.
20. Gonzalez C, Reuben RN. Ocular electromyography in the syndrome of median longitudinal fasciculus: patterns of inhibition and excitation. Am J Ophthalmol 1967; 64:916–26.

21. Haller KA, Miller-Meeks M, Kardon R. Early magnetic resonance imaging in acute traumatic internuclear ophthalmoplegia. Ophthalmology 1990; 97:1162–5.
22. Kommerell G. Unilateral internuclear ophthalmoplegia. The lack of inhibitory involvement in medial rectus muscle activity. Invest Ophthalmol Vis Sci 1981; 21:592–9.
23. Kommerell G, Jaedicke S. Dissoziierter Nystagmus Alssymptom des Naheinstellungsspasmus. Bericht über die 71. usammenkunft deer Deutschen Ophthalm. Gesellschaft in Heidelberg 1971. Munchen: JF Bergmann, 1972:478–81.
24. Kommerell G, Olivier D, Theopold H. Adaptive programming of phasic and tonic components in saccadic eye movements. Investigations in patients with abducens palsy. Invest Ophthalmol Vis Sci 1976; 15:657–60.
25. Kupfer C, Cogan DG. Unilateral internuclear ophthalmoplegia, a clinico-pathological case report. Arch Ophthalmol 1966; 75:484–9.
26. Leigh RJ, Zee DS. The neurology of eye movements. 2d ed. Philadelphia: Davis, 1991.
27. Loeffler JD, Hoyt WF, Slatt B. Motor excitation and inhibition in internuclear palsy. An electromyographic study. Arch Neurol 1966; 15:664–71.
28. Lutz A. Ueber die Bahnen der Blickwendung und deren Dissoziierung: (Nebst Mitteilung eines falles von Ophthalmoplegiainternuclearis anterior in Verbindung mit Dissoziierung der Bbogengange). Klin Monatsbl Augenheilkd 1923; 70:213–35.
29. Maciewicz RJ, Kaneko CRS, Highstein SM, Baker R. Morphophysiological identification of interneurons in the oculomotor nucleus that project to the abducens nucleus in the cat. Brain Res 1975; 96:60–5.
30. Marshall RS, Sacco RL, Kreuger R, Odel JG, Mohr JP. Dissociated vertical nystagmus and internuclear ophthalmoplegia from a midbrain infarction. Arch Neurol 1991; 48:1304–5.
31. Mehdorn E. Dissoziierter nystagmus bei internuklearer ophthalmoplegie—folge der internuklearen R. medialis-parese. Fortschr Ophthalmol 1987; 84:212–14.
32. Meienberg O, Müri R, Rabineay PA. Clinical and oculographic examinations of saccadic eye movements with diagnosis of multiple sclerosis. Arch Neurol 1986; 43:438–43.
33. Müri R, Meienberg O. The clinical spectrum of internuclear ophthalmoplegia in multiple sclerosis. Arch Neurol 1985; 42:851–5.
34. Mutschler V, Eber AM, Rumbach L, et al. Internuclear ophthalmoplegia in 14 patients. Clinical and topographic correlation using magnetic resonance imaging. Neuro-Ophthalmology 1990; 10:319–25.
35. Newman NJ and Lambert SR. Botulinum toxin treatment of supranuclear ocular motility disorders. Neurology 1992; 42:1391–3.
36. Nozaki S, Mukuno K and Ishikawa S. Internuclear ophthalmoplegia associated with ipsilateral downbeat nystagmus and contralateral incyclorotatory nystagmus. Ophthalmologica 1983; 187:210–16.
37. Optican LM, Zee DS, Chu FC. Adaptive responses to ocular muscle weakness in human pursuit and saccadic eye movements. J Neurophysiol 1985; 54:110–22.
38. Paton L. Ocular palsies. Br J Ophthalmol 1921; 5:250.
39. Pierrot-Deseilligny C, Chain F. L'ophtalmoplégie internucléure. Rev Neurol 1979; 135:485–513.

40. Pola J, Robinson DA. An explanation of eye movements seen in internuclear ophthalmoplegia. Arch Neurol 1976; 33:447–52.
41. Ranalli PJ, Sharpe JA. Vertical vestibulo-ocular reflex smooth pursuit and eye-head tracking dysfunction in internuclear ophthalmoplegia. Brain 1988a; 111:1299–317.
42. Ranalli PJ, Sharpe JA. Upbeat nystagmus and the ventral tegmental pathway of the upward vestibulo-ocular reflex. Neurology 1988b; 38:1329–30.
43. Remmel RS, Skinner RD, Pola J. Cat pontomedullary reticular neurons projecting to the regions of the ascending MLF and the vestibular nuclei. In: Baker A, Berthoz A, eds. Control of gaze by brain stem. Amsterdam: Elsevier/North Holland, 1977:163–6.
44. Rizzo M, Corbett J. Bilateral internuclear ophthalmoplegia reversed by Naloxone. Arch Neurol 1983; 40:242–3.
45. Sauvineau. Un nouveau type de paalysie associee des mouvements horizontaux des yeux. Bull Soc Fr Ophtalmol 1895; 13:524–34.
46. Smith JL, Cogan DG. Internuclear ophthalmoplegia. A review of fifty-eight cases. Arch Ophthalmol 1959; 61:687–94.
47. Smith JL, David NJ. Internuclear ophthalmoplegia: two new clinical signs. Neurology 1964; 14:307–9.
48. Spiller WG. Ophthalmoplegia internuclearis anterior. A case with necropsy. Brain 1924; 47:345–7.
49. Stroud MH, Newman NM, Keltner JL, Gay AJ. Abducting nystagmus in the medial longitudinal fasciculus (MLF) syndrome—internuclear ophthalmoplegia (INO). Arch Ophthalmol 1974; 92:2–5.
50. Thömke F, Hopf HC. Abduction saccades in unilateral internuclear ophthalmoplegia. Neuro-Ophthalmology 1990; 10:277–85.
51. Ventre J, Vighetto A, Bailly G, Prablanc C. Saccade metrics in multiple sclerosis: versional velocity disconjugacy as the best clue? J Neurol Sci 1991; 102:144–9.
52. Von Noorden GK, Tredici TD, Ruttum M. Pseudo-internuclear ophthalmoplegia after surgical paresis of the medial rectus muscle. Am J Ophthalmol 1984; 98:602–8.
53. Yee RD, Cogan DG, Zee DS, Baloh RW, Honrubia V. Rapid eye movements in myasthenia gravis. II. Electro-oculographic analysis. Arch Ophthalmol 1976; 94:571–5.
54. Zee DS, Hain TC, Carl JR. Abduction nystagmus in internuclear ophthalmoplegia. Ann Neurol 1987; 21:383–8.
55. Zee DS, Yamazaki A, Butler PH, Gücer G. Effects of ablation of flocculus and paraflocculus on eye movements in primate. J Neurophysiol 1981; 46:878–99.

33

Neurological Paraneoplastic Syndromes

Robert W. Baloh
University of California School of Medicine, Los Angeles, California

Neurological remote effects of cancer were first described at the end of the last century, but case reports were largely anecdotal, and since similar syndromes occurred without cancer, many questioned a cause and effect relationship (1). The mechanism by which a tumor can damage the nervous system without directly invading it is still not entirely clear; both viral and autoimmune etiologies have been suspected. Probably the best characterized paraneoplastic central nervous system syndrome is cerebellar degeneration associated with gynecological tumors in women (2,3). These patients have antibodies that bind with a specific antigen expressed by Purkinje cells and the tumor cells. If the gynecological tumor does not express the antigen, the patient does not develop cerebellar degeneration (4).

Cancer can have remote effects on the nervous system from the cortex to the peripheral nerves. Almost all tumors have been associated with such effects, but small cell carcinoma of the lung is most common. The characteristic pathological findings are perivascular cuffing by lymphocytes, activation of microglia with the formation of microglial nodules, and selective loss of neurons (1). The process is predominantly, although not exclusively, confined to gray matter. A dramatic neuro-ophthalmological paraneoplastic syndrome is the opsoclonus-myoclonus syndrome (5). This disorder is characterized by chaotic conjugate eye movements in all directions along with myoclonus of the trunk and limbs. It is usually seen in children with neuroblastoma. Pathological studies have identified perivascular mononuclear cell infiltrates of the brainstem and cerebellum in some patients but others show no abnormalities. Zee and Robinson (6) speculated that selective involvement of the omnipause neurons in the pontine reticular formation could account for these unusual ocular oscillations. Since the omnipause neurons provide inhibitory control of the presaccade burst neurons (also located in the pontine reticular formation), loss of omnipause neuron inhibition could lead to uncontrolled saccadic eye movements. However, so far, there is no convincing evidence for selective involvement of any neuron population in patients with the opsoclonus-myoclonus syndrome.

I. CEREBELLAR DEGENERATION

A. Diagnostic Workup

The findings on examination in patients with paraneoplastic cerebellar degeneration are no different from those of other patients with diffuse cerebellar lesions. The trunk and extremities are ataxic and the speech is usually slurred. The course is subacute, with most patients developing severe disability within 6 months of onset. Often intractable nausea and vomiting occur early. All types of spontaneous nystagmus are seen, but downbeat nystagmus is most common. Gaze-evoked and rebound nystagmus also are common. Eye movement recordings document impaired smooth pursuit, optokinetic nystagmus, and fixation-suppression of vestibular nystagmus. Saccades may be dysmetric, but peak velocity remains normal. Vestibular responses are normal or hyperactive.

Any patient with subacute cerebellar degeneration should be examined carefully for an occult malignancy (Fig. 1). Antineuronal antibodies are identified in approximately 50% of patients with paraneoplastic cerebellar degeneration (7). As noted earlier, the most specific antibody is the anti-Purkinje cell antibody found in woman with gynecological tumors [the so-called anti-Yo antibody in the classification of Furneaux et al. (4)]. With immunohistochemical staining, this antibody binds to the Purkinje cell cytoplasm producing a characteristic "ring of pearls" on microscopic examination of the cerebellum. It is so specific for gynecological tumors that surgical exploration of the pelvis is indicated in any woman with the antibody and without an obvious malignancy regardless of the outcome of other diagnositc studies. An antineuronal nuclear antibody (anti-Hu) (4) has been found in a few patients with small cell carcinoma of the lung and cerebellar degeneration, but this antibody is more commonly associated with paraneoplastic peripheral neuropathy. Its role in the pathophysiology of cerebellar degeneration is unknown. Neuroimaging studies are usually normal, although occasionally there can be some mild cerebellar atrophy. Cerebrospinal fluid examination may show a mild pleocytosis and elevated gamma globulin or may be completely normal.

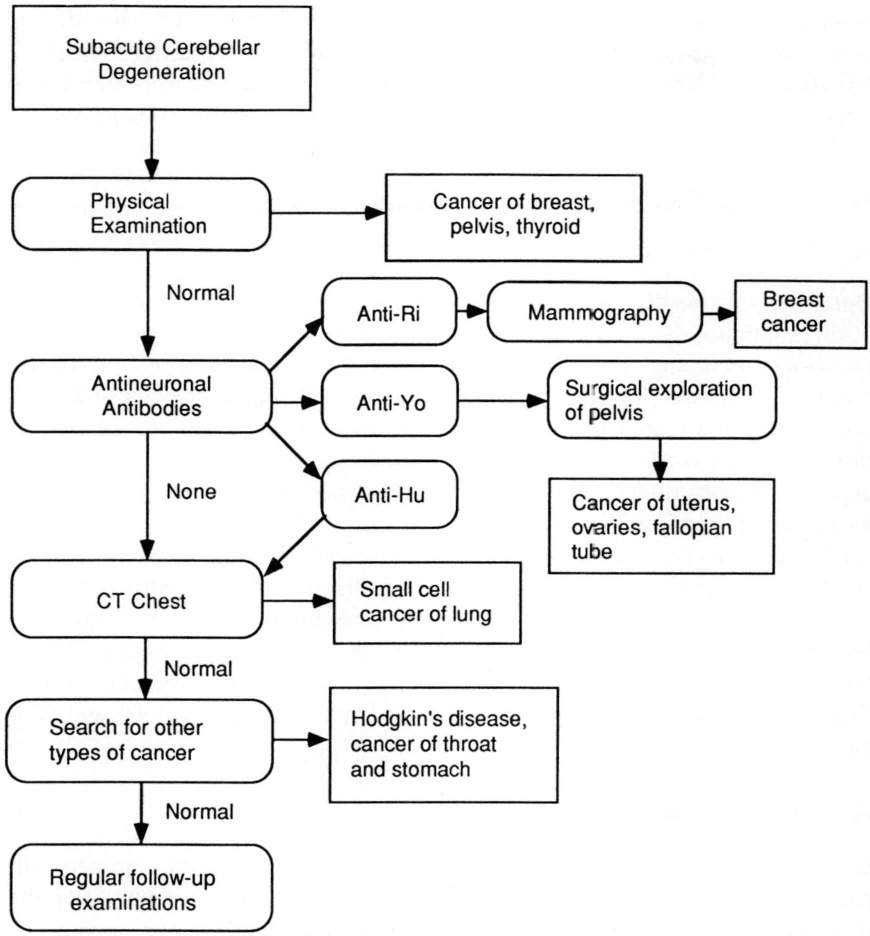

Figure 1 Diagnosis of paraneoplastic cerebellar degeneration.

B. Management

The first goal is to identify and remove the underlying neoplasm. Although infrequent, there are a few reports of clinical improvement after resection of the tumor (1). Most patients reach a "burnt-out stage" where they remain with a moderate to severe cerebellar deficit. We have followed a woman with paraneoplastic cerebellar degeneration for 2 years after a fallopian tube cancer was removed. Exploratory surgery was initiated after anti-Purkinje antibodies were identified in her serum. Despite complete removal of the tumor and tumor markers returning to normal, her clinical examination has been unchanged. Her severe nausea and vomiting have diminished, however. Plasmapheresis or immunosuppression is generally not effective (2,7), although there are a few isolated reports of improvement in the cerebellar deficit after plasmapheresis.

II. OPSOCLONUS SYNDROMES

A. Diagnostic Workup

Opsoclonus is readily identified, even by the uninitiated. Conjugate saccades occur continuously in all directions often with torsional components. Eye movement recordings document that the saccades have normal peak velocities for their amplitude. The combination of opsoclonus and myoclonus in a child should lead to a search for a neuroblastoma; in an adult, small cell carcinoma of the lung is most likely. A subgroup of adults with opsoclonus and cerebellar ataxia (primarily truncal) have an antineuronal nuclear antibody (anti-Ri) (8). Nearly all of these patients have cancer of the breast (8). So far, no antineuronal antibodies have been found in patients with opsoclonus and neuroblastoma or small cell carcinoma of the lung. A few patients with the anti-Ri–positive opsoclonus syndrome and a few with nonparaneoplastic opsoclonus have had lesions of the brainstem or cerebellum on magnetic resonance imaging (MRI), but most patients with opsoclonus have normal neuroimaging studies (8). Cerebrospinal fluid examination may show a lymphocytic pleocytosis and mild elevation of protein or may be normal.

B. Management

Unlike cerebellar symptoms and signs, spontaneous remissions are common with paraneoplastic opsoclonus. In some patients, the opsoclonus remits after the malignancy is removed. Some patients have exacerbations after months of remission. Several different medications have been reported to improve the opsoclonus associated with paraneoplastic syndromes (Table 1). Some children

Table 1 Treatment of Opsoclonus

Drug	Dosage	Reference
ACTH	20–40 U/day	9–11
Prednisone	60 mg/m^2/day	9,11
Thiamine	200 mg initially, then 10 mg/day	12
Clonazepam	0.5–2.0 mg/day	5,13

with opsoclonus-myoclonus and neuroblastoma have shown dramatic improvement with adrenocorticotropin (ACTH) or high-dose steroids (9–11). The improvement is so rapid that it is probably not a nonspecific anti-inflammatory effect. In adults, steroids, thiamine, and clonazepam may improve opsoclonus, but many patients do not respond to any of these medications (12,13).

III. BRAINSTEM ENCEPHALITIS

A. Diagnostic Workup

Paraneoplastic brainstem encephalitis is a diagnosis that can only be made at postmortem examination, although it should be suspected in any patient with cancer who develops a subacute progressive brainstem syndrome (with or without involvement at other levels of the nervous system). A few patients have been found to have antineuronal nuclear antibodies (anti-Hu) but most have no detectable antineuronal antibodies. Brainstem encephalitis often presents with oculomotor deficits, including nuclear and supranuclear gaze disorders (1,14). We recently reported two patients with a paraneoplastic brainstem syndrome associated with prostate cancer who presented with progressive loss of horizontal voluntary eye movements (15). Neither had antineuronal antibodies. As with the cerebellar degeneration syndromes, patients with paraneoplastic brainstem encephalitis usually have normal neuroimaging studies. The cerebrospinal fluid (CSF) may show some mild inflammatory response with pleocytosis and elevated gamma globulin. Although there are well-known viral syndromes associated with malignant disease and viral-like particles have been identified in a few isolated cases of paraneoplastic encephalomyelitis (1), no specific virus has ever been isolated or identified.

B. Management

As in the case of cerebellar degeneration, there is no effective treatment for paraneoplastic brainstem encephalitis. Removal of the underlying malignancy may stop the progression or even rarely lead to improvement, but in most cases, the neurological syndrome remains unchanged. Similarly, immunosuppression and plasmapheresis have not proved effective.

ACKNOWLEDGMENT

This work was supported by NIH Grants 09823 and AG 09693.

REFERENCES

1. Henson RA, Urich H. Cancer and the nervous system. The neurological manifestations of systemic malignant disease. Oxford, England: Blackwell Scientific, 1982:311–621.
2. Anderson NE, Rosenblum MK, Posner JB. Paraneoplastic cerebellar degeneration: clinical-immunological correlations. Ann Neurol 1988; 24:559–67.

3. Hetzel DJ, Stanhope CR, O'Neill BP, Lennon VA. Gynecologic cancer in patients with subacute cerebellar degeneration predicted by anti-Purkinje cell antibodies and limited in metastatic volume. Mayo Clin Proc 1990; 65:1558–63.
4. Furneaux HM, Rosenblum MK, Dalman J, Wong E, Woodruff P, Graus F, Posner J. Selective expression of Purkinje-cell antigens in tumor tissue from patients with paraneoplastic cerebellar degeneration. N Engl J Med 1990; 322:1844–51.
5. Dropcho E, Payne R. Paraneoplastic opsoclonus–myoclonus. Association with medullary thyroid carcinoma and review of the literature. Arch Neurol 1986; 43:410–15.
6. Zee DS, Robinson DA. A hypothetical explanation of saccadic oscillations. Ann Neurol 1979; 5:405–14.
7. Hammack JE, Kimmel DW, O'Neill BP, Lennon VA. Paraneoplastic cerebellar degeneration: a clinical comparison of patients with and without Purkinje cell cytoplasmic antibodies. Mayo Clin Proc 1990; 65:1423–31.
8. Luque FA, Furneaux HM, Ferziger R, Rosenblum MK, Wray SH, Schold SC, Glantz MJ, Jaeckle KA, Biran H, Lesser M, Paulsen WA, River ME, Posner JB: Anti-Ri. An antibody associated with paraneoplastic opsoclonus and breast cancer. Ann Neurol 1991; 29:241–51.
9. Kinsbourne M. Myoclonic encephalopathy of infants. J Neurol Neurosurg Psychiatry 1962; 25:271–6.
10. Dyken P, Kolar O. Dancing eyes, dancing feet: infantile polymyoclonia. Brain 1968; 91:305–20.
11. Boltshauser E, Deonna T, Hirt HR. Myoclonic cerebellopathy of infants, or dancing eyes syndrome. Helv Paediatr Acta 1979; 34:119–33.
12. Nausieda PA, Tanner CM, Weiner WJ. Opsoclonic cerebellopathy: A paraneoplastic syndrome responsive to thiamine. Arch Neurol 1981; 38:780–1.
13. Leigh RJ, Zee DS. The neurology of eye movements. Philadelphia: Davis, 1983.
14. Reddy RV, Vakila ST. Midbrain encephalitis as a remote effect of a malignant neoplasm. Arch Neurol 1981; 38:781–3.
15. Baloh RW, DeRossett SE, Kuncl RW, Miller NR, Cloughesy TF, Merrill J, Posner JB, Novel brainstem syndrome associated with prostate carcinoma. Neurology 1993; 43:2591–2596.

34

Neuro-Ophthalmology of Mitochondrial DNA Diseases

Donald R. Johns
Beth Israel Hospital, Massachusetts Eye and Ear Infirmary, and Harvard Medical School, Boston, Massachusetts

Kyle H. Smith
Texas A & M University School of Medicine, and Scott and White Clinic, Temple, Texas

A number of human diseases are caused by disorders of mitochondrial structure or function. The neuro-ophthalmologist may be the first physician to encounter patients with these "mitochondrial diseases" due to the prominent neuro-ophthalmological manifestations involving the afferent, cortical, and oculomotor visual systems.

Each of the mitochondrial diseases is a relatively rare entity, but as a group they appear surprisingly frequently in the referral neuro-ophthalmological population. Moreover, these diseases represent some of the first molecularly proven examples of many cardinal neurological diseases: myopathy (chronic progressive external ophthalmoplegia, CPEO), stroke (mitochondrial encephalomyopathy, lactic acidosis, and strokelike episodes, MELAS), seizures (myoclonic epilepsy and ragged red fibers, MERRF), and optic neuropathy (Leber's hereditary optic neuropathy, LHON). Our understanding of the molecular basis of these diseases has progressed rapidly since the first human diseases were definitively linked to mitochondrial DNA (mtDNA) abnormalities in 1988.

The main function of mitochondria is to produce sufficient adenosine triphosphate (ATP) to fuel the myriad energy-requiring cellular functions. Mitochondrial energy production can be deranged genetically by mutations in the nuclear DNA or mitochondrial DNA (mtDNA) genes that encode proteins involved in oxidative phosphorylation. The human mitochondrial diseases have been associated with a variety of pathogenetic mutations involving mtDNA encoded genes.

Unlike nuclear DNA that is inherited in equal proportions from both parents, mtDNA is inherited exclusively from the mother. This maternal inheritance occurs because the maternal oocyte contains hundreds of mitochondria within its cytoplasm, each with several copies of mtDNA, whereas the head of the sperm contributes no mitochondria during fertilization. Mutations of mtDNA are, therefore, transmitted from the mother to all of her children. Only the female offspring will then be able to pass the mutation on to their children.

Deletions of mtDNA, as opposed to point mutations, are generally not transmitted from one generation to the next. For this reason, diseases that are caused by mtDNA deletions (CPEO) are usually sporadic, whereas diseases that result from point mutations of mtDNA (MELAS, MERRF, and LHON) may demonstrate a maternal pattern of inheritance. Not all persons who harbor a pathogenic mtDNA point mutation will express the disease. Therefore, these mitochondrial diseases will often appear to occur sporadically despite the existence of the mutation in previous generations. The variable penetrance and expressivity of these diseases is, in part, a function of mtDNA heteroplasmy, which is a mixture of both normal and mutant mtDNA in tissue from a given patient.

Initiation of a diagnostic workup in patients with suspected mitochondrial disease depends on recognition of the phenotypic manifestations of the disease and referral for appropriate specialized testing. The simplest tests for mitochondrial dysfunction are serum or cerebrospinal fluid lactate concentrations that are often increased in patients with mitochondrial disease. Unfortunately, this increased concentration is rather insensitive and may only be present intermittently. Skeletal muscle, a relatively accessible tissue, is clinically involved in many of these disorders and is the focus of most diagnostic procedures. Electromyography can document the presence of a myopathy even in the absence of clinically overt symptoms. In vivo phosphorus magnetic resonance spectroscopy of resting muscle is a powerful tool that may detect associated metabolic abnormalities, but it is not 100% specific and is not yet widely available (1).

Skeletal muscle biopsy has remained the gold standard in the diagnosis of most mitochondrial diseases. Histochemical stains of muscle tissue may reveal evidence of abnormal proliferating mitochondria in the form of increased oxidative staining (succinic dehydrogenase, NADH dehydrogenase) or abnormal accumulations of mitochondrial membranes ("ragged red fibers" on Gomori trichrome), and they may also reveal focal areas of decreased oxidative activity (cytochrome oxidase). Light microscopy may also demonstrate specific histological features that suggest another primary etiology for the patient's muscle disease. Ultrastructural analysis may reveal more direct evidence of abnormal, proliferating mitochondria, including "parking lot" inclusions and other distinct features. Skeletal muscle is suitable for biochemical analysis by enzymatic, spectrophotometric, or oxygen electrode polarographic techniques that are available at a number of specialized centers. Most importantly, skeletal muscle biopsy provides appropriate material for the molecular genetic assays that have revolutionized the diagnostic workup of these diseases.

In this chapter, we review the basic clinical features of each of the major mitochondrial diseases with an emphasis on the molecular genetic testing now available for each of them.

I. CHRONIC PROGRESSIVE EXTERNAL OPHTHALMOPLEGIA

A. Clinical Features

One of the cardinal manifestations of human mtDNA disorders is chronic progressive external ophthalmoplegia (CPEO). CPEO manifests as a slowly progressive disorder of skeletal eye muscle that is typically symmetrical and unaccompanied by diplopia. The initial manifestation of this disorder is usually ptosis, which may bring the patient to the attention of the oculoplastic surgeon. The ophthalmoparesis is progressive and eventually results in total ophthalmoplegia. CEPO may occur in isolation or may be accompanied by a number of other ophthalmological, neurological, and systemic features: "ophthalmoplegia-plus" (2). Many patients with apparently isolated CPEO will have subtle manifestations of a limb myopathy on careful examination or electromyography. One subset of the ophthalmoplegia-plus disorders is the Kearns-Sayre syndrome, which is a disorder characterized by ophthalmoplegia, onset before 20 years of age, and pigmentary retinopathy plus at least one of the following: cardiac conduction defects, elevated cerebrospinal fluid (CSF) protein concentration (>100 mg/dl), or cerebellar ataxia (3). Many of the neurological signs in CPEO, other than ophthalmoplegia and ptosis, also are seen in other mtDNA diseases (Table 1).

Documentation of family history is crucial as oculopharyngeal dystrophy usually follows an autosomal dominant pattern of inheritance. The vast majority

Table 1 Common Neurological Manifestations of Mitochondrial Diseases

1. Sensorineural deafness
2. Myopathy with prominent fatiguability
3. Atypical pigmentary retinopathy
4. Cerebellar ataxia
5. Seizures
6. Vascular headache
7. Dementia
8. Myoclonus

of cases of CPEO occur sporadically, because mtDNA deletions, as opposed to mtDNA point mutations, are not transmissible. Exceptional cases of autosomal dominant CPEO have been documented that harbor multiple mtDNA deletions that are caused by a defective nuclear-encoded gene involved in maintaining mtDNA fidelity (4).

B. Diagnostic Tests

Laboratory evaluation of patients with presumed CPEO should include studies to evaluate other potential causes of ophthalmoplegia, including ocular myasthenia gravis (see Chap. 19), thyroid eye disease, and oculopharyngeal dystrophy. Laboratory abnormalities in CPEO include elevation in serum lactate concentration (inconsistent), myopathic potentials on electromyography of skeletal muscles, ragged red fibers on skeletal muscle biopsy, and oxidative phosphorylation defects on biochemical studies (Table 2).

C. Molecular Genetic Testing

Molecular genetic analysis of mtDNA from skeletal muscle will demonstrate large deletions in most patients with CPEO. The frequency of demonstrable mtDNA deletions depends on the presence of other features: 50% of patients with isolated CPEO harbor a deletion, whereas 80% of patients with CPEO and pigmentary retinopathy, and 90% of patients with the Kearns-Sayre syndrome have deletions. At least some of the deletion-negative patients harbor pathogenetic mtDNA point mutations in transfer RNAs (tRNAs), including the same tRNA-leucine (UUR) mutation seen in the majority of patients with MELAS syndrome (5). These deletions, which were the first proven examples of mtDNA abnormalities causing human disease, can be detected by Southern blot analysis (6) or by widely interspaced primer polymerase chain reaction (PCR) (7) (Table 3). The deletions vary markedly in size and location but 25–40% occur in the exact same location at a "hot spot" for mtDNA deletion formation (6,8). There is a poor correlation between size, location, and proportion of deleted mtDNA with the phenotypic expression or associated biochemical abnormalities.

Table 2 Laboratory Abnormalities in Mitochondrial Diseases

1. Sensorineural hearing loss on audiogram
2. Myopathic potentials on electromyography
3. Ragged red fibers in skeletal muscle biopsy
4. Cardiac conduction defects
5. Elevated serum and CSF lactate concentration
6. Oxidative phosphorylation defects on biochemical studies

Table 3 Molecular Genetic Testing for Mitochondrial Diseases

Disease	mtDNA abnormality	Tissue required	Methodology
CPEO	Deletion	Skeletal muscle biopsy (100 mg)	Southern blot (6), widely interspaced primer PCR (7)
MELAS	Point mutation at np 3243	Skeletal muscle, blood, urine	PCR-amplified mtDNA digested with: *ApaI* (5,11)
MERRF	Point mutation at np 8344	Skeletal muscle, blood, urine	Direct sequence analysis, mismatch PCR
LHON	Point mutation at a. np 11778 b. np 3460 c. np 15257 d. np 14484	Blood	PCR-amplified mtDNA digested with: a. *SfaNI/MaeIII* (29) b. *BsaHI* (22) c. *AccI* (19,29) d. Sau 3AI (23,28)

D. Management

Ptosis surgery should only be performed by a surgeon who is familiar with the special surgical limitations imposed by the facial and orbicularis oculi weakness seen in CPEO. A ptosis procedure that repositions the lid margin at a "normal" height may leave these patients with disabling exposure keratitis. Diplopia is rarely a problem due to the insidiously progressive and symmetrical nature of the CPEO.

Many patients with CPEO have systemic manifestations that may contribute to the morbidity of the disease. We recommend screening for cardiac conduction disease (electrocardiogram), diabetes mellitus, and hearing loss (audiogram). We have treated a number of patients with coenzyme Q10 (ubiquinone), 30–300 mg/day in divided doses, and have noted some anecdotal success in the treatment of limb weakness and fatiguability, but the ptosis and ophthalmoplegia have been less responsive. Patients are advised to remain physically active but to avoid exercising to the point of exhaustion to limit metabolic stress. Genetic counseling to reinforce the sporadic nature of CPEO also is important.

II. MITOCHONDRIAL ENCEPHALOMYOPATHY, LACTIC ACIDOSIS, AND STROKELIKE EPISODES SYNDROME

A. Clinical Features

The mitochondrial encephalomyopathy, lactic acidosis, and strokelike episodes (MELAS) syndrome is another mitochondrial disease that brings patients to neuro-ophthalmological attention (9). The strokelike episodes have a definite posterior preponderance, so that many patients develop cortical visual field defects (homonymous hemianopias) and cortical blindness. The strokelike episodes tend to occur in the setting of prolonged focal seizures or prolonged vascular headache. Episodic nausea and vomiting are noted intercurrently and is particularly severe at the time of the strokelike events. The strokes do not follow vascular territories and the strokes appear to be caused by an overwhelming defect in substrate utilization rather than the usual defect in substrate availability operative in occlusive vascular disease. The neurological deficits may be reversible despite demonstrable signal abnormalities on magnetic resonance imaging (MRI) studies. The availability of molecular genetic testing has broadened the clinical parameters of MELAS syndrome. The age of onset in our patients ranges from infancy to 45 years. Developmental delay and short stature may be noted in the early-onset cases. Seizures and vascular headache occur commonly. A host of other neurological accompaniments common to many mitochondrial diseases also occur, including sensorineural deafness, ataxia, pigmentary retinopathy, peripheral neuropathy, myopathy, and muscle fatiguability (see Table 1).

B. Diagnostic Tests

The laboratory evaluation of patients with possible MELAS syndrome should include studies to exclude other causes of stroke in the young. There is a mild, intermittent elevation of serum lactate concentration that may be normal between strokelike episodes. Preliminary studies suggest that an elevation of cerebrospinal fluid (CSF) lactate concentration may be a more consistent finding. Computed tomography (CT) may demonstrate basal ganglia calcification or evidence of tissue loss. MRI may reveal the signal abnormalities of new and old "infarcts" with a posterior predominance. Although less widely available, phosphorus magnetic resonance spectroscopy may demonstrate abnormalities in high-energy phosphate metabolism (10).

C. Molecular Genetic Testing

MELAS syndrome has been linked to two point mutations in the tRNA-leucine (UUR) mtDNA gene (5,11–12). The mutation at position 3243 accounts for 80–90% of patients with the MELAS phenotype and can be detected by molecular genetic analysis of PCR-amplified mtDNA that has been digested with the restriction enzyme *ApaI* (Table 3). The 3243 mutation is readily identified as it creates a restriction site for *ApaI*. The mutation was originally described in DNA extracted from muscle, but DNA derived from noninvasive tissues such as blood and urine also contains a detectable proportion of the mutation (5,13). We found the mutation in biopsied skeletal muscle in 20 families, all of whom also had the mutation in blood and urine. Analysis of skeletal muscle also provides histological confirmation of the mitochondrial abnormalities and allows determination of the associated biochemical defects.

C. Management

Recognition of the MELAS syndrome in a young stroke patient may dramatically alter the extent and nature of the diagnostic workup and management. The exercise limitations noted above for CPEO are even more important in this disease. Since many of the strokelike episodes occur in the setting of prolonged seizures, we recommend aggressive treatment of the seizure disorder with vigilant attention to anticonvulsant levels. Carbamazepine and valproate are commonly used, whereas phenytoin is used when parenteral therapy is required. We prefer calcium channel blockers, especially verapamil sustained release, for treatment of the commonly associated vascular headaches. Genetic counseling must be individualized in each family and can be supplemented with molecular genetic testing of noninvasive tissues from maternal relatives. The majority of cases are sporadic, but mild, oligosymptomatic manifestations may be seen in some maternal relatives. One important goal of genetic counseling is to assure an affected male proband that he will not pass the disorder to his offspring because of the strict maternal transmission of mtDNA. His maternal relatives are at risk for the disorder and the females may also act as carriers.

There is no definitive treatment available for the biochemical defect underlying the MELAS syndrome, but experimental agents are available that act as electron shuttles to bypass a blockage in the electron transport chain. Antioxidants, free radical scavengers, and enzyme cofactors of oxidative phosphorylation may also be useful. Evaluation of the efficacy of therapy is difficult, because the natural history of MELAS syndrome is notoriously variable with a propensity for spontaneous remissions.

III. MYOCLONIC EPILEPSY AND RAGGED RED FIBERS

Myoclonic epilepsy and ragged red fibers (MERRF) is the third major mitochondrial encephalomyopathy to have its molecular basis identified in recent years. The neuro-opthalmological features are less prominent than in the other mitochondrial diseases but can include pigmentary retinopathy and optic atrophy. The dominant clinical symptoms are progressive myoclonus epilepsy and ataxia. A peculiar form of respiratory insufficiency is seen in the most severe cases (14). Some of the associated neurological manifestations of mitochondrial diseases (see Table 1), including deafness, myopathy, and dementia, are also seen. Phosphorus magnetic resonance spectroscopy has demonstrated abnormalities in skeletal muscle but not in brain tissue of these patients (15). MERRF is caused by a point mutation in the tRNA-lysine gene at position 8344 that can be detected by molecular genetic methods in skeletal muscle, blood, and urine (14) (see Table 3).

IV. LEBER'S HEREDITARY OPTIC NEUROPATHY

A. Clinical Features

Leber's hereditary optic neuropathy (LHON) was the first human disease shown to be caused by a heritable defect in mtDNA (16). Four primary pathogenetic mtDNA mutations and several secondary mtDNA mutations have been associated with LHON (16–24). The core clinical phenotype is that of a painless optic neuropathy occurring in an otherwise healthy young person (25–28). Loss of central vision may occur rapidly or may slowly progress for several months. Visual symptoms often affect only one eye initially but virtually always involve both eyes within 1 year. Most patients become symptomatic in the third or fourth decade of life, with a mean age at onset of 23 years (range 6–70 years). Men are affected much more frequently than women (male:female ratio = 2–3:1). As most patients with molecularly proven LHON have no documented family history of visual loss, one should not be dissuaded from the diagnosis of LHON in the absence of a suggestive family history.

The visual loss is severe, with a nadir of visual acuity ranging from 20/200 to hand motions and is accompanied by central or cecocentral scotomas. The funduscopic findings at the onset of visual loss are variable. The classic triad of circumpapillary telangiectatic microangiopathy, "pseudoedema" of the peripapillary nerver fiber layer, and absence of leakage of the telangiectatic vessels on fluorescein angiography is often observed, but the ophthalmoscopic examination in the acute phase may also be entirely normal. Optic atrophy eventually supervenes in the chronic phase. Significant recovery of visual acuity is noted in some patients and is more commonly associated with certain LHON genotypes (26–28). Other neurological accompaniments are infrequent and include peripheral neuropathy and demyelinating disease.

B. Diagnostic Tests

The major diagnostic errors made in patients who are eventually molecularly proven to have LHON include atypical optic neuritis and "toxic-nutritional amblyopia." Therefore, LHON should be considered in any patient with an atypical optic neuritis (painless, bilateral, no recovery) or a presumed toxic or nutritional optic neuropathy. Other causes of acute optic neuropathy, including compressive lesions, should be evaluated with the appropriate laboratory and neuroimaging studies. In contrast to the other mitochondrial diseases discussed above, there is usually no overt biochemical or histological evidence of dysfunction of oxidative phosphorylation. The most important dictum for the workup of suspected LHON is to have a high index of suspicion and to order appropriate molecular genetic testing (see Table 3).

C. Molecular Genetic Testing

The availability of reliable molecular genetic testing has revolutionized the diagnosis of LHON. Three primary pathogenetic mtDNA mutations have been described to date in LHON, and each can be readily detected with molecular genetic techniques (see Table 3) The first mutation at nucleotide position 11,778 ("11,778 mutation") in the ND-4 gene accounts for 50% of our cases and can be detected with 100% sensitivity and specificity by the simultaneous loss of an *SfaNI* restriction site and gain of an *MaeIII* restriction site (29). These tests, like those described below for the other two primary mtDNA mutations, are performed on PCR-amplified mtDNA that is extracted from a routine blood sample. Although rare exceptions have been noted (30), the 11,778 mutation is a very poor prognostic sign for significant recovery of visual acuity.

The second pathogenetic mtDNA mutation occurs at nucleotide 3460 in the ND-1 gene and accounts for 8% of our cases of LHON (17–18,22). It is detected by the loss of a *BsaHI* restriction site. Our analysis of the clinical phenotype associated with this mutation revealed three major differences when compared with the phenotype of patients with the 11,778 mutation (26). Patients with the 3460 mutation have a much better prognosis for visual recovery (21% of eyes versus 4%), are more likely to have a positive family history of visual loss compatible with LHON (86 versus 43%) and have a high incidence of tobacco and alcohol abuse. Indeed, tobacco-alcohol amblyopia was the major source of diagnostic confusion in these patients. The use of tobacco and alcohol are the only known potentially modifiable risk factors for visual loss in this disease. However, preliminary data suggest that a variety of metabolic abnormalities, such as poorly controlled diabetes mellitus and hyperlipidemia, and other environmental factors may play a role in the pathogenesis of LHON.

A third pathogenetic mtDNA mutation has been identified at nucleotide 15,257 in the cytochrome *b* gene of complex III of oxidative phosphorylation, which makes this type of LHON the first known human disease involving a defect in complex III (19–20). It is readily detected by the loss of an *AccI* restriction site. Patients with this mutation appear to have a better prognosis for visual recovery than patients with the more common 11,778 mutation and have a higher incidence of neurological accompaniments, particularly spinal cord and peripheral nerve involvement (27). A secondary mutation at nucleotide 15,812 in cytochrome *b* occurs in about 50% of 15,257-positive families and appears to prevent significant recovery of visual acuity (27).

A fourth primary LHON-associated mtDNA mutation has been discovered at nucleotide 14,484 in ND-6 gene that appears to be the second most common primary mutation (23). This mutation is associated with the best prognosis for visual recovery among the primary LHON-associated mtDNA mutations, nearly 10-fold better than that associated with the 11,778 mutation (28). Two allelic mutations in the COX III gene at nucleotides 9438 and 9804 have also recently been reported in association with LHON (24).

Molecular genetic testing for each of the four primary mtDNA mutations had 100% specificity in our series of 200 families with the LHON phenotype but was only approximately 80% sensitive (29). One major thrust of LHON research is to discover the responsible pathogenetic mtDNA mutation in the remaining 20% of cases. Eventually molecular genetic testing for LHON should approach 100% sensitivity and specificity. This testing has proven useful in a number of different settings, including confirmation of the diagnosis in probable cases and establishment of the diagnosis in atypical or obscure cases. In addition to expediting the diagnostic workup of LHON, molecular genetic testing has implications for family counseling, risk factor intervention, prognosis for visual recovery, and therapy.

D. Management

Careful assessment of coexistent potential risk factors for visual loss by historical (tobacco, alcohol, illicit drug use, environmental exposures) and laboratory (hyperlipidemia, diabetes mellitus) means is the cornerstone of a rational intervention strategy. These strategies would be most useful when applied to at risk maternal relatives. Coexistent systemic abnormalities that are occasionally associated with LHON such as cardiac conduction defects, migraine, and peripheral neuropathy should be recognized and treated appropriately. Referrals for genetic counseling and low-vision assessment also are important in the management of patients with LHON. Although no therapeutic "magic bullet" is yet available, precise knowledge about the molecular etiology will guide future therapeutic developments and will allow us to avoid inappropriate treatment.

V. NOVEL MITOCHONDRIAL DISEASE PHENOTYPES

The four disorders discussed above were for many years thought to have a mitochondrial etiology due to inheritance patterns and morphological and biochemical characteristics. Recent advances in molecular genetics established their precise etiological basis. More recently, a number of novel mitochondrial disease phenotypes have been identified on the basis of mtDNA defects. Two of these syndromes have prominent neuro-ophthalmological features.

A family in England has been described with the phenotype of peripheral neuropathy, ataxia, retinitis pigmentosa, seizures, developmental delay, and dementia (NARP) (31). The retinal lesions mimicked those seen in classic retinitis pigmentosa and thus differed from the "atypical" pigmentary retinopathy seen in other mitochondrial diseases. The family was shown to harbor a heteroplasmic mutation at nucleotide 8993 in the ATPase 6 gene of complex V of oxidative phosphorylation. This mutation is readily detected in PCR-amplified mtDNA from blood or muscle by the creation of an *AvaI* restriction site.

We have identified a brother and sister who presented with a subacute optic neuropathy and myelopathy (32) at ages 10 and 14. Both eventually had recovery of visual acuity in each eye from 20/400 to 20/40 but were left with a residual spastic paraparesis. The brother had recurrence of a steroid-responsive cervical myelopathy, but his vision did not deteriorate further. There was no laboratory evidence of demyelinating disease and no family history of a similar disorder. In vitro analysis of mitochondria isolated from the brother's skeletal muscle showed an abnormality in mtDNA-encoded protein synthesis. Two mtDNA mutations of presumed pathogenetic significance were found in the tRNA-aspartate gene and second subunit of cytochrome oxidase (COX II) gene of complex IV of oxidative phosphorylation.

VI. CONCLUSIONS

Molecular genetic analysis of mtDNA in human disease has had a rapid and profound impact on a number of different diseases that are of primary interest to the neuro-ophthalmologist. These molecular genetic advances have been rapidly translated from the laboratory bench to the bedside of the patient with neuro-ophthalmological disease. Although the diseases covered in this chapter were discussed as separate entities, many of the patients have clinical and laboratory features that overlap (see Tables 1 and 2). The neuro-ophthalmologist is in a pivotal position to recognize these patients and guide their diagnosis and management. Many patients with mitochondrial diseases will present with partial or novel phenotypes and will require a high index of suspicion from an astute clinician. We anticipate that molecular genetic advances in the near future will allow us to definitively diagnose more of these challenging patients.

REFERENCES

1. Matthews PM, Allaire C, Shoubridge EA, Karpati G, Carpenter S, Arnold DL. In vivo muscle magnetic resonance spectroscopy in the clinical investigation of mitochondrial disease. Neurology 1991: 41:114–1201.

2. Drachman DA. Ophthalmoplegia-plus: the neurodegenerative disorders associate with progressive external ophthalmoplegia. Arch Neurol 1968; 18:654–674.
3. Rowland LP. Progressive external ophthalmoplegia. Handb Clin Neurol 1975; 22:177–202.
4. Zeviani M, Servidei S, Gellera C, Bertini E, DiMauro S, DiDonato S. An autosomal dominant disorder with multiple deletions of mitochondrial DNA starting at the D-loop region. Nature 1989; 339:309–11.
5. Johns DR, Hurko O. Mitochondrial leucine tRNA mutation in neurological diseases. Lancet 1991; 1:927–8.
6. Johns DR, Rutledge SL, Stine OC, Hurko O. Directly repeated sequences associated with pathogenic mitochondrial DNA deletions. Proc. Natl Acad Sci (USA) 1989; 86:8059–62.
7. Johns DR, Hurko O. Preferential amplification and molecular characterization of junction sequences of a pathogenetic deletion in human mitochondrial DNA. Genomics 1989; 5:623–8.
8. Moraes CT, DiMauro S, Zeviani M, et al. Mitochondrial DNA deletions in progressive external ophthalmoplegia and Kearns-Sayre syndrome. N Engl J Med 1989; 320:1293–9.
9. Pavlakis S, Phillips PC, DiMauro S, DeVivo DC, Rowland LP. Mitochondrial myopathy, encephalopathy, lactic acidosis, and strokelike episodes: a distinctive clinical syndrome. Ann Neurol 1984; 16:481–8.
10. Eleff SM,, Barker PB, Blackband SJ, Chatham JC, Lutz NW, Johns DR, Bryan RN, Hurko O. Phosphorus magnetic resonance spectroscopy of patients with mitochondrial cytopathies demonstrates decreased levels of brain phosphocreatine. Ann Neurol 1990; 27:626–30.
11. Goto Y, Nonaka I, Horai S. A mutation in the tRNA (leu) (UUR) gene associated with the MELAS subgroup of mitochondrial encephalomyopathies. Nature 1990; 348:651–3.
12. Goto Y, Nonaka I, Horai S. A new mtDNA mutation associated with mitochondrial myopathy, encephalopathy, lactic acidosis and stroke-like episodes (MELAS). Biochim Biophys Acta 1991; 1092:238–40.
13. Hammons SR, Sweeney MG, Brockington M, Morgan-Hughes JA, Harding AE. Mitochondrial encephalopathies: molecular genetic diagnosis from blood samples. Lancet 1991; 1:1311–3.
14. Shoffner JM, Lott MT, Lezza AM, et al. Myoclonic epilepsy and ragged red fiber disease (MERRF) is associated with a mitochondrial DNA tRNA (lys) mutation. Cell 1990; 931–7.
15. Matthews PM, Berkovic SF, Shoubridge EA, Andermann F, Karpati G, Carpenter S, Arnold DL. In vivo magnetic resonance spectroscopy of brain and muscle in a type of mitochondrial encephalomyopathy (MERRF). Ann Neurol 1991; 29:435–438.15.
16. Wallace DC, Singh G, Lott MT, Hodge JA, Schurr TG, Lezza AMS, Elsas LJ, Nikoskelainen EK. Mitochondrial DNA mutation associated with Leber's hereditary optic neuropathy. Science 1988; 242:1427–30.
17. Huoponen K, Vilkki J, Aula P, Nikoskelainen EK, Savontaus ML. A new mtDNA mutation associated with Leber hereditary optic neuroretinopathy. Am J Hum Genet 1991; 48:1147–53.

18. Howell N, Bindoff LA, McCullough DA, Dubacka I, Poulton J, Mackey D, Taylor L, Turnbull DM. Leber hereditary optic neuropathy: identification of the same mitochondrial ND1 mutation in six pedigrees. Am J Hum Genet 1991; 49:939–50.
19. Johns DR, Neufeld MJ. Cytochrome b mutations in Leber hereditary optic neuropathy. Biochem Biophys Res Commun 1991; 181:1358–64.
20. Brown MD, Voljavec AS, Lott MT, Torroni A, Yang CC, Wallace DC. Mitochondrial DNA complex I and III mutations associated with Leber's hereditary optic neuropathy. Genetics 1992; 130:163–73.
21. Johns DR, Berman J. Alternative, simultaneous Complex I mitochondrial DNA mutations in Leber's hereditary optic neuropathy. Biochem Biophys Res Commun 1991; 174:1324–30.
22. Johns DR. Mitochondrial ND-1 mutation in Leber hereditary optic neuropathy. Am J Hum Genet 1992; 50:872–4.
23. Johns DR, Neufeld MJ, Park RD. An ND-6 mitochondrial DNA mutation associated with Leber hereditary optic neuropathy. Biochem Biophys Res Commun 1992; 187:1551–57.
24. Johns DR, Neufeld MJ. Cytochrome *c* oxidase mutations in Leber hereditary optic neuropathy. Biochem Biophys Res Commun 1993; 196:810–15.
25. Newman NJ, Lott MT, Wallace DC. The clinical characteristics of pedigrees of Leber's hereditary optic neuropathy with the 11,778 mutation. Am J Ophthalmol 1991; 111:750–62.
26. Johns DR, Smith KH, Miller NR. Leber's hereditary optic neuropathy: clinical manifestations of the 3460 mutation. Arch Ophthalmol 1992; 110:1577–81.
27. Johns DR, Smith KH, Savino PJ, Miller NR. Leber's hereditary optic neuropathy: clinical manifestations of the 15257 mutation. Ophthalmology 1993; 100:981–86.
28. Johns DR, Heher KL, Miller NR, Smith KH. Leber's hereditary optic neuropathy: clinical manifestations of the 14484 mutation. Arch Ophthalmol 1993; 111:495–98.
29. Johns DR, Neufeld MJ. Pitfalls in the molecular genetic diagnosis of Leber's hereditary optic neuropathy. Am J Hum Genet 1993; 53:916–20.
30. Stone EM, Newman NJ, Miller NR, Johns DR, Lott MT, Wallace DC. Visual recovery in patients with Leber's hereditary optic neuropathy and the 11778 mutation. J Clin Neuro Ophthalmol 1992; 12:10–14.
31. Holt IJ, Harding AE, Petty RK, Morgan-Hughes JA. A new mitochondrial disease associated with mitochondrial DNA heteroplasmy. Am J Hum Genet 1990; 46:428–33.
32. Johns DR, Hurko O, Griffin JW, Attardi G. Molecular basis of a new mitochondrial disease: acute optic neuropathy and myelopathy. Ann Neurol 1991; 30:234.

35

Diseases of the Basal Ganglia

Christopher Kennard
Charing Cross and Westminster Medical School, London, England

The main clinical manifestations of diseases of the basal ganglia are disorders of axial and limb movement, and from a neuroophthalmological point of view, a wide variety of disturbances of eye movements have been reported (1) since Westphal reported oculomotor abnormalities in Huntington's disease in 1863 (2). Analysis of eye movements in, for example, a patient with a rigid-akinetic syndrome now forms an integral part of the overall clinical examination contributing to the final pathological diagnosis. Although eye movements are important to examine as they are frequently abnormal, other clinical features of relevance are facial expression, frequency of blinking, and visual function itself. The latter has only recently been shown to be disturbed in Parkinson's disease and may explain why these patients sometimes complain of deteriorating vision.

I. CLASSIFICATION OF BASAL GANGLIA DISEASES

The basal ganglia include the striatum (caudate nucleus and putamen), the subthalamic nucleus, and the outflow structures, the globus pallidus and substantia nigra. Recent anatomical and physiological findings have led to the concept that the basal ganglia serve to integrate inputs from widespread cortical areas and funnel these influences via the thalamus to the motor cortex. However, it appears that inputs are kept segregated, so there are specific circuits each serving different functions, such as somatomotor or oculomotor function (3). Although the precise role played by the basal ganglia in normal movement is still not fully understood, it is possible to distinguish two major motor outcomes of basal ganglia disease. These are the akinetic-rigid syndrome of parkinsonism and abnormal involuntary movements or dyskinesias. There are a large number of different diseases that can give rise to these two types of movement disorder (Table 1).

II. AKINETIC-RIGID SYNDROMES

Disturbances of the basal ganglia commonly give rise to inability to move (akinesia) and slowness of movement (bradykinesia) associated with muscular

Table 1 Causes of Akinetic-Rigid Syndrome and Dyskinesias

Akinetic-Rigid Syndrome
Pure parkinsonism
Parkinson's disease
Post-encephalitic parkinsonism
Drug-induced parkinsonism
Parkinsonism-plus
Progressive supranuclear palsy
Multiple system atrophy
Olivopontocerebellar atrophy
Strionigral degeneration
Shy-Drager syndrome
Corticobasal ganglionic degeneration
Basal ganglia calcification
Parkinsonism in Dementia
Alzheimer's disease
Lewy body disease
Cerebrovascular disease
Multi-infarct
Binswanger
Head injury
Anoxia
Hydrocephalus
Dyskinesias
Huntington's disease
Wilson's disease
Drug-induced
Cerebral palsy
Torsion dystonia
Myoclonus

rigidity. These features along with rest tremor are the hallmarks of ideopathic Parkinson's disease, in which there is an abnormal dopaminergic input to the striatum. Many other pathologies, however, can give rise to an akinetic-rigid syndrome. For example, extensive damage to the striatum, as in Wilson's disease and strionigral degeneration, or damage to the output zones of the basal ganglia, as in progressive supranuclear palsy and the progressive pallidal degenerations. Finally, diffuse cerebral conditions, as in Alzheimer's disease and diffuse cerebrovascular disease, can give rise to the same syndrome.

Unfortunately, there are no neuro-ophthalmological signs that allow precise differentiation between these various pathologies except for the intermittent oculogyric crises that are only seen in postencephalitic parkinsonism.

A. Facial Expression and Eyelid Function

Patients with all forms of parkinsonism often exhibit a lack of facial expression, which has been described as passive or "wooden." This may be associated with a prominent stare, probably due to a paucity of spontaneous eye movements. Normal individuals usually make on average about 16 blinks per minute, which in more severe Parkinson's disease may fall to as few as 2 per minute (4). The glabellar tap sign, in which there is an inability to suppress eye blinks in response to repeated glabellar taps, was once thought to be pathognomonic of Parkinson's disease but has now been shown to be a nonspecific sign found in a wide variety of conditions of generalized cerebral pathology.

Spontaneous blepharospasm is rare in Parkinson's disease but is common and disabling in postencephalitic disease when a patient's eye may remain shut for several seconds or even minutes, and the examiner may find it difficult to raise the lids with the fingers.

Some patients may have difficulty in voluntarily opening their eyes in the absence of any visible activity in the orbicularis oculi. Indeed, the brow may be raised sharply (Collier's sign) and the frontalis actively contracted in an effort to open the eyes. This condition has been called apraxia of eyelid opening, although using the term *apraxia* in the presence of a motor deficit seems inappropriate. It is considered to be due to a sustained inhibition of the levator palpabrae (5). This disorder is most commonly seen in progressive supranuclear palsy. A facial expression sometimes seen in this condition is one of surprise or perplexity due to widely opened eyes associated with a hyperactive frontalis muscle or a fixed smile or grin (6).

B. Eye Movements

1. Fixation and Convergence

Square wave jerks (SWJs) are saccadic intrusions observed during fixation. They are 1 degree or more in amplitude directed away from fixation, followed some

200 ms later by a saccade of equal but opposite direction returning gaze to the fixation point. They can be observed by clinical observation, and they occur in normal individuals at a rate of approximately 3/min. SWJs occur at an increased frequency in a number of diseases, including cerebellar disease, Huntington's disease, and Alzheimer's disease. An abnormally high frequency of SWJs has been found in patients with progressive supranuclear palsy and parkinsonism-plus (>10/min) but in very few of a large group of patients with ideopathic Parkinson's disease (7).

Convergence accommodation is often impaired from the early stages in Parkinson's disease and may cause disturbances of near vision, which may be aggravated by anticholinergic drugs. It may also cause diplopia for near objects, although there is no paresis of external ocular muscles.

2. *Vertical Gaze*

In attempting to differentiate a patient with Parkinson's disease from one with parkinsonism-plus or progressive supranuclear palsy, probably the most useful part of the bedside examination of eye movements is an evaluation of vertical gaze. Despite early studies that suggested up gaze was limited in Parkinson's disease (8), more recent studies (9) and clinical experience have shown that it is in fact normal. Disturbances of vertical gaze are, however, a common feature of other parkinsonian syndromes, in particular progressive supranuclear palsy. In this condition, there is usually an impairment of voluntary down gaze, with slow and then small amplitude saccades prior to involvement of up gaze saccades. This progresses with restricted vertical gaze of supranuclear type such that oculocephalic maneuvers give rise to a full range of ocular excursion. As the disease progresses, so horizontal movements are similarly involved, with an eventual oculomotor paralysis. Unfortunately, a number of the akinetic-rigid syndromes also give rise to impaired vertical gaze such as corticobasal degeneration, although in these cases usually up gaze is more impaired than down gaze.

The hallmark of postencephalitic parkinsonism is oculogyric crises, in which there are episodes of sustained involuntary upward and lateral gaze. The magnitude of the deviation varies from extreme to minimal. These episodes are associated with an increase in rigidity, marked diaphoresis, and tremor, they last for a few minutes or hours, and end spontaneously. Although never seen in ideopathic Parkinson's disease and now rarely seen in patients following encephalitis, oculogyric crises may be encountered in acute neuroleptic-induced extrapyramidal reactions.

3. *Horizontal Gaze*

Although examination of horizontal saccades and smooth pursuit may not be a helpful in differentiating Parkinson's disease from other akinetic-rigid syndromes, it nonetheless often reveals abnormalities. When tested at the bedside, it is often commented that in Parkinson's disease saccades between two targets are frequently of reduced amplitude (hypometric), with the main saccade being followed by a series of small saccades before fixation of the target is achieved. In laboratory conditions, however, in mild to moderately affected patients, reflexive saccades to the sudden appearance a target is normal. It is in more volitional saccadic paradigms, such as saccades to a remembered target or to a predictable target that have revealed hypometric saccades in Parkinson's disease (10). Unfortunately, it is not possible to reproduce these paradigms at the bedside.

One further paradigm that has recently been successfully transposed from the laboratory to the clinic is the antisaccade paradigm (11). In this task, a peripheral target (e.g., a raised finger) is presented to the subject, who has been instructed to direct the gaze to an equal and opposite (mirror image) position. Normal subjects, with a few instruction trials, are able to perform this task fairly accurately. About 10–15% of trials will, however, be errors in which the subject makes a saccade reflexively to the target rather than away from it. In Parkinson's disease, the error rate is not raised, but in progressive supranuclear palsy, the error rate may be as high as 90% (12). Raised error rates are, however, found in other disorders such as Huntington's disease and Alzheimer's disease and in patients with lesions of the prefrontal cortex.

Smooth pursuit in Parkinson's disease also is abnormal owing to a reduced gain resulting in catch-up saccades. This gives the pursuit a jerky appearance, and it has been described as "cogwheel pursuit" by analogy with the cogwheel rigidity found in the somatomotor system (8). Since the neurophysiological mechanisms for these two motor system abnormalities are entirely different, this analogy seems inappropriate. However, a similar abnormality of smooth pursuit is found in a number of different neurological disorders both of the basal ganglia and elsewhere.

A useful, but not absolute, pointer to the diagnosis of ideopathic Parkinson's disease, as opposed to other causes of the akinetic-rigid syndrome, is a beneficial response to treatment with L-dopa. Unfortunately, in clinical practice, it is unusual to note any improvement in pursuit eye movements unless the patient is profoundly akinetic or in an "off" state.

C. Visual Function

It is not uncommon for patients with Parkinson's disease, particularly in the later stages of the disease, to complain of difficulties with vision; for example, when reading. Since Parkinson's disease is considered a disorder of motor function, these complaints at first sight appear difficult to relate to the disease process. This view is further supported by finding no acuity changes after careful refraction. It is only since the introduction of tests of contrast sensitivity (CS) that hidden visual defects have been uncovered. These tests, using sinusoidal gratings as targets, have revealed that patients with Parkinson's disease have an impairment in their ability to detect patterns of a certain size, which does not have any effect on visual acuity. They show reduced sensitivity to gratings of intermediate frequency (13). Additional tests have shown that not only is there a defect in spatial tuning functions but also one of temporal function (14). These defects are probably related to disturbance of the dopamine amacrine cells in the retina, which is supported by abnormalities in the electroretinogram and visual evoked responses.

D. Conclusions

Although the neuro-ophthalmological examination can be most revealing in patients with Parkinson's disease and other akinetic-rigid syndromes, few of the abnormalities clearly differentiate one disease from another. Repeated examination, particularly of eye movements, over time may be rewarding and indicate that a previously diagnosed case of Parkinson's disease in fact has progressive supranuclear palsy or one of the multiple system atrophies.

III. THE DYSKINESIAS

Diseases of the basal ganglia also can give rise to a wide variety of abnormal involuntary movements. For clinical purposes, these dyskinesias can be divided into five categories: (1) tremors; (2) chorea and ballism; (3) myoclonus; (4) tics; and (5) dystonias. The differential diagnosis of patients presenting with various forms of dyskinesia is usually determined by the precise nature of the abnormal movements, age of onset, family and drug history, and laboratory tests. Apart from abnormal eye movements in Huntington's disease, the neuro-ophthalmological examination is usually unrewarding with the important exception of Wilson's disease, a disorder of copper metabolism, in which the Kayser-Fleischer (K-F) ring is a pathognomonic sign. This is a gray-brown ring of copper located at the periphery of the cornea in Descemet's membrane. It is best visualized with a slit lamp but may be recognized by direct illumination. The sunflower cataract is the other classic, but much less common, ocular abnormality in this condition. Since Wilson's disease is eminently treatable a search for a K-F ring in patients with unexplained movement disorders should always be performed, as it is almost always found in cases presenting with a neurological as opposed to a hepatic syndrome. Other tests, including serum caeruloplasmin and copper levels, confirm the diagnosis.

A. Facial Expression and Eyelid Function

Observation of facial movements and expression may be helpful in this group of disorders. Eye blinking occurs frequently as part of the upper facial involvement of chorea (the "seductive winking") in Huntington's disease, but the rigid variant often presents with a masklike wide-eyed facies. In fully developed Wilson's disease, the face is relatively expressionless except for a fixed snarling smile.

Cranial dystonia, known eponomously as either the syndrome of Meige or Breughel, consists of three recognizable components that may appear separately or in combination. They are blepharospasm, oromandibular dystonia, and laryngeal dystonia, but only blepharospasm will be discussed further. Blepharospasm consists of spasms of the orbicularis oculi that cause eye closure. At the beginning of the disease, blepharoclonus or repetitive excessive eye blinking may be all that is evident. As it progresses, true muscular spasms, sometimes only unilateral at first, occur intermittently. These spasms, which tend to occur later in the day, may be provoked by bright sunlight, television, reading, fatigue, crossing the road or driving, or by stress and anxiety. With time the spasms become more frequent and of longer duration and sometimes result in functional blindness. Some patients develop trick movements or actions such as touching an eyelid or the forehead that may suppress the spasms for a period of time. The treatment of this condition is dealt with in Chapter 30.

Patients with Giles de la Tourette syndrome may show blepharospasm and eye tics that include involuntary gaze deviations, but formal testing of eye movements have found them to be normal.

B. Eye Movements

1. Fixation and Accommodation

Patients with Huntington's disease often show impaired fixation due to saccadic intrusions, square wave jerks. This is particularly evident when the patients view a structured background. Larger irregular to-and-fro jerks of changing amplitude and direction have also been reported.

2. Vertical and Horizontal Gaze

A disturbance of voluntary gaze, particularly saccades, is often found in Huntington's disease. Saccades made on command may show a prolonged latency, and often an obligatory blink or head turn is used to start the eyes moving. The saccades, once initiated, are usually hypometric. Later in the course of the disease, they become slow, initially in the vertical plane and subsequently also in the horizontal plane (15). In cases of chorea due to nondegenerative conditions or tardive dyskinesia, such vertical slowing is not observed (16).

In Huntington's disease, laboratory testing of saccades has revealed a number of abnormalities (17,18), of which the excessively high error rate in the antisaccade task is the most notable.

Considering the degree of involvement of the basal ganglia in Wilson's disease, the extent of eye movement abnormality is relatively small. A few cases of slowed saccades and limitation of up gaze have been reported, but these cases are the exception rather than the rule.

There are no specific eye movement disorders that have been observed in other dyskinetic basal ganglia disorders such as torsion dystonia and myoclonus.

C. Conclusions

Despite the marked disturbances observed in the axial and limb musculature in the dyskinesias, there are surprisingly few well-documented abnormal neuro-ophthalmological features apart from the K-F rings in Wilson's disease and the ocular motor deficits in Huntington's disease.

REFERENCES

1. Kennard C, Lueck CJ. Oculomotor abnormalities in diseases of the basal ganglia. Rev Neurol (Paris) 1989; 145:587–95.
2. Westphal C. Ueber eine dem Bilde der Cerebrospinalen grauen Degeneration ähnliche Erkrankung des Centralen Nervensystems ohne Anatomischen Befund nebst Bemerkung über paradoxe Contraction. Arch Psych Nervenkrank 1883; 14:87–134.
3. Alexander GE. DeLong MR, Strick PL. Parallel organization of functionally segregated circuits linking basal ganglia and cortex. Ann Rev Neurosci 1986; 9:357–81.
4. Karson CN, LeWitt PA, Calne DB, Wyatt RJ. Blink rates in parkinsonism. Ann Neurol 1982; 12:580–83.
5. Lepore F, Duvoisin RC. "Apraxia" of eyelid opening. An involuntary levator inhibition. Neurology 1985; 35:423–27.
6. Jankovic J. Progressive supranuclear palsy; clinical and pharmacological update. Neurol Clin 1984; 2:473–86.
7. Rascol O, Sabatini U, Simonetta-Moreau M, Montastruc JL, Rascol A, Clanet M. Square wave jerks in parkinsonian syndromes. J Neurol Neurosurg Psychiatry 1991; 54:599–602.
8. Corin MS, Elizan TS, Bender MB. Oculomotor function in patients with Parkinson's disease. J Neurol Sci 1972; 15:251–65.
9. Tanyeri S, Lueck CJ, Crawford TJ, Kennard C. Vertical and horizontal saccadic eye movements in Parkinson's disease. Neuro-ophthalmology 1989; 9:165–77.
10. Crawford TJ, Henderson L, Kennard C. Abnormalities of non-visually guided eye movements in Parkinson's disease. Brain 1989; 112:1573–86.
11. Currie J, Ramsden B., McArthur C, Maruff P. Validation of a clinical antisaccade eye movement test in the assessment of dementia. Arch Neurol 1991; 48:644–48.
12. Pierrot-Deseilligny C, Rivaud S, Pillon B, Fournier E, Agid Y. Lateral visually-guided saccades in progressive supranuclear palsy. Brain 1989; 112:471–87.
13. Bulens C, Meerwaldt JD, Van der Wildt GJ, Keemink CJ. Contrast sensitivity in Parkinson's disease. Neurology 1986; 36:1121–5.

14. Bodis-Wollner I, Marx MS, Mitra S, Bobak P, Mylin L, Yahr M. Visual dysfunction in Parkinson's disease. Brain 1987; 110:1675–98.
15. Hotson JR, Louis AA, Langston EB, Moreno JA. Vertical saccades in Huntington's disease and nondegenerative choreoathetoid disorders. Neuro-ophthalmology 1984; 4:207–17.
16. Leigh RJ, Newman SA, Folstein SE, Lasker AG, Jenson BA. Abnormal ocular motor control in Huntington's disease. Neurology 1983; 33:1268–75.
17. Lasker AG, Zee DS, Hain TC, Folstein SE, Singer HS. Saccades in Huntington's disease: initiation defects and distractibility. Neurology 1987; 37:364–70.
18. Lasker AG, Zee DS, Hain TC, Folstein SE, Singer HS. Saccades in Huntington's disease: slowing and dysmetria. Neurology 1988; 38:427–31.

36

Progressive Supranuclear Palsy

Frederick E. Lepore
University of Medicine and Dentistry of New Jersey/Robert Wood Johnson Medical School, New Brunswick, New Jersey

I. DIAGNOSIS

Although superficially masquerading as Parkinson's disease (PD) to the unwary clinician, progressive supranuclear palsy (PSP) is a distinct degenerative disorder characterized by usual onset in the seventh decade of life, bradykinesia, postural instability, axial rigidity, pseudobulbar signs, cognitive slowing, and abnormal supranuclear regulation of ocular and eyelid movements (1). Men and women are affected with equal frequency. PSP is commonly heralded by progressive gait difficulties with falling. The median survival time from onset of symptoms is 6 years.

PSP can be distinguished from PD by absence of tremor and symmetrical onset. Patients with PSP differ from their PD counterparts, who exhibit facial hypomimia in contrast to the "startled" facial expression of PSP. The erect posture and neck hyperextension of patients with PSP is dissimilar to the stooped "simian" posture of PD. Unlike the short shuffling steps of patients with PD, those with PSP have a wide-based unsteady gait.

The progressive dysarthria, dysphagia, and, less frequently, emotional incontinence of PSP has been attributed to pseudobulbar palsy. Controversy surrounds the cognitive impairment of PSP, which has been variously described as bradyphrenia or a "subcortical" dementia lacking the classic cortical deficits of aphasia, apraxia, agnosia, or memory loss. Other investigators propose that neuropsychological impairment of PSP is confined to tasks dependent on acquiring visual information and is not a dementia.

Striking ophthalmoplegia underlies this impaired acquisition of visual information and readily identifies most patients with PSP. The earliest ocular symptoms include blurred vision, difficulty focusing, and inability to look downward. In their original description Steele, Richardson, and Olzewski established the supranuclear character of this disordered ocular motility by observing "a loss of conjugate vertical gaze to command and in following and attraction movements. The eyes moved fully when gaze was fixed and the head passively moved" (2). The initial vertical gaze deficit is the onset of slow and later hypometric downward saccades. Later, the saccadic palsy is apparent on upward and lateral gaze. Eventually nuclear ophthalmoplegia may ensue, and the eyes become immovable to any gaze strategy or reflex ocular movement, including Bell's phenomenon (3). Additional abnormalities of the clinical ocular motility examination include:

1. Frequent square wave jerks
2. Saccadic or jerky pursuit
3. Hypoactive vestibulo-ocular reflex
4. Abnormal cancellation of vestibulo-ocular reflex
5. Loss of convergence
6. Tonic deviation without nystagmus on caloric testing
7. Impaired optokinetic nystagmus

There is an abundance of eyelid abnormalities in PSP, beginning with the "startled" expression, which may reflect the combination of upward gaze paresis and intact lid elevation. Spontaneous blink rate is greatly reduced at three blinks/min. In 18% of patients with PSP, we found involuntary levator ("apraxia" of lid opening) inhibition characterized by:

1. Transitory inability to initiate lid opening
2. No evidence of ongoing orbicularis oculi contraction, such as descent of eyebrows beneath the superior orbital margins
3. Vigorous frontalis contractions during periods of inability to raise eyelids
4. No oculomotor or ocular sympathetic nerve dysfunction and no ocular myopathy

"Apraxia" of lid closure, consisting of inability to close eyes on command with preservation of normal reflex blinking, was observed in 8%, blepharospasm in 16%, and combinations of these supranuclear eyelid opening and closing disorders in 13% of patients with PSP (4).

It should be stressed that supranuclear ophthalmoplegia is not unique to PSP but can be found in over 10 other multisystem degenerative disorders, including olivopontocerebellar atrophy, Creutzfeldt-Jakob disease, corticobasal degeneration, and Guamanian amyotrophic lateral sclerosis/Parkinsonism–dementia complex (5). Conversely, absence of ophthalmoplegia does not unequivocally exclude the diagnosis of PSP, as exemplified by a patient with PSP with a 4-year history of extrapyramidal findings preceding onset of supranuclear ophthalmoparesis with square wave jerks (6).

Although mildly diffuse slowing on electroencephalography (EEG) and slightly elevated protein content of cerebrospinal fluid has been reported in PSP,

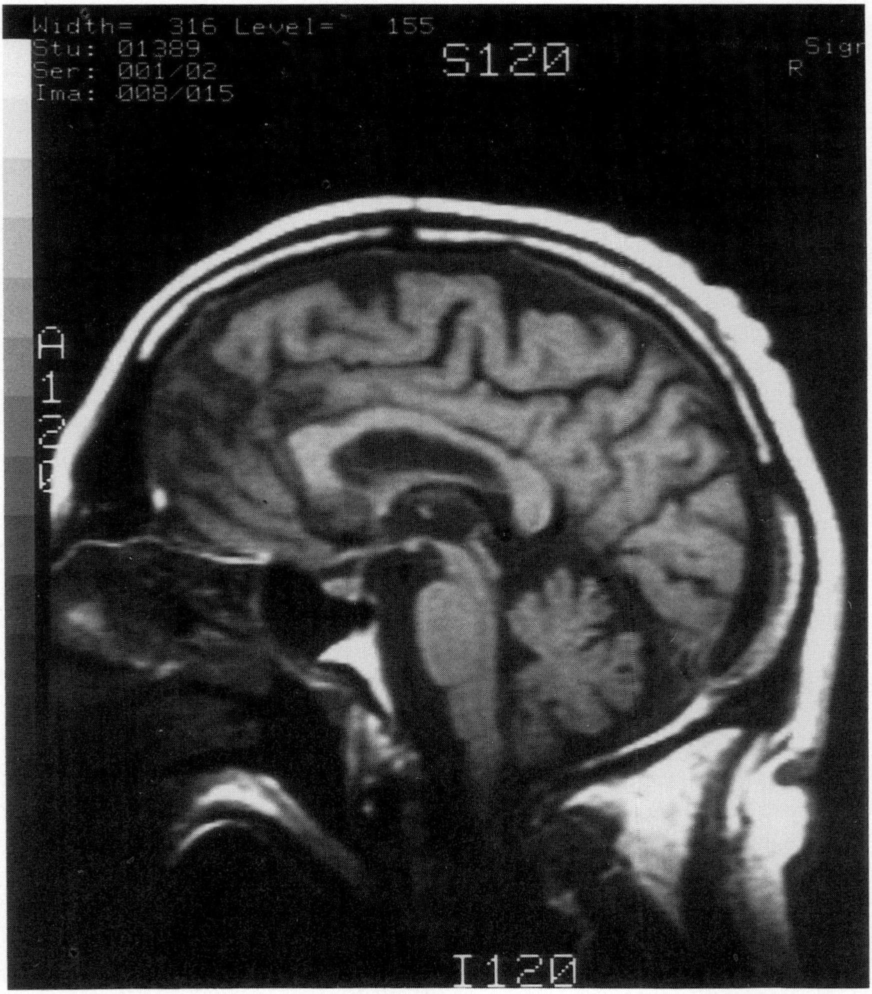

Figure 1 MRI of the head of a 67-year-old man with an 8-year history of PSP reveals marked midbrain atrophy. Midbrain measures 9 mm on sagittal images.

magnetic resonance imaging (MRI) (Fig. 1) and computed tomography (CT) of the brain remain the most useful ancillary investigations for PSP. CT midbrain anterior-posterior diameter of less than 15 mm indicates midbrain tegmentum atrophy—a salient feature of PSP (7).

At autopsy, the atrophy revealed by neuroimaging can be more precisely delineated as three major areas of neuronal damage:

1. Pallidosubthalamic complex
2. Zona compacta of substantia nigra
3. Superior colliculus, periaqueductal gray matter

In these areas, light microscopy reveals neuronal loss, gliosis, and neurofibrillary tangles composed mainly of straight filaments or, rarely, pairs of helical filaments.

II. MEDICAL TREATMENT

A definitive pharmacological therapy for PSP has not been forthcoming. The multiple disruptions of dopaminergic, cholinergic, and serotonergic neurotransmitter systems most readily account for the disappointing long-term response to a variety of neuropharmacological agents. Nevertheless, modest benefits can initially be produced by a variety of dopaminergic, anticholinergic, cholinergic, antiserotonergic, and tricyclic medications. One study of 87 PSP patients showed that the three most frequently used drugs were amitryptiline (32% of patients benefited), imipramine (28% of patients benefited), and levodopa-carbidopa (38% of patients benefited) (8). In a given patient, this certainly justifies a sequence of empiric trials with individual agents, bearing in mind that polypharmacy with these neurotropic agents increases the likelihood of undesirable cognitive side effects.

Many clinicians initiate treatment with dopaminergic agents such as levodopa-carbidopa (beginning at 25/100, containing 25 mg carbidopa and 100 mg levodopa tid). Other approaches include increasing dopamine release with amantadine (100 mg qd to bid) or direct dopamine receptor agonists such as bromocriptine (starting at 1.25 mg qd) or pergolide (starting at 0.05 mg qd). The efficacy of anticholinergic therapy in Parkinson's disease has led clinicians to treat PSP with trihexyphenidyl (beginning at 1 mg qd) or benzotropine (beginning at 0.5 mg qd). Benefits are modest and evanescent. In comparison to Parkinson's disease, both dopamine agonists and cholinergic antagonists are less effective, and this is attributed to loss of basal ganglionic cholinergic interneurons in PSP. These neurons are postsynaptic to dopamine cells, and their loss may underlie the lack of tremor in PSP (9).

The tricyclic antidepressant, amitriptyline (50 mg qhs) produced overall clinical improvement in patients with PSP, and this has been attributed to more potent inhibition of serotonin reuptake as compared with the less efficacious tricyclic desipramine. Similarly, fluoxetine (starting at 20 mg qd) has modestly benefited PSP by presumably blocking serotonin reuptake. A rational basis for serotonergic therapy becomes elusive when trying to account for the efficacy of the serotonin antagonist methylsergide (starting at 2 mg qd), which improve quality of life, dysphagia, and possibly extraocular movements and mental function in PSP (10). These salutary effects of an antiserotonergic agent are not easily reconciled with the degeneration of serotonergic raphe nuclei found in PSP. Long-term methylsergide therapy can be complicated by retroperitoneal, cardiac, and pleuropulmonary fibrosis, and this necessitates a 3- or 4-week drug-free interval following each 6-month course of therapy.

The selective alpha-2 presynaptic antagonist, idazoxan, is a centrally acting noradrenergic agent that may be able to bypass the denervated basal ganglia in PSP and directly stimulate alpha receptors in sensory-motor cortex, cerebellum, brainstem, and spinal cord. A double-blind study of this experimental drug demonstrated significant improvement of mobility, balance, gait, and digital dexterity in nine PSP patients (11). Expected side effects of increased norepinephrine transmission included tachycardia, systolic blood pressure elevation, facial flushing, and sense of warmth.

Most clinicians attest that the modest improvement of mobility conferred by dopaminergic or anticholinergic medications is not mirrored by improvement of ophthalmoplegia in PSP; however, methylsergide has been reported to improve spontaneous eye movements, fixation, vertical tracking, and optokinetic nystagmus in vertical and horizontal directions. With loss of volitional eye movements in general and downward gaze in particular, patients may not be able to look downward through the "add" segment of bifocals, and a separate pair of reading glasses will be more practical for close work. Difficulties with accommodation may be increased by the anticholinergic effects of many medications for PSP and can be offset by stronger convex lenses for reading. Close work is further hampered by loss of convergence in PSP—a situation that may be ameliorated with base-in prism. The visual deficits of ophthalmoplegia in PSP may be augmented by abnormal orienting responses and spatial attention. These latter findings have been shown to improve with methylsergide and physostigmine. Although cognitive deficits in PSP are not caused by cholinergic cortical deficits similar to those of Alzheimer's disease, the improvement of visuospatial attention with a centrally acting anticholinesterase agent implies that the cholinergic deficiency in PSP may play a role in visual cognition.

Uncontrolled eyelid closure will frequently incapacitate a patient with PSP. Although about one third of patients with blepharospasm will respond to various pharmacological agents, including trihexyphenidyl, amantadine, carbidopa-levodopa, clonazepam, bromocriptine, pergolide, haloperidol, baclofen, and lithium, the most effective current therapy is periorbital and eyelid injection of botulinum A toxin (12). Involuntary levator inhibition can occur in isolation or concurrently with blepharospasm in PSP, and it remains a difficult treatment problem, although improvement has been reported with desipramine (13). Botulinum toxin injections have helped involuntary levator inhibition (14). possibly by suppressing blepharospasm that may act as a "trigger." Patients with PSP may develop exposure keratitis from infrequent spontaneous blinking, and this can decrease visual acuity as well as initiate or exacerbate blepharospasm due to local corneal irritation. Methylcellulose or polyvinyl alcohol eye drops four or five times daily or an ocular lubricating ointment of white petrolatum and mineral oil applied to the inferior cul-de-sac of both eyes at bedtime will facilitate healing and prevention of exposure keratitis.

PSP is a relentlessly progressive condition, and although the foregoing therapeutic armamentarium provides limited respite, the physician will all too frequently confront a bedbound, terminally dysphagic, severely dysarthric, and totally ophthalmoplegic patient less than 7 years after onset of the disease. Severe dysphagia may be helped by cricopharyngeal myotomy in some cases but a feeding tube frequently is necessary. Akinesia and loss of postural reflexes confine the patient to bed and mandate physical therapy. In the most advanced stages, optimal management of PSP must be based on education of family members and expert nursing care.

REFERENCES

1. Duvoisin RC, Golbe LI, Lepore FE. Progessive supranuclear palsy. Can J Neurol Sci 1987; 14:547–554.
2. Steele JC, Richardson JC, Olszewsky J. Progressive supranuclear palsy. Arch Neurol 1964; 10:121–130.
3. Troost BT, Daroff RB. The ocular motor defects in progressive supranuclear palsy. Ann Neurol 1977; 2:397–403.
4. Golbe LI, Davis PD, Lepore FE. Eyelid movement abnormalities in progressive supranuclear palsy. Movement Disorders 1989; 4:297–302.
5. Lepore FE, Steele JC, Cox TA, Tillson G, Calne DB, Duvoisin RC, Lavine L, Mc Darby JV. Supranuclear disturbances of ocular motility in Lytico-Bodig. Neurology 1988; 38:1849–1853.
6. Nuwer MR. Progressive supranuclear palsy despite normal eye movements. Arch Neurol 1981; 38–784.
7. Schonfeld SM, Golbe LI, Sage JI, Safer JN, Duvoisin RC. Computed tomographic findings in progessive supranuclear palsy: correlation with clinical grade. Movement Disorders 1987; 2:263–278.
8. Nieforth KA, Golbe LI. Retrospective study of drug response in 87 patients with progressive supranuclear palsy. Clin Neuropharmacol 1993; 4:338–346.
9. Young AB. Progressive supranuclear palsy: postmortem chemical analysis. Ann Neurol 1985; 5:521–522.
10. Rafal RD, Grimm RJ. Progessive supranuclear palsy: functional analysis of the response to methylsergide and antiparkinsonian agents. Neurology 1981; 31:1507–1518.
11. Ghika J, Tennis M, Hoffman E, Schoenfeld D, Growdon J. Idazoxan treatment in progressive supranuclear palsy. Neurology 1991; 41:986–991.
12. Scott AB, Kennedy RA, Stubbs MA. Botulinum A toxin injection as a treatment for blepharospasm. Arch Ophthalmol 1985; 103:347–350.
13. Newman GC. Treatment of progressive supranuclear palsy with tricyclic antidepressants. Neurology 1985; 35:1189–1193.
14. Katz B, Rosenberg JH. Botulinum therapy for apraxia of eyelid opening. Am J Ophthalmol 1987; 103:718–719.

37

Ocular/Neurosyphilis Update

J. Lawton Smith
University of Miami School of Medicine, Bascom Palmer Eye Institute, Miami, Florida

"Undoubtedly syphilis is the single illness which produces more ocular and nervous system involvement than any other, and consequently the neuro-ophthalmologist must have an intimate knowledge of syphilis." This statement, which was made by Dr. Frank B. Walsh in 1957 (1), would hardly merit that emphasis by many practitioners today considering the fact that a whole generation of physicians has received little exposure to this subject in medical school curricula since the discovery of penicillin in 1943. The problem of syphilis, however, has not only not disappeared but the number of cases has been growing at an alarming rate, as is seen in Tables 1–3. These tables show the dramatic rise in the number of reported cases of syphilis in the 5 most recent years that data are available from the Centers of Disease Control and Prevention (CDC) (2).

Syphilis has not only been increasing rapidly in incidence but has in many respects gone underground. Between 1977 and 1982, one half of all patients in the United States with early syphilis were homosexual and bisexual men. Associated with the AIDS epidemic, however, the proportion of early syphilis cases has changed, so that the disease currently is occurring predominantly in black and Hispanic heterosexual men and women, with a peak incidence in the 15 to 34-year age group. Infectious syphilis is often correlated with exchange of sex for crack cocaine. The highest case rates are now found in large urban areas as New York City, parts of Florida and Texas, Los Angeles, and the District of Columbia.

A dramatic evidence of the epidemic is seen in the number of cases of

Table 1 Reported Cases of Syphilis in the United States (All Stages, 1987–1991)

1987	1988	1989	1990	1991
89,833	107,489	117,659	136,433	130,648

congenital syphilis being reported. This reflects the rate of infectious syphilis in females, and the incidence of congenital syphilis has gone from 4.3 cases per 100,000 live births in 1983 to 103.4 in 1991—an astounding increase.

Syphilis has gone underground in that primary lesions previously were readily seen in heterosexual males, whereas perirectal and anal chancres are often invisible in homosexual males. Furthermore, the effects of the acquired immunodeficiency syndrome (AIDS) in suppressing serological responses has also rendered the diagnosis of syphilis more difficult. It is universally recognized that many cases of syphilis are not reported, so that the problem is significantly larger than the statistics document. There has been a resurgence of patients presenting to ophthalmology clinics in large urban teaching hospitals with acute ocular manifestations of early, infectious syphilis. It will thus be only a matter of time until later manifestations of the disease (syphilitic optic atrophy and neurosyphilis) will likewise increase in frequency. Therefore, with the combination of a rapidly increasing incidence of sexually transmitted disease, early infectious lesions being more difficult to detect, and the role of AIDS in confusing serodiagnosis, it is evident that increasing attention must be paid to the diagnosis and treatment of syphilis by the medical profession in general and by ophthalmologists and neurologists in particular.

I. CLINICAL DESCRIPTION

Syphilis is a chronic generalized infectious disease caused by *Treponema pallidum*, a thin, delicate spiral-shaped organism that propels itself by spinning

Table 2 Reported Cases of Late and Late Latent Syphilis in the United States (1987–1991)

1987	1988	1989	1990	1991
22,988	27,363	22,032	25,713	27,500

Table 3 Reported Cases of Congenital Syphilis in the United States (1987–1991)

1987	1988	1989	1990	1991
444	658	1,807	3,272	4,322

along its longitudinal axis. The organism has 6–14 spirals, a total length of 6–15 μm, and its unique spiral structure is maintained by six fibrils, three arising at each end of the organism. Electron microscopy has identified six laminas surrounding the cytoplasm. The disease is usually sexually transmitted, and the organism can rapidly penetrate intact mucous membranes or abraded skin and within a few hours enters the lymphatics and blood stream even before the appearance of the primary lesion. The organism divides every 30–33 h, and the incubation period of syphilis is inversely proportional to the number of organisms inoculated. In experimental infection in rabbits, a single treponeme can initiate infection that leads to a discernible lesion only after 6 weeks, whereas intradermal injection of 10,000,000 organisms usually produces a lesion within 72 h. The primary lesion appears at the inoculation site within 2–6 weeks and then heals spontaneously. In heterosexual men, the chancre is usually on the penis, but in homosexual men and in women, the primary lesion is often not seen and may be entirely missed by the patient. Regional lymphadenopathy accompanies the primary lesion and appears within 1 week of onset of the lesion. The nodes are firm, nonsuppurative, and painless. The chancre heals within 6 weeks on its own. About 6 weeks later, generalized symptoms of secondary syphilis usually appear. These consist of a maculopapular cutaneous rash, often involving the face, scalp, palms, and soles. Constitutional symptoms of a flulike illness may be present. Some patients, however, enter the latent stage without ever developing secondary lesions. The untreated patient then enters a latent period of subclinical infection, and in about one third of untreated cases, a tertiary stage develops—most commonly involving the central nervous system, eye, and aorta.

Although there are ranges to the data presented, a helpful mnemonic for the ophthalmologist is seen in Table 4.

II. SEROLOGICAL DIAGNOSIS

There are so many blood tests for syphilis that this often causes confusion. There are two basic types of antibodies found in this disease—*nonspecific* (reagin) and *specific* (treponemal) antibody. The most common reagin tests used are the rapid plasma reagin (RPR) agglutination test, and the Veneral Disease Research

Table 4 The Rules of Sixes in Syphilis

1. *Treponema pallidum* has six spirals
2. The organism is 6 μm long
3. The organism is made up of six fibrils
4. Each fibril is made up of six laminas
5. The primary lesion appears within 6 weeks of exposure
6. Primary lesion persists for 6 weeks and heals spontaneously
7. Six weeks after healing of primary, secondary manifestations appear
8. The initial 2-degree lesions are 6-mm macules
9. After 6 weeks, 6-mm papules appear
10. 2-degree lesions subside on their own within 6 weeks
11. Symptomatic neurosyphilis occurs in about 6.5% of cases
12. 16% of cases develop benign tertiary disease
13. Aortitis occurs in up to 60% of cases at autopsy
14. There are six letters in FTA-ABS test—the most important blood test in syphilis

Laboratory (VDRL) flocculation test. It is important to emphasize that the VDRL test is negative in nearly one third of patients with primary or late syphilis. Obtaining a serum RPR or VDRL test is *not* sufficient in evaluating a patient suspected of having ocular or neurosyphilis. The more specific and sensitive fluorescent treponemal antibody absorption (FTA-ABS) test should be *routinely* obtained in suspected late syphilis. Reactivity of various serological tests in untreated syphilis is seen in Table 5.

The importance of getting a serum FTA-ABS test in patients with eye and neurological involvement was seen in the following study. At the Bascom Palmer Eye Institute in Miami, Florida, blood tests were evaluated on 1985 patients seen between 1957 and 1963 (3). Of these, 718 patients showed reactive serum FTA-ABS tests. However, only 441 patients had reactive serum VDRL tests. Thus, 39% of the cases of late syphilis would have been overlooked if only a

Table 5 Stage of Disease—% Positive

	Stage			
Test	1	2	Latent	3
VDRL	72	100	73	77
FTA-ABS	91	100	97	100
TPI	46	98	95	95
TPHA	69	100	98	100

serum reagin test had been obtained. Furthermore, the FTA-ABS test was found to be reactive in 41% of the 1985 sera studied.

A more recent confirmation of this was presented by Spoor et al. (4). They drew serum FTA-ABS tests on 227 patients prior to ambulatory outpatient oculoplastic surgery in Detroit, Michigan. They found that 55% of these patients had reactive serum FTA-ABS tests. Some studies have shown an incidence of 25–40% of the eye clinic population in Miami, Atlanta, Georgia, St. Louis, Missouri, and Los Angeles, California, as well as Detroit, having reactive serum FTA-ABS tests. The FTA-ABS test is preferred to the MHA-TP, HATTS, or TPHA tests in my experience. The TPI (*Treponema pallidum* immobilization) test is also an excellent test but is not commercially available in the United States.

III. OCULAR SYPHILIS

Involvement of the eye (with the rare exception of periocular chancre) often occurs in both secondary and tertiary stages of acquired syphilis and usually presents as two quite different clinical pictures in these two groups. A broad classification of ocular syphilis is given in Table 6 (5):

IV. NEUROSYPHILIS

Syphilitic optic atrophy occurs often in predominantly ocular syphilis but also may be the presenting clinical entity (6). It also occurs so commonly in association with neurosyphilis that it may be considered as a clinical bridge between ocular and neurosyphilis and thus has been cited in the classification of both ocular and neurosyphilis.

V. NEURO–OPHTHALMOLOGICAL EXAMINATION

Points to emphasize on neuro-ophthalmological examination of patients with late ocular/neurosyphilis are:

Pupil: Look for anisocoria, sluggish light reactions; light-near dissociation; miosis; unequal pupils; poor response to mydriatics, iris atrophy, transillumination defects, Krukenberg's spindle, posterior synechiae.

Uvea: Look for nongranulomatous or granulomatous iridocyclitis, secondary glaucoma, retinitis pigmentosa–like changes in fundi, perivasculitis.

Cornea: Look for interstitial keratitis. A mirrorlike sheen near Descemet's membrane with clear cornea anterior to it is an indication for an FTA-ABS test.

Table 6 Classification of Ocular Syphilis

1. Brows: alopecia of outer third of the eyebrow occurs transiently in second stage syphilis; is often permanent in late disease.
2. Lids and conjunctiva: chancre, and lesions of second stage syphilis may involve lides and conjunctiva. Conjunctival syphilis and chronic syphilis tarsitis are rare.
3. Orbit: orbital periostitis and gumma (rare).
4. Sclera: scleritis and episcleritis.
5. Cornea: interstitial keratitis of congenital syphilis, interstitial keratitis of acquire syphilis (rare), Mauthner's keratitis punctata profunda, keratitis pustuliformis profunda, deep stromal infiltrates with hypopyon, Kraupa's corneal infiltration in late syphilis, keratitis linearis migrans, gumma of cornea, corneal dystrophy in syphilis with vitamin deficiency, probably same as keratitis linearis migrans of Fuchs, corneal marginal ulcers in syphilis (malnutrition).
6. Iris: iritis (Zeeman's type of syphilitic iritis consists of roseola, fibrinous iritis, iritis papulosa, and severe diffuse iridocyclitis).
7. Pupil: Stokes and Brehmer found in 126 cases of neurosyphilis the following: abnormal pupils 63%, Argyll Robertson pupils 35%; slow pupillary reflexes 23%; irregular pupils 21%; unequal pupils 19%. To these should be added: light-near dissociation (Argyll Robertson–like pupils); dilated and fixed pupils (typically seen in paresis); pseudo–Argyll Robertson pupil (seen in aberrant regeneration of III).
8. Lens: secondary cataracts with syphilitic uveitis, traumatic dislocation of lens—about two thirds of these cases have reactive serum FTA-ABS tests.
9. Uvea: choroiditis of congenital syphilis, iritis and/or chorioretinitis of acquired syphilis, uveitis in late syphilis, gumma of choroid or ciliary body (rare).
10. Retina and choroid (acquired syphilis): diffuse syphilitic chorioretinitis of Forster, disseminated choroiditis, areolar choroiditis (Forster), syphilitic retinitis and neuroretinitis, neuritis papulosa of Fuchs, juxtapapillary retinochoroiditis gummatous lesions of retina. Syphilis of retinal blood vessels: thrombosis of central vein or branches, embolism or thrombosis of central artery or branches, neovascularization in vitreous, perivasculitis.
11. Congenital syphilis: salt and pepper fundus (Sidler-Huguenin type I), circumscribed chorioretinitis (Sidler-Huguenin type II), syphilitic pseudoretinitis pigmentosa, syphilitic retinal perivasculitis.
12. Optic nerve syphilis: syphilitic perioptic neuritis, optic neuritis (papillitis) and neuroretinitis, syphilitic retrobulbar neuritis, primary optic atrophy (tabetic optic atrophy), secondary optic atrophy, papilledema in syphilis, gumma of optic nerve.

Fundus: Look for salt and pepper fundus, granulomatous chorioretinitis, perivascular sheathing in periphery, old branch artery or vein occlusions.
Optic atrophy: Any type.
Optic disc: Swollen disc with intact acuity—think of luetic perioptic neuritis in second stage syphilis, or papilloedema in luetic meningitis, or atypical anterior ischemic optic neuropathy in second stage syphilis.
Visual field defects: Irregular contraction of peripheral isopters frequent marked contraction of color peripheral isopters, nerve fiber bundle defects, altitudinal defects, enlarged blind spots in perineuritis, bitemporal and homonymous defects in chiasmatic arachnoiditis and meningovascular syphilis.

An abbreviated outline of the most common type encountered and the things the clinician should look for follows.

A. Ocular Syphilis

Cornea: interstitial keratitis
Pupil: light dissociation
Uvea: anterior and posterior uveitis
Retina: a retinitis pigmentosa–like fundus
Optic nerve: disc swelling and optic atrophy

B. Neurosyphilis

1. Asymptomatic neurosyphilis: spinal fluid examination in a patient with reactive serum RPR or VDRL
2. Meningeal neurosyphilis: spinal fluid examination in a patient with meningitis
3. Vascular neurosyphilis: spinal fluid examination in a patient with a stroke
4. Tabes dorsalis: locomotor ataxia, AR pupils, pale optic discs
5. Paresis (dementia paralytica): dementia, abnormal pupils, tremors, release phenomena
6. Syphilitic optic atrophy: pale optic discs

When any of the above processes are considered in the differential diagnosis, a careful and complete cerebrospinal fluid examination should be done. A common error in our hospital is to fail to record the opening pressure, which should always be done. A cerebrospinal fluid (CSF) VDRL should always be obtained. The usefulness of an FTA-ABS test on CSF is debated, and it is preferred to obtain this test on the serum. The colloidal gold test was a very helpful test in my experience, but it is virtually unobtainable at this time. One should get an electrophoretic pattern of the CSF protein, which will help in interpretation of mild or borderline protein elevations.

VI. AIDS AND SYPHILIS

AIDS is caused by HIV, a human retrovirus of the lentivirus group. AIDS was first recognized in the United States in the summer of 1981 when the CDC reported the unexplained occurrence of *Pneumocystis carinii* pneumonia in five previously healthy homosexual men in Los Angeles and Kaposi's sarcoma in 26 previously healthy homosexual men in New York City and Los Angeles. (By mid 1990, approximately 120 cases among adults and adolescents and approximately 2000 cases among children less than 13 years old had been reported in the United States.) AIDS is a global epidemic with virtually every country in the world reporting cases. Sexual contact is the major mode of transmission of HIV worldwide. In the United States, 60% of adult cases are in homosexual or bisexual men who do not use intravenous drugs. The next largest group (20%) consists of heterosexual men and women who are IV drug users and is related to sharing of needles. Seven percent of cases are men who are homosexual or bisexual and who also use IV drugs. One percent are hemophiliacs with no other risk factors. An additional 2% are nonhemophiliacs who have received transfusions of blood or blood products. Approximately 80% of all pediatric cases (<13 years of age) are infected by their mothers. The remainder are among blood transfusion recipients (11%) and hemophiliacs (5%).

It is interesting that commonly encountered opportunistic infections in AIDS are listed as: *Pneumocystis*, cytomegalovirus, *Candida albicans*, *Mycobacterium avium-intracellulare*, *Mycobacterium tuberculosis*, *Cryptococcus neoformans*, *Toxoplasma gondii*, herpes simplex, herpes zoster, *Cryptosporidium*, *Isopora belli*, and *Salmonella*. Yet in a textbook published in 1991 (7), *T. pallidum* is not even included in this list.

The interrelationship between syphilis and HIV infection is clinically a very important one. Berger (8), in a prospective study of neurosyphilis in HIV^+ individuals, found that a history of syphilis was obtained in 18.8% of 69 HIV^- control subjects compared with 40.5% of 257 HIV^+ subjects. A reactive serum FTA-ABS test was obtained in 46% of 254 HIV^+ subjects compared with 17.4% of 69 HIV^- control subjects. It is important to note from Berger's prospective study that a reactive serum RPR was detected significantly less often in all groups, ranging from 5.6% of HIV controls in 9.6% of the HIV^+ subjects.

Berger's study confirmed a high prevalence of prior syphilis, as determined by history (40%) or the presence of a reactive serum FTA-ABS (36%) among HIV^+ subjects. When either of these two criteria was accepted as diagnostic of syphilis, the rate increased to 46% among HIV^+ subjects. Among neurologically asymptomatic HIV^+ subjects, the rate of neurosyphilis was 1.8%. For the purposes of Berger's study, neurosyphilis was defined as the presence of a reactive CSF VDRL in a person not previously treated for neurosyphilis or the presence of a reactive CSF FTA-ABS occurring in an association with an illness consistent with neurosyphilis that responded clinically to penicillin therapy.

The requirement of having a reactive CSF VDRL test may have excluded some patients with neurosyphilis. Lukehart et al. (9) demonstrated the presence of viable *T. pallidum* in the CSF in the absence of a reactive CSF VDRL. Two HIV^+ patients with neurosyphilis had an initially nonreactive CSF VDRL but converted to reactive 12 days and 3 months, respectively, after beginning treatment with IV penicillin. Berger wrote an interesting editorial (10) pointing out the difficulties involved in diagnosing neurosyphilis and the invalidity of relying solely on the CSF VDRL test.

Berger also emphasized that there is significant overlap between the neurological spectrum of disease caused by HIV-1 and that caused by *T. pallidum* (8). Acute and chronic meningitis, cranial neuropathies, dementing encephalopathy, ischemic cerebrovascular disease, and myelopathy may be caused by either organism. The conclusions are evident: (1) any HIV^+ person with a history of syphilis or a reactive serum FTA-ABS test should have a lumbar puncture if it has not been performed recently; (2) HIV testing should be obtained in all patients with ocular or neurosyphilis; (3) serum RPR and FTA-ABS tests should be obtained in all patients clinically suspect for AIDS or who are HIV seropositive.

The interrelationship between HIV infection and syphilis with regard to the serological responses is a particularly interesting one. There have been reports of extremely high titered serological responses seen in association with early infectious syphilis in patients who are HIV^+, but it also is now well documented that HIV infection can cause the loss of previously positive serological tests (both reagin and treponemal tests) in patients with documented syphilis. The importance of recognizing these two different serological patterns is illustrated by the following two cases.

Case 1 (LE)

A 68-year-old white male, reported in detail elsewhere (11), noted the onset of painless transient obscurations of vision in the right eye in November 1988. He was found to have extensive optic disc edema in that eye and an extensive workup up to and including MRI of the brain was negative. Within 2 weeks of onset, he noted photophobia and floaters in the left eye, and was then found to have iritis and vitritis, more marked in the left eye.

Neuro-ophthalmological examination revealed good acuity in both eyes and normal fields but for an enlarged right blind spot, and ophthalmoscopy disclosed a highly choked disc on the right (Fig. 1) with a normal optic disc on the left. Ultrasonography showed that the right optic nerve sheath was enlarged owing to

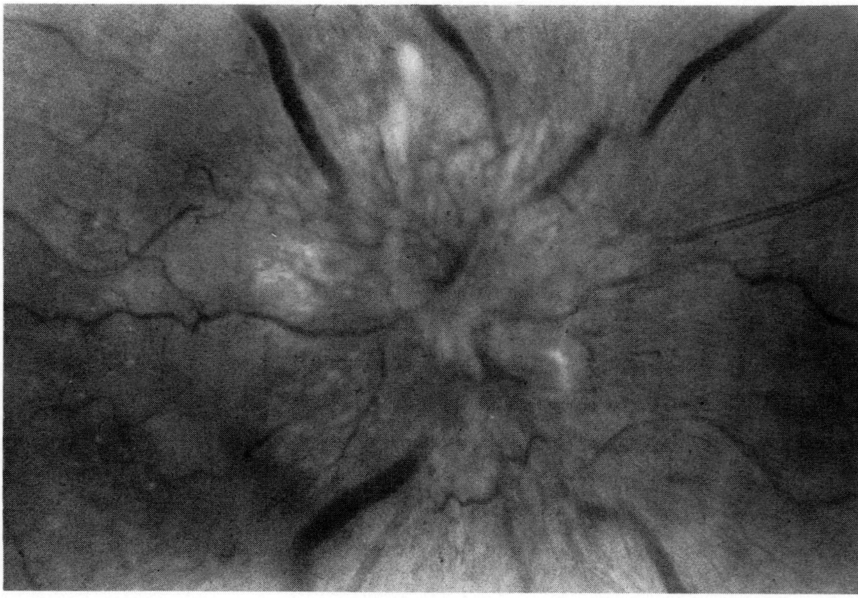

Figure 1 Right optic disc of case 1 on January 9, 1989, showing extensive disc edema in a patient with a syphiloma/gumma of optic nerve.

a solid, noncomprehensible lesion. As the patient had previously had a colon carcinoma, the possibility of a metastatic lesion was considered. Routine serological testing revealed a reactive serum RPR 1:1024 and a 4+ serum FTA-ABS test. Lumbar puncture disclosed a clear acellular fluid under normal pressure with protein of 83 mg% and a reactive CSF VDRL. The impression was syphiloma or gumma of the right optic nerve with bilateral asymmetrical syphilitic uveitis.

The patient received 200 million units of IV aqueous penicillin and had a dramatic clearing of both the optic disc swelling and uveitis. Because of the diagnosis of ocular syphilis in this patient, a serum HIV test was drawn, which was repeatedly positive and confirmed in an additional laboratory, and he showed a decreased T4/T8 ratio.

Comment. This case emphasizes three points: (1) a routine RPR or VDRL should be obtained—this had not been obtained in the initial extensive workup; (2) ultrasound with 30-degree test is helpful in evaluating optic nerve swelling to differentiate between a mass lesion versus increased subarachnoid fluid; (3) a routine HIV test should be obtained for every patient with syphilis.

Case 2 (FB)

A 36-year-old white male was first seen in neuro-ophthalmological consultation November 22, 1991, for evaluation of advisability of antibiotic therapy for late syphilis. In July 1987, he had developed flulike illness with fever and sweats for several weeks. Some fatigue and depression persisted, and he was found to be HIV^+ in November 1987. The patient did well until May 1989, when he developed oral candidiasis and a skin lesion near the left knee. The latter was biopsied and found to be Kaposi's sarcoma. The patient was started on azidothymidine (AZT) therapy, which was stopped in late 1990 because of muscle weakness. In early 1991, the patient developed severe watery diarrhea and the Kaposi's sarcoma began to spread diffusely over the body. A stormy course of AIDS ensued thereafter, including thrombophlebitis, staphylococcal bacteremia, and repeated courses of antibiotics and chemotherapy. The patient was seen in California where serum VDRL, MHATP, and FTA-ABS tests were performed and all were reported as nonreactive. Family history revealed that his father died of AIDS.

Of particular interest here was the fact that the patient had been admitted to Jackson Memorial Hospital in Miami, Florida, on March 9, 1983, at age 28. He gave a history then of admitted homosexual activities for 12 years with multiple sexual partners. In April 1982, the patient developed fever, weakness, and malaise lasting a month. He had recently developed oral candidiasis. In February 1983, a skin rash was noted on the hands and trunk with papules. Prior to that, the patient gave a history of hepatitis at age 17, conjunctivitis in 1982, and a questionable history of nonspecific urethritis.

Examination revealed prominent submandibular, cervical, axillary, and occipital lymph nodes that were rubbery and nontender. A residual maculopapular rash was noted over the extremities and upper chest. Two lymph nodes were biopsied to rule out a lymphoma and both showed only mixed hyperplasia. The patient was found to have a reactive serum RPR with a titer of 1:513 and a 4+ serum FTA-ABS test (confirmed on two occasions). He was treated with erythromycin for a 15-day course and received nystatin for oral thrush. Discharge diagnoses were (1) acquired immune deficiency syndrome, (2) oral candidiasis, (3) secondary syphilis, and (4) diffuse lymphadenopathy.

Eye examination on November 22, 1991, 8 years later, revealed a chronically ill 36-year-old young man with multiple foci of disseminated Kaposi's sarcoma with literally hundreds of lesions over the entire body (face, trunk, back, and extremities) (Fig. 2). The vision was 20/15 in each eye and the pupils were within normal limits. Cogwheel following movements were present in all directions of gaze. Slit lamp and peripheral fields were normal. A dilated fundus examination revealed normal optic discs but typical white spots of AIDS were seen in both eyes (Fig. 3).

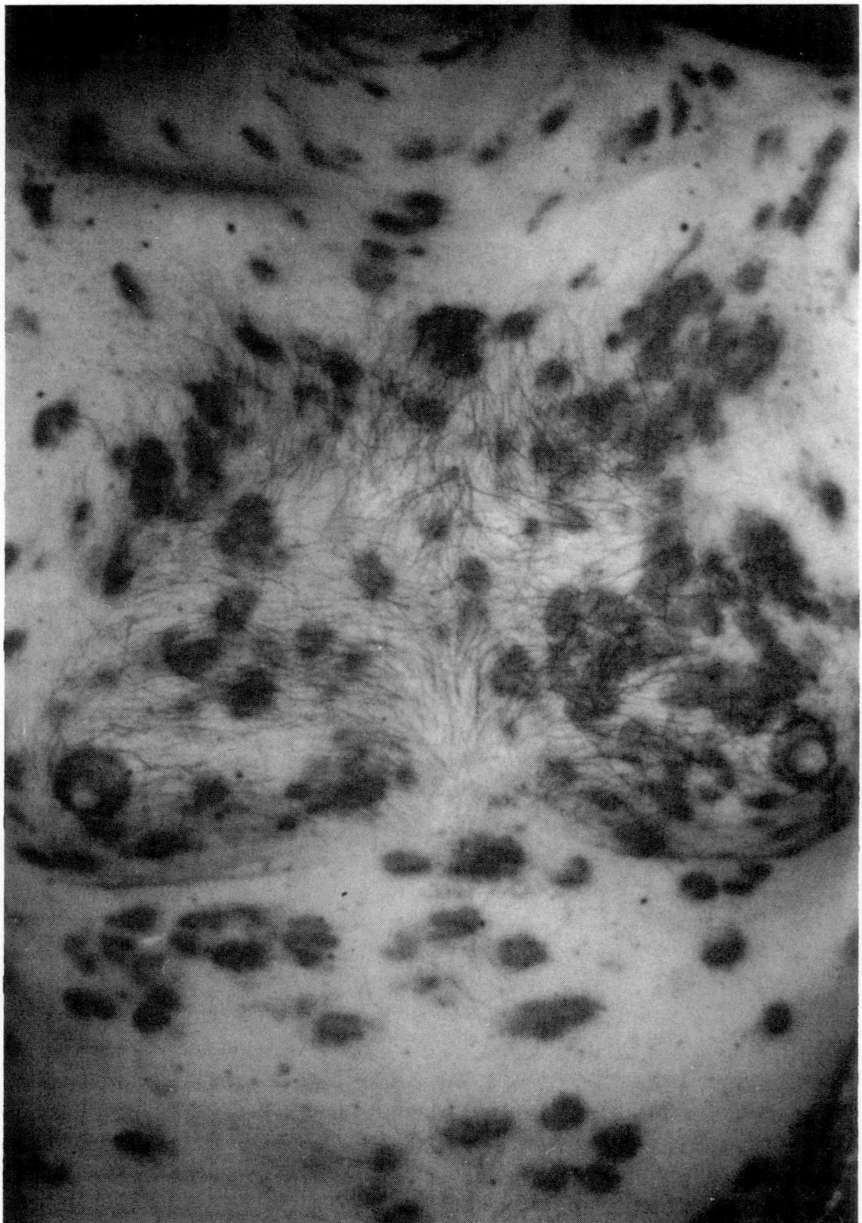

Figure 2 Chest of case 2 on November 12, 1991, showing myriad Kaposi's sarcoma lesions.

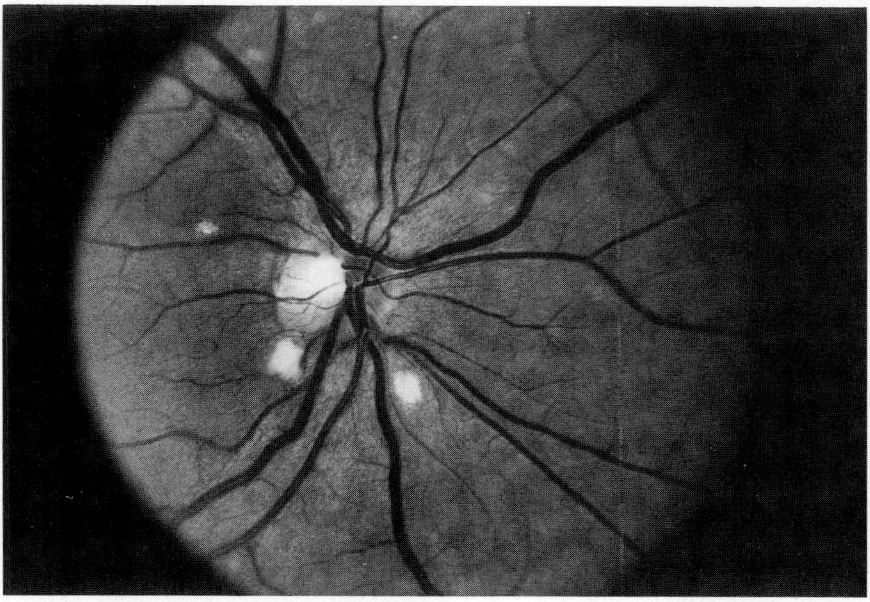

Figure 3 Right eye of case 2 on December 12, 1991, showing classic white spots in retina seen with AIDS.

Total white blood count was 2900; CD4 (T-helper) lymphocytes were 1% (normal 32–62%) and CD8 (T-suppressor) lymphocytes were 71% (normal 17–44%) with a T-helper/T-suppressor ratio of 0.001 (normal 0.9–3.5).

Serum RPR at Smith-Kline laboratories on February 26, 1991, was nonreactive. Serum RPR was nonreactive and serum FTA-ABS was reactive at the Microbiology Reference Laboratory. Two months earlier, serum VDRL, MHATP, and FTA-ABS tests in California had been reported as nonreactive. Accordingly, serum was sent to the Pasteur Institute in Paris, who reported VDRL, TPHA, FTA-ABS, SPHA, and FTA-ABS immunoglobulin M were all nonreactive and quantitative TPI showed 0% immobilization.

Because of a remote history of penicillin allergy, the patient was skin tested to penicillin and found to be negative. He was admitted to a hospital in another county shortly thereafter for pneumonia, and despite large doses of antibiotics, he died of complications of AIDS about 3 days later. A postmortem examination was not performed.

Comment. Haas et al. (12) reported that 38% of a group of symptomatic HIV^+ homosexual men who had a documented history of treated syphilis lost seroreactivity to syphilis. The patient here reported is the best documented instance of this phenomenon that I have seen.

This patient thus documents a clinically and serologically documented classic case of secondary syphilis who was violently seropositive for syphilis in 1983 but who with the subsequent progression of AIDS was seen in 1991 and was totally seronegative to both reagin and treponemal testing. Any clinician seeing this patient in 1991, who did not have this former history, would not have been able to make the diagnosis of former syphilis or to determine activity of the disease or assess adequacy of treatment by serological criteria. This patient illustrates the extreme importance of getting a very careful history for sexually transmitted diseases in these patients, of documenting that information to the best of one's ability, and of obtaining RPR and FTA-ABS tests on all patients who are HIV^+ and also of obtaining an HIV test on all patients with reactive RPR and/or FTA-ABS tests. In an interesting paper by Katz et al. (13), a study of 46 hospitalized patients with neurosyphilis seen in Jackson Memorial Hospital in Miami, Florida, between January 1984 and April 1989 was done. The diagnosis of neurosyphilis was accepted only in the presence of a reactive CSF VDRL test coupled with a reactive RPR or FTA-ABS test in serum. These investigators emphasized that ocular syphilis frequently accompanied other primary classes of neurosyphilis. Thirty-six percent of HIV^+ patients and 31% of patients with AIDS gave a prior history of syphilis as compared with 14% of HIV^- patients. Two patients with AIDS had received the CDC recommended regimen of high-dose intravenous aqueous penicillin 4 and 6 months earlier for neurosyphilis. They were diagnosed with active neurosyphilis on the basis of increasing abnormalities in the CSF, persistently high RPR titers, and progressive neurological symptoms.

Ocular complaints were present in 19% of HIV^+ patients as compared with 9% of HIV^- patients. Syphilitic eye disease was associated with syphilitic meningitis in five HIV-infected patients; with meningovascular syphilis in 1 HIV^- and 4 HIV^+ patients, and with general paresis in 1 HIV^- patient. Ocular syphilis associated with skin rash was significantly more common the HIV^+ group (21%) as compared with no HIV-uninfected patients. This study firmly established that there are differences in neurosyphilis occurring with HIV infection. Forty-six percent of the HIV-infected group had syphilitic meningitis, with frequent signs of secondary syphilis, including skin rash, fever, lymphadenopathy, and syphilitic uveitis.

Katz et al. (13) emphasized that the diagnosis of syphilitic eye disease requires a high index of suspicion. In one literature review (14), 85% of patients with ophthalmic syphilis also had neurosyphilis. Katz' study showed the converse also is true; a high percentage (43%) of HIV^+ patients with neurosyphilis also have ophthalmic syphilis. Ocular syphilis may be the earliest clue for the presence of both neurosyphilis and HIV infection.

Becerra et al. (15) reported that none of 12 HIV^+ patients with syphilitic uveitis had meningeal or neurological symptoms indicative of central nervous

Table 7 Classification of Neurosyphilis

1. Asymptomatic neurosyphilis
2. Meningovascular syphilis
    A. Meningeal syphilis
        Diffuse basal meningitis
        Diffuse syphilitic spinal arachnoiditis
        Pachymeningitis cervicalis hypertrophica
        Meningeal gumma
    B. Syphilitic meningomyelitis
    C. Erb's syphilitic spastic paraplegia
    D. Amyotrophic syphilitic myelitis
    F. Amyotrophic meningomyelitis
    G. Syphilitic amyotrophy
    H. Hydrocephalus due to syphilis
    I. Vascular neurosyphilis (hemiplegia; Heubner's arteritis; Lissauer's dementia paralytica)
3. Parenchymatous neurosyphilis
    A. Tabes dorsalis
    B. Paresis (dementia paralytica) (GPI)
    C. Taboparesis
    D. Paresis sine paresi (asymptomatic latent preparetic neurosyphilis of Stokes)
4. Syphilitic optic atrophy (also see ocular syphilis)
5. Congenital
    congenital tabes (juvenile tabes)
    congenital paresis (juvenile paresis)
    hydrocephalus
    congenital dementia, epilepsy, cerebral palsy due to syphilis

system (CNS) involvement, yet all had abnormal CSF examinations and 6 had a reactive CSF VDRL.

In a study of CSF changes in 200 patients with asymptomatic neurosyphilis, Merritt et al. (16) noted that 60% had fewer than 5 WBC/mm^3 and 58% had CSF proteins less than 40 mgm%. Radiological findings in neurosyphilis are nonspecific, but increased meningeal enhancement seen on brain CT in HIV^{++} patients may reflect the increased incidence of syphilitic meningitis in this group.

VII. THERAPY OF OCULAR AND NEUROSYPHILIS

Because of the frequent association of ocular and neurosyphilis, the following workup and management is recommended. All patients showing clinical signs of ocular or neurosyphilis should have a serum RPR or VDRL test with titer and a serum FTA-ABS test ordered. A careful history for prior infection with any sexually transmitted disease should be taken by the physician after having established a caring, professionally responsible relationship with the patient. It is often the case that the history becomes positive after the blood test does! Any patient with a history of previous venereal infection showing these clinical signs or with a reactive FTA-ABS test should have serological testing for HIV infection (enzyme-linked immunosorbent assay [ELISA] and confirmatory Western blot).

If a diagnosis of active ocular or neurosyphilis is established, a course of high-dose intravenous aqueous penicillin is advised. Usually 3 million units of aqueous penicillin every 4 h is given. Most investigators believe that the total daily dose should be 20 million units or less to avoid any possibility of penicillin toxicity (e.g., seizures). I have had no personal problems of penicillin overdosage in using this regimen in patients who are not allergic to penicillin. The patient should be given about 18–20 million units a day for a total of 10 days (200 million units total).

A lumbar puncture is indicated in every young patient with ocular and neurosyphilis. This decision can be individualized in the elderly patient who presents a totally different problem. For example, if routine blood testing before cataract surgery in a 75-year-old woman reveals a nonreactive serum RPR but a reactive FTA-ABS test, one may elect simply to give this patient 1 g of erythromycin po daily for 30 days and not do a lumbar puncture if the patient is otherwise well. If one is going to give the patient the same treatment for ocular syphilis as one would give for neurosyphilis, and I believe that is advisable, then a lumbar puncture may in some cases not be done. If there is any question, however, a careful and complete spinal fluid examination should be done, and certainly spinal fluid examination is required in any HIV^+ patient.

In the patient who is allergic to penicillin, there is a dilemma. Erythromycin in a total course of 30 g (e.g., 250 mg q6h for 30 days) has been advocated in early (primary or secondary) syphilis for these patients. In a patient with confirmed penicillin allergy, doxycycline 100 mg po bid for 2 weeks is now often advised for early syphilis (17). I prefer to use doxycycline, 100 mg po tid, to help penetration across the blood ocular/brain barrier. Penicillin allergy should be confirmed by skin testing. One can desensitize patients and treat with penicillin if active neurosyphilis is found, but I have had no personal experience with this. For the patient with a definite history of penicillin allergy, I would personally recommend either a course of intravenous Rocephin 2 g/day for 10 days or doxycycline, 100 mg tid PO for 4 weeks, in a patient with active ocular or neurosyphilis at this time depending on the clinical urgency and patient compliance. These patients should be monitored carefully for evidence of a Jarisch-Herxheimer reaction. The simplest way is to take the temperature every hour for 4 h before starting the antibiotic therapy, and then take it every hour for 8 h after commencing antibiotic therapy, and then every 2–4 h for the next 24 h. This is not usually a reaction of clinical consequence, but one should be aware of it.

Finally, for the busy reader who looks at the end of a journal article or book chapter but who does not have time to read the whole thing, the following list may be helpful in closing.

A. Most Common Errors in Management of Ocular/Neurosyphilis

1. Forget to get a *titer* on a reactive VDRL or RPR test and forget to follow titer after treatment.
2. Forget to order an FTA-ABS test when VDRL or RPR test is nonreactive in a patient with clinical signs suspicious for ocular/neurosyphilis.
3. Physician orders a serum FTA-AVS\\BS but *lab refuses* to do it because of nonreactive serum VDRL or RPR test.
4. Physician orders an FTA-ABS test on *spinal fluid but does not* order an FTA-ABS test on the blood.
5. Forget to get an RPR or VDRL on a patient with a reactive FTA-ABS test.
6. Remember that *Lyme* borreliosis can give a *false-positive* FTA-ABS test (22%) but a false-positive VDRL or RPR test has *not* been reported with Lyme disease. Take a careful history for Lyme borreliosis and consider a Lyme IFA and ELISA test when appropriate.
7. Remember that a beaded FTA-ABS response can be seen in patients with *lupus* (rare).
8. Forget to take a careful *history* for sexually transmitted diseases and details of prior treatment. This is best done at the end of a careful examination when rapport and patient confidence have been established.
9. *Treat* a patient with reactive serum FTA-ABS test without appropriate history or inquiry as to timing and amount of prior treatment.
10. Forget to get a serum *HIV* test in a patient with ocular or neurosyphilis.
11. Forget to order RPR and FTA-ABS in every HIV^+ patient.
12. Omit getting a lumbar puncture in patients with active ocular syphilis.

Space does not allow a complete coverage of this subject, but the references may help the interested reader who needs further to explore this fascinating neuro-ophthalmological subject that bridges every medical specialty.

REFERENCES

1. Walsh FB. Clinical neuro-ophthalmology. 2d ed. Baltimore: Williams & Wilkins, 1957:541.
2. United States Centers for Disease Control and Prevention, Division of STD/HIV Prevention, Atlanta, GA (data through the courtesy of Francoise Hamers, MD, MPH).

3. Harner RE, Smith JL, Israel CW. The FTA-ABS test in late syphilis. A serological study of 1,985 cases. JAMA 1968; 203:545–8.
4. Spoor TC, Ramocki JM, Nesi FA, Sorscher M. Ocular syphilis 1986. Prevalence of FTA-ABS reactivity and cerebrospinal fluid findings. J Clin Neuro Ophthalmol 1987; 7:91–5.
5. Smith JL. Spirochetes in late seronegative syphilis, penicillin notwithstanding. Springfield, IL: Charles C Thomas, 1969.
6. Bruetsch WL. Syphilitic optic atrophy. Springfield, IL: Charles C Thomas, 1953.
7. Wilson JD, Braunwald E, Isselbacher KJ, Petersdorf RG, Martin JB, Fauci AS, Root RK, eds. Harrison's principles of internal medicine. 12th ed. New York: McGraw-Hill, 1991.
8. Berger JR. Neurosyphilis in human immunodeficiency virus type 1–seropositive individuals. Arch Neurol 1991; 48:700–2.
9. Lukehart SA, Hook EW III, Baker-Zander SA, Collier AC, Critchlow CW, Handsfield NH. Invasion of the central nervous system by Treponema pallidum: implications for diagnosis and treatment. Ann Intern Med 1988; 109:855–62.
10. Berger JR. Diagnosing neurosyphilis. The value of the cerebrospinal fluid VDRL or lack thereof. J Clin Neuro Ophthalmol 1989; 9:234–5.
11. Smith JL, Byrne SF, Cambron CR. Syphiloma/gumma of the optic nerve and human immunodeficiency virus seropositivity. J Clin Neuro Ophthalmol 1990; 10:175–84.
12. Haas JS, Bolan G, Larsen SA, Clement MJ, Bacchetti P, Moss AR. Sensitivity of treponemal tests for detecting prior treated syphilis during human immunodeficiency virus infection. J Infect Dis 1990; 162:862–6.
13. Katz DA, Berger JR, Duncan RC. Neurosyphilis: a comparative study of the effects of infection with human immunodeficiency virus. Arch Neurol 1993; 50:243–9.
14. Levy JH, Liss RA, Maguire AM. Neurosyphilis and ocular syphilis in patients with concurrent human immunodeficiency virus infection. Retina 1989; 9:175–80.
15. Becerra LI, Ksiazek SM, Savino PJ, et al. Syphilitic uveitis in human immunodeficiency virus infected and noninfected patients. Ophthalmology 1989, 96:1727–30.
16. Merritt HH, Adams RD, Solomon HC. Neurosyphilis. New York: Oxford University Press, 1946.
17. Margo CE, Hamed LM. Ocular syphilis. Surv Ophthalmol 1992; 37(3):203–20.

38

Neuro-Ophthalmic Lyme Disease in Perspective

Jacqueline M.S. Winterkorn
Cornell University Medical College, New York, and North Shore University Hospital–Cornell University Medical College, Manhasset, New York

Lyme disease has been the subject of considerable medical interest in the United States during the past 15 years, but the inventory of symptoms and signs attributable to this previously little known disease has yet to be fully defined. In their efforts to avoid missing the diagnosis, physicians have included it in the differential diagnosis of many etiological dilemmas. As a result, they have diagnosed Lyme disease in patients who have syndromes of unknown cause (1), especially with neurological and ocular manifestations. Overdiagnosis of Lyme disease (2) has been a problem, particularly in geographical areas endemic for the disease, where symptoms and signs of unknown etiology occurring in patients with blood tests showing antibodies to the Lyme organism often have been attributed to Lyme disease without adequate justification. After over a decade of vigilance for sequelae of Lyme borreliosis, the striking aspect of the neuro-ophthalmic literature is how few cases of Lyme disease are accompanied by any ocular findings and how rarely there are any long-term sequelae (3). This chapter is written at a time when physicians are beginning to place Lyme disease more appropriately in the order of differential diagnosis of neurological and ophthalmic disorders.

I. HISTORY

Lyme disease was identified in the United States in 1977, after two astute Connecticut mothers urged investigation of an epidemic of joint swelling and pain that had been diagnosed as "juvenile rheumatoid arthritis" in youngsters of Old Lyme and surrounding towns in Connecticut. After studying the outbreak, Dr. Allen Steere identified the disease as "Lyme arthritis" (4,5), which he described as an infection spread by the bite of the tiny deer tick, *Ixodes dammini*.

In 1982, Dr. Willy Burgdorfer identified the infectious agent as a spirochete, now known as *Borrelia burgdorferi* (6), which resembles the treponeme causing syphilis. As its dermatological, rheumatological, cardiological, and neurological manifestations were elucidated, Lyme disease was recognized as a multisystem disorder and, likened to syphilis, has been referred to as "the new great imitator" (7).

However, Lyme disease is not a new entity. A strikingly similar syndrome characterized by a skin rash following tick bite was described in Germany in 1883 (8) and has been observed in Europe for over 100 years. In the early 1900s, Afzelius (9) described erythema migrans, the bull's-eye rash that heralds Lyme infection, and concluded that the lesion was caused by a tickborne spirochete. A neurological presentation of the disease, including lymphocytic meningitis and painful radiculopathy, was reported in 1922 by Garin and Bujadoux (10) and described more fully in 1941 by Bannwarth (11). Shortly after *Borrelia burgdorferi* was isolated in the United States, the same or a very similar spirochete was acknowledged to be the cause of the European borreliosis (12).

II. EPIDEMIOLOGY

Although Lyme disease occurs worldwide and throughout the United States, it tends to be concentrated in geographical areas where its vector, the *Ixodes* tick, is exposed to large populations of deer and rodents infected by *Borrelia* (13). The endemic areas in the United States comprise the Northeast coastal area from Maine to Maryland; the northern Midwest, including Minnesota, Wisconsin, and Michigan; and the Pacific coastal states of Oregon and California. In the years immediately after surveillance for Lyme disease was initiated by the Centers for Disease Control and Prevention, epidemiological studies showed a steady rise in the incidence of Lyme borreliosis, with an 18-fold increase from 497 cases in 1982 to 8803 cases in 1989 (14). New York state, which has reported more than half of the cases in the United States, experienced a sevenfold increase in Lyme cases between 1986 and 1989, which was partly attributed to the burgeoning deer population and the increasing proportion of *Ixodes* ticks infected by borreliae. Although the number of cases reported annually leveled off after 1990, over 10% of the population in high-prevalence areas has been estimated to have antibodies suggesting exposure to Lyme borreliosis (15).

III. COURSE OF DISEASE

Lyme borreliosis usually is contracted in late spring or summer, less often in autumn, and rarely in winter, reflecting the 2-year life cycle and feeding patterns of the *Ixodes* tick (16). Tick eggs hatch in spring and the larvae seek a blood meal during the summer. Those that survive the winter molt into nymphs that feed the following spring. The mature ticks feed from late summer through fall. Transmission of Lyme borreliosis occurs while the tick is having a blood meal and requires about 12–24 h of contact between tick and host.

Within 3–30 days after the tick bite, a red macule or papule appears. The red spot expands centrifugally, with partial central clearing, forming a light center within a reddened ring—the distinctive lesion recognizable as *erythema migrans*, the pathognomonic rash of Lyme disease (Fig. 1).

Although clinical manifestations of Lyme disease, like syphilis, are divided into chronological stages, the symptoms and signs in each stage are variable, the stages may overlap in time, and not all patients exhibit each stage. Early and late manifestations can develop in several organ systems (18,19).

Early Lyme disease includes stages I and II (Table 1). Stage I is the period of acute localized infection manifested by the diagnostic annular rash. The erythema migrans rash is usually asymptomatic and may be ignored by the

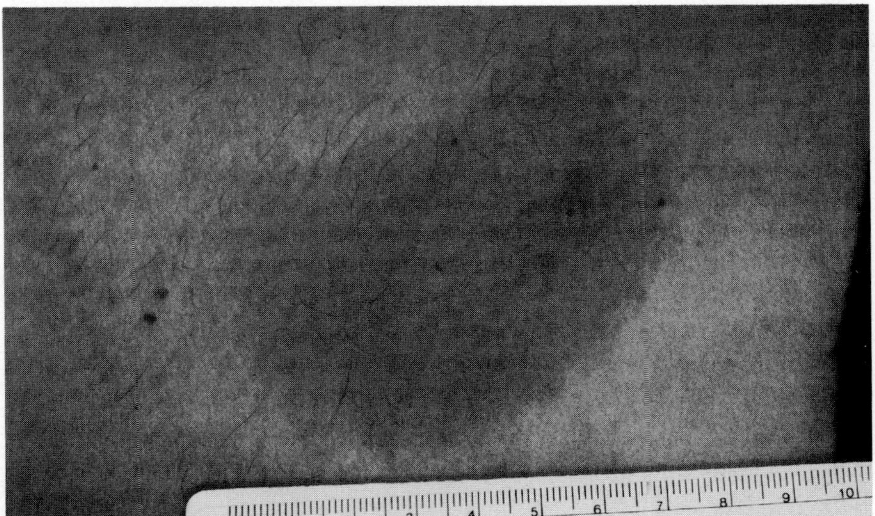

Figure 1 Erythema migrans. Pathognomonic bull's eye rash heralding Lyme disease is seen on patient's thigh. (Illustration courtesy of Dr. J. J. Halperin.)

Table 1 Manifestations of Lyme Disease

	Early Lyme disease		Late Lyme disease
	Stage I	Stage II	Stage III
Possible Pathology	Infection	Dissemination	Immune reaction
Skin	Erythema migrans	Erythema migrans	Acrodermatitis chronica and atrophicans
Rheumatological		Arthralgia	Lyme arthritis
Cardiac		Arrythmia, AV Block	
Neurological	Headache, meningismus	Meningitis, cranial neuritis VII > III, IV, VI, radiculopathy	Encephalopathy, neuropathy, fatigue, leukencephalitis
Ocular	Conjunctivitis, photophobia	Choroiditis,[a] uveitis,[a] neuroretinitis,[a] Vascular occlusion,[a] Postpap atrophy	Keratitis, Episcleritis[a]

[a]Rare case reports only.

patient, but on occasion it can be itchy, burning, tender, or painful. Erythema migrans usually resolves spontaneously without treatment, and it is recalled by as few as half of those patients with Lyme borreliosis. In rare cases, the rash may persist for weeks or months, but with appropriate antibiotic therapy, it fades in days (17).

Stage II, reflecting dissemination of the infection, can occur days, weeks, or months later. The initial lesion can be accompanied by a flulike syndrome with lymphadenopathy, fever, and myalgias. Neurological symptoms include headache and stiff neck. Ocular manifestations include photophobia, conjunctivitis, and periorbital edema. Typically about 4 weeks after infection, the untreated patient may develop prominent dermatological, rheumatological, cardiac, or neurological complaints. Although the initial skin lesion fades, between 10 and 50% of untreated patients will develop multiple secondary annular skin lesions that also tend to be asymptomatic and gradually fade and disappear. Antibiotic therapy at this stage leads to more rapid resolution of the lesions. Migratory pains in joints, tendons, muscles, and bone develop in more than half of untreated patients. A minority of patients, fewer than 10%, suffer a brief period of cardiac involvement and can have atrioventricular block, left ventricular arrhythmia, or myocarditis. This usually resolves without residual damage. The triad of neurological presentations known as Garin-Bujadoux-Bannwarth syndrome, comprising lymphocytic meningitis, cranial neuropathy, and painful radiculopathy, has been reported to develop in 15% of untreated cases of Lyme disease

Table 2 Frequency of Occurrence in UNTREATED Lyme Disease

Lyme stage	Manifestation	Frequency (%)
Early Lyme infection dissemination	Erythema migrans	75
	Secondary skin lesions	50
	Arthralgias	50
	Stiff neck	40
	Lymphocytic meningitis	15
	Conjunctivitis	11
	AV nodal block	8
	Facial palsy	7
Late (chronic) Lyme disease	Arthritis	60
	Encephalomyelitis	1
	Keratitis	<4

(20). Although ocular manifestations are uncommon, case reports have associated almost every kind of ocular inflammation with Lyme disease.

Late or chronic Lyme disease can begin within days of infection or may become apparent many years later. Although this stage may involve immune reactivity, many of its signs and symptoms still resolve on treatment with antibiotics. Late dermatological, rheumatological, neurological, and ocular manifestations of Lyme disease have been described (3,25). The most common manifestation is "Lyme arthritis," which consists of recurrent bouts of inflammatory oligoarthritis or synovitis, and typically affects large joints such as the knee (21). Unlike juvenile rheumatoid arthritis, for which it was initially mistaken, Lyme arthritis seems to develop preferentially in individuals with the HLA-DR4 allele (22,23). Other HLA groups may influence susceptibility to developing late effects in different organs. This in part may explain the very variable expression of Lyme disease (24).

IV. DIAGNOSIS

A patient in an endemic area who recalls a tick bite, observes the pathognomonic rash, has associated flulike symptoms, and subsequently develops rheumatological complaints may require no further evaluation for the physician to be confident of the diagnosis of Lyme disease. However, if the patient has overlooked the tick bite and rash, the diagnosis may be elusive. Various criteria have been suggested to support a clinical diagnosis of Lyme disease, including exposure in an endemic area and rapid improvement in symptoms after specific antibiotic therapy.

Laboratory confirmation of the diagnosis of Lyme disease is increasingly important. Although the spirochete *Borrelia burgdorferi* has been identified in the skin, retina, vitreous, brain, and other organs of patients and experimental animals, and has been isolated from blood and synovial and cerebrospinal fluids, it remains notoriously difficult to culture. Laboratory tests for diagnosing Lyme borreliosis most commonly attempt to identify specific antibodies in a patient's blood. Both the immunofluorescence assay (IFA) and the more reliable enzyme-linked immunoabsorbant assay (ELISA) measure blood levels of immunoglobulins (Ig) M and G against *Borrelia burdorferi*. The IFA is considered positive when fluorescent antihuman immunoglobulin signals the presence of antibody to Lyme spirochetes at a dilution of the patient's serum above some arbitrary threshold. In the ELISA, a comparison is made between spectrophotometric measurements of a colored enzyme preparation reacting with antibody in the patient's serum and with uninfected control sera, and the result is expressed as the ratio of the optical densities. Unfortunately, these tests are imperfect and provide at times falsely negative and more frequently falsely positive results (25) even on the same blood sample when tested in different laboratories. Sources of variability include the lack of standardization of control sera among laboratories; differing surface antigenicity among strains of *Borrelia*; and cross-reactivity of a patient's autoantibodies with antibodies to the organism itself (26). Although early antibiotic treatment can result in subsequent negative tests (so-called seronegative Lyme disease), a much more frequent diagnostic pitfall is the persistence of immune positivity raising undue concern about active disease long after adequate treatment had led to its complete resolution. When the results of serological testing are positive but not definitive, a Western blot technique can confirm the diagnosis by isolating antigenic responses to Lyme-specific surface proteins. This test also may be helpful in discriminating Lyme disease from syphilis, since their cross-reactivity provides continuing controversy (27,28).

Testing for syphilis should always accompany testing for Lyme disease; and in endemic areas, tests for Lyme should be taken whenever syphilis is suspected. Considerable cross-reactivity has been demonstrated between the FTA-ABs and the Lyme ELISA in either direction. In the setting of a negative VDRL with a positive FTA-ABs as well as a positive Lyme titer, Lyme disease should be considered. However, a positive serological test for Lyme disease is more likely to signal syphilis than vice versa except in locales highly endemic for Lyme disease.

Newer diagnostic methods under investigation include IgM capture techniques, lymphocyte antigen stimulation, polymerase chain reaction, urine antigen testing, and silver staining of organisms.

A spinal tap should always be performed and the patient's cerebrospinal fluid (CSF) evaluated whenever chronic neurological sequelae are considered possibly due to Lyme disease. Although Lyme spirochetes occasionally have been cultured from CSF, the diagnosis of neuroborreliosis usually is based on a positive CSF ELISA. Antibody titers in CSF are not always high in early stages of Lyme disease, but significant intrathecal antibody is considered a reliable marker for chronic Lyme disease in the central nervous system (24,29). When antibodies to Lyme disease are not found, serious consideration must be given to diagnosis of other conditions that have varied systemic manifestations, including other spirochetal diseases, such as syphilis and leptospirosis; other bacterial infections, including Rocky Mountain spotted fever and brucellosis, disseminated gonococci, subacute bacterial endocarditis; viral infections, including mononucleosis; autoimmune diseases, including systemic lupus, rheumatoid arthritis, fibromyalgia, and polymyalgia rheumatica; and systemic maladies, including thyrotoxicosis, Reiter's syndrome, sarcoidosis, and multiple sclerosis (30).

V. NEUROLOGICAL MANIFESTATIONS

The neurological manifestations typical of Lyme disease are meningitis or meningoencephalitis with cranial and radicular neuropathies (20,31).

A. Meningitis

Lymphocytic meningitis occurs in about 15% of untreated patients with Lyme disease and is characterized by headache, backache, stiff neck, nausea, vomiting, photophobia, fever, and fatigue (30). Examination of CSF shows a lymphocytic or plasma cell pleocytosis, with over 100 cells-cm^3, mildly elevated protein, and normal glucose. However, the broad differential diagnosis of other causes of aseptic meningitis must be considered before attributing such signs and symptoms to Lyme disease.

Papilledema commonly occurs in Lyme meningitis and can be accompanied by transient visual obscurations. A failure to recognize that papilledema is a sign of Lyme meningitis has resulted in several case reports misinterpreting neuro-ophthalmic sequelae of Lyme disease. Thus, an association between "pseudotumor cerebri" and Lyme disease has been suggested in reports involving three children (32,33); but the CSF profile in each case revealed lymphocytosis or elevated protein indicating that these children had meningitis and not pseudotumor cerebri.

B. Cranial Neuropathy

Cranial nerve palsies and radicular pain with weakness often accompany the aseptic meningitis of Lyme disease (31,34). The facial nerve is the cranial nerve most commonly affected by Lyme disease (35,36). Unilateral or bilateral facial nerve palsy is seen in about half the cases of Lyme meningitis, but it also can occur in the absence of meningitis. Seventh nerve palsy may be the presenting sign of Lyme disease (30). Although as many as a fourth of patients presenting with facial palsy during the summer months in one Lyme-endemic area were found to have positive Lyme serology (37), Lyme disease remains an infrequent cause of isolated facial neuropathy (38). Ischemia is a more common cause than Lyme disease, especially in an older patient, and sarcoid is more likely than Lyme disease to cause bilateral facial nerve weakness. The differential diagnosis of acquired seventh nerve palsy should also include syphilis, Guillian-Barré syndrome, and lymphoreticular disorders. Diplopia caused by a cranial nerve (III, IV, VI) palsy as a manifestation of Lyme disease occurs much less frequently than a facial nerve palsy. Neurosensory hearing impairment reflecting damage to the auditory-vestibular nerve can also occur (36). Involvement of the trigeminal nerve may cause facial paresthesias, numbness or pain (39), and involvement of cranial nerves IX and X occasionally leads to loss of taste and difficulty swallowing (24). Case reports have associated serologically confirmed Lyme disease with other unusual peripheral cranial neuropathies, for example, an isolated paralysis of the recurrent laryngeal nerve (40) as well as with intracranial polyneuropathy (41), although causality is difficult to establish in anecdotal cases.

C. Radiculopathy

The radiculopathies associated with Lyme disease are characterized by mixed motor and sensory loss (39,42), with motor abnormalities confirmed by electromyography (42,44), and sensory impairment demonstrated by formal testing (39). Neuropathic pains, including dysesthesias and paresthesias (44), may be localized initially to the level of the tick bite but become widely distributed. The peripheral neuropathies of Lyme disease can take many forms but most represent an expression of mononeuropathy multiplex (45–47).

D. Pupils

Evidence has been presented that Lyme disease causes efferent pupillary abnormalities, but it is not conclusive. A single case report has described the development of Horner's syndrome that became apparent shortly after the patient was bitten by a tick and resolved when he received antibiotic treatment (48). The occurrence of a tonic pupil (49) as well as Argyll Robertson pupils (31) has been mentioned in reports on other neurological sequelae of Lyme disease.

E. Optic Neuropathy

Unlike syphilis, Lyme disease has not been convincingly shown to cause isolated optic neuritis. Most optic neuropathies reported in the neurological literature on Lyme disease have described visual defects resulting from optic disc edema during meningitis (28,29,49,50–52) and optic atrophy, probably reflecting postpapilledema atrophy following Lyme meningoencephalitis (53–56) rather than a primary optic neuropathy.

Optic neuropathies characterized by monocular papillitis, including anterior ischemic optic neuropathy (52,57–59) and demyelinating optic neuritis (31,49,60,61), have been reported to occur in patients coincidentally found to have positive serology for Lyme disease but without a demonstrated causal relationship. Co-occurrence of a positive Lyme titer and a common syndrome such as demyelinating optic neuritis or anterior ischemic optic neuropathy is not an unusual event in an area endemic for Lyme borreliosis and must not be interpreted as an association unless CSF titers are positive for Lyme disease. Since these cases have reported blood titers and not CSF titers, the presence of active Lyme disease cannot be assumed. In some of the reported cases there has even been inadequate evidence of serological positivity to confirm the past occurrence of Lyme disease. For example, a 53-year-old patient has been described (57) who suffered optic disc swelling and altitudinal visual field loss sequentially in both eyes, without recovery despite treatment with antibiotics and steroids. Although this investigator has suggested an association between nonarteritic anterior ischemic optic neuropathy and Lyme disease, a causal relationship was not established. The diagnosis of Lyme disease seems similarly unwarranted in the case of a 71-year-old man living in an area hyperendemic for Lyme disease who suffered visual loss but who had negative Lyme serology and a positive temporal artery biopsy (59). A report entitled "Lyme Disease and Optic Neuritis" (61) described a 39-year-old woman from a nonendemic region who developed a papillitis following a rash and aseptic meningitis. Since this patient had positive tests for syphilis (FTA-ABS and MHA-TP) at the same time as a positive Lyme ELISA, the diagnosis of Lyme disease is in doubt.

Optic neuritis has been described in patients with additional neurological signs of demyelination and with serological tests positive for Lyme disease, but unless the CSF produces evidence of antibodies to Lyme disease, these patients are more likely to have an underlying demyelinating diathesis. In locations where Lyme disease is endemic, a significant proportion of the residents have blood tests that remain positive for Lyme disease even without clinical history of infection. In clinical practice, although a course of antibiotic therapy may prudently be offered to a patient with a positive Lyme titer, only many years of prospective observation of patients with positive Lyme titers and optic neuritis will prove whether they have demyelinating disease unrelated to their positive

Lyme titers or optic neuritis caused by Lyme disease. So far, no case has been reported in which the afferent pupillary defect resolved and the vision rapidly improved in response to antibiotic treatment suggesting that the presence of a positive serology for Lyme disease was unrelated to the optic neuritis (30,49,59). A definitive case of an isolated optic neuropathy caused by Lyme disease still remains to be demonstrated.

F. Encephalitis

Lyme disease, like syphilis, may affect the central nervous system parenchyma as well as the meninges and cranial and peripheral nerves. Nonfocal symptoms of encephalopathy, including lethargy, memory loss, and emotional lability, have been reported by Reik et al. (52) to occur in two thirds of their patients with Lyme meningitis. The encephalopathy tends to be mild and self-limited, perhaps reflecting an inflammatory reaction without invasion of the CNS by spirochetes (24). Only very rarely, focal encephalitis of the CNS indicated by reports of transverse myelitis, ataxia, chorea, seizures, and hemiparesis (36,60) has implied parenchymal involvement.

G. Chronic Neurological Sequelae

Late manifestations of Lyme disease in the nervous system have been carefully documented in several studies (24,29,34,41) and consist of distinctive patterns and combinations of peripheral polyneuropathy, mild encephalopathy, and rarely a progressive leukoencephalomyelitis. Chronic neurological dysfunction has been apparent between 1 month and 14 years after initial diagnosis (29).

Peripheral nerve involvement is characterized by polyneuropathy with paresthesias. The prominent symptoms of Lyme encephalopathy include fatigue, weakness, headache, depression, and memory impairment. These nonspecific complaints are virtually identical to those of patients with fibromyalgia and fatigue syndromes ascribed to chronic viral infection (1).

In the progressive encephalomyelitis of chronic Lyme disease, the nonspecific mental status alterations of encephalopathy are compounded by multifocal signs, including ataxia, sensory loss, hemiparesis, and rarely seizures. This syndrome often mimics multiple sclerosis and even is associated with similar white matter lesions on magnetic resonance imaging of the brain (Fig. 2) (51,52). Similarities between these infrequent cases of Lyme encephalomyelitis and the far more commonly occurring cases of multiple sclerosis (MS) have led to confusion between these two diagnoses, especially in locales where Lyme disease is endemic and patients with multiple sclerosis are likely to have positive Lyme serology. Infection with *B. burgdorferi* has even been hypothesized to underlie development of MS (61,62). However, that hypothesis has been disproven by comparing the presence of Lyme antibodies in patients with MS and in controls

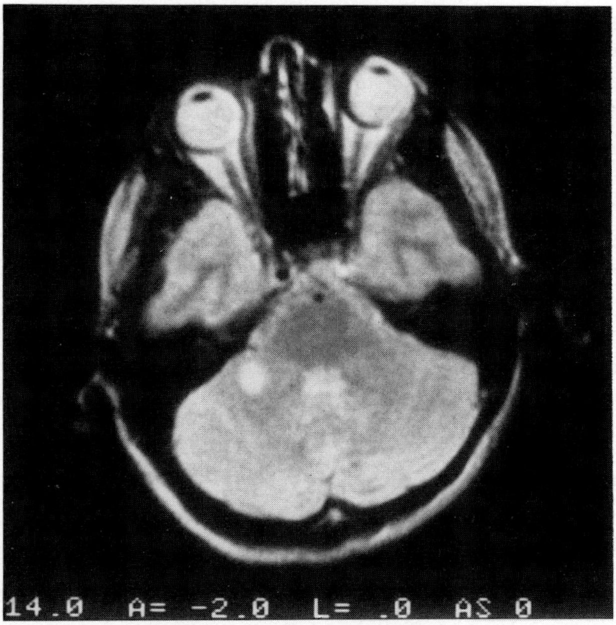

Figure 2 MRI in Lyme encephalomyelitis. MRI of 23 year old woman with Lyme disease confirmed by CSF titers shows lucencies on T2. (Illustration courtesy of Dr. J. J. Halperin).

and finding positive serology in similarly low frequency in both groups (62,63). Furthermore, recent studies of clinical and laboratory findings in patients with chronic Lyme disease (1,24,29,71) have pointed out that Lyme encephalomyelitis can be readily distinguished from MS accompanied by positive Lyme titers on the basis of (1) a history of other systemic signs and complications indicative of active Lyme disease; (2) the presence of Lyme antibodies in the CSF; and (3) dramatic response of Lyme disease to treatment with intravenous ceftriaxone.

In an enthusiastic but uncritical search for new manifestations of Lyme disease, many other neurological syndromes have been attributed to Lyme borreliosis when only co-occurrence has been demonstrated. Case reports have suggested associations between Lyme disease and amyotrophic lateral sclerosis (64), Parkinson's disease (65), Alzheimer's dementia (66), space-occupying lesions (67,68), CNS vasculitis (69,70), recurrent strokes (70), and psychiatric disorders ranging from anorexia nervosa to depression (71).

Although the spectrum of neurological disease actually attributable to Lyme disease may have seemed difficult to define because of uncertainty about whether a clinical syndrome signaled Lyme disease or merely represented an unrelated finding in a patient with Lyme antibodies, active neuroborreliosis has been shown to be consistently recognizable (24,29,72). Neurological Lyme disease can be defined by a limited set of symptoms and signs, and most importantly by the presence of intrathecal antibodies that can be demonstrated reliably in almost every case with CNS manifestations. Cases with only peripheral manifestations may not have significant intrathecal antibody (43), but most cases of chronic Lyme disease have had an unequivocal past history of Lyme infection, including either tick bite, rash, rheumatological manifestations, or positive serology (24,29). Late Lyme disease does not seem to present mysteriously without history (1,72).

Finally, despite chronicity, neurological symptoms of Lyme disease are usually relieved or improved by a 2- or 3-week course of antibiotic therapy. Indeed, Steere (1) has emphasized that the major reason that patients diagnosed as having Lyme disease fail to respond to appropriate antibiotic therapy is that they do not have Lyme disease.

VI. OCULAR MANIFESTATIONS

Unlike the characteristic cutaneous, cardiac, rheumatologic, and neurologic manifestations of Lyme disease, ocular findings are not prominent. Summaries of the literature have alerted ophthalmologists to ocular symptoms and signs seen in patients with positive Lyme serology, without emphasizing the need for critical evaluation in order to avoid overdiagnosis of the disease. Since most reports have been anecdotal summaries of a case or two, comprehensive lists of every ophthalmic finding associated with Lyme disease are subject to misinterpretation unless they indicate that a causal relationship has not been substantiated (see Table 1). Case reports have described a variety of common ocular syndromes occurring in individual patients from Lyme-endemic areas, with a positive blood test for Lyme disease usually discovered during extensive evaluation for possible causes of the idiopathic syndrome. Such reports have not always employed adequate criteria to establish the cause of a patient's ocular symptoms and signs. Although many different forms of ocular inflammation have been seen in patients with serology positive for Lyme disease, the absence of multiple similar cases consistently developing a specific ocular sign raises doubts about the ocular sign being a significant or direct manifestation of Lyme disease. A critique of a case report in which a branch retinal artery occlusion was attributed to Lyme disease (73) pointed out "that a co-occurrence is not an association" (74).

> Among patients with positive Lyme titers have been cases of keratoconus, meningioma, diabetic neuropathy, and biopsy-proven propionbacter vitritis. In most cases, the patients have an ocular symptom and Lyme disease, not an ocular symptom from Lyme disease (74).

Skepticism seems appropriate in interpreting reports of ocular sequelae of Lyme disease.

A. Conjunctivitis

Conjunctivitis and periorbital edema (75–77) probably accompany the flulike illness in stage I Lyme disease with even greater regularity than suggested by Steere et al. (75), who recognized it in 11% of their initial patients.

If the tick bite is on or near the eyelids, the erythema migrans rash may be seen on the eyelid and associated with local edema.

B. Keratitis

Keratitis is the single best documented and most characteristic ocular manifestation of late Lyme disease (1–3,78–84). It has been seen in the cornea between 6 months and 6 years after initial infection. Although keratitis is the only ocular manifestation reported in long-term studies of patients with untreated Lyme disease, it nevertheless remains a relatively rare manifestation of Lyme disease overall. In a large series of 788 adults referred for possible manifestations of Lyme disease, *keratitis was the only ocular finding*, and it occurred in one patient (1). Keratitis was the only ocular sequela reported in a study of the long-term course of children with untreated Lyme arthritis and it occurred in only 2 (4%) of 47 youngsters (3).

The keratitis characteristic of Lyme disease is a bilateral corneal infiltration with multiple focal opacities at all depths of the corneal stroma (78–82) (Fig. 3). The nummular opacities extend from limbus to limbus but frequently spare the visual axis (79). Occasionally mild neovascularization is seen that is reminiscent of the more severe interstitial keratitis of syphilis (79). Lyme keratitis seems to represent an immune reaction rather than an active infection of the cornea, and it responds to treatment with steroids rather than antibiotics (3,80–86). Two cases of episcleritis attributed to late Lyme disease (76,82) and an orbital myositis attributed to Lyme disease without justification (2,83) also have responded to corticosteroid therapy.

Patients have been described with other forms of keratitis (84,85) of less certain causation by Lyme disease. A patient with positive blood tests for Lyme disease had both keratitis and hearing loss, which together were interpreted as a form of Cogan's syndrome (84); and an ulcerative keratitis (85) was seen in a woman who subsequently developed an autoimmune vasculitis that eventually required treatment with azathioprine. This seems unlikely to have been related to Lyme disease.

C. Uveitis

Uveitis encompasses a variety of ocular conditions for which an etiology rarely is identified despite extensive medical evaluation for immunological, infectious, neoplastic, and granulomatous diseases, including specific tests for sarcoid and syphilis. Positive Lyme titers have been found in patients with diverse uveitic syndromes, including anterior uveitis (iritis, granulomatous iritis, and iridocy-

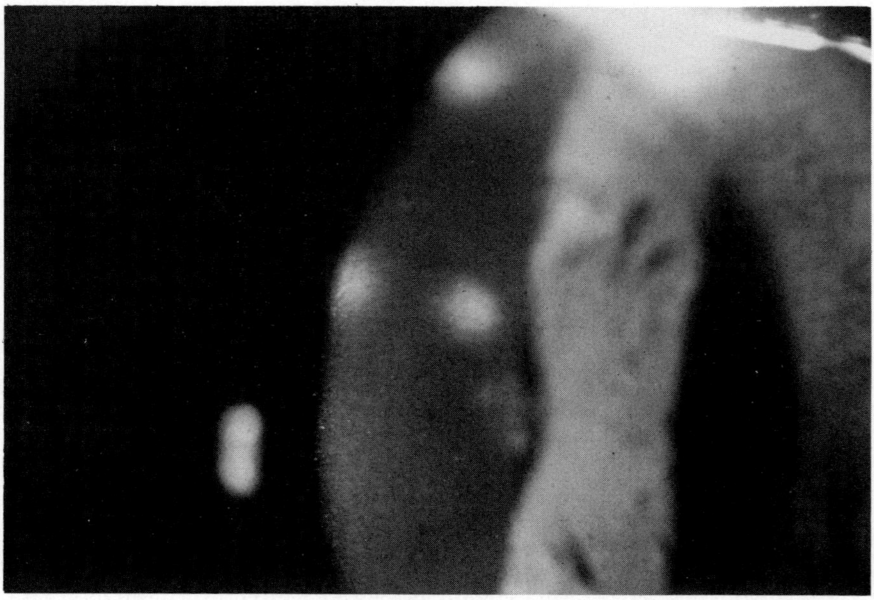

Figure 3 Lyme keratitis: Note multiple nummular hazy opacities at varying levels of the cornea from limbus to limbus. (Illustration courtesy of Dr. E. W. Kornmehl.)

clitis) (86–88), intermediate uveitis (pars planitis) (89), posterior uveitis (vitritis) (90,91), and panophthalmitis (75,92–94).

A patient reported soon after Lyme disease became popular (75,92) was a 42-year-old woman with well-documented Lyme disease who developed iritis 1 month after antibiotic treatment for erythema migrans. Iritis progressed to vitritis, and after steroids were given and vitrectomy performed, the patient developed a panophthalmitis, which despite further use of antibiotics deteriorated to phthisis and monocular blindness. Although not cultured from the initial vitrectomy specimen, *B. burgdorferi* was identified microscopically in the vitreous debris after enucleation. More recently, *B. burgdorferi* has been isolated from an iridectomy specimen taken from a uveitis patient (95).

On the other hand, another case illustrates the danger of concluding that a vitritis is caused by Lyme disease just because a patient with vitritis has positive Lyme serology. A 62-year-old man presented with chronic vitritis and bilateral facial palsy and was found to have positive Lyme titers in both blood and CSF. The vitritis did not respond to multiple courses of IV ceftriaxone. A vitreous biopsy was done, which in this case revealed *Propionibacterium acnes* (99).

Despite the possibility that Lyme disease is responsible for some cases of uveitis, evaluation of large series of uveitis patients has shown that false-positive Lyme titers are not uncommon in patients with uveitis caused by sarcoid and Behçet's, Vogt-Koyanagi-Harada, and Reiter's syndrome or associated with HLA B27. Lyme borreliosis overall is an extremely rare cause of uveitis and tests for Lyme disease should not even be obtained in a nonendemic area (96,97).

D. Neuroretinitis

Neuroretinitis is another ocular syndrome for which usually no etiology is demonstrated despite extensive medical evaluation. Four cases of neuroretinitis associated with Lyme disease, in which treatment with ceftriaxone produced a rapid resolution, certainly suggests causality. However, this is not definitive proof since neuroretinitis characteristically resolves rapidly even without treatment (2,40,99,100).

Other retinal signs observed in single cases include retinal vasculitis, macular edema associated with posterior uveitis, retinal granuloma, and a focal retinitis (75,87,92,93,102.)

E. Choroiditis

Different examples of choroiditis (99–104) have been reported in patients with positive Lyme serology, but causality is difficult to establish. Since several cases have involved retinal pigmented epithelium or the inner choroid, which share a common blood supply from the short posterior ciliary vessels, a common vasculitis mechanism could be hypothesized. However, such a variety of different choroiditis has been described without a consistent or repeated pattern of presentation that it is tempting to consider most of these casual associations. Lyme disease has been associated with multifocal choroiditis, birdshot chorioretinopathy, serpiginous choroiditis, pigment epitheliopathy, and acute multifocal placoid pigment epitheliopathy (100–106). The etiology of choroiditis remains a mystery. Positive Lyme titers have been found in some cases of choroiditis suggesting that Lyme disease may be a contributing factor in rare cases. However, even when positive Lyme serology has been found in cases of choroiditis, many of the patients have had no other evidence of having had Lyme disease and the possibility exists that false-positive Lyme serology may be a measure of these patients' underlying autoimmune diatheses (104).

Lyme disease has been associated with such a broad spectrum of ocular diseases that it has been compared with syphilis. However, after a decade on the alert for significant ocular manifestations, individual case reports still constitute the bulk of the medical literature on ocular sequelae of Lyme disease. The paucity of patients with ocular consequences of Lyme disease is striking in contrast to reports of large numbers of patients with dermatological, rheumatological, cardiological, and neurological sequelae of Lyme disease. Furthermore, although the manifestations in skin, joints, heart, and nervous system present in characteristic and consistent patterns, very few ocular signs and symptoms have been seen with enough consistency to be linked with Lyme borreliosis as the definitive cause. Even if Lyme disease is causative in some of the anecdotal reports, ocular sequelae of Lyme disease are rare.

VII. TREATMENT

Therapeutic regimens recommended for Lyme disease have evolved and changed several times during recent years. In the early years, treatment was aggressive because of fears of failure; but recently, treatment for Lyme disease has become more conventional with the recognition that Lyme disease probably responds to treatment as well as other bacterial disorders and poses a less severe threat than anticipated. For most adult patients, permanent resolution of symptoms and signs of Lyme infections can be achieved by oral administration of either doxycycline (100 mg twice per day) or amoxicillin (250–500 mg three times per day). For children, since tetracycline and doxycycline are contraindicated during tooth development, the recommended oral therapy is amoxicillin, 50 mg/kg day in three divided doses (26).

In the most severe cases of arthritis, cardiac symptoms, or central nervous system manifestations, a course of intravenous ceftriaxone is suggested. Failure to improve or recover after a course of antibiotics is not an indication for yet another course, since in all likelihood it reflects a misdiagnosis of the underlying cause of the patient's syndrome.

Lyme disease, like most other infectious diseases, should be treated effectively by a single, limited course of antibiotic therapy. Protracted therapy for an infectious disease is required only in cases where the infection is sequestered from the bloodborne antibiotic, as in endocarditis or osteomyelitis, or where the organism itself has the capacity to "hide" intracellularly. But even in those examples, therapeutic protocols do not call for repeated courses of therapy. For example, successful treatment of endocarditis requires 6 weeks of a single antibiotic or 2 weeks of multiple antibiotics administered intravenously; CNS syphilis is adequately treated by 21 days of intravenous therapy. Only Hansen's disease and tuberculosis require a year's course of oral therapy. The common practice of administering recurrent courses of oral and/or intravenous antibiotics to treat symptoms attributed to Lyme disease has been advocated by Lyme community action and self-help groups and may be based more on fear than on scientific principles for treating infectious disease.

Corticosteroid therapy in Lyme disease has been a source of controversy. Systemic steroids can be helpful in treating transient myocarditis. Topical steroids are sufficient in treating keratitis and have been advocated in the treatment of uveitis, which remains of uncertain etiology.

VIII. CONCLUSIONS

Lyme disease is a tickborne spirochetal infection with well-documented effects on the skin, joints, and heart. The characteristic pattern of involvement of the nervous system produces an early meningitis accompanied by painful radiculopathy and by cranial neuritis frequently affecting the facial nerve. When treated promptly, Lyme disease can be a mild and limited disease.

If untreated, a small percentage of patients progress to chronic sequelae, especially arthritic and neurological conditions. Lyme arthritis is the most characteristic chronic manifestation. Late reaction in the peripheral nervous system results in polyneuropathy with sensory loss and in the central nervous system is most often characterized by a mild nonspecific encephalopathy with memory loss and fatigue and only extremely rarely by focal signs of encephalomyelitis. Ophthalmic manifestations of Lyme disease are rare; the only late manifestation occurring consistently is keratitis. A wide variety of neurological and ophthalmic syndromes have been described in patients with positive serology suggesting either a past or current infection, but are almost certainly not caused by Lyme disease. Since the proven spectrum of neurological and ocular symptoms and signs of Lyme disease remains to be established, the physician's skepticism about the diagnosis of Lyme disease in endemic areas will help in defining the appropriate priority for this infection in differential diagnosis.

REFERENCES

1. Steere AC, Taylor E, McHugh GL, et al. The overdiagnosis of Lyme disease. JAMA 1993; 269:1812–16.
2. Winterkorn, JMS. Lyme disease: neurologic and ophthalmic manifestations Surv Ophthalmol 1990; 35:191–204.
3. Szer IS, Taylor E, Steere AC. The long-term course of Lyme arthritis in children. N Engl J med 1991; 325:159–63.
4. Steere AC, Malawista SE, Snydam DR, et al. Lyme arthritis: an epidemic of oligoarthritis in children and adults in three Connecticut communities. Arthritis Rheum 1977; 20:7–17.
5. Steere AC, Malawista SE, Hardin JA, et al. Erythema chronicum migrans and Lyme arthritis: the enlarging spectrum. Ann intern Med 1977; 685–98.
6. Burgdorfer W, Barbour AG, Hayes SF, et al. Lyme disease—a tick-borne spirochetosis? Science 1982; 216:1317–9.
7. Pachner AR. Borrelia burgdorferi in the Nervous System: the New Great Imitator. In: Lyme disease and related disorders. Ann NY Acad Med 1988; 539:56–64.

8. Weber K, et al. Erythema migrans and related disorders. Yale J Biol Med 1984; 57:13–21.
9. Afzelius A. Erythema chronicum migrans. Acta Derm Venereol (Stockh) 1921; 2:120–5, 1921.
10. Garin CH, Bujadoux C. Paralysie par les tiques. J Med Lyons 1922; 3:765–7.
11. Bannwarth A. Chronische lymphocytare meningitis, entzundliche polyneuritis and rheumatismus: ein Beitrag zum problem allergie und Nervensystem. Arch Psychiatr Nervenkr 1941; 113:284–376.
12. Asbrink E, Hovmark A, Hederstedt B. The spirochetal etiology of acrodermatitis chronica atrophicans Herxheimer. Acta Derm Venereol (Stockh) 1984; 64:506–12.
13. White DJ, Chang HG, Benach JL, et al. The geographic spread and temporal increase of the Lyme disease epidemic. JAMA 1991; 266:1230–6.
14. MWR Lyme disease surveillance—United States, 1989–1990. Morb Mortal Wkly Rep 1991; 40:417–21.
15. Alpert B, Esin J, Sivak SL, Wormser GP. Incidence and prevalence of Lyme disease in a suburban Westchester county community. NY State J Med 1992; 92:5–8.
16. Spielman A, Wilson ML, Levine JF. Ecology of Ixodes borne babesiosis and Lyme disease. Ann Rev Entomol 1985; 30:439–61.
17. Malane MS, et al. Diagnosis of Lyme disease based on dermatologic manifestations. Ann Intern Med 1991; 114:490–8.
18. Steere AC. Lyme disease. N Engl J Med 1989; 321:586–96.
19. Steere AC, Bartenhagen NH, Kraft JE, et al. The early clinical manifestations of Lyme disease. Ann Intern Med 1983; 99:76–82.
20. Pachner AR, Steere AC. The triad of neurologic manifestations of Lyme disease: meningitis, cranial neuritis, and radiculoneuritis. Neurology 1985; 35:47–53.
21. Steere AC, Schoen RT, Taylor E. The clinical evolution of Lyme arthritis. Ann Intern Med 1987; 107:7.
22. Ruberti G, Begovich AB, Steere AC, Klitz W, Erlich HA, Fathman CG. Molecular analysis of the role of the HLA class genes DRB1 DQA1 DQB1 and DPB1 in susceptibility to Lyme arthritis. Hum Immunol 1991; 31:20–7.
23. Steere AC, Dwyer E, Winchester. Association of chronic Lyme arthritis with HLA-DR4 and HLA-DR2 alleles. N Engl J Med 1990; 323:219–23.
24. Halperin JJ, Volkman DJ, Wu P. Central nervous system abnormalities in Lyme neuroborreliosis. Neurology 1991; 41:1571–82.
25. MacDonald AB. Ambiguous serologies in active Lyme borreliosis. J Clin Neuro Ophthalmol 1988; 8:79–80.
26. Rahn DW, Malawista SE. Lyme disease: recommendations for diagnosis and treatment Ann Intern Med 1991; 114:472–81.
27. Magnarelli LA. Laboratory diagnosis of Lyme disease. Rheum Dis Clin North Am 1989; 15:735–45.
28. Fawcett PT, Gibney KM, Rose CD, Dubbs Doughty RA. Frequency and specificity of antibodies that cross react with Borrelia burgdorferi antigens. J Rheumatol 1992; 19:582–7.
29. Logigian EL, Kaplan RF, Steere AC. Chronic neurologic manifestations of Lyme disease. N Engl J Med 1990; 323:1438–44.

30. Scully RE, Mark EG, McNeely BU. Case reports of the MGH. N Engl J Med 1984; 311:172–181.
31. Reik L, Steere AC, Bartenhagen NH, Shope RE, Malawista SE. Neurologic abnormalities of Lyme disease. Medicine 1979; 58:281–94.
32. Raucher HS, Kaufman DM, Goldfarb J, et al. Pseudotumor cerebri and Lyme disease: a new association. J Pediatr 1985; 107:931–33.
33. Jacobsen DM, Frens DB. Pseudotumor cerebri syndrome associated with Lyme disease. Am J Ophthalmol 1989; 107:81–2.
34. Ackermann R, Rehse-Kupper B, Gollmer E, Schmidt R. Chronic neurologic manifestations of erythema migrans borreliosis. Ann NY Acad Sci 1988; 539:16–23.
35. Clark JR, Carlson RD, Sasaki CT, et al. Facial paralysis in Lyme disease. Laryngoscope 1985; 95:1341–5.
36. Pachner AR. Spirochetal diseases of the central nervous system. Neurol Clin 1986; 4:207–22.
37. Halperin JJ, Golightly M. Lyme borreliosis in Bell's palsy. Neurology 1992; 42:1268–70.
38. Kuiper H, Devriese PP, Jongh BM, Vos K, Dankert J. Absence of Lyme borreliosis among patients with presumed Bell's palsy. Arch Neurol 1992; 49:940–3.
39. Halperin JJ. Nervous System manifestations of Lyme. Rheum Dis Clin North Am 1989; 15:635–47.
40. Schroeter V, Belz GG, Blenk H. Paralysis of recurrent laryngeal nerve in Lyme disease. Lancet 1988; 2:1245.
41. Schmutzhard E, Stanek G, Pohl P. Polyneuritis cranialis associated with Borrelia burgdorferi. J Neurol Neurosurg Psychiatry 1985; 18:1182–4.
42. Logigian EL, Steere AC. Clinical and electrophysiologic findings in chronic neuropathy of Lyme disease. Neurology 1992; 42:303–12.
43. Halperin JJ, Kaplan GP, Brazinsky S, Tsai TF, Cheng T, Ironside A, Wu P, Delfiner J, Golightly M, Brown RH. Immunologic reactivity against Borrelia burgdoferi in patients with motor neuron disease. Arch Neurol 1990; 47:586–94.
44. Halperin JJ, Little BW, Coyle PK, Dattwyler RJ. Lyme disease: cause of a treatable peripheral neuropathy. Neurology 1987; 7:1700–6.
45. Wokke JHJ, DeKoning J, Stanek G, Jennekens FGI. Chronic muscle weakness caused by Borrelia burgdorferi meningoradiculitis. Ann Neurol 1987; 22:389–92.
46. Halperin JJ, Luft BJ, Volkman DJ, Dattwyler RJ. Lyme neuroborreliosis: peripheral nervous system manifestations. Brain 1990; 113:1207–21.
47. Rousseau JJ, Lust C, Langerle PF, Bigaignon G. Acute transverse myelitis as presenting neurological feature of Lyme disease. Lancet 1986; 2:1222–3.
48. Glauser TA, Brennan PJ, Galetta SL. Reversible Horner's syndrome and Lyme disease. J Clin Neuro Ophthalmol 1989; 9:225–8.
49. Lesser RL, Kornmehl EW, Pachner AR, Kattah J, Hedges TR, Newman NM, Ecker PA, Glassman MI. Neuro-ophthalmologic manifestations of Lyme disease. Ophthalmology 1990; 97:699–706.
50. Wu G, Lincoff H, Ellsworth RM, Haik BG. Optic disc edema and Lyme disease. Ann Ophthalmol 1986; 18:252–5.
51. Bendig JW, Ogilvie D. Severe encephalopathy associated with Lyme disease Lancet 1987; 1:681–2.

52. Reik L, Burgdorfer W, Donaldson JO. Neurologic abnormalities in Lyme disease without erythema chronicum migrans. Am J Med 1986; 41:73–8.
53. Halperin JJ, Luft BJ, Anand AK, et al. Lyme neuroborreliosis: central nervous system manifestations. Neurology 1989; 39:753–9.
54. Bertuch AW, Rocco E, Schwartz EG. Eye findings in Lyme disease. Conn Med 1987; 51:151–2.
55. Winward KE, Smith JL, Culbertson WW, Paris-Hamelin AJ. Ocular Lyme borreliosis. Am J Ophthalmol 1989; 108:651–7.
56. Stiernstedt G, Gustaffson R, Karlsson M, et al. Clinical manifestations and diagnosis of neuroborreliosis. Ann NY Acad Sci 1988; 539:46–56.
57. Schechter SI. Lyme disease associated with optic neuropathy. Am J Med 1986; 81:143–5.
58. Smith JL, Parsons TM, Paris-Hamelin AJ, Porschen RK. The prevalence of Lyme disease in a non-endemic area J Clin Neuro-ophthalmology 1989; 9:148–55.
59. Pizzarello LD, MacDonald AB, Semlear R, et al. Temporal arteritis associated with Borrelia infection: a case report. J Clin Neuro Ophthalmol 1989; 9:3–6.
60. Finkel MF. Lyme disease and its neurologic complications. Arch Neurol 1988; 45:99–104.
61. Farris BK, Webb RM. Lyme disease and optic neuritis. J Clin Neur-Ophthalmol 1988; 8:73–8.
62. Schmutzhard E, Pohl G, Stanek G. Borrelia burgdorferi antibodies in patients with relapsing/remitting form and chronic progressive form of multiple sclerosis. J Neurol Neurosurg Psychiatry 1988; 41:1215–21.
63. Coyle PK. Borrelia burgdorferi antibodies in multiple sclerosis patients. Neurology 1989; 39:765.
64. Waisbren BA, Cashman N, Schell RF, Johnson R. Borellia burgdorferi antibodies and amyotrophic lateral sclerosis. Lancet 1987; 1:332–7.
65. Kohlhepp W, Kuhn W, Kruger H. Extrapyramidal features in central Lyme borreliosis. Eur Neurol 1989; 29:150–5.
66. MacDonald AB, Miranda JM. Concurrent neocortical borreliosis and Alzheimer's disease. Hum Pathol 1987;18:750–61.
67. Mokry M, Flaschka G, Kleinert G, Kleinert R, Fazekas F, Kopp W. Chronic Lyme disease with an expansive granulomatous lesion in the cerebellopontine angle. Neurosurgery 1990; 27:446–51.
68. Murray R, Morawetz R, Kepes J, et Gammal T, LeDoux M. Lyme neuroborreliosis manifesting as an intracranial mass lesion. Neurosurgery 1992; 30:768–73.
69. Brogan GX, Homan CS, Viccellio P. The enlarging clinical spectrum of Lyme disease: Lyme cerebral vasculitis, a new disease entity. Ann Emerg Med 1990; 19:575–6.
70. Veenendaal-Hilbers JH, Perquin WVM, Hoogland PH, Doornbos L. Basal meningovasculitis and occlusion of the basilar artery in two cases of Borrelia burgdorferi infection. Neurology 1988; 38:1317–9.
71. Kaplan RF, Meadows ME, Vincent LC, Logigian EL, Steere AC. Memory impairment and depression in patients with Lyme encephalopathy: comparison with fibromyalgia and non-psychotically depressed patients. Neurology 1992; 42:1263–7.

72. Finkel MJ, Halperin JJ. Nervous system Lyme borreliosis revisited. Arch Neurol 1992; 49:102–7.
73. Lightman DA, Brod RD. Branch retinal artery occlusion associated with Lyme disease. Arch Ophthalmol 1991; 109:1198–9.
74. Winterkorn JMS. Lyme disease? Arch Ophthalmol 1992; 110:794.
75. Steere AC, Duray PH, Kaufmann DJH, Wormser GP. Unilateral blindness caused by infection with the Lyme spirochete Borrelia burgdorferi. Ann Intern Med 1985; 103:383–5.
76. Flach AJ, Lavoie PE. Episcleritis, conjunctivitis and keratitis as ocular manifestations of Lyme disease. Ophthalmology 1990; 97:973–5.
77. Mombaerts IM, Maudgal PC, Knockaert DC. Bilateral follicular conjunctivitis as a manifestation of Lyme disease. Am J Ophthalmol 1991; 112:96–7.
78. Baum J, Barza M, Weinstein P. Bilateral keratitis as a manifestation of Lyme disease. Am J Ophthalmol 1988; 105:75–7.
79. Kornmehl EW, Lesser RL, Jaros P, Rocco E, Steere AC. Bilateral keratitis in Lyme disease. Ophthalmol 1989; 96:1194–7.
80. Orlin SE, Lauffer JL. Lyme disease keratitis. Am J Ophthalmol 1989; 107:678.
81. Bertuch R, Schwartz EG. Lyme disease: ocular manifestations Ann Ophthalmol 1988; 20:376–8.
82. Zaidman GW. Episcleritis and symblepharon associated with Lyme keratitis. Am J Ophthalmol 1990; 109:487–8.
83. Seidenberg KB, Leib ML. Orbital myositis with Lyme disease. Am J Ophthalmol 1990; 109:13–6.
84. Fox GM, Heiskov Smith JL. Cogan's syndrome and seroreactivity to Lyme borreliosis. J Clin Neuro Ophthalmol 1990; 10:83–7.
85. DeLuise VP, O'Leary MJ. Peripheral ulcerative keratitis related to Lyme disease. Am J Ophthalmol 1991; 111:244–5.
86. Wokke JHJ, VanGijn J, Elderson A, Stanek G. Chronic forms of Borrelia burgdorferi infections of the nervous system. Neurology 1987; 37:1031–4.
87. Winward KE, Smith JL. Ocular disease in Caribbean patients with serologic evidence of Lyme borreliosis. J Clin Neuro Ophthalmol 1989; 9:65–70.
88. Eichenfeld AH, Goldsmith DP, Benach JL, et al. Childhood Lyme arthritis: experience in an endemic area. J Pediatr 1986; 109:753–8.
89. Breeveld J, Rothova A, Kuiper H. Intermediate uveitis and Lyme borreliosis. Br J Ophthalmol 1992; 76:181–2.
90. Kuiper H, Koelman JHTM, Jager MJ. Vitreous clouding associated with Lyme borreliosis. Am J Ophthalmol 1989; 108:453–4.
91. Rothova A, Kuiper H, Spanjaaed L, Dankert J, Breebart A. C Spiderweb vitritis in Lyme borreliosis. Lancet 1991; 337:490.
92. Kauffmann DJH, Wormser GP. Ocular Lyme disease: case report and review of the literature. Br J Ophthalmol 1990; 74:325–7.
93. Wiegand W. Augenbefunde bei Borreliose-bilaterale Panuveitisit exsudativer Amotio. Fortschr Ophthalmol 1989; 86:659–62.
94. Zierhut M, Kreissig I, Pickert A. Panuveitis with positive serological tests for syphilis and Lyme disease. J Clin Neuro Ophthalmol 1989; 9:71–75.
95. Preac-Mursic V, Pfister HW, Spiegel H, Burke H, Wilske B, Reinhardts, Bohmer

R. First isolation of Borrelia burgdorferi from an iris biopsy. J Clin Neuro-ophthalmol 1993; 13:155–161.
96. Isogai E, Isogai H, Kotake S, Yoshikawa K, et al. Detection of antibodies against Borrelia burgdorferi in patients with uveitis. Am J Ophthalmol 1991; 112:23–30.
97. Rosenbaum JT, Rahn DW. Prevalence of Lyme disease among patients with uveitis. Am J Ophthalmol 1991; 112:462–3.
98. Winterkorn JMS, Svitra P. Mimicking Lyme disease: facial palsy, Guillian Barre, and vitritis from other causes. (In preparation).
99. Schonherr U, Lang GE, Meythaler FH. Bilaterale Leber'sche Neuroretinitis stellata bei Borrelia burgdorferi serokonversion. Klin Monatsbl Augenheilkd.
100. Miller NR. Case described in Walsh and Hoyt's Clinical Neuro-Ophthalmology, Volume 5, 1995, pp 3657–3658. In press.
101. Wilk CM, Bialasiewicz AA, Ruprecht KW, Naumann G. Bilaterale akute konfluierende choroiditis disseminata bei Borrelia Burgdorferi-infekton. Klin Mbl Augenheilk 1986; 194:88–96.
102. Bialasiewicz AA, Ruprecht KW, Naumann GOH, Blenk H. Bilateral diffuse choroiditis and exudative retinal detachment with evidence of Lyme disease. Am J Ophthalmol 1988; 105:419–20.
103. Bodine SR, Marino J, Camisa TJ, Salvate AJ. Multifocal choroiditis with evidence of Lyme disease. Ann of Ophthalmol 1992; 124:169–73.
104. Suttorp-Schulten M, Luyendijk L, van Dam AP, deKeizer R, Baarsma G, Box P, Rothova A. Birdshot chorioretinopathy and Lyme borreliosis. Am J Ophthalmol 1993; 115:149–53.
105. Tonjes W, Mielke U, Schmidt HJ, Haass A, Holzer G. Akute multifokale plakoide pigmentepitheliopathie mit entzundlichem liquorbefund. Sonderform einer Borreliose? Dtsch Med Wochenschr 1989; 114:793–5.
106. Wolf MD, Folk JC, Nelson JA, Peeples ME. Acute posterior multifocal placoid pigment epitheliopathy and Lyme disease Arch Ophthalmol 1992; 110:750.

39

Diagnosis, Diagnostic Pitfalls, and Treatment of Giant Cell Arteritis

Michael L. Slavin
Long Island Jewish Medical Center, New Hyde Park, and Albert Einstein College of Medicine, Bronx, New York

Temporal, cranial, or giant cell arteritis (GCA) is a systemic vasculitis of the elderly that in the textbook case presents with stereotypical symptoms of headache, scalp tenderness, jaw claudication, polymyalgia rheumatica, weight loss, and visual loss. The erythrocyte sedimentation rate (ESR) is typically elevated and histological confirmation of the diagnosis can be made in most cases with biopsy of the superficial temporal artery. Treatment of GCA will quickly relieve most systemic symptoms, but more importantly will forestall bilateral irreversible visual loss that may occur in up to 60% of untreated patients (1). The mainstay of treatment for GCA is high-dose corticosteroids early on followed by lower doses over a period of many months to years. The weaning of corticosteroids is often based on clinical symptoms and the ESR. Adverse effects of treatment unfortunately are not uncommon and include weight gain, irritability, and hyperglycemia, hypertension, as well as severe and sometimes irreversible ones such as systemic infection, perforation of the bowel, gastrointestinal bleed, pronounced proximal myopathy, osteoporosis and vertebral collapse, and ischemic necrosis of the femoral head(s) or other bones.

Although the textbook case of GCA is straightforward to diagnose (and tragic when misdiagnosed because of ensuing visual loss), other (and often frequent!) clinical cases will be among the most challenging cases to diagnose. The physician must constantly weigh risks and benefits of treatment, with the false-negative cases running the risk of devastating visual loss and the false-positive ones suffering the side effects of therapy. In this chapter, I review the systemic, ophthalmic, and neuro-ophthalmological symptoms and signs of GCA and illustrate with clinical examples some pitfalls of diagnosis and therapy.

I. NONVISUAL SYMPTOMS AND SIGNS

Two series of cases with GCA will be described in order to demonstrate the sensitivity and specificity of various nonvisual symptoms and signs, laboratory results, and biopsy of the superficial temporal artery (TAB) (Table 1). *Sensitivity* will refer to the percentage of cases of GCA (which were confirmed with a positive TAB) that manifest that particular feature, whereas *specificity* refers to the percentage of cases in the control population (with a negative TAB) *not* manifesting that feature. Series I was reported by Chmelewski and associates in 1992 and describes 98 patients who had undergone TAB in a general hospital setting over the period from 1985 to 1990 (2). Series II, reported by Hedges et al. in 1983, retrospectively described 91 patients who underwent TAB in an eye infirmary over a 10-year period (3). Obviously, the different population studied in each series may account for fluctuation in the incidence of any particular feature. As can be seen from Table 1, the symptom of jaw claudication is highly specific for GCA both in the ophthalmic and in the general hospital group. Therefore, a patient presenting with jaw claudication has a very strong possibility of having GCA. Jaw claudication, of course, needs to be distinguished from poorly fitting dentures, tooth abscess, and temporomandibular joint dysfunction (4), and it may rarely be caused by amyloidosis or other vasculitides affecting the facial artery (5). Interestingly, most of my dental colleagues are unaware of either jaw claudication or GCA! Although its specificity as a symptom of GCA is high, its sensitivity was only 50% in series I and 28% in series II. Other studies indicate that tongue and swallowing claudication are unusual symptoms but also are highly specific (6).

Polymyalgia rheumatica (PMR) (early morning pain and stiffness of the neck, shoulders, and hips) although having 91.7% specificity in series II, showed only 28% specificity in series I. It can be concluded from the former study that patients with visual dysfunction who have concomitant PMR have an extraordinarily high probability of having GCA. On the other hand, series I reflects the fact that PMR itself may be a distinct disorder (7). Many investigators think that PMR is a limited form of GCA, but there is no unanimity of opinion in that regard. We know from the literature that anywhere from 15 to 41% of cases of PMR may have a positive TAB (8). False-positive symptoms of PMR may stem from cervical arthritis, diffuse osteoarthritis, fibromyalgia, polymyositis, and functional aches and pains. In the past, I recall one patient, later diagnosed with GCA, who presented with severe visual loss from bilateral incomplete central

Table 1 Clinical Features in Biopsy Proven GCA[a]

No. of Cases with Biopsy-Proven GCA	Series I (General Hospital Setting) 30 (Mean Age 73.1 Years)	Series II (Eye Infirmary) 28 (All Older Than 61 Years)
No. of Cases with Negative TAB	68 (Mean Age 67.5 Years)	60 (Only 14 (23%) Older Than 61 Years
No. of Cases with "Biopsy Negative" GCA	14[b]	3
Nonvisual Features (Sensitivity/Specificity)[c]		
JAM Claudication	50/82	28/98.3
PMR	80/28	25.8/91.7
Headache	93/62	71/36
Scalp ABN Inc. Tenderness	47/69	53/85 (Tenderness Only)
Fever	57/72	—
Visual Symptoms	60/53	—[d]
Visual Signs	23/78	—
ESR <50	17/85	—
ESR >100	12/75	—
ESR >60	—	77.4/66.7

[a]GCA is giant cell arteritis, TAB is temporal artery biopsy, ESR is Westergren erythrocyte sedimentation rate, PMR is polymyalgia rheumatica.
[b]14 of 68 cases (at with least 2 year follow-up) were diagnosed as having GCA despite negative TAB. In this group, the clinical features were similar to the cases with positive TAB.
[c]Sensitivity = cases with sign or symptom or cases of biopsy proven GCA × 100. Specificity = cases without sign or symptom or cases with negative biopsy × 100.
[d]Since this study was done at an eye infirmary, most cases had visual signs and symptoms.

retinal artery occlusion who had been treated with a neck collar for several months with the erroneous diagnosis of "cervical arthritis."

Headache was evident in 93 and 71% of cases with GCA in series I and II, respectively, but was not a highly specific symptom. Although headache is most commonly localized to the temporal area in the vicinity of the superficial temporal arteries, no specific headache location can be defined. Thus, some headaches may occur exclusively in the occipital or cervical area. The duration and type of headache also are variable; that is, headache may be intermittent or constant or described as throbbing, stabbing, or dull. Other causes of headache, including migraine, musculoskeletal/tension, and intracranial tumor with/without increased intracranial pressure, should be excluded. It is often difficult to distinguish a new-onset headache or a change in headache pattern in some patients with long-standing headaches (see illustrative case 5 below). Other constitutional symptoms of GCA include weight loss, malaise, and fever.

Nonvisual clinical signs of GCA include tenderness, cordlike changes, and decreased pulse in the superficial temporal artery. I find that patients who state that their scalp vessels have recently "become prominent" have a good chance of having GCA, although this finding is not totally specific. I have recently seen a case in which "prominence" and "tenderness" of the scalp vessels were secondary to severe migraine. Although GCA most commonly affects the superficial temporal artery, ophthalmic artery, central retinal artery, and facial artery, almost any organ system may be affected (9,10). As opposed to other cases of systemic vasculitis, symptomatic involvement of the lung and kidney are uncommon. Table 2 lists some less familiar ways GCA might present to our medical colleagues in various subspecialties (11–20).

Laboratory signs that aid in the diagnosis of GCA include the hemoglobin level, the time-honored Westergren erythrocyte sedimentation rate (ESR), C-reactive protein level, plasma viscosity, serum fibrinogen level, and serum alkaline phosphatase and aspartate aminotransferase levels (6,21–25). Anemia is a nonspecific finding in both PMR and GCA, with approximately 35% of patients collectively in one series having a hemoglobin below 12 g/dl (22).

In series I (see Table 1), the ESR in patients with positive TAB ranged from 14 to 134 mm/h (mean 83.1 mm/h) and was below 50 mm/h in 17%. The ESR was below 60 mm/h in 23% in series II. Thus cases of GCA with low or "normal" ESR may certainly occur (26–28). (Normal reference ranges given in most laboratories are from 0 to 10 mm/h for men and up to 20 mm/h for women. Most investigators, however, define *normal* using the formula: age/2 for men, and (age + 10)/2 for women. Thus a 70-year-old woman with an ESR of 40 mm/h would have a borderline result.) In a report by Wong and Korn of 37 patients with biopsy-proven temporal arteritis and *normal* ESR, 17 had an ESR less than 20 mm/h, and 20 had an ESR between 20 and 40 mm/h (26). In that group, the incidences of temporal artery, visual, and systemic symptoms were similar to a group of 22 patients with

Table 2 Systemic Features of GCA[a]

Ophthalmological	Psychiatric	Neurological (11)	Mouth	Heart (14,15)
See Text	Psychosis	Mononeuropathy (Tibial Neuritis)	Tongue Infarction (16)	Angina Pectoris
	Depression	Peripheral Neuropathy	Tongue Mass	MI
	Confusion	TIA[b]	Tongue Numbness	CHF
		Cerebral/Brainstem Infarction[b] (12)	Macroglossia	
		Vertigo		
		Tremor		
		Seizures		
		Dementia (13)		
		Hearing Loss		
		Carpal Tunnel Syndrome		
Gynecological	**Abdominal**	**Dermatological (17)**	**Other**	
Breast Mass (20)	Ischemic Bowel	Lower Extremity Nodules	Upper Limb Claudication[d] (19)	
Ovarian Mass [c] (18)	GI Bleed	Vesicles	Supraclavicular Lymphadenopathy	
		Ulcer		
		Gangrene		
		Scalp Necrosis (16)		

[a]GCA is giant cell arteritis, MI is myocardial infarction, CHF is congestive heart failure, GI is gastrointestinal.

[b]Intracranial infarction is thought to result more often from *extracranial* involvement of vessels. Embolism due to thrombus from an arteritic vertebral artery or internal carotid artery may be etiologic in many cases. Postmortem evidence of GCA affecting the *intracranial* carotid, vertebral and basilar arteries however has been reported.

[c]The palpated mass was an ovarian cyst. Coincidentally GCA of the ovarian and myometrial arteries was detected.

[d]For larger vessel arteritis, also think of Takayasu's arteritis, another cause of giant cell arteritis often seen in young patients.

GCA and high ESR. Jaw claudication and headache, however, were more commonly seen in the group with a high ESR. The ESR may also be falsely high in patients with anemia, since a decreased red cell volume will offer less resistance to the relative upward displacement of plasma and thus faster overall sedimentation of erythrocytes (28). On the other hand, polycythemia would lead to the opposite situation. The "zeta sedimentation rate" is a test that presumably corrects for concomitant anemia (29). A handy formula (that I use) that provides a reasonable degree of correction in the standard Westergren ESR is: Corrected ESR = ESR – (standard hematocrit – actual hematocrit) × 1.75. Standard hematocrit is 45 for males and 42 for females (30). For example, the corrected ESR in a man with a hematocrit of 30 and a Westergren ESR of 60 mm/h is 33.75 mm/h.

Serum C-reactive protein is another acute-phase reactant that may be elevated in an inflammatory process (22–24). *Unlike the ESR, it will not vary with anemia*, red blood cell morphology, or concentration of plasma proteins. In a report by Eshaghian and Goeken (24), 11 patients with biopsy-proven temporal arteritis had increased ESR (defined in that series as greater than or equal to 50 mm/h), whereas 10 of 11 had increased C-reactive protein (in the one case where C-reactive protein [CRP] was normal, the ESR was 50 mm/h). During the period when corticosteroids were being tapered, however, a normal ESR but an elevated CRP were seen in patients with recrudescence of symptoms! For example, one patient developed visual loss late in the course of GCA with an ESR of 14 mm/h but an elevated C-reactive protein. In 32 patients with negative temporal artery biopsy that truly did not have GCA, the ESR was greater than 50 mm/h in 18 of 32 (56%), whereas the CRP was positive in only 14 of 32 (44%) patients (i.e., the false-positive rate of these tests). Although it has not been definitively shown that CRP or other serum tests are more sensitive than the ESR, I believe that the CRP and ESR are complementary tests and I use both of them to guide treatment, especially while weaning patients from corticosteroids.

What was the eventual diagnosis of the negative biopsy cases in series I and II above, and in how many cases was it thought likely that GCA was the correct diagnosis despite negative biopsy? (In other words, how good is the TAB in diagnosing GCA?) Out of 68 cases with negative TAB in series I, 15 (22%) were subsequently diagnosed with neurological disorders thought to have resulted in symptoms in common with GCA, including migraine, transient ischemia, and other optic neuropathies. Fourteen patients (21%) were later diagnosed with "pure" PMR, 10 (15%) had other vasculitides (e.g., systemic lupus erythematosus, rheumatoid arthritis), 4 (6%) had malignancies, and 14 (21%) were thought to have "biopsy-negative" GCA. Those with biopsy-negative GCA shared a similar incidence of symptoms and signs with those with biopsy-positive GCA. In series II, of 60 patients with negative biopsy followed over a minimum period of 2 years, 13 (22%) were discovered to have cancer (mainly of the breast and colon), 10 (17%) had chronic inflammatory disease (including rheumatoid arthritis, scleroderma, and systemic lupus erythematosus), and 30 (50%) had cerebral or cardiac vascular disease, whereas only 3 (5%) were thought to have "biopsy-negative" GCA. Thus TAB was positive in only 30 of 44 patients (68%) with clinical GCA in series I but in 90% of patients in series II. Other reports have indicated an incidence of false-negative biopsies of approximately 10% (31,32).

What accounts for negative biopsies in GCA? The main reason for a false-negative biopsy seems to be that GCA is segmental in nature resulting in skip areas of involvement (33,34). It also is plausible that the superficial temporal artery is not involved in every case. Most investigators recommend taking a biopsy of a "long" segment (at least 2 cm) of superficial temporal artery or biopsy the fellow artery if the first side is negative (5,35). Biopsy of the occipital artery has also been shown to be positive in cases of GCA in which cervical headache was present and has also been reported to be positive in a case in which a previous superficial temporal biopsy was negative (36,37)! False-positive biopsies, on the other hand, are rare but have been described with polyarteritis nodosa (38), Wegener's granulomatosis (39), and herpes zoster ophthalmicus (40). In GCA and Wegener's granulomatosis, as opposed to polyarteritis nodosa and herpes zoster arteritis, the biopsy will show a panarteritis most often accompanied by giant cells or epithelioid cells. In addition, GCA will show disruption or loss of the internal elastic lamina (41). The clinical presentation and course should allow differentiation of these vasculitides.

An additional diagnostic sign of GCA often used by neurologists and rheumatologists is the response of various symptoms to corticosteroids (42). Thus, if the symptoms of headache and PMR in a patient with anterior ischemic optic neuropathy respond rapidly and dramatically to corticosteroids (usually within 48 h), a diagnosis of GCA is made irrespective of ESR or TAB. I believe that one must exercise extreme caution in interpreting this sign! A patient of mine with new-onset diplopia, "cervical arthritis," and a borderline ESR was given corticosteroids in preparation for a temporal artery biopsy. The neck pain that was previously treated with nonsteroidal anti-inflammatory agents with quick relief also abated quickly after corticosteroids. The TAB was negative for GCA. The patient was thought to have an isolated ischemic (atherosclerotic) fourth nerve palsy. Other causes of headache such as inflammatory orbital pseudotumor and Tolosa-Hunt syndrome are extremely corticosteroid sensitive. Cluster and sometimes migraine headaches will respond to corticosteroids. In addition, a placebo effect of the corticosteroids might even occur!

II. VISUAL SYMPTOMS AND SIGNS

Visual symptoms occurred in 60% and visual signs in only 23% of patients with GCA in series I above. Visual loss is the most feared complication of GCA and in some series may occur in up to 60% of *untreated* cases! (1)

Visual loss from GCA may occur from five distinct syndromes: anterior ischemic optic neuropathy, complete or incomplete central retinal artery occlusion, posterior ischemic optic neuropathy, choroidal ischemia, or amaurosis fugax. Diplopia may accompany any of the above or be a presenting sign. When any of the above signs are present in the elderly, GCA should *always* be suspected. If any of the constitutional symptoms or signs of GCA as outlined above are present concomitantly, GCA should be the diagnosis until proven otherwise. Unfortunately, cases of GCA may present with visual loss only, and patients may actually down play their less noticeable systemic symptoms ["occult" giant cell arteritis (43)]. Careful questioning is mandatory in this group.

III. ANTERIOR ISCHEMIC OPTIC NEUROPATHY

The syndrome of anterior ischemic optic neuropathy (AION) may be idiopathic in nature (nonarteritic AION, NAION) or caused by GCA (arteritic AION, AAION). In series II above, AION was seen in approximately 70% of all patients with GCA, and it does represent the most common cause of visual loss in this disease. NAION may be seen in patients aged 40 years or older (mean age approximately 55 years) (44), whereas AAION is again most often seen in the elderly population. Clinical features that help differentiate these two types include (45) the following.

A. Laterality (46)

When the headache of GCA is not evident, both NAION and AAION will typically present with painless unilateral visual loss. Bilateral but *simultaneous* visual loss is a feature that strongly suggests GCA. In up to 40% of cases of NAION, the fellow eye may become involved months to years later by a similar process (some patients may first present only after the fellow eye is affected [44]). Hayreh had described cases of NAION with typical unilateral visual loss in which simultaneous swelling of the optic disc of the *asymptomatic* fellow eye was present (47). Typically, such patients develop the fullblown syndrome of NAION in the second eye months later.

B. Progressive Visual Loss from AION

Although GCA will more commonly result in devastating or progressive unilateral visual loss and early involvement of the fellow eye, it has been recognized that a minority of nonarteritic cases may show unilateral progression in the first month (48). At this time, a randomized, controlled study investigating the use of optic nerve sheath fenestration in this condition is underway. All progressive cases of AION, however, should be *carefully* reviewed for other signs of GCA.

C. Premonitory Ophthalmic Symptoms

Episodes of transient visual loss (amaurosis fugax) preceding AION are uncommon in NAION, and AAION should be carefully excluded. Other transient symptoms of GCA include unilateral or bilateral "flashing lights," which are often erroneously attributed to migraine equivalents. A history of recent or concurrent diplopia also suggests arteritis.

D. Funduscopic Signs

A swollen disc is always evident in both AAION and NAION during the acute phase. NAION may present with pale or hyperemic swelling. Focal or diffuse narrowing of the retinal arterioles will be either present initially or will develop over the next several weeks. During the ensuing 1–2 months, optic atrophy will replace optic disc swelling. If the fellow eye is affected later on, a "pseudo–Foster Kennedy syndrome," that is, optic atrophy in one eye and optic disc edema in the other, will be detected. The presence of marked, chalky white (like a cumulus cloud) disc edema (Fig. 1), concomitant retinal swelling, marked cotton-wool

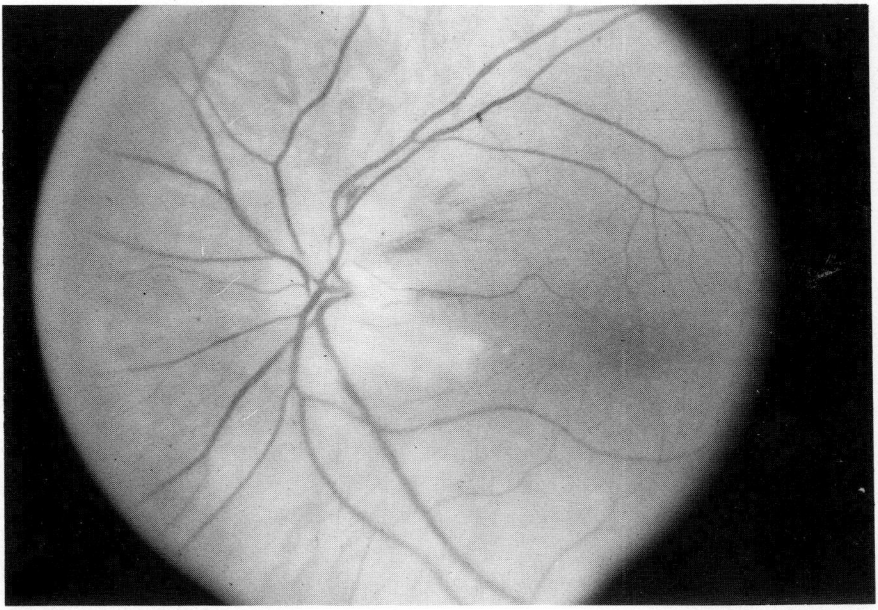

(a)

Figure 1 (a) Pale chalklike inferior swelling of the left optic disc with accompanying retinal edema in a patient with GCA. (b) In another case, note the markedly pale, cloudlike disc edema.

spots, or a serous retinal detachment should strongly suggest arteritis (45). In such cases, choroidal ischemia may be evident on fluorescein angiography (see below).

The cup-to-disc ratio (CDR) of the involved and the fellow eye in cases of NAION has been shown to be smaller than in those of an age-matched population (the so-called "disc at risk"). In two combined series with 78 cases of NAION, only one fellow eye showed a CDR of greater than 0.4 (46 cases showed either no cup or a cup less than 0.1) (49,50). In addition, Hayreh has shown that in his series of NAION of 26 eyes, the mean CDR in the fellow eye was 0.065 (51). In a similar study, Feit and associates reported 30 cases with the largest CDR of the fellow eye being 0.55 [mean 0.21 (52)]. Thus a diagnosis of NAION should be made with caution in a patient with a CDR in the fellow eye greater than 0.5. Think GCA!

E. Other Ocular Signs Accompanying AAION

Ophthalmoplegia (see below) or ptosis most likely reflects ischemia to the intraorbital nerves or the orbital muscles themselves (53). Concurrent ciliary body ischemia may result in relative ocular hypotension. Other unusual signs of GCA include the ischemic ocular syndrome (54) (conjunctival injection, corneal

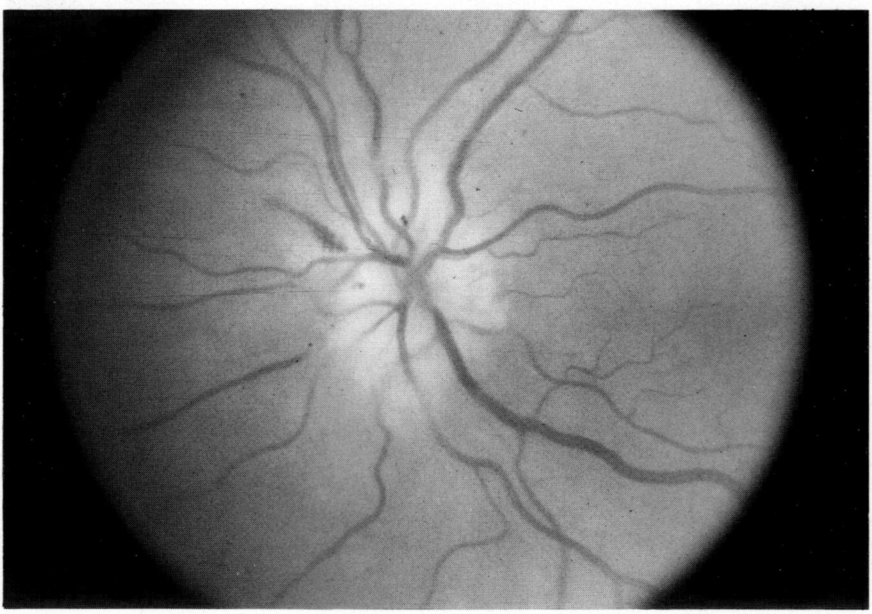

(b)

Figure 1 (Continued)

edema, ocular hypotension, anterior chamber cells and flare, rubeosis iridis, cataract, "venous stasis" retinopathy), scleritis, peripheral corneal melting, and the tonic pupil (55).

F. Fluorescein Angiography

It has been shown recently in two series that eyes with AAION will show a delay in the choroidal filling on fluorescein angiogram compared with those with NAION or normal individuals (56,57). In the report of Siatkowski et al. (56), it was concluded that GCA be strongly suspected in cases of AION in which complete choroidal filling was evident 18 s or longer after fluorescein dye instillation (Fig. 2). I think that this sign is very valuable in the diagnosis of GCA, although its sensitivity and specificity have yet to be firmly established.

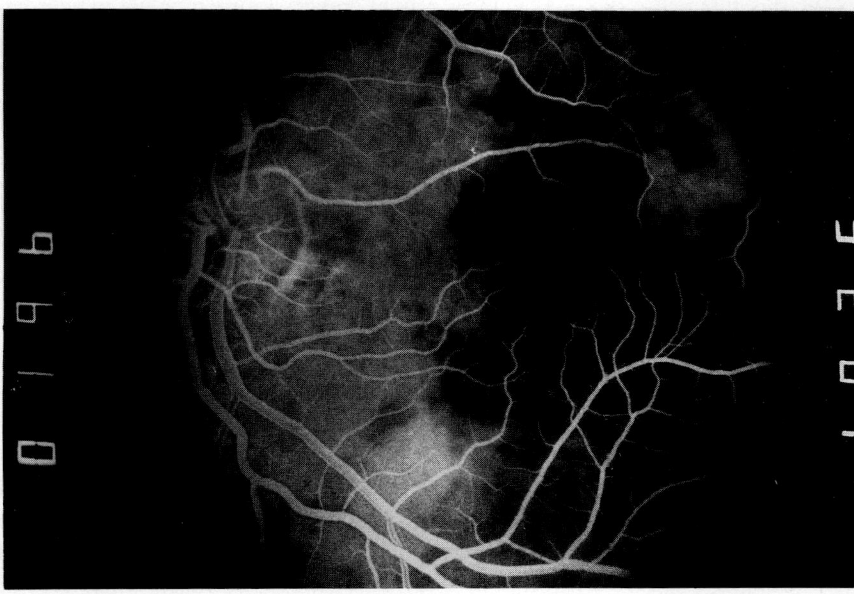

Figure 2 Fluorescein angiogram of the left eye (20 s after dye administration) showing choroidal ischemia, nasal and temporal to the macula. Note the prominence of the retinal capillaries in the area of choroidal ischemia (double arrowheads). The distal part of the superior cilioretinal artery (single arrow) is also not filled. This patient developed typical AION just 24 h later and was found to have GCA.

In sum, a flowchart showing my approach to the diagnosis of AION (in cases without systemic signs of GCA) is depicted in Figure 3.

IV. CENTRAL RETINAL ARTERY OCCLUSION

GCA as a cause of complete or incomplete central retinal artery occlusion (CRAO) is not uncommon. Since the elastic lamina (which is consistently abnormal in GCA) is usually not present within the branch retinal arterioles, branch artery occlusion is uncommon. The most common cause of CRAO in the elderly, however, is embolic, with its source being an ipsilateral atheromatous plaque at the carotid bifurcation in the neck, the heart itself, or thrombi in the vessels of the aortic arch or the intracavernous carotid siphon. Cardiac conditions that may result in emboli include, for example, intermittent or chronic atrial fibrillation, an abnormal or prosthetic valve, a previous myocardial infarction with or without ventricular aneurysm, subacute bacterial or marantic endocarditis, cardiac myxoma, and patent foramen ovale. GCA should always be *considered* as the possible cause of CRAO unless retinal emboli are seen or the patient has a known cardiac risk factor. ESR and CRP levels should be evaluated. Of course, a careful history listening for nonocular symptoms of GCA is mandatory. I think that a fluorescein angiogram should be done in every case of CRAO, since the finding of concomitant choroidal ischemia strongly suggests GCA. A TAB will often be the deciding factor in equivocal cases (e.g., CRAO with no definite risk factors for emboli in a case of vague long-standing headaches and a normal ESR and CRP level). Case 5 (see below) illustrates some of the possible frustrations involved when pursuing the correct etiology of CRAO.

V. POSTERIOR ISCHEMIC OPTIC NEUROPATHY/CHOROIDAL ISCHEMIA

The diagnosis of posterior ischemic optic neuropathy (PION) should be made with extreme caution. An elderly patient with acute unilateral visual loss showing an afferent pupil defect but a *normal* optic nerve and fundus should be diagnosed as having retrobulbar "optic neuropathy," with PION being a diagnosis of exclusion. Another cause of these signs is choroidal ischemia (58,59). I have reported three such cases in which an erroneous diagnosis of retrobulbar optic neuropathy was first made (60). Fluorescein angiography, however, showed marked choroidal ischemia in all cases. Each patient shortly went on to develop further visual loss with typical findings of AION in the next several days and were shown to have biopsy-proven GCA. Systemic symptoms were lacking in two of those cases but the ESR was markedly elevated in both. Thus, my initial workup of isolated retrobulbar neuropathy

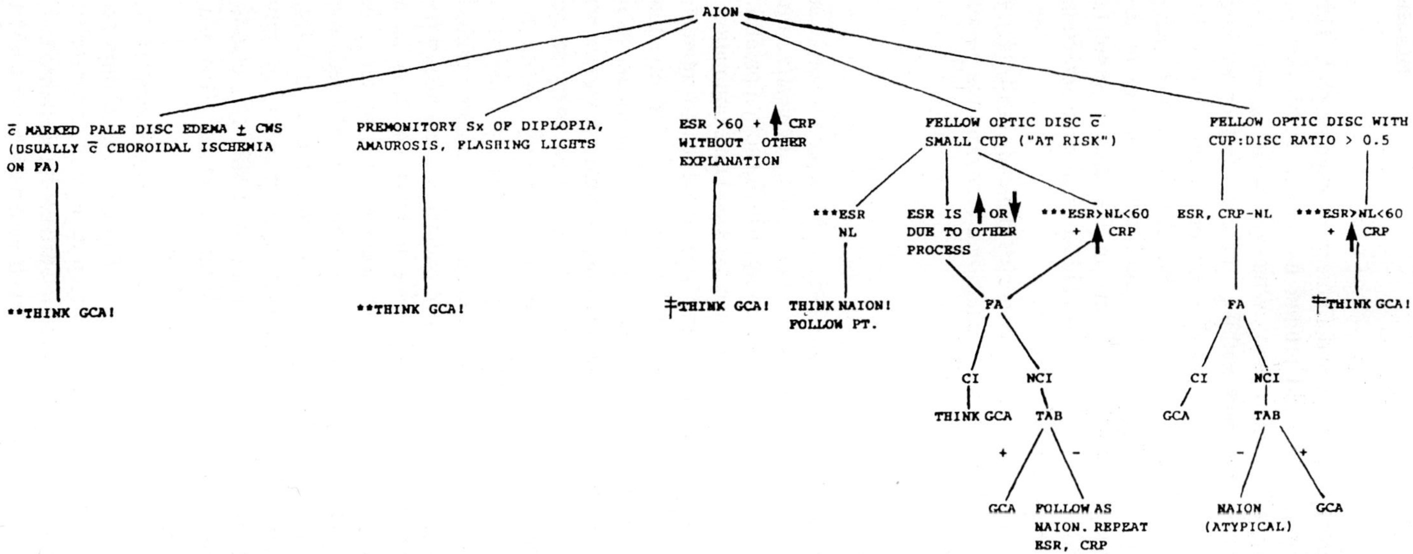

Figure 3 Workup of isolated AION*‡.

*AION is anterior ischemic optic neuropathy *without* systemic features of giant cell arteritis; NAION is nonarteritic ischemic optic neuropathy; GCA is giant cell arteritis; CWS is cotton wool spots; FA is fluorescein angiogram; TAB is temporal artery biopsy; ESR is Westergren erythrocyte sedimentation rate; Sx is symptoms; CRP is C-reactive protein.

†Most cases with "occult" GCA that present with AION *will* have subtle systemic symptoms!

**At this point, the clinical features strongly suggest GCA. I would proceed with further workup as outlined in text but *consider* treating for GCA (on an individual basis!) regardless of latter results.

‡The ESR elevation must be reproducible and not due to another cause. A complete workup for GCA is necessary. If the latter is negative, *consider* "biopsy-negative" GCA!

***NL ESR:(Age +10) % 2 for females; age%2 for males). If elevated it must be *reproducible*!

in the elderly includes an emergency ESR and fluorescein angiography. The finding of an abnormality in either should prompt the urgent instillation of high-dose corticosteroids (see treatment below). When choroidal ischemia is absent (i.e., when a true retrobulbar neuropathy is present), further workup should also include magnetic resonance imaging to rule out compressive optic neuropathy (e.g., supraclinoid carotid aneurysm, meningioma, pituitary adenoma, mucocele, lymphoma, glioblastoma of the optic nerve/chiasm) or inflammatory or infectious neuritides (optic neuritis in the elderly (another diagnosis of exclusion), syphilis, Lyme disease, sarcoidosis, and sinus infection with orbital apex extension (e.g., aspergillosis).

In conclusion, the diagnosis of GCA, must be suspected clinically in all elderly patients with visual loss. The TAB and ESR are *additional* corroborative pieces of a sometimes complex puzzle.

VI. DIPLOPIA

The causes of double vision in the elderly are legion. Most commonly, an ischemic, probably atherosclerotic mechanism is responsible. Typically, the presenting sign will be that of a cranial mononeuropathy, which is often painful. A sixth, fourth, or pupil-sparing third nerve palsy may be found on examination. The diplopia usually improves spontaneously after several weeks to months. It is uncommon for the pain (usually in the distribution of the first division of the trigeminal nerve on the same side as the neuropathy) to last longer than 10 days. An acute third nerve palsy involving the pupil should be viewed as a neuro-ophthalmological emergency and aneurysm of the carotid artery at the junction of the posterior communicating artery or basilar artery should be excluded expeditiously. In the vast majority of cases, ipsilateral pain is a distinct symptom. Other causes of painful diplopia include inflammatory orbital pseudotumor, Tolosa-Hunt syndrome (a diagnosis of exclusion), and aneurysm of the intracavernous carotid artery. It is imperative to think of GCA as a possible cause of diplopia with pain. Diplopia has been reported to occur in up to 15% of cases of GCA (1,61). Most likely, the stereotypical syndrome of an ischemic mononeuropathy will not be present (62). If questioned carefully, the patient will often reveal that the headache is not acute in onset nor only ipsilateral to the neuropathy. Accompanying symptoms of PMR, jaw claudication, scalp tenderness, malaise, or weight loss strongly suggest GCA. An ESR and C-reactive protein level are prudent tests to order.

Painless diplopia would be more a feature of ocular myasthenia than GCA, although the latter should be excluded in atypical cases. Painless vertical diplopia from skew deviation may be due to a brainstem infarction or rarely metastasis. I have seen cases of intermittent diplopia in the elderly attributed to vertebrobasilar insufficiency in which more subtle symptoms such as headache and PMR were overlooked. The diplopia in those cases may have been due to orbital muscle ischemia or vertebral arteritis. Remember that vertebral arteritis may result in symptoms of vertebrobasilar insufficiency (i.e., transient vertigo, diplopia, drop attack(s), brainstem stroke, homonymous hemianopia, or cortical blindness (11,12).

VII. TREATMENT

Corticosteroids are the mainstay of treatment for GCA. If the diagnosis of GCA is made when the patient has constitutional or transient visual symptoms only, permanent visual loss may be forestalled in almost every case! Unfortunately, the diagnosis of GCA is made too often *after* visual loss has occurred. Two facts should be kept firmly in mind: (1) Only the occasional patient will show visual recovery, even when aggressive treatment is started emergently (63–65) and (2) emergency treatment will hopefully halt progression of further visual loss in the affected or fellow eye, but I have seen several cases in which visual loss was relentless despite megadose intravenous corticosteroids (60,66).

Unfortunately, there are no reliable treatment guidelines to follow once the diagnosis of GCA is made, because we still do not have specific answers to the following questions:

1. In which cases should megadose intravenous therapy be given, and how much and for how long?
2. How long should treatment with "high"-dose oral corticosteroids be continued (3–6 weeks or 3 months?) and what constitutes "high" dose (8)?
3. For how long in total should the patient be kept on steroids (1 year or longer) (7,67–70)?
4. What if the patient is intolerant of corticosteroids or develops devastating side effects? Treated patients are at a risk of developing, for example, severe proximal myopathy, hypertension, diabetes, avascular necrosis of bone, gastrointestinal bleed, bowel perforation (in two of my cases colon perforation occurred), concomitant systemic infection, and osteoporosis. For example, in one study, the incidence of symptomatic vertebral fracture after long-term therapy was 26% (71). Should alternative medications be instituted in such cases?

Although no specific "rules" may be stated, I will usually proceed under the following *general* guidelines (Table 3):

If a patient has acute AION, CRAO, PION, choroidal ischemia, amaurosis fugax, or diplopia due to GCA, emergency treatment should be instituted. Intuitively, high-dose corticosteroids with the fastest means of delivery should

Table 3 A Treatment Regimen of GCA[a]

	AION	
GCA	PION	IV Methylprednisolone
	CRAO	500 mg q 6h × 5 Days
	Choroidal Ischemia	
	Amaurosis Fugax	
	Diplopia	
Then:[b]		
Prednisone Daily		100 mg for 1 week
In Divided Doses:		80 mg for 1 week
		70 mg for 1 week
		60 mg for 1 week
		50 mg for 1 week
		40 mg for 1 week
		30 mg for 2 weeks
		25 mg for 2 weeks
		20 mg for 1 month
		17.5 mg for 1 month
		15 mg for 1 month
		12.5 mg for 1 month
		10.0 mg for 1 month
		7.5 mg for 2 months
		5 mg for 2 months
		Then stop treatment[c]

[a]GCA is giant cell arteritis, AION is anterior ischemic optic neuropathy, PION is posterior ischemic optic neuropathy, CRAO is central retinal artery occlusion.
[b]The weaning schedule given here is predicated on visual and systemic symptoms. ESR and CRP are drawn before treatment, at 6 weeks of treatment and then monthly. Ophthalmic examination takes place weekly until the 80 mg level, biweekly until the 40 mg level, and then monthly. Recrudescence of symptoms warrants re-evaluation.
[c]Follow patient monthly × 3, then bimonthly for 1st year. Follow ESR/CRP levels.

be begun. This will best insure against further visual loss, and in occasional cases may result in recovery of vision. Each patient, however, will need to be *individualized* and their specific risk/benefit ratio of treatment evaluated (72). Both the physician and the patient should be comfortable with the arrange-ments. If possible, I will hospitalize the patient and begin intravenous methylprednisolone, 500 mg (to run in over a 30-min period) every 6 h for 5 days. The patient will concomitantly receive an antacid or medication to decrease gastric acid secretion. Serum glucose and electrolytes will be measured daily. While hospitalized, a TAB will be performed. Remember again that GCA is a clinical diagnosis. A negative biopsy should, however, reopen the thought processes toward a *possible* alternative diagnosis. After discharge, the patient is begun on oral prednisone, 100 mg daily for 1 week and 80 mg for the second week. If the patient is stable visually and improved systemically at the 2-week mark, further weaning occurs at the rate of 10 mg each week until the 40-mg level.

If the patient notices further visual or constitutional symptoms anytime during this process (and in my experience this is unusual), they are instructed to contact me urgently. At the 6- to 7-week mark, an ESR and CRP will be redrawn. If the ESR and CRP were elevated to begin with, they may be helpful to use as markers for further weaning. The weaning schedule will continue as follows: 40 mg daily for 1 week, 30 mg daily for 2 weeks, 25 mg daily for 2 weeks. The patient will be examined again at this time (approximately after 10 weeks). A repeat ESR and CRP level may help determine further weaning, which is typically: 20 mg daily for 1 month, 17.5 mg daily for 1 month, 15 mg daily for 1 month, 12.5 mg daily for 1 month, 10 mg daily for 2 months, 7.5 mg daily for 2 months, and then 5 mg daily for 2 months. During that period of time, monthly examinations by both me and by the internist (e.g., to check blood pressure, serum glucose, stool guaiac) will take place. ESR and CRP also are checked monthly. Although moderately elevated levels of the latter will usually not warrant slowing the weaning process, recrudescence of symptoms in the face of rising levels will make me sit back and take another look. Again, each case needs to be individualized.

After 2 months on 5 mg daily, I will *attempt* to stop treatment. I have been successful in the vast majority of cases in that regard. Although, it is true that GCA may be evident for several years, with late recurrences noted, I feel the risk/benefit ratio favors an attempt at stopping medication at the 1-year mark. Of course, these patients should then be followed carefully: first monthly and then every 2–3 months for the first year. Recrudescence of symptoms should be sought and ESR and CRP followed.

In sum, I believe that megadose corticosteroids are indicated emergently in cases of acute visual loss from GCA followed by high-dose therapy as outlined above. After the 6-week mark, I think that lower chronic doses may be employed without a significant threat of visual loss. Careful follow-up is mandatory both by the ophthalmologist and the internist. Although GCA may linger on for many years in some cases, I usually attempt to stop treatment at the 1-year mark if possible. Again, careful follow-up is necessary with specific questioning regarding constitutional symptoms. It seems clear from the literature and from my own experience, that systemic symptoms will most often precede recrudescence of frank visual symptoms. In addition, I do *not* think that alternate day dosing is appropriate at any time with GCA.

What about the patient "intolerant" of corticosteroids or one who has suffered an early severe complication? In most cases, treatment of the adverse effect while lowering of the dose of corticosteroids is appropriate. Cytotoxic agents (i.e., cyclophosphamide [Cytoxan (73)], methotrexate (74), or azathioprine [Imuran (75)] have been employed in some cases, but no specific data are available to allow recommendation of any particular regimen. The risk/benefit ratio of these drugs needs to be carefully assessed before their use. Methotrexate has been shown to be effective in the long-term therapy of rheumatoid arthritis (76). Several reports have described dapsone as being useful as a corticosteroid-"sparing" agent in GCA and PMR but side effects include anemia and agranulocytosis (77,78). The above case reports, however, should be read with extreme care before drawing any conclusions. For instance, Krall and associates in 1989 reported three patients with GCA treated with prednisone and methotrexate. In each case, corticosteroids alone were the initial treatment (74). When the corticosteroids were weaned, however, symptoms recurred. Methotrexate (mean 12.5 mg weekly) was then added that allowed further weaning of corticosteroids in the face of a stable clinical course. After careful analysis of their cases, however, it is clear that the initial daily dose of prednisone used was *too low* and the rate of weaning was *too rapid* (in case 1 with GCA and visual symptoms, prednisone, 60 mg, was begun. Medication was weaned and stopped after only 5 months; in case 2, the highest dose used was prednisone, 60 mg, in the face of transient visual loss and was weaned to 12.5 mg in just 3 months; and in case 3 with GCA, corticosteroids were tapered from 40 to 10 mg over only 4 months). The best treatment of *truly* "corticosteroid-resistant" GCA remains to be determined.

VIII. ILLUSTRATIVE CLINICAL CASES AND COMMENTS

Case 1

An 85-year-old female physician developed visual loss in the right eye 1 week earlier. There was a history of at least 3 weeks of headaches and jaw claudication.

On examination, visual acuity was light perception right eye and 20/60 left eye. A 4+ right afferent pupil defect was present. She saw five and a half of six American Optical Hardy Rand Rittler color vision test plates with the left eye and none with the right. Goldmann visual fields were concentrically constricted in the left eye with no focal scotomas seen. Only a small superotemporal island of vision remained on the right. Ophthalmoscopy revealed pale edema of the right nerve with a normal fellow optic nerve. Retinal pigment epithelial changes in the left macula were thought to be consistent with the stated vision. Superficial temporal arteries were "prominent" and "cordlike" without pulses. The ESR was 110 mm/h. A clinical diagnosis of GCA was made.

The patient was begun on prednisone, 100 mg daily. Three days later, she noted visual loss on the left. Although the visual acuity was still 20/60, the visual field revealed marked nasal field loss as well as constriction of the temporal isopters. The patient was hospitalized and started on intravenous methylprednisolone, 1 g daily. By the next morning, the visual field further diminished in size, with only a 30-degree inferior altitudinal island respecting the horizontal meridian remaining. In desperation, heparin sulfate was added and methylprednisolone was increased to 1500 mg daily. The patient was kept in a supine position to increase circulation to the eyes. Despite this therapeutic regimen, vision fell slowly to 20/200, with a 10-degree inferior island of vision noted 3 days later. Two days later, left vision was no light perception.

Comment. Once visual loss begins with GCA, it may be inexorable despite high-dose corticosteroids. In retrospect, I would have performed a fluorescein angiogram on the left eye when I first examined her to look for choroidal ischemia and thus establish bilaterality of involvement. I would have begun intravenous methylprednisolone, 2 g, immediately rather than high-dose oral medication.

Case 2

A 71-year-old man with a 7-year history of PMR on low-dose corticosteroids complained of seeing "flashing lights" in each eye over a 7- to 10-day period. He also noted transient vertical and then horizontal diplopia. Soon after, inferior visual field loss in the right eye ensued. Although the patient admitted to "slight" headache, there was no jaw claudication, weight loss, or scalp tenderness. He felt that the blood vessels in the temples became "dilated" lately.

On examination, visual acuity was hand movements on the right and 20/20 on the left. Color vision was normal on the left but nil on the right. Goldmann visual fields were normal on the left with the right showing an inferior altitudinal scotoma. Ophthalmoscopy revealed pale disc swelling on the right with slight narrowing of retinal arterioles. The left fundus was normal. The ESR was 58 mm/h. The patient was begun on prednisone, 100 mg daily, by his rheumatologist. A long segment of superficial temporal artery was biopsied and sent for histopathology. The initial reading was negative for GCA. The pathologists were asked to cut more sections and review the existing sections. A diagnosis of GCA was made after reviewing the *additional* material. The patient has remained stable after a full course of corticosteroids.

Comment. A clinical diagnosis of AAION and not NAION was obvious based on (1) the past history of PMR, (2) the transient visual symptoms preceding irreversible unilateral visual loss, (3) a history of "slight" headache with dilation of superficial arteries, and (4) a mild elevation in the ESR. Still and all, the TAB was initially "normal." The clinician must urge the pathologist to do a careful examination of *all* tissue submitted. Remember that the diagnosis of GCA should rest on the clinical evidence alone even if the biopsy is truly negative.

In retrospect, I would have performed a fluorescein angiogram to look for choroidal ischemia in the involved and uninvolved eye. The finding of choroidal ischemia in the involved eye would have shored up the diagnosis of GCA. Choroidal ischemia in the fellow eye would have persuaded me to treat this patient in a more aggressive fashion from scratch.

Case 3 (60)

A 78-year-old man complained of painless visual field loss below fixation in the left eye for 3 days. He denied all constitutional symptoms of GCA.

On examination by a retinologist, visual acuity was 20/25+ on the right and 20/25 on the left. Goldmann visual fields showed an inferior altitudinal defect on the left. A questionable left afferent pupil defect was noted. Fundus examination was normal. A fluorescein angiogram was performed that demonstrated a choroidal filling defect in the superior and inferior portions of the left macula that persisted until the late stages of the study. There was also delayed filling of a cilioretinal arteriole branch to the superior macula (Fig. 2).

The next day further left visual loss ensued. On neuro-ophthalmological examination, visual acuities were 20/20 on the right and 20/30– on the left. Visual fields now showed only a central 5-degree island remaining on the left. A 2+ left afferent pupil defect was noted. Swelling of the left optic nerve was now evident. The ESR was 150 mm/h. The TAB was consistent with GCA. After a course of intravenous methylprednisolone and high-dose oral prednisone, the patient was weaned to the 5-mg level after 9 months. Although he was visually and systemically stable, the ESR was then 77 mm/h. Prednisone was increased to 10 mg daily.

Comment. This challenging patient without symptoms or signs of GCA presented with an inferior altitudinal defect with a normal fundus. Either retrobulbar neuropathy or choroidal ischemia could account for this picture. The finding of choroidal ischemia on fluorescein angiography should strongly suggest GCA in patients without concomitant cardiac hypoperfusion or carotid stenosis (*Note*: In either of those conditions, the retinal filling time would also be markedly delayed.) Here is a case of "occult" GCA in which choroidal ischemia was a prelude to AION. The weaning of oral prednisone was slightly too rapid, as seen by a pronounced elevation of the ESR. The precise time one should stop treatment in a case like this is unknown.

Case 4

A 69-year-old woman noted the acute onset of blindness in the left eye and visual "blurring" on the right. There was at least a 5-month history of headache and jaw claudication. On examination, visual acuity was 20/20 on the right and no light perception on the left. The left pupil was nonreactive, whereas a 2+ response was noted on the right. A 3+ left afferent pupil defect was noted. Goldmann visual field showed minor nasal depression of the I2e isopter on the right. Humphrey static perimetry, however, revealed an inferior altitudinal defect with a mean deviation of −5.14 DB. Fundus examination was normal on the right, whereas the left showed pale swelling of the optic disc and two areas of retinal infarction in the posterior pole. The ESR was first found to be 24 mm/h but on repeat was 46 mm/h. A clinical diagnosis of GCA was made and confirmed histopathologically. The patient was treated with the usual intravenous and oral regimen and has done well.

Comment. The clinical diagnosis of GCA was again inescapable even if just visual signs were considered. The bilaterality and the presence of retinal and posterior ciliary artery ischemia were glaring signs. Note that here again the ESR was normal. The repeat ESR, however, was mildly elevated.

Case 5

A 67-year-old woman complained of chronic seasonal headaches (which she was having presently) over a 7-year period without recent change. There was no PMR, jaw claudication, weight loss, nor fever. Three weeks earlier, the patient noted diminished central vision in the left eye. One year ago, she noted an episode of left-sided amaurosis fugax.

On examination, visual acuity was 20/25 on the right and 20/30 on the left. The patient saw five of six color vision plates on the right but only two of six on the left. Goldmann visual fields revealed a small central scotoma on the left. A 1.5 log unit left afferent pupil defect was noted. Ophthalmoscopy was normal on the right. The left optic disc was normal. Just inferior and superior to the disc were large areas of retinal infarction. In addition, mild retinal opacity throughout the posterior pole and a macular cherry red spot were noted. Superficial temporal arteries were nontender with normal pulses. The ESR was 30 mm/h. A diagnosis of incomplete central retinal artery occlusion was made and the patient was started on low-dose aspirin. The echocardiogram was normal.

On follow-up 10 days later, the patient insisted that her headache was getting worse and that she developed jaw pain while chewing. When I suggested that perhaps I had "put words in her mouth" during the prior examination, she became upset. I felt behooved to perform a TAB! To my surprise, the biopsy was positive for GCA. She was begun on corticosteroids and has been doing well. The headache completely went away after several days of treatment.

Comment. A clinical diagnosis of GCA in this case was not immediately made. After all, there was (1) a long-standing history of headaches that was unchanged, (2) a normal ESR, and (3) a history of previous amaurosis fugax 1 year earlier. Despite this, the patient developed additional symptoms of GCA 10 days later. The rapid response of the headache to corticosteroids is a clinical sign used by many neurologists and rheumatologists in diagnosing GCA (see text above). In each case of CRAO, GCA should be carefully excluded (i.e., ESR, fluorescein angiogram looking for concomitant choroidal ischemia, TAB as necessary) unless retinal emboli are seen or an embolic source is likely (e.g., as in a patient with atrial fibrillation).

Case 6

A 79-year-old hypertensive man developed progressive right visual loss over a 4-day period. There was no associated headache, jaw claudication, PMR, scalp tenderness, or weight loss.

On examination, visual acuity was light perception on the right and 20/15 on the left. Pupils showed a 3+ response to light on the left with no response on the right. A large right afferent pupil defect was noted. Left visual fields were normal. Severe chalky white, cloudlike, left optic disc edema was noted. The right fundus was unremarkable. Fluorescein angiography showed marked choroidal ischemia with incomplete filling still seen in the late phases of the study. The ESR was 32 mm/h and on repeat was 26 mm/h. Bilateral TABs (with a generous specimen taken from each side) were negative. Despite the negative ESR and TABs, high-dose oral prednisone, 100 mg, was begun. Magnetic resonance angiography (MRA) of the head and neck ruled out other causes of choroidal ischemia.

Comment. This case illustrates the frustration that may arise in trying to abide by established criteria for the diagnosis of GCA. In this case, two signs highly suggestive of AAION, that is, chalky white optic disc edema and choroidal ischemia, were evident. The risk of corticosteroids as well as the risk of visual loss in the fellow eye were completely explained to the patient. Both the patient and the physician felt comfortable with the initiation of treatment despite the negative TABs and ESR.

REFERENCES

1. Keltner JL. Giant-cell arteritis. Signs and symptoms. Ophthalmology 1982; 89:1101–10.
2. Chmelewski WL, McKnight KM, Agudelo CA, Wise CM. Presenting features and outcomes in patients undergoing temporal artery biopsy. Arch Intern Med 1992; 152:1690–5.
3. Hedges TR, Gieger GG, Albert DM. The clinical value of negative temporal artery biopsy specimens. Arch Ophthalmol 1983; 101:1251–4.
4. Austin D, O'Donnell F, Attanasio P. Temporal arteritis mimics TMJ/myofascial pain syndrome. Ohio Dent J 1992; 66:44–7.
5. Hall S, Hunder GG. Is temporal artery biopsy prudent? Mayo Clin Proc 1984; 59:793–6.

6. Hunder GG, Bloch DA, Michel BA, Stevens MB, Arend WP, Calabrese LH, Edworthy SM, Fauci AS, Leavitt RY, Lie JT, Lightfoot RW Jr, Masi AT, McShane DJ, Mills JA, Wallace SL, Zvaufker NJ. The American College of Rheumatology 1990 criteria for the classification of giant cell arteritis. Arthritis Rheum 1990; 33:1122–8.
7. Delecoeuillerie G, Joly P, Cohen de Lara A, Paolaggi JB. Polymyalgia rheumatica and temporal arteritis: a retrospective analysis of prognostic features and different corticosteroid regimens (11 year survey of 210 patients). Ann Rheum Dis 1988; 47:733–9.
8. Lundberg I, Hedfors E. Restricted dose and duration of corticosteroid treatment in patients with polymyalgia rheumatica and temporal arteritis. J Rheumatol 1990; 17:1340–5.
9. Sendino A, Barbado FJ, Gonzalez-Anglada I, Anton E, Lopez-Barea F, Vazquez JJ: Temporal arteritis: a form of systemic panarteritis. Ann Rheum Dis 1992; 51:1082–4.
10. Spiera H. Giant cell arteritis and polymyalgia rheumatica. Hosp Pract 1990; Nov 15:71–88.
11. Reich KA, Giansiracusa DF, Strongwater SL. Neurologic manifestations of giant cell arteritis. Am J Med 1990; 89:67–72.
12. Caselli RJ, Hunder GG, Whisnant JP. Neurologic disease in biopsy-proven giant cell (temporal) arteritis. Neurology 1988; 38:352–9.
13. Caselli RJ. Giant cell (temporal) arteritis: a treatable cause of multi-infarct dementia. Neurology 1990; 40:753–5.
14. Cherin P, Awada H, Cattan S, Amor B. Inflammatory arteritis with reversible coronary localization in an 70 year-old woman. Eur Heart J 1989; 10:577–80.
15. Molloy DW, Brooymans MA, Borrie MJ. Acute chest pain in an elderly woman. Can J Cardiol 1988; 4:144–5.
16. Pye M. Lingual and scalp infarction as a manifestation of giant cell arteritis: delay in diagnosis leading to blindness. J Rheumatol 1988; 15:1597–8.
17. Hitch JM, Raleigh NC. Dermatologic manifestations of giant-cell (temporal, cranial) arteritis. Arch Dermatol 1970; 101:409–15.
18. Lhote F, Mainguene C, Griselle-Wiseler V, Fior R, Feintuch MJ, Royer I. Giant cell arteritis of the female genital tract with temporal arteritis. Ann Rheum Dis 1992; 51:900–3.
19. Walz-Leblanc BA, Ameli FM, Keystone EC. Giant cell arteritis presenting as limb claudication. Report and review of the literature. J Rheumatol 1991; 18:470–2.
20. McKendry RJ, Guindi M, Hill DP. Giant cell arteritis (temporal arteritis) affecting the breast: report of two cases and review of published reports. Ann Rheum Dis 1990; 49:1001–4.
21. Ellis ME, Ralston S. The ESR in the diagnosis and management of the polymyalgia rheumatica/giant cell arteritis syndrome. Ann Rheum Dis 1983; 42:168–70.
22. Berlit P. Clinical and laboratory findings with giant cell arteritis. J Neurol Sci 1992; 111:1–12.
23. Kyle V, Cawston TE, Hazleman BL. Erythrocyte sedimentation rate and C reactive protein in the assessment of polymyalgia rheumatic/giant cell arteritis on presentation and during follow up. Ann Rheum Dis 1989; 48:667–71.

24. Esphaghian J, Goeken JA. C-reactive protein in giant cell (cranial, temporal) arteritis. Ophthalmology 1980; 87:1160–6.
25. Brittain GPH, McIlwaine GG, Gibson JM. Plasma viscosity or erythrocyte sedimentation rate in the diagnosis of giant cell arteritis. Br J Ophthalmol 1991; 75: 656–9.
26. Wong RL, Korn JH. Temporal arteritis without an elevated erythrocyte sedimentation rate. Case report and review of the literature. Am J Med 1986; 80:959–64.
27. Biller J, Asconape J, Weinblatt ME, Toole JF. Temporal arteritis associated with normal sedimentation rate. JAMA 1982; 247:486–7.
28. Jacobson DM, Slamovits TL. Erythrocyte sedimentation rate and its relationship to hematocrit in giant cell arteritis. Arch Ophthalmol 1987; 105:965–7.
29. Bull BS, Brecher G. An evaluation of the relative merits of the Wintrobe and Westergren sedimentation methods, including hematocrit correction. Am J Clin Pathol 1974; 62:502–10.
30. Ravel R. Clinical laboratory medicine. Clinical application of laboratory data. 4th ed. Chicago: Year Book, 1984:235–6.
31. Wagener HP, Hollenhorst RW. The ocular lesions of temporal arteritis. Am J Ophthalmol 1958; 45:617–30.
32. Fauchald P, Rygvold O, Oystese B. Temporal arteritis and polymyalgia rheumatica: clinical and biopsy findings. Ann Intern Med 1972; 77:845–52.
33. Albert DM, Ruchman MC, Keltner JL. Skip areas in temporal arteritis. Arch Ophthalmol 1976; 94:2072–7.
34. Klein RG, Campbell RJ, Hunder GG, Carney JA. Skip lesions in temporal arteritis. Mayo Clin Proc 1976; 51:504–10.
35. Ponge T, Barrier JH, Grolleau JY, Ponge A, Vlasak A-M, Cottin S. The efficacy of selective unilateral temporal artery biopsy versus bilateral biopsies for diagnosis of giant cell arteritis. J Rheumatol 1988; 15:997–1000.
36. Weems JJ. Diagnosis of giant cell arteritis by occipital artery biopsy. Am J Med 1992; 93:231–2.
37. Kattah JC, Cupps T, Manz HJ, El Khodary A, Caputy A. Occipital artery biopsy: a diagnostic alternative in giant cell arteritis. Neurology 1991; 41:949–50.
38. Coppeto JR, Miller D. Polyarteritis nodosa diagnosed by temporal artery biopsy. Am J Ophthalmol 1986; 102:541.
39. Small P, Brisson M-L. Wegener's granulomatosis presenting as temporal arteritis. Arthritis Rheum 1991; 34:220–3.
40. Behari M, Mishra NK, Sarkar C, Roychowdhery D, Prasad K, Maheshwari MC. Contralateral hemiplegia in herpes zoster ophthalmicus. Role of temporal artery biopsy. J Assoc Physicians India 1989; 37:606–9.
41. McDonnell PJ, Moore GW, Miller NR, Hutchins GM, Green R. Temporal arteritis. A clinicopathologic study. Ophthalmology 1986; 93:518–30.
42. Allsop CJ, Gallagher PJ. Temporal artery biopsy in giant-cell arteritis. A reappraisal. Am J Surg Pathol 1981; 5:317–23.
43. Cullen JF. Occult temporal arteritis. A common cause of blindness in old age. Br J Ophthalmol 1967; 51:513–25.
44. Boghen DR, Glaser JS. Ischaemic optic neuropathy. The clinical profile and natural history. Brain 1975; 98:689–708.

45. Hayreh SS. Anterior ischaemic optic neuropathy. Differentiation of arteritic from non-arteritic type and its management. Eye 1990; 4:25–41.
46. Beri M, Klugman MR, Kohler JA, Hayreh SS. Anterior ischemic optic neuropathy. VII. Incidence of bilaterality and various influencing factors. Ophthalmology 1987; 94:1020–8.
47. Hayreh SS. Anterior ischemic optic neuropathy V. Optic disc edema as an early sign. Arch Ophthalmol 1981; 99:1030–40.
48. Sergott RC, Cohen MS, Bosley TM, Savino PJ. Optic nerve decompression may improve the progressive form of nonarteritic ischemic optic neuropathy. Arch Ophthalmol 1989; 107:1743–54.
49. Beck RW, Savino PJ, Repka MX, Schatz NJ, Sergott RC. Optic disc structure in anterior ischemic optic neuropathy. Ophthalmology 1984; 91:1334–7.
50. Doro S, Lessell S. Cup-disc ratio and ischemic optic neuropathy. Arch Ophthalmol 1985; 103:1143–4.
51. Hayreh SS. Anterior ischemic optic neuropathy. New York: Springer-Verlag, 1975:66.
52. Feit RH, Tomsak RL, Ellenberger C Jr. Structural factors in the pathogenesis of ischemic optic neuropathy. Am J Ophthalmol 1984; 98:105–8.
53. Barricks ME, Traviesa DB, Glaser JS, Levy IS. Ophthalmoplegia in giant cell arteritis. Brain 1977; 100:209–21.
54. Hamed LM, Guy JR, Moster ML, Bosley T. Giant cell arteritis in the ocular ischemic syndrome. Am J Ophthalmol 1992; 113:702–5.
55. Rabinowich L, Mehler MF. Parasympathetic pupillary involvement in biopsy-proven temporal arteritis. Ann Ophthalmol 1988; 20:400–2.
56. Siatkowski RM, Gass JDM, Glaser JS, Smith JL, Schatz NJ, Schiffman J. Fluorescein angiography in the diagnosis of giant cell arteritis. Am J Ophthalmol 1993; 115:57–63.
57. Mack HG, O'Day J, Currie JN. Delayed choroidal perfusion in giant cell arteritis. J Clin Neuro Ophthalmol 1991; 11:221–7.
58. Fastenberg DM, Feldon SE. Reversible choroidal vascular insufficiency without infarction in temporal arteritis. Graefe's Arch Ophthalmol 1982; 218:327–30.
59. Spolaore R, Gaudric A, Coscas G, De Margerie J. Acute sectorial choroidal ischemia. Am J Ophthalmol 1984; 98:707–16.
60. Slavin ML, Barondes MJ. Visual loss due to choroidal ischemia as a prelude to anterior ischemic optic neuropathy in giant cell arteritis: a report of three cases. Am J Ophthalmol (submitted for publication)
61. Dimant J, Grob D, Brunner NG. Ophthalmoplegia, ptosis, and miosis in temporal arteritis. Neurology 1980; 30:1054–8.
62. Jay WM, Nazarian SM. Bilateral sixth nerve pareses with temporal arteritis and diabetes. J Clin Neuro Ophthalmol 1986; 6:91–5.
63. Schneider HA, Weber AA, Ballen PH. The visual prognosis in temporal arteritis. Ann Ophthalmol 1971; 3:1215–30.
64. Rosenfeld SI, Kosmorsky GS, Klingele TG, Burde RM, Cohn EM. Treatment of temporal arteritis with ocular involvement. Am J Med 1986; 80:143–5.
65. Matzkin DC, Slamovits TL, Sachs R, Burde RM. Visual recovery in two patients after intravenous methylprednisolone treatment of central retinal artery occlusion secondary to giant-cell arteritis. Ophthalmology 1992; 99:68–71.

66. Slavin ML, Margolis A. Progressive anterior ischemic optic neuropathy due to giant cell arteritis despite high-dose intravenous corticosteroids. Am J Ophthalmol 1988; 106:1167.
67. Friedman G, Friedman B. Prolonged corticosteroid treatment in the management of temporal arteritis. Klin Wochenschr 1988; 66:1167–70.
68. Kyle V, Hazleman BL. Treatment of polymyalgia rheumatica and giant cell arteritis. I. Steroid regimens in the first two months. Ann Rheum Dis 1989; 48:658–61.
69. Kyle V, Hazleman BL. Treatment of polymyalgia rheumatica and giant cell arteritis. II. Relation between steroid dose and steroid associated side effects. Ann Rheum Dis 1989; 48:662–6.
70. Kyle V, Hazleman BL. Stopping steroids in polymyalgia rheumatica and giant cell arteritis. Treatment usually lasts for two to five years. Br Med J 1990; 300: 344–5.
71. Huston KA, Hunder GG, Lie JT, Kennedy RH, Elveback LR. Temporal arteritis. A 25 year epidemiologic, clinical, and pathologic study. Ann Intern Med 1978; 88:162–7.
72. Buchbinder R, Detsky AS. Management of suspected giant cell arteritis: a decision analysis. J Rheumatol 1992; 19:1220–8.
73. Utsinger PD. Treatment of steroid nonresponsive giant cell arteritis (GCA) with cytoxan. Arthritis Rheum 1982; 25:S31 (abst).
74. Krall P, Mazanec DJ, Wilke WS. Methotrexate for corticosteroid-resistant polymyalgia rheumatica and giant cell arteritis. Cleveland Clin J Med 1989; 56:253–7.
75. De Silva M, Hazleman BL. Azathioprine in giant cell arteritis/polymyalgia rheumatica: a double-blind study. Ann Rheum Dis 1986; 45:136–8.
76. Kremer JM, Lee JK. The safety and efficacy of the use of methotrexate in long term therapy for rheumatoid arthritis. Arthritis Rheum 1986; 26:822–31.
77. Spiera H, Swerdlow F. Dapsone as a steroid-sparing agent in giant cell arteritis (GCA). Arthritis Rheum 1987; 30:S62 (abstr).
78. Boesen P, Dideriksen K, Stentoft J. Dapsone in temporal arteritis and polymyalgia rheumatica. J Rheumatol 1988; 15:879–80.

40

Vascular Insults—Eye Movements

B. Todd Troost
Bowman Gray School of Medicine, Winston-Salem, North Carolina

Most of what we know about the supranuclear control of eye movements in humans has derived from observation and clinicopathological correlation of patients with strokes. This chapter reviews some of the eye movement abnormalities caused by cerebrosvascular disease with some recommendations regarding management.

I. GAZE DEVIATIONS AND PALSIES

Most hemispheric and unilateral brainstem lesions cause disturbances of horizontal gaze. Midbrain disturbances or bihemispheric disorders affect vertical gaze. Acute cerebral infarcts may cause tonic deviations which are usually temporary. Irritative deviations caused by seizure activity or acute intracerebral hemorrhage cause the eyes to deviate tonically to the opposite side. The contralateral ocular deviations caused by acute hemorrhage have been called "wrongway deviation" (1). So-called paralytic deviations are toward the side of the hemispheric lesion and are associated with impaired gaze toward the opposite side. These are usually the result of middle cerebral artery distribution infarcts and are associated with contralateral hemiparesis, hemisensory deficit, and visual field defects. Large lesions also impair pursuit. With a small lesion sparing the posterior hemisphere and brainstem, an isolated unilateral saccadic deficit may occur. Initially the eyes are deviated toward the side of the lesion without the ability to make saccades to the opposite side. An alert, cooperative patient fixing on a target may be able to pursue in both directions. Usually the supranuclear character of the disorder may be revealed by the ability to move the eyes reflexly to the opposite side with caloric or oculocephalic stimuli. The tonic ocular deviation is often casually referred to as a "gaze preference" but is indeed the result of the saccadic palsy with the eyes presumably deviated toward the side of the lesion by the opposite normal saccadic system. When the contralateral hemisphere is intact, the saccadic palsy is transient, manifest initially by an increasing ability to make large saccades beyond midposition toward the direction of the paresis. The eccentric contralateral gaze position cannot be maintained and the eyes tend to drift back toward the center. Such slow ocular drifts back toward center alternating with saccades toward the direction of intended gaze result in a irregular slow nystagmus termed gaze paretic nystagmus. Gradually the magnitude of saccades toward the defective side increases and the ability to make fast eye movements in both directions recovers. It is believed that the recovered ability to make bilateral saccades results from the ability of each hemisphere to make saccades in both directions, which suggests that there is indeed an uncrossed motor saccadic pathway. Recovery from an acute paresis of saccades is usually a matter of days. Failure to recover from a cerebral saccadic palsy suggests that there is a coexisting contralateral lesion. When a hemisphere that has assumed the initiation of saccades in both directions is subsequently damaged, a persistent bilateral saccadic palsy ensues (2).

Bilateral infarcts of the frontomesencephalic eye movement pathway cause saccadic palsy or paresis in both horizontal directions with intact pursuit, oculocephalic responses, and a slow phase of vestibular nystagmus. Vertical saccades may also be defective. This condition has been termed global saccadic palsy.

II. SMOOTH PURSUIT DEFECTS

Many conditions affect the ability of the smooth pursuit system to match target velocity. The clinically impaired difficulty with pursuit is manifested by lack of smooth pursuit of a slowly moving target. Pursuit attempts are replaced by "catch-up" saccades to regain fixation. This is termed saccadic or cogwheel pursuit and occurs with drowsiness, sedative drugs, inattention, fatigue, and impaired levels of consciousness. Vascular disease that produces diffuse cerebral, cerebellar, or brainstem disease such as a multiinfarct state may produce bilateral cogwheel pursuit. Thus, cogwheel pursuit in both directions is not localizing or specific. True complete pursuit defect with absolute inability to track a moving target at any speed with a patient who has completely normal refixation saccades is rare.

Unidirectional horizontal paresis pursuit occurs with unilateral posterior hemispheric infarcts and is clinically manifest by broken up, cogwheeled, or fragmented pursuit while tracking is attempted in a direction toward the damaged hemisphere. Since the pursuit attempt is broken up by saccades, it is often termed "saccadic pursuit." There is usually a contralateral homonymous visual field defect.

III. OPTOKINETIC DEFECTS

Optokinetic nystagmus (OKN) is a complicated reflex response (3). There are two types of optokinetic response—one with full field visual stimuli and the other type, employed at the bedside, with a tape or rotating drum when the stimulus is primarily applied to the central visual field. Patients with unilateral, posterior hemispheric infarcts, contralateral hemianopia, and ipsilateral pursuit defects also demonstrate an impairment in OKN when targets are moved in the direction of the damaged hemisphere (4). The clinical usefulness of optokinetic testing at the bedside is limited. Most often information about the patient's neurological state is more readily apparent by testing other functions such as the visual fields, pursuit, and saccadic eye movements. On rare occasions there may be intact pursuit in the presence of impaired OKN or impaired pursuit with intact OKN (5).

Acute unilateral hemispheric frequently cause a combined contralateral gaze palsy involving both saccadic and pursuit eye movements. The saccadic component of the palsy is secondary to interruption of the frontomesencephalic pathway. With a large lesion producing optundation or poor attention, there is usually an associated bilateral pursuit abnormality. Normal pursuit tracking may recover as the patient becomes more alert depending on the size of the lesion leaving an isolated unidirectional defect in saccadic eye movement that, as previously described, usually recovered in a matter of days.

The decussating frontomesencephalic saccadic pathway and the ipsilaterally functioning smooth pursuit pathway converge anatomically at subthalamic and upper brainstem levels. Bilateral lesions in these areas cause a global paralysis of horizontal eye movements. Vertical gaze may also be paralyzed. Reflex eye movements such as those produced by oculocephalic maneuvers or caloric irrigation produce tonic deviation without the fast phases of nystagmus. With acute cerebral infarcts, these reflex eye movements may also be lost temporarily reflecting bilateral brainstem dysfunction from supratentorial lesions analogous to spinal shock (6).

IV. BRAINSTEM DEFECTS

Many of the classic vascular brainstem syndromes as well as those more recently described have prominent eye movement abnormalities. Some features are summarized in Table 1 and described in the following paragraphs.

Table 1 Brainstem Syndromes

Syndromes	Location of lesion	Signs/symptoms		
		Ipsilateral	Contralateral	Bilateral
		Midbrain		
Weber	3rd cranial nerve; corticospinal and corticobulbar tracts	3rd nerve palsy	Paresis of lower face, tongue, and extremities	
Benedikt	3rd cranial nerve; red nucleus	3rd nerve paralysis	Intention tremor, hemichorea, hemiathetosis	
Claude	3rd cranial nerve; brachium conjuctivum; red nucleus	3rd nerve paralysis	Intention tremor, ataxia, dysmetria	
Nothnagel	3rd cranial nerve; red nucleus, corticospinal tract	3rd nerve palsy	Ataxia, tremor, hemiparesis	
Parinaud	Pretectal nuclei, riMLF			Paralysis of upward gaze, paralysis of convergence, variable pupillary areflexia
Pretectal sylvian aqueduct, Koeber-Salius-Elschnig, dorsal midbrain	Pretectal nuclei, periaqueductal gray matter, riMLF			Impairment of vertical gaze, convergence-retraction nystagmus, convergence spasm, variable vertical nystagmus, variable pupillary areflexia
MLF syndrome	Ipsilateral MLF	Monocular paralysis of adduction on gaze away from lesion	Nystagmus of abducting eye on gaze away from lesion	

WEBINO (Wall-eyed bilateral internuclear ophthalmoplegia)	Bilateral MLF			Bilateral paralysis of adduction with abduction nystagmus of each eye on attempted lateral gaze
Down gaze palsy	medial riMLF			Bilateral paralysis of downward gaze
Supranuclear monocular elevation paresis	Unilateral riMLF upgaze efferents	Monocular elevator palsy (either)	Monocular elevator palsy (or)	Elevation palsy may be ipsilateral or contralateral depending upon lesion location
Vertical one and one half down syndrome	Bilateral medial riMLF, plus unilateral riMLF upgaze efferents			Selective downgaze palsy plus monocular elevator palsy
Top of the basilar	Midbrain; mesial temporal lobe			Vertical gaze abnormality; disorders of convergence; dorsal midbrain syndrome; behavioral abnormalities, including somnolence and hallucinations
		Pons		
Foville	7th nerve, PPRF, corticobulbar tract, corticospinal tract	7th nerve palsy, ipsilateral gaze paralysis	Hemiparesis	
Millard-Gübler	7th nerve, nucleus or fasciculus, corticospinal tract	7th nerve paralysis	Hemiparesis	
Medial pontine syndrome	Medial armniscus, corticospinal tract		Hemiparesis; position & vibratory loss	
Locked-in syndrome	Ventral pons			Horizontal gaze paralysis, bilateral hemiplegia, preserved vertical gaze

Table 1 (*Continued*)

Syndromes	Location of lesion	Signs/symptoms		
		Ipsilateral	Contralateral	Bilateral
One and one half syndrome	PPRF, ipsilateral MLF	Monocular paralysis of adduction on gaze away from lesion plus ipsilateral gaze paralysis on gaze to side of lesion	Nystagmus of abducting eye on gaze away from lesion	
		Medulla		
Wallenberg	Lateral medulla	Homer's syndrome, loss of cutaneous sensation on the face, ataxia, lateropulsion, or hypometria of eye movements	Loss of pain and temperature of limbs and trunk, hypometria of eye movements	Nystagmus, nausea, hiccups

Unilateral midbrain tegmentum lesions may produce a loss of saccades in the opposite direction. Associated injury medial longitudinal fasciculus and oculomotor complex usually complicates the picture. Therefore, isolated gaze palsy from unilateral midbrain disease is rare. Ipsilateral, but not contralateral, pursuit defects also accompany isolated midbrain reticular formation lesions (7). Because of the proximity of the riMLF unilateral midbrain disease is often associated with a variety of disturbances of vertical gaze (see below).

Keane has discussed midbrain vertical gaze paresis and has suggested the name pretectal syndrome for what in the past has been called the dorsal midbrain syndrome, Parinaud syndrome, Koerber-Salus-Elschnig syndrome, sylvian aqueduct syndrome, posterior commissural syndrome, and collicular plate syndrome. The most common causes of the pretectal syndrome are midbrain infarction and pineal region tumors. There is almost always an associated pupillary abnormality, with the pupils being large with poor light reaction and relatively preserved near reaction. Among the constellation of neuro-ophthalmological signs are vertical gaze paresis, pathological lid retraction (Collier's sign), lid lag, and globe retraction during attempts at upward saccades producing convergence retraction nystagmus.

Selective down gaze palsy can occur with infraction involving the medial portions of the riMLF bilaterally (8). Isolated down gaze palsy has also been described with bilateral infarcts of the dorsal lateral periaqueductal gray matter (9) with interruption of fibers entering or exiting the riMLF. The vergence system that links accommodation, convergence, and pupillary constriction (the near triad) also has its final prenuclear way station in the midbrain reticular formation, which is dorsal and lateral to the oculomotor nucleus in the monkey. Hyperconvergence may be one sign of the top of the basilar syndrome (10).

Monocular elevation paresis may be caused by a ipsilateral or contralateral midbrain infarct or tumor. It is now believed to be caused by interruption of up gaze efferents from the riMLF (11). When combined with a selective palsy of down gaze from bilateral riMLF infarcts, a so-called vertical one and one half (down) syndrome may be produced consisting of total palsy of down gaze and monocular paralysis of up ward gaze.

The descending pathways for horizontal eye movements decussate in the lower midbrain and upper pons, descend in the brainstem, and terminate in the pontine paramedian reticular formation (PPRF) at the level of the abducens nuclei. The PPRF is then the final prenuclear anatomical substrate for ipsilateral saccades. With acute pontine infarction there is an ipsilateral paralysis of gaze that is usually permanent in contrast to the transient palsies associated with hemispheric infarction. The eyes tend to remain in the midline rather than deviate as with cerebral disease. In patients who do have ocular deviations, the eyes would tend to deviate away from the side of the lesion in contrast to most acute hemispheric gaze palsies when the eyes deviate toward the side of the lesion.

When a PPRF lesion is combined with a lesion of the MLF on the same side of the brainstem, a condition termed by Fisher (12) as the one and one half syndrome may be produced. It is characterized by an ipsilateral gaze palsy (the one) on attempted gaze toward the side of the lesion and an internuclear ophthalmoplegia paralyzing adduction of the ipsilateral eye (the half). The eye on the side of the lesion producing the one and one half syndrome cannot move laterally because of the gaze palsy and cannot move medially because of interruption of excitatory fibers to the medial rectus carried in the medial longitudinal fasciculus. Hitchings and Troost described a patient with a relatively isolated one and one half syndrome who had focal brainstem disease produced by a small hemorrhage (13). With acute brainstem infarcts, the patients may develop a marked exotropia termed paralytic pontine exotropia (14).

The clinical characteristic of internuclear ophthalmoplegia (INO) is failure of adduction of the eye on the side of the medial longitudinal fasciculus lesion and abduction nystagmus in the opposite eye. Brainstem vascular disease is the usual cause of unilateral internuclear ophthalmoplegia in adults. Sometimes patients with bilateral INO show exotropia that has been termed the WEBINO (walleyed bilateral INO) syndrome (15).

Lateral medullary infarcts may produce eye movement abnormalities. The nystagmus tends to be a gaze-evoked horizontal rotary jerk nystagmus. Other ocular motor abnormalities involve gaze-evoked eyelid and ocular nystagmus inhibited by the near reflex and horizontal gaze-evoked monocular downbeat nystagmus.

A type of eye movement abnormality known as saccadic lateropulsion has been described in association with medullary infarction (16). Saccades to the side of the medullary lesion show overshoot (hypermetria), whereas those in the opposite direction show undershoot (hypometria). As pointed out by Daroff, et al. (17), pure cerebellar lesions are rarely encountered in clinical practice, as most lesions (infarcts, multiple sclerosis, tumors, and spinocerebellar degenerations) also affect the brainstem. Therefore, it is better to speak of the cerebellar system when considering the variety of eye signs.

In addition to nystagmus, poor pursuit, and dysmetria, other clinical signs of cerebellar system disease include an inability to suppress vestibulo-ocular reflex during combined head and eye movements and multiple-step saccadic refixations (hypometric saccades). Lateropulsion of saccadic eye movements may occur with unilateral cerebellar infarcts or with lateral medullary syndrome (18,19).

The phase *skew deviation* denotes a vertical misalignment of the eyes secondary to an acquired supranuclear or vestibulo-ocular lesion. It is a relatively nonspecific sign indicating brainstem or cerebellar system disease without specific localizing value (20). Acquired monocular elevation palsy is one form of skew that may represent a focal midbrain lesion immediately rostral to the oculomotor nuclei (11).

Brainstem syndromes involving the nuclear or fascicular portion of the sixth nerve usually have accompanying neurological signs, including a gaze paresis if the sixth nerve nucleus is involved and contralateral hemiparesis. Further discussion of vascular brainstem syndromes is provided elsewhere (16,21).

The oculomotor nerve may be involved in the brainstem at the nuclear or fascicular level. Usually associated brainstem signs and symptoms will lead to the proper diagnosis, particularly with magnetic resonance (MR) imaging available for confirmation. Even in the absence of associated brainstem signs, isolated complete or partial third nerve palsies may be from intrinsic brainstem vascular disease. Recent evidence suggests that there may be a segregation of exiting parasympathetic fibers from the Edinger-Westphal nucleus. The observation is based on the fact that in some diabetic patients with isolated pupil-sparing third nerve palsy small mesencephalic lesions have been demonstrated by MRI (22).

Fascicular lesions within the brainstem involving the exiting fibers of the oculomotor complex in the brainstem are usually identified by the associated brainstem signs (16,21). Third nerve palsy with a contralateral hemiplegia is known as the Weber syndrome indicating involvement of the ipsilateral corticospinal tract. Contralateral ataxia with an ipsilateral third nerve palsy suggests involvement of the crossing superior cerebellar peduncle and is known as Benedikt's syndrome.

V. MANAGEMENT

Management of vascular diseases causing eye movement abnormality depends on identification of the etiology. Hemispheric strokes primarily originate from thromboembolic disease in the carotid circulation. High-resolution noninvasive imaging of the carotid system should determine whether there is extensive plaque formation or stenotic disease in the appropriate carotid artery. If greater than 75% stenosis is found in the appropriate carotid artery, surgical therapy has proven to be better than medical therapy. Only then should angiography be undertaken prior to consideration of carotid endarterectomy. In the absence of identifiable carotid disease, further investigations would include transesophageal echocardiography and a search for less common causes of stroke such as blood dyscrasia, vasculitis, and coagulation disorder. With posterior circulation distribution strokes, surgery is usually not indicated and, after evaluation of the patient for risk factors such as lipid abnormality, vasculitis, and clotting disorder, standard management includes antiplatelet therapy, including aspirin and ticlopidine (23). In the presence of a cardiac arrythmia such as atrial fibrillation, the use of warfarin therapy should be considered. Other risk factors, particularly in younger patients include migraine and the use of hormonal drugs in women.

In addition to standard medical therapy and supportive care, acute stroke management includes the use of calcium channel-blocking drugs and free oxygen radical scavengers now under investigation. Acute anticoagulation with either heparin or heparin followed by warfarin is not of proven benefit (23). Anticoagulation for recurrent transient ischemic attacks (TIAs) and evolving stroke is poorly documented and must be individualized on a patient by patient basis (23).

The management of patients with isolated cranial nerve palsies effecting eye movements is again individualized. Acute isolated abducent palsies should be thoroughly investigated. In many large reviews (24–26), approximately one third were found to be nonspecific "vascular" or undetermined. It is noteworthy that all three of these series showed a small number of patients with multiple sclerosis. The extent of the workup in an adult patient with an isolated sixth nerve palsy has been long debated. Even in the presence of hypertension or diabetes, all such patients should have MRI, especially if the condition is painful. Even though "vascular" sixth nerve palsy may be accompanied by pain, such patients must be followed carefully. Usually "medical" sixth nerve palsy clears within 4–12 weeks. Failure to improve indicates the need for more diligent search, including repeat MRI and spinal fluid examination.

Fascicular interpeduncular or subarachnoid involvement of the third nerve may provide difficult problems in diagnosis and management. The key question is whether a new acute isolated third nerve palsy is caused by a posterior communicating artery aneurysm. This is particularly true when the pupil is spared or relatively spared. The normal pupil does not completely exclude the possibility of aneurysm. Trobe (27,28) proposed that (1) patients with normal pupillary sphincter and completely palsies extraocular muscles should not have cerebral angiography if they are age 50 or more; (2) patients with normal pupillary sphincter and incompletely palsied extraocular muscles should have angiography; and (3) patients with subnormal pupillary sphincter and completely palsied extraocular muscles ("relative pupil sparing") should have angiography. The phrase *medical third nerve palsy* refers to isolated third nerve palsies believed to be due to ischemia in hypertensive or diabetic patients when the pupil is either totally or relatively spared. The clinical onset in such patients is usually with moderate pain in and around the eye that may proceed the ophthalmoplegia and be painful enough to suggest the possibility of aneurysm. Pain is not a good distinguishing feature between aneurysmal third nerve palsy and medical third nerve palsy; however, the presence of partial or significant pupillary involvement should always raise the specter of aneurysm. The ophthalmoplegia may be partial, particularly at onset, with some muscles entirely spared. Recovery almost always occurs, with the pain disappearing in a matter of weeks and the ophthalmoplegia recovering gradually within 3–4 months. Persistence of pain or failure of recovery should lead to more aggressive reevaluation, as should the additional involvement of cranial nerves IV, V, or VI. Then attention should be drawn to the skull base or area of the cavernous sinus.

In general, the evaluation and management of each patient should be individualized depending on the clinical situation, the age of the patient, and concomitant risk factors.

REFERENCES

1. Sharpe JA, Bondar RL, Fletcher WA. Contralateral gaze deviation after frontal lobe hemorrhage. J Neurol Neurosurg Psychiatry 1985; 48:86–92.
2. Steiner I, Melamed E. Conjugate eye deviation after acute hemispheric stroke: delayed recovery after previous contralateral frontal lobe damage. Ann Neurol 1984; 16:509–11.
3. Troost BT. An overview of the ocular motor neurophysiology. Ann Otol Rhinol Laryngol 1981; 90:29–36.
4. Baloh RW, Yee RD, Honrubia V. Optokinetic nystagmus and parietal lobe lesions. Ann Neurol 1980; 7:269–76.
5. Barratt H, Gresty MA, Page NGR. Neurological evidence for dissociation of pursuit and optokinetic systems. Acta Otolaryngol 1985; 100:89–98.
6. Rosenberg M, Sharpe J, Hoyt WF. Absent vestibulo-ocular reflexes and acute supratentorial lesions. J Neurol Neurosurg Psychiatry 1975; 38:6–12.
7. Zackon DH, Sharpe JA. Midbrain paresis of horizontal gaze. Ann Neurol 1984; 16:495–504.
8. Pierrot-Deseilligny CH, Chain F, Gray F. Parinaud's syndrome. Brain 1982; 105:667–96.
9. Jacobs L, Heffner RR, Newman RP. Selective paralysis of downward gaze caused by bilateral lesions of the mesencephalic periaqueductal gray matter. Neurology 1985; 35:516–21.
10. Caplan LR. "Top of the basilar" syndrome. Neurology 1980; 30:72–9.
11. Ford CS, Schwartze GM, Weaver RG, et al. Monocular elevation paresis caused by an ipsilateral lesion. Neurology 1984; 34:12647.
12. Fisher CM. Some neuro-ophthalmologic observations. J Neurol Neurosurg Psychiatry 1967; 30:383–92.
13. Hitchings LP, Crum A, Troost BT. Isolated one-and-one-half syndrome from focal brainstem hypertensive hemorrhage: precise localization with MRI. Neurology 1988; 38:1501.
14. Sharpe JA, Rosenberg MA, Hoyt WF. Paralytic pontine exotropia. Neurology 1974; 24:107681.
15. McGettrick P, Eustace P. The w.e.b.i.n.o. syndrome. Neuro-Ophthalmology 1985; 5:109–12.
16. Troost BT. Signs and symptoms of stroke syndromes of the brain stem. In: Hofferberth B, Brune GG, Sitzer G, et al., eds. Vascular brain stem diseases. Basel: Karger, 1990: 112–24.
17. Daroff RB, Troost BT, Leigh RJ. Supranuclear disorders of eye movements. In: Glass JS, ed. Neuro-ophthalmology. 2nd ed. Philadelphia: Lippincott, 1990:299–23.
18. Ranalli PJ, Sharpe JA. Contrapulsion of saccades and ipsilateral ataxia: a unilateral disorder of the rostral cerebellum. Ann Neurol 1986; 20:311.

19. Benjamin EG, Zimmerman CF, Troost BT. Lateropulsion and upbeat nystagmus are manifestations of central vestibular dysfunction. Arch Neurol 1986; 43:962–4.
20. Keane JR. Ocular skew deviation. Arch Neurol 1975; 32:185–90.
21. Troost BT. Ophthalmic aspects of cerebrovascular disease. In: Vinken PJ, Bruyn CW, Klawans HL, eds. Handbook of clinical neurology. Vol. 55: Vascular diseases, Part III. Amsterdam: Elsevier, 1989:107–28.
22. Hopf HC, Gutmann L. Diabetic 3rd nerve palsy: evidence for a mesencephalic lesion. Neurology 1990; 40:10415.
23. Rothrock JF, Hart RG. Antithrombotic therapy in cerebrovascular disease. Ann Intern Med 1991; 115:885–9.
24. Shrader EC, Schlezinger NS. Neuro-ophthalmologic evaluation of abducens nerve paralysis. Arch Ophthalmol 1960; 63:84.
25. Rucker CW. The causes of paralysis of the third, fourth and sixth cranial nerves. Am J Ophthalmol 1966; 61:1294302.
26. Rush JA, Younge BR. Paralysis of cranial nerves III, IV, and VI: Cause and prognosis in 1000 cases. Arch Ophthalmol 1979; 11:209–14.
27. Trobe JD. Isolated pupil-sparing third nerve palsy. Ophthalmology 1985; 92:58–61.
28. Trobe JD. Isolated third nerve palsies. Semin Neurol 1986; 6:135–41.

41

Treatment of Headaches and Facial Pain

Robert B. Daroff
Case Western Reserve University School of Medicine and University Hospitals of Cleveland, Cleveland, Ohio

Christina M. Whitney-Rainbolt
Montana State University College of Nursing, Bozeman, Montana

This chapter outlines strategies for the symptomatic and prophylactic treatment of the most common recurrent head and face pain syndromes—trigeminal neuralgia, tension-type headaches, migraine, and cluster headache—as defined in the International Headache Society Classification (IHS) (1).

Trigeminal neuralgia and tension-type headaches have the fewest therapeutic options.

I. TRIGEMINAL NEURALGIA

Trigeminal neuralgia requires prophylactic treatment, and the anticonvulsants carbamazepine and phenytoin are the most effective monotherapy agents. We begin treatment with carbamazepine, which is used in the same manner as in epilepsy. If clinical toxicity emerges before an adequate therapeutic response, we lower the dose below the toxicity level and add gradually increasing doses of baclofen. If this regimen is unsuccessful, we discontinue these drugs and start phenytoin, which is increased, if necessary, to clinical toxicity.

When there is an adequate therapeutic response, we maintain the dose for approximately 3 months and then attempt a gradual taper. Many patients with trigeminal neuralgia temporarily remit and may have long intervals without any need for treatment. When drug therapy fails, surgical treatment with either microvascular decompression or a radio-frequency ablative procedure is indicated, except in the elderly or frail in whom nerve blocks are preferable.

The pain in trigeminal neuralgia lasts only seconds, but occasionally a patient will be incapacitated by repeated paroxysms. Intravenous phenytoin (250 mg given over 5 min) often breaks these repetitive paroxysms (2).

II. TENSION-TYPE HEADACHE

Infrequent tension-type headaches can be treated with whatever nonnarcotic analgesic is effective. We never prescribe anxiolytics because of the strong likelihood of habituation. Physicians and patients should be aware that the IHS Classification (1) defines "drug overuse" as 45 g aspirin per month or equivalent (four 325-mg tablets of acetylsalicyclic acid [ASA] or acetaminophen daily) or requirement for narcotic analgesics more than twice a month. We are not enthusiastic about caring for patients with tension-type headaches who either "overuse" drugs and we insist that they take prophylactic tricyclics, enroll in a biofeedback-behavioral modification program, or both, during our attempts to decrease overused medications.

Although amitriptyline has been the most studied antidepressant for treating tension-type and migraine headaches, all the tricyclics are effective and the choice depends on the desired sedating or anxiolytic properties (Table 1). The doses required are less than those needed for treating depression; 75–100 mg daily of amitriptyline or imipramine would be high for headaches. We start with the smallest size tablet with daily increases as tolerated. In occasional refractory patients who have failed biofeedback, we use phenelzine. In our experience, antidepressants, other than tricyclics and monoamine oxidase inhibitors, are not effective in headache treatment; this is particularly true for fluoxetine.

Table 1 Tricyclics in Order of Decreasing Sedation

Doxepin
Amitriptyline
Nortriptyline
Imipramine
Desipramine
Protriptyline

III. MIGRAINE

A. General Measures

The simplest treatment option is avoidance of known headache precipitants. Patients who get a migraine after drinking red wine or beer or eating lunch meats may benefit from a tyramine- and nitrate-restricted diet (Table 2). We allow women with migraine *without* aura to take oral contraceptives, but if the headaches are refractory to antimigrainous therapy, we will suggest discontinuation for at least 6 months. Patients with "weekend migraine" should maintain their weekday routine on weekends, including arising at the same hour and consuming similar amounts of caffeine. These measures usually require coexisting pharmacological management for optimal results.

B. Symptomatic Treatment (Table 3)

Daily use of any analgesics or ergotamine can cause chronic daily headaches that are refractory to prophylactic medications (3,4).

Unless contraindicated, we give all patients a trial of ergotamine, using the

Table 2 Vascular Headache Diet: Food and Beverages to Avoid[a]

Ripe avocados, bananas, and figs	
Bean curd (soy bean paste, soy sauces, miso soup)	
Beer (including nonalcoholic beer), ale, wine	
All cheeses except cottage and cream cheese	
Chocolate	
Liver	
Meat or fish that has undergone aging, fermenting, pickling, or smoking. This includes:	
bologna	pickled herring
hot dogs	salami
lox	sausage
mortadellas	smoked salmon
pepperoni	
Pizza	
Pods of broad beans (Fava beans, Italian green beans, Chinese pea pods, lima and navy beans)	
Shrimp paste	
Yogurt, homemade	
Yeast extractions (e.g., Marmite, a dietary supplement) [yeast in baked goods is permitted]	

[a]Avoid all other foods that convincingly provoke headaches.

Table 3 General Symptomatic Treatment of Migraine

1.	Aspirin
2.	Acetaminophen
3.	Ergotamine preparations
4.	"Midrin"
5.	Naproxen sodium (825 mg + 550 mg)
6.	Naproxen (750 mg + 250 mg)
7.	Ibuprofen (800 mg + 400 mg)
8.	Sumatriptan SC
9.	DHE (0.5–1 mg IM or 0.75–2.0 mg SQ)
10.	Analgesic-barbiturate combinations
11.	Narcotic analgesics
12.	Biofeedback/behavioral modification

sublingual form if the headache rapidly peaks in severity, the oral form if there is a build-up of an hour or more, and the suppository form if nausea and vomiting are a problem or the other routes are ineffectual. Raskin (5) recommends an ergotamine suppository "tolerance test" when the patient is headache free to determine the highest dose (one quarter to one suppository) below the nausea threshold. Unfortunately, all ergotamine suppository preparations contain caffeine, which may cause insomnia if taken in the evening.

The nonsteroidal anti-inflammatory drugs are effective abortive agents. For example, we advise 825 mg of naproxen sodium (naproxen in patients on salt restriction) at the headache onset followed by 550 mg in 1 h if the headache persists. We restrict narcotics and analgesic-barbiturate combinations to patients with no more than one migraine per month. Parenteral sumatriptan is extremely effective VIA. A user-friendly injection kit (6). Dihydroergotamine (DHE) requires intramuscular or subcutaneous injection by the patient or a family member and usually provides rapid relief. We recommend DHE when biofeedback and other methods have failed.

Biofeedback/behavior modification taught by a specialist can be an effective adjunct to migraine therapy. Patients must, however, be willing to commit the time to learn the principles and practice the techniques.

For emergency room treatment of a migraine (Table 4), prochlorperazine, DHE, or a combination of the two, or sumatriptan should obviate the need for narcotics.

For the treatment of status migrainosus (Fig. 1), we use Raskin's intravenous DHE protocol (5). This requires a 3-day hospitalization during which we administer a subnauseating dose of DHE every 8 h; daily analgesics are discontinued and a prophylactic agent started during the DHE infusion.

Table 4 Emergency Room Treatment of Migraine

1. DHE 0.75 mg IV
2. Prochlorperazine, 10 mg IV
3. Prochlorperazine, 5 mg IV, + DHE, 0.75 mg IV; may repeat DHE, 0.5 mg, in 30 min
4. Sumatriptan SC

C. Prophylactic Treatment

The indications for prophylactic treatment of migraine are (1) migraine sufficiently severe and frequent to interfere with the patient's ability to function at work, school, or home; (2) daily use of analgesics; (3) use of more than 10 mg of ergotamine per week; and (4) migraine with prolonged aura ("complicated" migraine). There are a variety of effective medications for migraine (Table 5). Propranolol is the most widely used beta blocker and is generally well tolerated when started at a low dose (20 mg tid) and gradually increased; the most troublesome side effects are depression, exercise intolerance, and weight gain. Anecdotal reports of strokes in patients with "complicated" migraine taking propranolol are probably mere coincidence but raise concerns for the prudent, defensive physician, particularly since many other "safe" drugs are available.

Naproxen sodium, used prophylactically, precludes the use of ASA or nonsteroidals for symptomatic therapy. If the patient is depressed or has both migraine and tension-type headaches, the drug of choice is a tricyclic antidepressant, the only class of drugs effective for both types of headache. As stated earlier, the tricyclics vary in their sedative properties (see Table 1). Thus, a patient with insomnia is better treated with doxepin or amitriptyline, whereas one with considerable daytime sleepiness should receive desipramine or protriptyline. As with tension-type headaches, the drug should be started at a low dose and gradually increased. Verapamil has particular theoretical appeal in "complicated" migraine but may take 6–8 weeks to take effect. Methysergide (up to 8 mg per day) is the only specific prophylactic antimigrainous drug. Complaints, such as leg cramps or "psychic" disturbances should prompt discontinuation. We have not observed complications of retroperitoneal or pleuropulmonary fibrosis as long as the patient is given a 1-month methysergide "holiday" every 6 months. We lack extensive personal experience with valproic acid (divalproex sodium). Cyproheptadine is limited in value because of sedation and appetite stimulation.

Phenelzine, a monoamine oxidase inhibitor, may be the most effective drug for treatment of migraine. We use it only when the patient has been refractory to all other agents and is willing to adhere strictly to medication

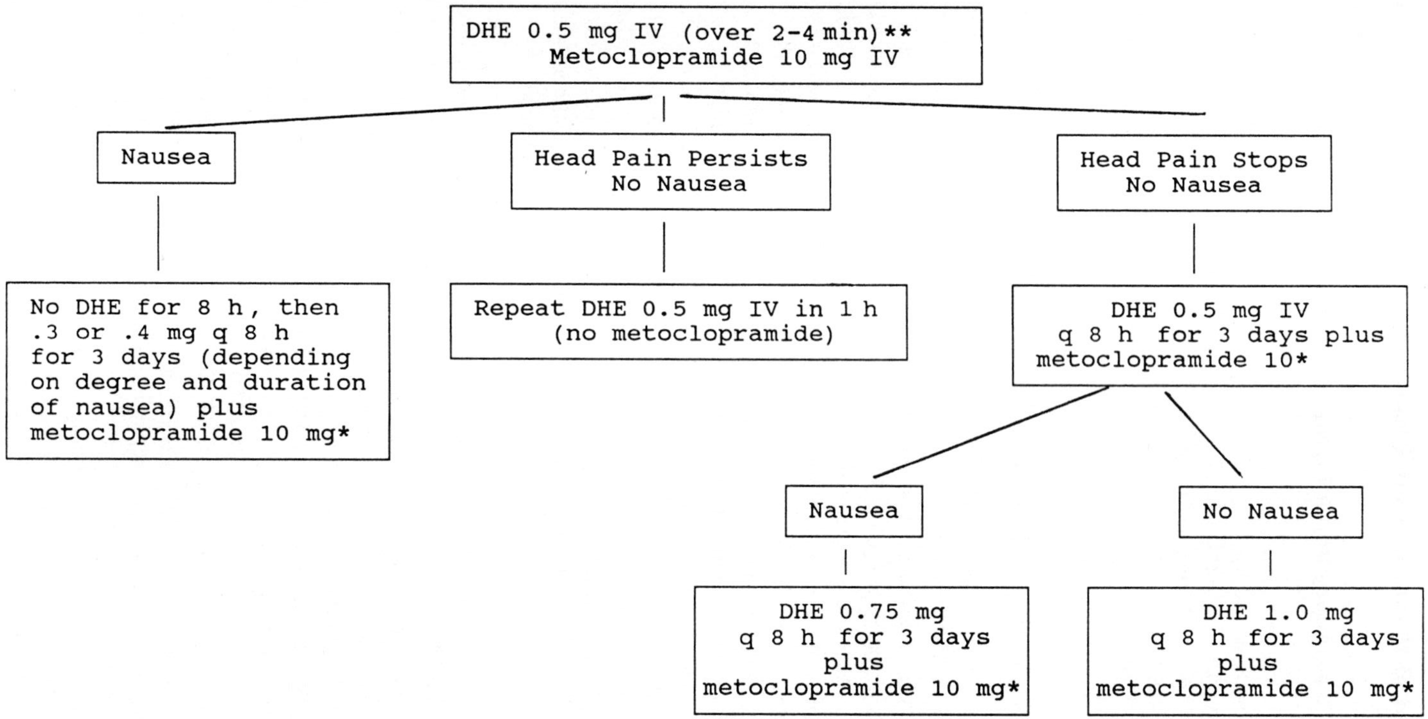

Figure 1 Raskin DHE protocol for status migrainosus. *D/C metoclopramide after sixth DHE dose. **If over 60 years, monitor cardiac status during first two doses of DHE.

Table 5 Prophylactic Treatment of Migraine with[a] or Without Aura

Beta blockers
propranolol
nadolol
atenolol
timolol
metoprolol
Naproxen sodium (550 mg bid)
Tricyclic antidepressants
Verapamil
Methysergide
Valproic acid (divalproex sodium 500–2000 mg qd)
Cyproheptadine
Phenelzine sulfate

[a]Plus 1 ASA qd.

and dietary restrictions. A medication card is available from the pharmaceutical company and should be given to patients taking phenelzine.

The treatment of menstrual migraine constitutes a vexing problem (7). The medications listed in Table 6 should be taken 1 week prior to menses and continued for 5 days after onset. Even with this anticipatory therapy, we abort menstrual migraine in only 30% of patients and often resort to a prophylactic drug (see Table 5), necessitating daily drug use to prevent the one monthly headache. When the headaches are exclusively perimenstrual, refractory to standard therapy, and disabling, we refer the patient to a gynecologist for suppression of cycling with medications.

IV. CLUSTER HEADACHES

A. Symptomatic Treatment

The "specific" symptomatic treatment (Table 7) for cluster headaches should be used until a prophylactic drug takes effect. Ergotamine suppositories, as used in

Table 6 Prophylactic Treatment of Menstrual Migraine

1. Fenoprofen calcium (600 mg bid)
2. Naproxen sodium (550 mg bid)
3. Naproxen (500 mg bid) + ergotamine/caffeine qd

Table 7 Specific Symptomatic Treatment of Cluster Headache

1. 100% oxygen (7–9 L for 10–15 min)
2. DHE (0.75 mg IV or 1.0 mg IM)
3. 4% intranasal lidocaine drops (preceded, if necessary, by decongestant drops)
4. Occipital nerve injection (for chronic cluster)
   betamethasone 6 mg/ml (1 ml)
   lidocaine 2% (1 ml)

migraine, may also be helpful, but the effect tends to diminish after the first week. Breathing 100% oxygen should be limited to 5 days a week. Raskin (2) provides the techniques for intranasal lidocaine and occipital nerve injection for chronic cluster headaches.

B. Prophylactic Treatment

All patients with cluster and chronic cluster headaches should be on prophylactic treatment. The drugs used (Table 8) overlap with antimigrainous drugs (8), but beta blockers and the tricyclics are not particularly effective.

Prednisone (60–80 mg qd) provides rapid relief from the cluster headaches, which then recur as the steroids are tapered. To minimize the duration of steroid therapy, we simultaneously start another agent, such as methysergide, valproic acid, or verapamil, that will hopefully begin to take effect as the steroids are reduced and discontinued. Treatment is continued for the duration of the cluster interval.

With chronic cluster headaches, lithium carbonate may be used and may even abort the attack allowing withdrawal after 6 months. The only other type of headache for which lithium seems "specific" is "hypnic headaches" (9).

Table 8 Prophylactic Treatment of Cluster Headache

1. Prednisone
2. Methysergide
3. Valproic acid (divalproex sodium)
4. Verapamil
5. Phenelzine sulfate
6. Lithium carbonate (for chronic cluster)

Table 9 Indomethacin-Responsive Headache Syndromes

1. Chronic paroxysmal hemicrania
2. Effort and exertional migraine
3. Benign coital cephalgia
4. Benign cough headache
5. Ice-pick headaches ("jabs and jolts," "needle in the eye syndrome")
6. Hemicrania continua

C. Indomethacin-Responsive Headache Syndromes

Chronic paroxysmal hemicrania, classified as a cluster variant (IHS), responds to indomethacin, as do the other unusual types of headaches (2) listed in Table 9.

REFERENCES

1. Headache Classification Committee of the International Headache Society. Classification and diagnostic criteria for headache disorders, cranial neuralgias and facial pain. Cephalalgia 1988; 8(Suppl 7):9–96.
2. Raskin NH. Headache. 2d ed., New York: Churchill Livingstone, 1988.
3. Mathew NT. Drug-induced headache. Neurol Clin 1990; 8:903–11.
4. Mathew NT, Kurman R, Perez F. Drug induced refractory headache—clinical features and management. Headache 1990; 30:634–38.
5. Raskin NH. Modern pharmacotherapy of migraine. Neurol Clin 1990; 8:857–65.
6. The Subcutaneous Sumatriptan International Study Group. Treatment of migraine attacks with sumatriptan. N Engl J Med 1991; 325:316–21.
7. Silberstein SD, Merriman GR. Estrogens, progestines, and headache. Neurology 1991; 41:786–93.
8. Solomon S, Lipton RB, Newman LC. Prophylactic therapy of cluster headaches. Clin Neuropharm 1991; 14:116–30.
9. Newman LC, Lipton RB, Solomon S. The hypnic headache syndrome: a benign headache disorder of the elderly. Neurology 1990; 40:1904–5.

Index

About the Editors

RONALD J. TUSA is Director of the Dizziness and Eye Movement Center and a Professor of Otolaryngology, Ophthalmology, and Neurology at the University of Miami School of Medicine, Florida. The author, coauthor, editor, or coeditor of over 15 books and monographs as well as numerous professional papers, Dr. Tusa is a member of the American Neurological Association, the American Academy of Neurology, the Association for Research in Vision and Ophthalmology, and the Society for Neuroscience, among others. He received the B.A. degree (1972) in biology from the University of California at Irvine and the Ph.D. degree (1978) in anatomy and the M.D. degree (1979) from the University of Pennsylvania, Philadelphia.

STEVEN A. NEWMAN is an Associate Professor of Ophthalmology and Neurological Surgery at the University of Virginia Health Sciences Center, Charlottesville. The author or coauthor of over 50 professional papers and an editorial reviewer for several scientific journals, Dr. Newman is a Fellow of the North American Neuro-Ophthalmology Society; a founding member of the North American Skull Base Society; and a member of the International Perimetric Society, the American Ophthalmic History Society, and the Association for Research in Vision and Ophthalmology, among others. Dr. Newman received the A.B. degree (1969) in physics from Princeton University, New Jersey, and the M. D. degree (1973) from the Albert Einstein College of Medicine, New York, New York.